Nursing Interventions Classification (NIC)

The NIC Logo

The NIC logo of a leaf and tree appears below and on the cover of this book. This leaf is an exact replica of one from a tree in the Linnaeus Botanical Garden in Uppsala, Sweden. The leaf was picked several years ago by an artist who lived next door to the garden for an imprint on a vase she was making. The vase was a present to a team member just when the research team was looking for a logo. Since the leaf came from the Linnaeus garden, the team thought this a meaningful logo. Carl Linnaeus (1701-1778) was the great classifier who brought order to the plant and animal kingdoms. In the logo, the leaf is joined with the tree, the universal symbol of taxonomy.

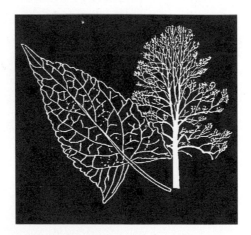

Nursing Interventions Classification (NIC)

Fourth Edition

Editors

Joanne McCloskey Dochterman, PhD, RN, FAAN
Distinguished Professor
Director of the Center for Nursing Classification and Clinical Effectiveness
Chair of Organizations, Systems and Community Area Study
College of Nursing
Professor, Health Management and Policy
College of Public Health
Adjunct Director of Nursing
The University of Iowa Hospital and Clinics
The University of Iowa
Iowa City, Iowa

Gloria M. Bulechek, PhD, RN, FAAN
Professor
College of Nursing
The University of Iowa
Iowa City, Iowa

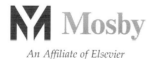

An Affiliate of Elsevier

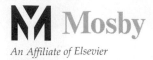

An Affiliate of Elsevier

11830 Westline Industrial Drive
St. Louis, Missouri 63146

NURSING INTERVENTIONS CLASSIFICATION (NIC),
FOURTH EDITION   ISBN 0-323-02392-4

Previous editions copyrighted 1992, 1996, 2000

Library of Congress Cataloging-in-Publication Data

Nursing interventions classification (NIC)/editors, Joanne McCloskey Dochterman,
    Gloria M. Bulechek.—4th ed.
      p. cm.
    Includes bibliographical references and index.
    ISBN 0-323-02392-4
      I. Nursing—Classification. I. Dochterman, Joanne McCloskey. II. Bulechek, Gloria M. III.
    [DNLM: 1. Nursing Process—classification. WY 15 N974 2004]
    RT42.N858 2004
    610.73'01'2—dc21   2003056210

Executive Publisher: Barbara Cullen
Developmental Editor: Julie Vitale
Publishing Services Manager: Deborah L.Vogel
Design Manager: Bill Drone

Printed in the United States of America

Last digit is the print number: 9   8   7   6   5   4   3   2

Preface

In 2002 we celebrated the tenth anniversary of NIC. This is the fourth edition of the *Nursing Interventions Classification (NIC)*; the first edition was published in 1992, the second edition in 1996, and the third edition in 2000. NIC is a comprehensive standardized language that describes the treatments that nurses perform. We have expanded and revised the Classification with continued research efforts and input from the professional community. The features of this edition are as follows:

- Three updated chapters introduce the classification: Chapter One gives an overview of NIC and addresses 20 questions sometimes asked about NIC; Chapter Two describes the beginning of NIC in 1987 and addresses the need for NIC and then describes the research to develop and maintain NIC; and Chapter Three focuses on implementation and use of NIC and features many forms that demonstrate use in both practice and education. Each of these chapters will be of interest to both the novice and experienced user of NIC.

- There are a total of 514 interventions in this edition compared with 486 in the third edition, 433 in the second edition, and 336 in the first edition. Twenty-nine of the interventions are new, and 94 of the previously included interventions have been revised for this edition. (See Appendix A for the list of new, revised, and deleted interventions.) The format for each of the interventions is the same as in previous editions. Each intervention has a label name, a definition, a list of activities that a nurse might do to carry out the intervention in the logical order that she or he might do these, and a short list of background readings. The standardized language is the label name and the accompanying definition. The activities can be selected or modified as necessary to meet the specific needs of the population or individual. Thus NIC can be used to communicate a common meaning across settings but still provide a way for nurses to individualize care. The background readings for many of the interventions have been updated for this edition with changes in activities made as indicated. The readings do not include, by any means, a complete reference list for any intervention. Rather, they are "places to start." They represent a few of the sources that were used in the development of the intervention's definition and activity list and provide support that this intervention is used by nurses. Each of the interventions has a unique code number to assist in computerization of NIC and facilitate reimbursement to nurses.

- The NIC taxonomy, which was included for the first time in the second edition, has been updated to include all of the new interventions. The taxonomy in this edition as in the previous edition includes 7 domains and 30 classes. NIC interventions have also been placed in a second taxonomy, the "Taxonomy of Nursing Practice" developed in 2002 to provide a common structure for nursing diagnoses, interventions, and outcomes. The taxonomies help nurses to locate and choose an intervention and provide structures that can assist with curriculum design. (See the overview of the NIC taxonomy on p. 110 and the introduction to the Taxonomy of Nursing Practice on p. 979 for more details.)

- In the second and third editions, linkages were provided between NIC interventions and NANDA diagnoses. These linkages have been updated for this edition, including the new interventions in this edition and the new diagnoses in the 2001-2002 NANDA publication. Although one can use NIC without NANDA, for those who are NANDA users, this list of linkages facilitates the selection of an intervention. These linkages also facilitate computerization of NIC and assist new nurses with clinical decision making. (See the introduction to the linkages on p. 783 for more information.)

- A new feature in the third edition was specialty area core interventions (those that define the nature of the specialty) as identified by 39 specialty organizations. These lists of core interventions have been updated and expanded for this edition to include core interventions for 43 specialties. (See the introduction to the core interventions on p. 905 for more information.)

- Entirely new to this edition is estimated performance time and level of education that a provider needs to safely and competently administer the intervention. This information was previously published in monograph form for only the interventions in the third edition of NIC; in this edition, times and education levels are included for all 514 interventions.

- This edition, like all previous editions, includes a form to submit suggestions for new or revised interventions (see Appendix B). This is provided to assist users of NIC to help in the refinement and expansion of the classification. Many of the new additions and revisions in this edition have resulted from users of NIC submitting suggestions to improve the classification.

In summary, NIC captures the interventions performed by all nurses. As in the past, all of the interventions included in NIC are meant to be clinically useful, although some are more general than others. Because the interventions encompass a broad range of nursing practice, no nurse could be expected to perform all interventions listed here, or even a major portion. Many of the interventions require specialized training, and some cannot be performed without appropriate certification. Other interventions describe basic hygiene and comfort measures that, in some instances, may be delegated to assistants but still need to be planned and evaluated by nurses.

The use of NIC:

- helps demonstrate the impact that nurses have on the system of health care delivery

- standardizes and defines the knowledge base for nursing curricula and practice

- facilitates the appropriate selection of a nursing intervention

- facilitates communication of nursing treatments to other nurses and other providers

- enables researchers to examine the effectiveness and cost of nursing care

- assists educators to develop curricula that better articulate with clinical practice

- facilitates the teaching of clinical decision making to novice nurses

- assists administrators in planning more effectively for staff and equipment needs

- promotes the development of a reimbursement system for nursing services

- facilitates the development and use of nursing information systems

- communicates the nature of nursing to the public

NIC is useful either by itself or linked with other classifications. NIC interventions have been linked with North American Nursing Diagnosis Association (NANDA) nursing diagnoses, Omaha System problems, Nursing Outcomes Classification (NOC) outcomes, resident assessment protocols (RAP) used in nursing homes, and OASIS (Outcome and Assessment Information Set) currently mandated for collection for patients who are covered by Medicare or Medicaid and are receiving skilled home care. NIC is recognized by the American Nurses Association (ANA) and is included as one data set that will meet the uniform guidelines for information system vendors in the ANA's Nursing Information and Data Set Evaluation Center (NIDSEC). NIC is included in the National Library of Medicine's *Metathesaurus for a Unified Medical Language*. The *Cumulative Index to Nursing Literature (CINAHL)* includes NIC interventions in its indexes. NIC is included in the Joint Commission on Accreditation of Healthcare Organizations' (JCAHO) accreditation requirements as one nursing classification system that can be used to meet the standard on uniform data. Alternative Link has included NIC in its ABC codes for reimbursement for alternative providers. NIC is registered in HL 7 (Health Level 7), the U.S. standards organization for health care. NIC is also licensed for inclusion in SNOMED (Systematized Nomenclature of Medicine). Interest in NIC has been demonstrated in several other countries, and translations into Chinese, Dutch, French, Icelandic, German, Japanese, Korean, Spanish, and Portuguese are completed or underway (see Appendix E, Selected Publications for translations of previous editions).

When standardized language is used to document practice, we can compare and evaluate the effectiveness of care delivered in multiple settings by different providers. The use of standardized language does not inhibit our practice; rather, it communicates the essence of nursing care to others and helps us improve our practice through research. The development and use of this classification help to advance nursing knowledge by facilitating the clinical testing of nursing interventions. We believe the continued development and use of this classification help in the advancement of nursing knowledge and in the efforts of nursing to gain greater voice in the health policy arena. We continue to welcome your feedback and look forward to your continued input.

Joanne McCloskey Dochterman
Gloria M. Bulechek

Strengths of the Nursing Interventions Classification

- **Comprehensive**—NIC includes the full range of nursing interventions from general practice and specialty areas. Interventions include physiological and psychosocial; illness treatment and prevention; health promotion; those for individuals, families, and communities; and indirect care. Both independent and collaborative interventions are included; they can be used in any practice setting regardless of philosophical orientation.

- **Research based**—The research, begun in 1987, uses a multimethod approach; methods include content analysis, questionnaire survey to experts, focus group review, similarity analysis, hierarchical clustering, multidimensional scaling, and clinical field testing. The research has been partially funded (7 years of support) by the National Institutes of Health, National Institute of Nursing Research.

- **Developed inductively based on existing practice**—Original sources include current textbooks, care planning guides, and nursing information systems from clinical practice, augmented by clinical practice expertise of team members and experts in specialty areas of practice. The new additions and refinements are the result of suggestions from users.

- **Reflects current clinical practice and research**—All interventions are accompanied by a list of background readings that support the development of the intervention. All interventions have been reviewed by experts in clinical practice and by relevant clinical practice specialty organizations. A feedback process is used to incorporate suggestions from users in practice.

- **Has easy-to-use organizing structure** (domains, classes, interventions, activities)—All domains, classes, and interventions have definitions. Principles have been developed to maintain consistency and cohesion within the Classification; interventions are numerically coded.

- **Uses language that is clear and clinically meaningful**—Throughout the work, the language most useful in clinical practice has been selected. The language reflects clarity in conceptual issues (e.g., what is an intervention versus a diagnosis or an assessment to make a diagnosis or an outcome).

- **Has established process and structure for continued refinement**—The Classification continues to be developed by researchers at the College of Nursing, the University of Iowa; commitment to the project is evident by years of work and continued involvement. The continued refinement of NIC is facilitated by the Center for Nursing Classification and Clinical Effectiveness, established in the College of Nursing at the University of Iowa in 1995 by the Iowa Board of Regents.

- **Has been field tested**—The process of implementation was initially studied in five field sites representing the various settings where nursing care takes place; hundreds of other clinical and educational agencies are also implementing the Classification. Steps for implementation have been developed to assist in the change process.

- *Accessible through numerous publications*—In addition to the Classification itself, approximately five dozen articles and chapters have been published by members of the research team since 1990. Book and article reviews and publications by others about the use and value of NIC attest to the significance of the work. A video has been made about the development of NIC. A newsletter published two times a year keeps people abreast of recent developments.

- *Linked to NANDA nursing diagnoses, Omaha System problems, NOC outcomes, RAP in long-term care, OASIS for home health care*—A linkage list of NIC interventions linked to NANDA diagnoses is included in this edition; linkages with NOC outcomes are available in a book and software form published by Mosby. Other linkages are available in monograph form from the Center for Nursing Classification and Clinical Effectiveness.

- *Recipient of national recognition*—NIC is recognized by the American Nurses Association, is included in the National Library of Medicine's *Metathesaurus for a Unified Medical Language,* is included in indexes of CINAHL, is listed by JCAHO as one classification that can be used to meet the standard on uniform data, is the focus of a video by the National League for Nursing, is included in Alternative Link's ABC codes for reimbursement by alternative providers, is registered in HL 7, and is included in SNOMED.

- *Developed at same site as outcomes classification*—The *Nursing Outcomes Classification (NOC)* of patient outcomes sensitive to nursing practice has also been developed at Iowa; both NIC and NOC are housed in the Center for Nursing Classification and Clinical Effectiveness.

- *Included in a growing number of vendor software clinical information systems*—The Systematized Nomenclature of Medicine (SNOMED) has included NIC in its multidisciplinary record system. Several vendors have licensed NIC for inclusion in their software, targeted at both hospital and community settings, as well as at practitioners in either general or specialty practice.

- *Translated into several languages*—Although NIC has been developed for applicability to nursing in the United States, nurses in several other countries are finding the Classification useful. Translations are complete or in the process for the following languages: Chinese, Dutch, French, German, Icelandic, Japanese, Korean, Portuguese, and Spanish.

Acknowledgments

Nothing of this magnitude is done alone. As with past editions, we wish to acknowledge help from a variety of sources:

The individuals and groups who submitted suggestions for new interventions or revised interventions and the individuals who reviewed submissions. These include the "Center Fellows" who provide a variety of expertise. This Classification is continuously improved to better reflect clinical practice and best practices through the participation of many. The names of individuals who contributed changes to this edition are in the preliminary pages.

The University of Iowa College of Nursing, University Provost Office, and University Office of the Vice President for Research for support of the Center for Nursing Classification [and Clinical Effectiveness], founded in 1995 to facilitate ongoing development of NIC and NOC. In 2002, the Center's name was expanded to the Center for Nursing Classification and Clinical Effectiveness. The work of the Fundraising Advisory Board and support from individual contributors are creating an endowment at the University of Iowa Foundation, which will provide permanent support for continued upkeep of the Classification.

Our editor, Barbara Cullen, at Mosby/Elsevier, who has shepherded this Classification through several editions and facilitated many of the advances in several arenas. We also thank her associates: Julie Lawley, Permissions Supervisor; Kathy Mantz, Marketing Manager; Michael Wisniewski, Director of Licensing Sales; and our developmental editor for this edition, Julie Vitale, as well as Claire Kramer, Project Manager, and Ruth Kaufman, Copy Editor. We thank Mosby for the sponsorship of the NIC/NOC Letter, which helps us to bring new information to more than 1500 subscribers.

The assistance of Shawn Gibbs, the former Coordinator, Center for Nursing Classification and Clinical Effectiveness at the College of Nursing, the University of Iowa, who assisted in the word processing and formatting of the original manuscript. This was a complicated and time-consuming job that he managed well.

The North American Nursing Diagnosis Association (NANDA) and the Nursing Outcomes Classification (NOC) researchers for their ongoing cooperation through the NNN Alliance to work together to facilitate linkages between NANDA diagnoses, NIC interventions, and NOC outcomes and to implement standardized language in practice. The NNN Alliance has promoted a joint conference every other year and the draft of a common structure for NANDA, NIC, and NOC.

The enthusiastic response to the Classification from many of the nurses in the United States and around the world who are using NIC in a variety of ways: to document their practice, to help students to learn how to plan nursing care, to organize nursing textbooks, and to conduct research studies. The requests of practitioners and students are resulting in the inclusion of standardized language in clinical and educational software.

Recognition List, Fourth Edition

The following individuals contributed to this edition of NIC in multiple ways. Some submitted new interventions for consideration or suggested revisions to existing interventions. Some assisted in the review process of additions, revisions, or deletions to the Classification. Others submitted examples of how they have implemented NIC in practice or education. All have made a valuable contribution to the users of NIC.

- **Ibtihal Almakhzoomy**, Doctoral Student, College of Nursing, The University of Iowa, Iowa City, Iowa
- **DeAnn Ambrosen**, Post-Doctoral Student, College of Nursing, The University of Iowa, Iowa City, Iowa
- **Sylviann Baldwin,** Clinical Informatics Nurse, Mason General Hospital, Shelton, Washington
- **Hope Barton**, Librarian, Hardin Health Science Library, The University of Iowa, Iowa City, Iowa
- **Patricia Beilke**, Staff Nurse, Immanuel St. Joseph–Mayo Health System, Austin, Minnesota
- **Lisa Burkhart**, Assistant Professor, Marcella Niehoff School of Nursing, Loyola University, Chicago, Illinois
- **Tania Couto Machado Chianca**, Associate Professor, School of Nursing, Federal University of Minas Gerais, Brazil
- **M. Kathleen Clark**, Associate Professor, College of Nursing, The University of Iowa, Iowa City, Iowa
- **Mary Clarke**, Doctoral Student, College of Nursing, The University of Iowa, Iowa City, Iowa
- **Martha Craft-Rosenberg**, Professor, College of Nursing, The University of Iowa, Iowa City, Iowa
- **Laura Cullen**, Advanced Practice Nurse, The University of Iowa Hospitals and Clinics, Iowa City, Iowa
- **Cindy Dalton**, Research Assistant, McGill University Health Center, Montreal, Quebec, Canada
- **Mary Date**, Clinical Nurse Specialist, Immanuel St. Joseph–Mayo Health System, Austin, Minnesota
- **Judith Donahue**, Director of Nursing Education, Iowa Lakes Community College, Emmetsburg, Iowa
- **Gloria Dorr**, Informatics Nurse Specialist, The University of Iowa Hospitals and Clinics, Iowa City, Iowa
- **Janice Denehy**, Associate Professor Emerita, College of Nursing, The University of Iowa, Iowa City, Iowa
- **Raeda Fawzi Abu Al Rub**, Doctoral Student, College of Nursing, The University of Iowa, Iowa City, Iowa
- **Sara Frisch**, Researcher, McGill University Health Center, Montreal, Quebec, Canada
- **Debbie Frost**, Staff Nurse, Integris Mental Health, Norman, Oklahoma
- **Janet Geyer**, Advanced Practice Nurse, Children's Hospital of Iowa, The University of Iowa Hospitals and Clinics, Iowa City, Iowa
- **Barbara Head**, Assistant Professor, College of Nursing, University of Nebraska Medical Center, Omaha, Nebraska

- **Martha Hernandez**, Advanced Practice Nurse, Baptist Counseling Association, Shawnee, Oklahoma
- **Keela Herr**, Professor, College of Nursing, The University of Iowa, Iowa City, Iowa
- **Jan Hootman**, President, National Association of School Nurses, Portland, Oregon
- **Amy Hovey**, Graduate Student, College of Nursing, The University of Iowa, Iowa City, Iowa
- **Carole E. Johnson**, Former Geriatric Care Manager, Vista Eldercare, Victory Memorial Hospital, Waukegan, Illinois
- **Lorraine M. Jordan**, Director of Research, American Association of Nurse Anesthetists Foundation, Park Ridge, Illinois
- **Mary Kanak**, Doctoral Student, College of Nursing, The University of Iowa, Iowa City, Iowa
- **Sherry Kelchen**, Graduate Student, College of Nursing, The University of Iowa, Iowa City, Iowa
- **Peg Kerr**, Doctoral Student, College of Nursing, The University of Iowa, Iowa City, Iowa
- **Mary Killeen**, Associate Professor, University of Michigan, Flint, Michigan
- **Jennifer Kneip**, Graduate Student, College of Nursing, The University of Iowa, Iowa City, Iowa
- **Vicki Kraus**, Advanced Practice Nurse, The University of Iowa Hospitals and Clinics, Iowa City, Iowa
- **Sharon LaDuke**, Patient Documentation Analyst, Claxton-Hepburn Medical Center, Ogdensburg, New York
- **Scott Chisholm Lamont**, Specialty Nurse III, University of New Mexico Health Sciences Center, Albuquerque, New Mexico
- **Margaret Lunney**, Professor, College of Staten Island, City University of New York, New York, New York
- **Kathy Marlow**, Graduate Student, College of Nursing, The University of Iowa, Iowa City, Iowa
- **Eleanor McClelland**, Associate Professor Emerita, College of Nursing, The University of Iowa, Iowa City, Iowa
- **Sue Moorhead**, Associate Professor, College of Nursing, The University of Iowa, Iowa City, Iowa
- **Michael Morgan**, Assistant Professor, Wayne State University, Detroit, Michigan
- **Madj Mrayyan**, Doctoral Student, College of Nursing, The University of Iowa, Iowa City, Iowa
- **Sherri Mummy**, Advanced Practice Nurse, The University of Iowa Hospitals and Clinics, Iowa City, Iowa
- **Leslie Myers**, Research Assistant, McGill University Health Center, Montreal, Quebec, Canada
- **Joanne O' Gava**, Inservice Director, Alverno Health Care Facility, Clinton, Iowa
- **Pamela Pfeiffer**, Clinical Business Systems Analyst, St. John's Mercy Health Care, St. Louis, Missouri
- **Jeanne Popson**, RN-BSN Student, College of Nursing, The University of Iowa, Iowa City, Iowa
- **Susan Powell,** Clinical Informatics, Mason General Hospital, Shelton, Washington
- **Annette Ray**, RN-BSN Student, College of Nursing, The University of Iowa, Iowa City, Iowa
- **Sally Reavely**, Nurse Attorney, Davis, Brown, Koehn, Shors & Roberts, P.C., Des Moines, Iowa
- **Cindy Scherb**, Associate Professor, Winona State University, Rochester, Minnesota
- **Martha E. Schmitz**, Undergraduate Student, College of Nursing, The University of Iowa, Iowa City, Iowa

- **Deb Schoenfelder**, Clinical Associate Professor, College of Nursing, The University of Iowa, Iowa City, Iowa
- **Larry Schumacher**, Doctoral Student, College of Nursing, The University of Iowa, Iowa City, Iowa
- **Margaret Simons**, Advanced Practice Nurse, Veterans Administration Medical Center, Iowa City, Iowa
- **Darinda Sutton**, Director of Nursing Informatics, University of Pittsburgh, Pittsburgh, Pennsylvania
- **Mary Tarbox**, Professor and Chair, Department of Nursing, Mount Mercy College, Cedar Rapids, Iowa
- **Magdalena Turnacova**, Staff Nurse, Specialized Therapeutic Institute of Tuberculosis and Respiratory Disease, Nitra Zobor, Slovak Republic
- **Sally Twedt**, Graduate Student, College of Nursing, The University of Iowa, Iowa City, Iowa
- **Rose Utley**, Assistant Professor, Southwest Missouri State University, Springfield, Missouri
- **Barbara Van de Castle**, Instructor, Johns Hopkins University, School of Nursing, Baltimore, Maryland
- **Rosalind Willis**, Staff Nurse, Good Samaritan Hospital, Puyallup, Washington

Fellows—(2002-2005) Center for Nursing Classification and Clinical Effectiveness

The Center for Nursing Classification and Clinical Effectiveness at the College of Nursing, the University of Iowa, has established a fellows program. An appointment of *Fellow, Center for Nursing Classification and Clinical Effectiveness* is designated for individuals who contribute significantly to the ongoing upkeep and implementation of NIC and NOC. Such individuals are nonstudents who are actively contributing to the Center and may include research team members, retired professors, staff at cooperating agencies, and visiting scholars.

Fellows donate a portion of their time to some work activity of the Center. They are available as resource persons for such activities as providing ad hoc reviews of proposed new interventions and outcomes, participating in team or other meetings, serving on a planning committee for a conference, reviewing drafts of monographs, and participating in grant writing activities. An appointment of a fellow is for a 3-year period, or shorter time, depending on need (e.g., Visiting Scholar).

The following individuals have been appointed as 2002-2005 Fellows:
- **Mary Ann Anderson**, Associate Professor, College of Nursing, University of Illinois
- **Ida Androwich**, Professor, Loyola University, Chicago
- **Terri Boese**, Lecturer, College of Nursing, University of Iowa
- **Veronica Brighton**, Lecturer, College of Nursing, University of Iowa
- **Gloria Bulechek**, Professor, College of Nursing, University of Iowa
- **Howard Butcher,** Assistant Professor, College of Nursing, University of Iowa
- **Pearl Slavik Cowen**, Professor, College of Nursing, University of Iowa
- **Sister Ruth Cox**, President and CEO, Alverno Health Care Facility, Dubuque
- **Martha Craft-Rosenberg**, Professor, College of Nursing, University of Iowa
- **Jeanette Daly**, Research Assistant, Family Medicine, University of Iowa
- **Connie Delaney,** Professor, College of Nursing, University of Iowa
- **Janice Denehy**, Associate Professor Emerita, College of Nursing, University of Iowa
- **Joanne Dochterman**, Distinguished Professor, College of Nursing, University of Iowa
- **Gloria Dorr**, Advance Practice Nurse, Informatics, University of Iowa Hospitals and Clinics
- **Teresa Gibbs**, Advance Practice Nurse, Informatics, University of Iowa Hospitals and Clinics
- **Barbara Head**, Assistant Professor, College of Nursing, University of Nebraska
- **Keela Herr,** Professor, College of Nursing, University of Iowa
- **Larry Hertel,** President and Founder, Professional Home Health Services, Cedar Rapids
- **Marion Johnson**, Professor Emerita, College of Nursing, University of Iowa
- **Gail Keenan,** Assistant Professor, College of Nursing, University of Michigan
- **Vicki Kraus**, Advanced Nurse Practitioner, University of Iowa Hospitals and Clinics
- **Meridean Maas**, Professor, College of Nursing, University of Iowa
- **Eleanor McClelland**, Associate Professor Emerita, College of Nursing, University of Iowa

- **Sue Moorhead**, Associate Professor, College of Nursing, University of Iowa
- **Aleta Porcella**, Clinical Nurse Specialist–Informatics, University of Iowa Hospitals and Clinics
- **David Reed**, Assistant Research Scientist/Statistician, College of Nursing, University of Iowa
- **Cindy Scherb**, Associate Professor, Winona State University, Rochester, Minnesota
- **Janet Specht**, Assistant Professor, College of Nursing, University of Iowa
- **Elizabeth Swanson**, Associate Professor, College of Nursing, University of Iowa
- **Mary Tarbox**, Professor and Chair, Department of Nursing, Mt. Mercy College
- **Joanne Tigges**, Alumna, College of Nursing, University of Iowa
- **Marita Titler**, Senior Associate Director of Nursing and Director, Nursing Research, Quality and Outcomes Management, University of Iowa Hospitals and Clinics
- **Toni Tripp-Reimer**, Professor, College of Nursing, University of Iowa
- **Bonnie Wakefield**, Associate Chief, Nursing Research, Veterans Administration Medical Center, Iowa City
- **Pamela Willard**, Clinical Assistant Professor, College of Nursing, University of Iowa
- **Janet Williams,** Associate Professor, College of Nursing, University of Iowa
- **Marilyn Willits**, Standards Nurse Specialist, Genesis Health Care, Davenport

Iowa Intervention Project Research Team: First, Second, and Third Editions (1987-2000)

FOUNDING TEAM MEMBERS

- Joanne C. McCloskey, Co-Principal Investigator
- Gloria M. Bulechek, Co-Principal Investigator
- Marlene Cohen
- Martha Craft-Rosenberg
- John Crossley
- Janice Denehy
- Orpha Glick
- Meridean Maas
- Colleen Prophet
- Toni Tripp-Reimer

ADDITIONAL TEAM MEMBERS

- Laurie Ackerman
- Ida Androwich
- Mary Aquilino
- Jean Barry-Walker
- Hope Barton
- Terri Boese
- Pat Button
- Mary Clarke
- Laura Cullen
- Jeanette Daly
- Gloria Dorr
- Deb Eganhouse
- Barbara Head
- Keela Herr
- Mary Kanak
- Charlotte Kelley
- Vicki Kraus
- Tom Kruckeberg
- Kara Logsden
- Eleanor McClelland
- Peg Mehmert
- Paula Mobily
- Sue Moorhead
- Mary Jane Oakland
- Maria Pringle
- Michelle Robnett
- Margaret Simons
- Vicki Steelman
- Mary Tarbox
- Marita Titler
- Bonnie Wakefield

STUDENT ASSISTANTS

- Raeda Al Ad Rub
- Joan Carter
- Claire Cheng
- Linda Chlan
- Joan Chohan
- Dottie Doolittle
- Peg Kerr
- Charmaine Kleiber
- Enjoo Lee
- Debra Nelson
- Debra Pettit
- Barbara Rakel
- Debby Renner
- Cindy Scherb
- Fran Vlasses
- Young-Hee Yom
- Huibin Yue

STAFF AND OFFICE ASSISTANTS

- Gael Amabile
- Raquel Ambriz
- Sally Blackmon
- Marci Cordaro
- William Donahue
- Chris Forcucci
- Karen Hines
- Kara Logsden
- Holly Tapper

CONSULTANTS AND ADVISORS

- Connie Delaney
- David Evans
- Marjory Gordon
- Norma Lang
- Maxine Loomis
- Karen Martin
- Judy Ozbolt
- Mark Raymond
- Virginia Saba
- Frederick Suppe
- Harriet Werley
- George Woodworth

Organizations That Have Contributed to the Development of NIC

Nurses from a variety of specialty organizations have participated in the development and validation of NIC since its beginning. These organizations are:

Academy of Medical-Surgical Nurses
Advocates for Child Psychiatric Nursing
American Academy of Ambulatory Care Nursing
American Association of Critical-Care Nurses
American Association of Diabetes Educators
American Association of Neuroscience Nurses
American Association of Nurse Anesthetists
American Association of Occupational Health Nurses
American Association of Spinal Cord Injury Nurses
American Board of Neuroscience Nurses
American College of Nurse-Midwives
American Holistic Nurses Association
American Nephrology Nurses Association
American Nurses Association
ANA Council on Gerontological Nursing
ANA Council on Maternal-Child Nursing
ANA Council on Psychiatric and Mental Health Nursing
American Psychiatric Nurses Association
American Radiological Nurses Association
American Society of Ophthalmic Registered Nurses, Inc.
American Society of Pain Management Nurses
American Society of Post-Anesthesia Nurses
American Urological Association Allied
Association for Practitioners in Infection Control
Association for Professionals in Infection Control and Epidemiology, Inc.
Association of Child and Adolescent Psychiatric Nurses, Inc.
Association of Community Health Nursing Educators
Association of Nurses in AIDS Care
Association of Operating Room Nurses, Inc.
Association of Pediatric Oncology Nurses
Association of Rehabilitation Nurses
Association of Women's Health, Obstetric and Neonatal Nurses
Dermatology Nurses Association
Developmental Disabilities Nurses Association
Drug and Alcohol Nursing Association, Inc.
Emergency Nurses Association

International Association for the Study of Pain
International Society of Nurses in Genetics
Intravenous Nurses Society
Midwest Nursing Research Society
NAACOG: The Organization for Obstetric, Gynecologic, Neonatal Nurses
National Association of Hispanic Nurses
National Association of Neonatal Nurses
National Association of School Nurses, Inc.
National Consortium of Chemical Dependency Nurses
National Flight Nurses Association
National Gerontological Nursing Association
National Nurses Society on Addictions
North American Nursing Diagnosis Association
Oncology Nursing Society
Society for Education and Research in Psychiatric-Mental Health Nursing
Society for Peripheral Vascular Nursing
Society for Vascular Nursing
Society of Gastroenterology Nurses and Associates, Inc.
Society of Otorhinolaryngology and Head-Neck Nurses, Inc.
Society of Pediatric Nurses
Society of Urologic Nurses and Associates

Definitions of Terms

Nursing Intervention

Any treatment, based upon clinical judgment and knowledge, that a nurse performs to enhance patient/client outcomes. Nursing interventions include both direct and indirect care; those aimed at individuals, families, and the community; and those for nurse-initiated, physician initiated and other provider-initiated treatments.

A *direct care intervention* is a treatment performed through interaction with the patient(s). Direct care interventions include both physiological and psychosocial nursing actions and include both the "laying on of hands" actions and those that are more supportive and counseling in nature.

An *indirect care intervention* is a treatment performed away from the patient but on behalf of a patient or group of patients. Indirect care interventions include nursing actions aimed at management of the patient care environment and interdisciplinary collaboration. These actions support the effectiveness of the direct care interventions.

A *community (or public health) intervention* is targeted to promote and preserve the health of populations. Community interventions emphasize health promotion, health maintenance, and disease prevention of populations and include strategies to address the social and political climate in which the population resides.

A *nurse-initiated treatment* is an intervention initiated by the nurse in response to a nursing diagnosis. It is an autonomous action based on scientific rationale that is executed to benefit the client in a predicted way related to the nursing diagnosis and projected outcomes. These actions would include those treatments initiated by advanced nurse practitioners.

A *physician-initiated treatment* is an intervention initiated by a physician in response to a medical diagnosis but carried out by a nurse in response to a "doctor's order." Nurses may also carry out treatments initiated by other providers, such as pharmacists, respiratory therapists, or physician assistants.

Nursing Activities

The specific behaviors or actions that nurses do to implement an intervention and that assist patients/clients to move toward a desired outcome. Nursing activities are at the concrete level of action. A series of activities is necessary to implement an intervention.

Classification of Nursing Interventions

The ordering or arranging of nursing activities into groups or sets on the basis of their relationships and the assigning of intervention labels to these groups of activities.

Taxonomy of Nursing Interventions

A systematic organization of the interventions based on similarities into what can be considered a conceptual framework. The NIC taxonomy structure has three levels: domains, classes, and interventions.

xxiii

Patient

A patient is any individual, group, family, or community who is the focus of nursing intervention. The terms *patient, individual,* and *person* are used in this book, but in some settings, *client* or another word may be the preferred term. Users should feel free to use the term that is most relevant to their care setting.

Family

Two or more individuals related by blood or by choice with shared responsibility to promote mutual development, health, and maintenance of relationships.

Community

A group of people and the relationships among members of the group that develop as they share in common a physical environment and some agencies and institutions (e.g., school, fire department, voting place).

How to Find an Intervention

This edition of the Classification contains 514 interventions listed alphabetically. For clinical use there are several methods available for finding the desired intervention:

Alphabetically: if one knows the name of the intervention and desires to see the entire listing of activities and background readings

NIC Taxonomy: if one wishes to identify related interventions in particular topic areas

Taxonomy of Nursing Practice: a second option for locating related interventions by topic area

Linkages with NANDA diagnoses: if one has a NANDA diagnosis and would like to have a list of suggested interventions

Core Interventions by Specialty: if one is designing a course or information system for a particular specialty group, this is a good place to start

An individual should not be overwhelmed by the size of the classification, which is intended to be comprehensive for all specialties and all disciplines. It does not take long to become familiar with the Classification and to locate the interventions most relevant to one's own practice. The selection of a nursing intervention for a particular patient is part of the clinical decision making of the nurse. Six factors should be considered when choosing an intervention: desired patient outcomes, characteristics of the nursing diagnosis, research base for the intervention, feasibility for doing the intervention, acceptability to the patient, and capability of the nurse. These are explained more fully in Chapter Three.

Contents

Detailed Contents

PART FOUR   *NIC Interventions Linked to NANDA Diagnoses,* 781

PART ONE

Construction and Use of the Classification

CHAPTER ONE

An Overview of the Nursing Interventions Classification (NIC)

A DESCRIPTION OF THE NURSING INTERVENTIONS CLASSIFICATION

The Nursing Interventions Classification (NIC) is a comprehensive standardized classification of interventions that nurses perform. It is useful for clinical documentation, communication of care across settings, integration of data across systems and settings, effectiveness research, productivity measurement, competency evaluation, reimbursement, and curricular design. The Classification includes the interventions that nurses do on behalf of patients, both independent and collaborative interventions, both direct and indirect care. An *intervention* is defined as *any treatment, based upon clinical judgment and knowledge, that a nurse performs to enhance patient/client outcomes.* Although an individual nurse will have expertise in only a limited number of interventions reflecting his or her specialty, the entire Classification captures the expertise of all nurses. NIC can be used in all settings (from acute-care intensive care units, to home care, to hospice care, to primary care) and all specialties (from critical care to ambulatory care and long-term care). The entire Classification describes the domain of nursing; however, some of the interventions in the Classification are also done by other providers. Other health care providers are welcome to use NIC to describe their treatments.

NIC interventions include both the physiological (e.g., Acid-Base Management) and the psychosocial (e.g., Anxiety Reduction). Interventions are included for illness treatment (e.g., Hyperglycemia Management), illness prevention (e.g., Fall Prevention), and health promotion (e.g., Exercise Promotion). Most of the interventions are for use with individuals, but many are for use with families (e.g., Family Integrity Promotion) and some are for use with entire communities (e.g., Environmental Management: Community). Indirect care interventions (e.g., Supply Management) are also included. Each intervention as it appears in the Classification is listed with a label name, a definition, a set of activities to carry out the intervention, and background readings.

In this edition, there are 514 interventions and more than 12,000 activities. The portions of the intervention that are standardized are the intervention labels and the definitions: these **should not** be changed when they are used. This allows for communication across settings and comparison of outcomes. Care can be individualized, however, through the activities. From a list of approximately 10 to 30 activities per intervention, the provider selects the activities that are appropriate for the specific individual or family and can then add new activities if desired. All modifications or additions to activities should be congruent with the definition of the intervention. For each intervention, the activities are listed in logical order, from what a nurse would do first to what he or she would do last. For many activities, the placement is not crucial, but for others, the time sequence is important. The lists of activities are fairly long because the Classification must meet the needs of multiple users; students and novices need more concrete directions than experienced nurses. The activities are not standardized because this would be nearly impossible with more than 12,000 of them and would also defeat the purpose of using these to individualize care. The short lists of background readings at the end of each intervention are those found most helpful in developing the intervention or supporting some of the activities in the intervention. They are a beginning place to start reading if one is new to the intervention, but they are by no means a complete reference list, nor are they inclusive of all the research on the intervention. For this edition, as in the past, we have updated the background readings for some of the interventions.

While the lists of activities are very helpful for the teaching of an intervention and for implementation of the delivery of the intervention, they are not the essence of the Classification. The intervention label names and definitions are the key to the Classification; the names provide a summary label for the discrete activities and allow us to identify and communicate our work. Prior to NIC, we only had long lists of discrete activities; with NIC, we can easily communicate our interventions with the label name, which is accompanied by both a formal definition and a list of implementation activities.

The interventions are grouped into 30 classes and 7 domains for ease of use. The 7 domains are Physiological: Basic, Physiological: Complex, Behavioral, Safety, Family, Health System, and Community (see pp. 112-125). A few interventions are located in more than one class, but each has a unique number (code) that identifies the primary class, and this code is not used for any other intervention. The NIC taxonomy was coded for several reasons: (1) to facilitate computer use, (2) to facilitate ease of data manipulation, (3) to enhance articulation with other coded systems, and (4) to allow for use in reimbursement. The codes for the 7 domains are 1 to 7; the codes for the 30 classes are A to Z, a, b, c, d. Each intervention has a unique number consisting of four spaces. If desired, activities can be coded sequentially after the decimal by using two digits (numbers are not included in the text so as not to distract the reader). An example of a complete code is 4U-6140.01 (Safety domain, Crisis Management class, Code Management intervention, first activity: "Ensure that the airway is open, artificial respirations are administered, and cardiac compressions are being delivered").

The interventions in this edition are also grouped into a second organizing structure, the Taxonomy of Nursing Practice, developed by a collaborative group working toward a common structure for North American Nursing Diagnosis Association (NANDA) diagnoses, NIC interventions, and Nursing Outcomes Classification (NOC) outcomes.[8] Readers may use either or both structures for locating interventions. The Taxonomy of Nursing Practice containing NIC interventions appears in Appendix D.

NIC interventions have been linked with NANDA nursing diagnoses, Omaha System problems,[11] NOC outcomes,[13] resident assessment protocols used in nursing homes,[3] and Outcome and Assessment Information Set (OASIS)[4] currently mandated for collection for Medicare/Medicaid-covered patients receiving skilled home care. The linkages with NANDA diagnoses are included in this volume; the linkages with Omaha, resident assessment protocols, and OASIS are available from the Center for Nursing Classification and Clinical Effectiveness at the University of Iowa College of Nursing. NIC is linked to NANDA diagnoses and NOC outcomes in a book published by Mosby in 2001.[13]

The language used in the Classification is clear and consistently worded and reflects language used in practice. Responses to surveys by clinicians, as well as 10 years of use of the Classification, have demonstrated that all of the interventions are used in practice. Although the overall listing of 514 interventions may seem overwhelming at first to the practitioner or nursing student, we have seen that nurses soon discover those interventions that are used most often in their particular specialty or with their patient population. Other ways to locate the desired interventions are the taxonomy, the linkages with diagnoses, and the core interventions for specialties also contained in this edition.

The Classification is continually updated and has an ongoing process for feedback and review. In the back of this book are instructions for users to submit suggestions for modifications to existing interventions or to propose a new intervention. Many of the changes in this edition have come about as a result of researchers and clinicians taking the time to submit suggestions for modifications based on their research and use. These submissions are then put through a two-level review process, first by selected individuals and then by a larger group. Interventions that need more work are sent back to the author for revision. All contributors whose changes are included in the next edition are acknowledged in the book. New editions of the Classification are planned for approximately every 4 years. Work that is conducted during intervals between editions and other relevant publications that enhance the use of the Classification are available from the Center for Nursing Classification and Clinical Effectiveness at the University of Iowa.

The research to develop NIC began in 1987 and has progressed through four phases, each with some overlap in time:

Phase I: Construction of the Classification (1987-1992)
Phase II: Construction of the Taxonomy (1990-1995)
Phase III: Clinical Testing and Refinement (1993-1997)
Phase IV: Use and Maintenance (1996-ongoing)

Work conducted in each of these phases is described in the next chapter. The research was begun with 7 years of funding from the National Institutes of Health, National Institute of Nursing. Ongoing work is supported by the Center for Nursing Classification and Clinical Effectiveness at the College of Nursing at the University of Iowa, financed partly by the College of Nursing and the University of Iowa and partly by earnings from licenses and related products. NIC was developed by a large research team whose members represented multiple areas of clinical and methodological expertise. In 2002, members of this team, as well as others who contribute to the continued development of NIC, were appointed to 3-year terms as "fellows" in the Center. For more information about the Center for Nursing Classification and Clinical Effectiveness, which houses NIC and NOC, please see the web site: http://www.nursing.uiowa.edu/cnc.

Multiple research methods have been used in the development of NIC. An inductive approach was used in Phase I to build the Classification based on existing practice. Original sources were current textbooks, care planning guides, and nursing information systems. Content analysis, focus group review, and questionnaires to experts in specialty areas of practice were used to augment the clinical practice expertise of team members. Phase II was characterized by deductive methods. Methods to construct the taxonomy included similarity analysis, hierarchical clustering, and multidimensional scaling. Through clinical field testing, steps for implementation were developed and tested; and the need for linkages between NANDA, NIC, and NOC was identified. Over time, more than 1000 nurses have completed questionnaires, and approximately 50 professional associations have provided input about the Classification. The next chapter gives more information about the research conducted to construct and validate NIC; more details can be found in chapters in the earlier editions of NIC and in numerous articles and chapters. A video made by the National League of Nursing and now available for rent from the Center for Nursing Classification and Clinical Effectiveness at the University of Iowa is a good documentary of the early work. Current information is available on the Center's web page.

Several tools that assist in the implementation of the Classification are available. Included in this book are the taxonomic structure to assist a user in finding the intervention of choice, linkages with NANDA diagnoses to facilitate decision support with these diagnostic languages, the core intervention lists for areas of specialty practice, and the amount of time and level of education needed to perform each intervention. Chapter 3 contains multiple examples of forms and computer screens submitted by users in practice and education. In addition, an anthology of early publications and an education monograph to demonstrate one program's implementation and use of NIC and NOC in an undergraduate curriculum are available from the Center for Nursing Classification and Clinical Effectiveness, as well as the linkage monographs described earlier. The Center maintains a LISTSERV, and a newsletter (*The NIC/NOC Letter*), produced twice a year, disseminates current information. A 4-hour web course on the basics of standardized language, NANDA, NIC, and NOC is available from the Center. All of these resources are explained further on the web site.

One indication of usefulness is national recognition. NIC is recognized by the American Nurses Association (ANA) and is included as one data set that will meet the uniform guidelines for information system vendors in the ANA's Nursing Information and Data Set Evaluation

Center (NIDSEC). NIC is included in the National Library of Medicine's *Metathesaurus for a Unified Medical Language*. The *Cumulative Index to Nursing Literature (CINAHL)* includes NIC interventions in its indexes. NIC is included in the Joint Commission on Accreditation of Healthcare Organizations' (JCAHO) accreditation requirements as one nursing classification system that can be used to meet the standard on uniform data. Alternative Link[1] has included NIC in its ABC codes for reimbursement for alternative providers. NIC is registered in Health Level 7 (HL7), which is the U.S. standards organization for messaging in health care. NIC is also licensed for inclusion in the Systematized Nomenclature of Medicine (SNOMED). Interest in NIC has been demonstrated in several other countries; and translations into Chinese, Dutch, French, Icelandic, German, Japanese, Korean, Spanish, and Portuguese have been completed or are underway (see Appendix E, Selected Publications, for translations of previous editions).

The best indication of usefulness, however, is the growing list of individuals and health care agencies that use NIC. Many health care agencies have adopted NIC for use in standards, care plans, competency evaluation, and nursing information systems; nursing education programs are using NIC to structure curricula and identify competencies for nursing students; vendors of information systems are incorporating NIC in their software; authors of major texts are using NIC to discuss nursing treatments; and researchers are using NIC to study the effectiveness of nursing care. Permission to use NIC in publications, information systems, and web courses should be sought from Mosby (see the inside front cover). Part of the money to purchase a license is returned to the Center to help with ongoing development of the Classification. Some common questions about NIC are addressed later in this chapter.

RELATED PROJECTS: NURSING OUTCOMES CLASSIFICATION, NURSING DIAGNOSIS EXTENSION CLASSIFICATION, NNN ALLIANCE, NURSING MANAGEMENT MINIMUM DATA SET

NIC research has "spun off" several other projects, most notably NOC and the Nursing Diagnosis Extension Classification (NDEC). Another project, the Nursing Management Minimum Data Set (NMMDS), although not a direct spin-off from NIC, was related and highly supported by some of the NIC investigators who had helped to identify the need. The NNN Alliance represents an effort to enhance collaboration among NANDA, NIC, and NOC. These related projects and efforts are briefly explained here because we often get questions about them and they are relevant for use of NIC.

NOC: Nursing Outcomes Classification

The realization soon came that, in addition to diagnoses and interventions, a third classification, patient outcomes, was also needed to complete the requirements for documentation of a nursing clinical encounter. One of the NIC team members, Meridean Maas, sought out another colleague, Marion Johnson, who had long expressed interest in outcomes, and together they decided to form another research team to develop a classification of patient outcomes. They attempted to recruit different individuals so as not to dilute the strength of the NIC team, but some of the NOC team members were also NIC team members. This has been a strength, providing for continuity and understanding between the two groups. In the early years of NOC, McCloskey and Bulechek served as consultants to the new team. The NOC team researchers were able to use, or modify and use, many of the research approaches and methods that were developed by the NIC team. The NOC team was begun in 1991, and the first edition of NOC was published in 1997. The name of the classification and the acronym of NOC were deliberately selected so that there would be association with NIC.

Nursing Outcomes Classification (NOC) was first published by Mosby in 1997 with 190 outcomes listed in alphabetical order. The second edition, with 260 outcomes and a taxonomic structure, was published in 2000,[12] at the same time as the third edition of NIC. Each outcome has a definition, a list of indicators that can be used to evaluate patient status in relation to the outcome, a five-point Likert scale to measure patient status, and a short list of references used in the development of the outcome. (See Chapter 3 for one example of a NOC outcome.) Examples of scales used with the outcomes are 1, extremely compromised, to 5, not compromised; and 1, never demonstrated, to 5, consistently demonstrated. The outcomes are developed for use across the care continuum and therefore can be used to monitor patient outcomes throughout an illness episode or over an extended period of care. The third edition of NOC is being published at the same time as this fourth edition of NIC. NOC, like NIC, is housed in the Center for Nursing Classification and Clinical Effectiveness at the University of Iowa College of Nursing. Although NOC has been in existence only since 1997, there have been numerous translations into other languages and multiple adoptions in both education and practice.

NDEC: Nursing Diagnosis Extension Classification

As work on NIC and NOC progressed, several of the NIC team members who had been active in NANDA over the years began to discuss the need to revise and expand the NANDA classification. The initial attitude about NIC is frequently influenced by the attitude about NANDA: a positive attitude about NANDA lends itself to adoption of NIC, but a negative or neutral attitude about NANDA results in a reluctance to pay serious attention to NIC. Although NIC (and NOC) can be used without NANDA, it is desirable in any patient encounter to know the diagnoses and the interventions and outcomes.

The use of standardized language in nursing began with the development of the NANDA classification in the 1970s. The use of NANDA diagnoses in practice and education spread rapidly in the 1980s. NANDA has been translated into multiple languages and is used in more than 20 countries throughout the world. However, in the United States and to some extent in Europe, some have become disenchanted with the language, the taxonomic structure, and the slow process of change. During the 1980s, interest in NANDA waned, with organizational membership and resources shrinking. Another member of the NIC research team, Martha Craft-Rosenberg, decided to take action to help improve the NANDA classification. She and another colleague at the University of Iowa, Connie Delaney, formed the Nursing Diagnosis Extension and Classification (NDEC) research team in November 1993. A year or so later, they made a written contract with the NANDA governing board to refine existing diagnoses and develop new diagnoses. This team—led by Craft-Rosenberg, Delaney, and Janice Denchy—submitted a large number of refined diagnoses and some new diagnoses for discussion at the 1998 NANDA convention. The 1999 to 2000 edition of the NANDA classification[18] includes a portion of these updates, and the proceedings from the 1998 conference[5] describe the NDEC work in full. In 2002 Martha Craft-Rosenberg became president-elect and in 2004, president of NANDA.

NNN Alliance

The NNN Alliance (pronounced *the 3N Alliance*), formed in 2001, represents a virtual and collaborative relationship between NANDA and the Center for Nursing Classification and Clinical Effectiveness (CNC) at the University of Iowa. The goal of this alliance is to advance the development, testing, and refinement of nursing language. The co-chairs of the Alliance are the Director of the Center for Nursing Classification and Clinical Effectiveness and the President of NANDA, with the governing boards of each organization serving as the governing board of the Alliance. To date, two central projects have been completed by the Alliance: the NNN conference and the Taxonomy of Nursing Practice. Although NANDA, NIC, and NOC had held two joint conferences in the 1990s, the first official NNN conference was held in Chicago in spring 2002 as a result of planning by an Alliance committee working with Nursecom. The conference, which in 2002 and in the future replaces the biennial NANDA conference, was very successful with more than 300 participants from many countries. The second NNN conference will be held in 2004 with the hope that this can continue in the future.

The NNN Alliance has also created a common organizing structure, the Taxonomy of Nursing Practice. This was created through support of a conference grant from the National

Library of Medicine[7] for an invitational conference held in August 2001. During this meeting, participants studied existing language classifications, nomenclatures, and data sets. At the completion of the conference, a small task force compiled the work of the conference attendees and created the first draft of a common unifying structure for diagnoses, interventions, and outcomes (NANDA, NIC, and NOC). The proposed structure was then disseminated among conference participants and exposed to the nursing community for feedback at the NNN Conference in April 2002 and on the NANDA and CNC web sites. Revisions to the document were based on feedback and the manuscript, *Collaboration in Nursing Classification: The Creation of a Common Unifying Structure for NANDA, NIC and NOC,* was prepared by Dochterman and Jones and is the first paper in the monograph *Unifying Nursing Languages: The Harmonization of NANDA, NIC, and NOC* published by the ANA in 2003.[8] In this edition in Appendix D, NIC interventions are placed in this common taxonomy.

NMMDS: Nursing Management Minimum Data Set

The purpose of the NMMDS is to develop a standardized management data set that can be used by nurse managers to extend and augment the clinical data set. Diane Huber and Connie Delaney, working with various others over the years, have taken the lead in developing variables and definitions for the NMMDS. In 1995 they received funding from the American Organization of Nurse Executives (AONE) to conduct an invitational conference to refine the previous work. The results were published in monograph form by AONE the following year.[6] The NMMDS consists of 17 variables that cluster into three dimensions: environment, nurse resources, and financial resources. The variables in the environment dimension consist of type of nursing delivery unit/service, patient population, volume of nursing delivery unit/service, nursing delivery unit/service accreditation, centralization, complexity, patient accessibility, method of care delivery, and complexity of clinical decision making. The variables in the nurse resources dimension include the management demographic profile, nursing staff/client care support personnel, nursing care staff demographic profile, and staff satisfaction. The variables in the financial resources dimension include payer type, reimbursement, nursing delivery unit/service budget, and expenses. Definitions and measures for each variable are published in the monograph.

QUESTIONS SOMETIMES ASKED ABOUT NIC

In this section we have tried to answer some of the common questions about NIC. Understanding the reasons that things have been done in a certain way (or not done) will assist in better use of the Classification. We began this section in the second edition of NIC and have added to it; the order of the questions, to some extent, reflects the order in which we have encountered them and the evolving types of concerns as use becomes more extensive. Those new to NIC will find it helpful to read through all the questions; questions new to this edition are numbers 16, 17, 18, 19, and 20.

   1. Why are certain rather basic activities included in the activity list for some interventions but not others? For example, why should an activity related to documentation be included in the labels Discharge Planning and Referral and not in every label? Or, why should an activity related to evaluation of outcomes be included in Discharge Planning and not in all intervention labels? Or, why should an activity on establishing trust be included in the labels Reminiscence Therapy and Support Group but not in other intervention labels?
   Basic activities are included *when they are critical* (i.e., absolutely essential to communicate the essence of the intervention) for the implementation of that intervention. They are not included when they are part of the routine but not an integral piece of the intervention. For example, hand washing is a routine part of many physical interventions but is not critical to interventions such as Bathing or Skin Care. (We are not saying that washing your hands should not be done for these interventions, just that it is not a critical activity.) Hand washing is a critical part, however, of such interventions as Infection Control and Contact Lens Care.

2. How do I decide which intervention to use when one intervention includes an activity that refers to another intervention? In some NIC interventions there is reference in the activity list to another intervention. For example, the intervention of Airway Management contains an activity that says "Perform endotracheal or nasotracheal suctioning, as appropriate." There is another intervention in NIC, Airway Suctioning, which is defined as "Removal of airway secretions by inserting a suction catheter into the patient's oral airway and/or trachea" and has 25 activities listed under it. Another example is the intervention of Pain Management, which contains an activity that says "Teach the use of nonpharmacologic techniques (e.g., biofeedback, TENS, hypnosis, relaxation, guided imagery, music therapy, distraction, play therapy, acupressure, hot/cold application, and massage) before, after, and, if possible, during painful activities; before pain occurs or increases; and along with other pain relief measures." Nearly all of the techniques listed in parentheses for this activity are listed in NIC as interventions, each with a definition and a set of defining activities. The two examples demonstrate that the more abstract, more global interventions sometimes refer to other interventions. Sometimes one needs the more global intervention; sometimes, the more specific one; and sometimes, both. The selection of nursing interventions for use with an individual patient is part of clinical decision making by the nurse. NIC reflects all possibilities. The nurse should choose the intervention(s) to use for a particular patient using the six factors discussed in Chapter 3.

3. When is a new intervention developed? Why do we believe that each of our interventions is different from others in the Classification? Maybe they are the same but are called something different? We developed the guiding principle, *a new intervention is added if 50% or more of the activities are different from those listed with another related intervention.* Thus each time a new intervention is proposed, it is reviewed against other existing interventions. If 50% or more of the activities are not different, it is not viewed as significantly different and therefore is not added to the Classification.

With interventions that are types of a more general intervention (e.g., Sexual Counseling is a type of Counseling; Tube Care: Gastrointestinal is a type of Tube Care), the most pertinent activities are repeated in the more concrete intervention so that this intervention can stand alone. This should not be all the activities, just those that are essential to carrying out the intervention. In addition, the intervention must have at least 50% new activities.

4. Does NIC include the important monitoring functions of the nurse? Very definitely yes. NIC includes many monitoring interventions (e.g., Electronic Fetal Monitoring: Antepartum, Health Policy Monitoring, Intracranial Pressure [ICP] Monitoring, Neurologic Monitoring, Newborn Monitoring, Surveillance, Surveillance: Late Pregnancy, Surveillance: Safety, Vital Signs Monitoring). These interventions consist mostly of monitoring activities but also include some activities to reflect the clinical judgment process, or what nurses are thinking and anticipating when they monitor. These interventions define what to look for and what to do when an anticipated event occurs. In addition, all interventions in NIC include monitoring activities when these are done as part of the intervention. *Monitor* and *identify* are the words we use to mean assessment activities that are part of an intervention. We have tried to use these words rather than the word *assess* in this intervention classification because *assessment* is the term used in the nursing process to refer to those activities that take place before diagnosis.

5. Does NIC include interventions that would be used by a primary care practitioner, especially interventions designed to promote health? Yes indeed. Although these are not grouped together in one class, NIC contains all of the interventions nurses use to promote health. Examples include Anticipatory Guidance, Decision-Making Support, Developmental Enhancement, Exercise Promotion, Health Education, Immunization/Vaccination Administration, Learning Facilitation, Nutrition Management, Weight Management, Oral Health Promotion, Parent Education, Risk Identification, Smoking Cessation Assistance, Substance Use Prevention, and Self-Responsibility Facilitation.

6. Does NIC cover treatments used by advanced practice nurses practicing in specialty areas? Definitely yes. Many of the interventions in NIC require advanced education and experience in a clinical practice. For example, the following interventions may reflect the practice of an advanced practice nurse working in obstetrics: Amnioinfusion, Birthing, Electronic Fetal Monitoring: Antepartum, Grief Work Facilitation: Perinatal Death, High-Risk Pregnancy Care, Labor Induction, Labor Suppression, Reproductive Technology Management, and Ultrasonography: Limited Obstetric. A similar list can be identified for most specialties. Medication Prescribing is an intervention used by many nurses in advanced practice.

7. Does NIC include alternative therapies? We assume this question refers to treatments that are not part of mainstream medical practice in this country. Interventions in NIC that might be listed as alternative therapies include Autogenic Training, Biofeedback, Calming Technique, Hypnosis, Meditation, Simple Guided Imagery, Simple Relaxation Therapy, and Therapeutic Touch. Many of these interventions are located in the class Psychological Comfort Promotion. Other alternative therapies will be added to NIC as they become part of accepted nursing practice; in this edition we have included, for the first time, Aromatherapy. NIC interventions are also included in Alternative Link's ABC codes[1] for use by alternative providers (providers other than allopathic physicians) to document care for reimbursement.

8. How do I find the interventions I use when there are so many interventions in NIC? At first glance, NIC, with more than 500 interventions, may seem overwhelming. Remember, however, that NIC covers the practice domain of *all nurses*. An individual nurse will use only a portion of the interventions in NIC on a regular basis. These can be identified by reviewing the classes in the taxonomy that are most relevant to an individual's practice area. In those agencies with nursing information systems, the interventions can be grouped by taxonomy class, nursing diagnosis, patient population (e.g., burn, cardiac, maternity), nursing specialty, or unit. Many computer systems will also allow individual nurses to create and maintain a personal library of most used interventions. We have been told by nurses using the Classification that they quickly identify a relatively small number of interventions that reflect the core of their practice.

9. Can I change the activities in an intervention when I use it with my patient? Yes. The standardized language is the label name and the definition, and these should remain the same for all patients and all situations. The activities can be modified to better reflect the needs of the particular situation. These are advantages of NIC: it provides both a standardized language that will help us communicate across settings about our interventions and it allows for individualized care. The NIC activities use the modifiers "as appropriate," "as needed," and "as indicated" to reflect the fact that individuals are unique and may require different approaches. The NIC activities include all ages of patients, and, when used with adults, some of the activities directed toward children may not be appropriate (and vice versa). In this case, these can be omitted from an agency's list of activities. Also, the NIC interventions are not at the procedure level of specificity, and some agencies may wish to be more specific to reflect particular protocols developed for their populations. The activities can easily be modified to reflect this. At the same time that we believe that the activities can and should be modified to meet individual needs, we *caution that activities should not be changed so much that the original NIC list is unrecognizable.* If this is done, then the intervention may, in fact, not be the same. Any modified or new activities should fit the definition of the intervention. In addition, when an activity is being added consistently for most patients and populations, then it may be needed in NIC's general listing of activities. In this case, we would urge the clinician to submit the proposed activity addition or change. In this way the activity list continues to reflect the best of current practice and is most useful in teaching the interventions to new practitioners.

10. How does NIC contribute to theory development in nursing? The intervention labels are concepts that name the treatments that nurses provide. The definitions and activities that accompany the labels provide for definition and description of the interventions. Clarification of intervention concepts contributes to the development of nursing knowledge and facilitates communication within the discipline. As nursing's ability to link diagnoses, interventions, and outcomes grows, prescriptive theory for nursing practice will evolve. NIC is a crucial development because it provides the lexical elements for middle-range theories in nursing that will link diagnoses, interventions, and outcomes. Interventions are the key elements in nursing. All other aspects of nursing practice are contingent upon, and secondary to, the treatments that identify and delineate our discipline. This intervention-centric approach does not diminish the importance of the patient; but from a disciplinary perspective, the phenomenon of interest of the patient is important because it can be affected by nursing action. We believe that use of standardized languages for nursing diagnoses, interventions, and outcomes heralds a new era in the development of nursing theory, moving from the past focus on grand theory to the development and use of nursing middle-range theories. (See the articles with first authors of Blegen or Tripp-Reimer in the publications list in Appendix E for further discussion about this.) Although we believe that, in the future, nursing grand theories will be replaced by nursing middle-range theories, for the present, NIC can be used with any existing grand theory. NIC can be used by any institution, nursing specialty, or care delivery model, regardless of philosophical orientation.

11. Does the Classification include administrative interventions? The Classification includes indirect care interventions done by first-line staff or advance practice nurses but does *not* include, for the most part, those behaviors that are administrative in nature. An *indirect care intervention* is a treatment performed by a direct care provider away from the patient but on behalf of a patient or group of patients; an *administrative intervention* is an action performed by a nurse administrator (nurse manager or other nurse administrator) to enhance the performance of staff members in order to promote better patient outcomes. Some of the interventions in NIC, when used by an administrator to enhance staff performance, would then be administrative interventions. Most of these are located in the taxonomy in the Health System domain. It should be noted that the borders between direct, indirect, and administrative interventions are not firm and some NIC interventions may be used in various contexts. For example, the nurse in the hospital may provide Caregiver Support as an indirect intervention administered to a relative of the patient being cared for, but the nurse in the home, treating the whole family, may provide this intervention as direct care. With the addition of more interventions for communities, we have added interventions that are more administrative in nature, for example, Cost Containment and Fiscal Resource Management. These are, however, delivered by the primary care nurse in the community setting or by the case manager, both of whom have a larger administrative role.

12. Does my health care agency need to be computerized to use NIC? No, NIC can be used in a manual care planning and documentation system. If the system is manual, nurses unfamiliar with NIC will need ready access to the NIC book. The book should also be available for nurses working in agencies that have computerized NIC (we think every unit should have a book and encourage individual nurses to have their own copies), but, with a computer, NIC can be stored and accessed electronically. Computers make it easy to access NIC interventions in a variety of ways (for now, by taxonomic classes and nursing diagnoses, but it is also possible by patient population, unit type, outcome, clinical path, etc.). Computers can easily accommodate a variety of clinical decision support screens for nurses. Documenting what we do for patients using a standardized language on computers makes it possible for nursing to build agency, state, regional, and national databases to do effectiveness research. If your agency is not computerized, help it to become computerized. But you do not have to wait for the computer to use NIC. NIC is helpful in the communication of nursing care with or without a computer.

13. When do I need to obtain a license? Other related questions include: **Why do I need a license? Why isn't NIC in the public domain? Why is the copyright for NIC held by a publisher?** A license is needed if you put NIC on a nursing information system or if you will use a substantial part of the Classification for commercial gain or advantage. NIC is published and copyrighted by Mosby, Inc., a part of Elsevier Science. Mosby, not the NIC authors or the Center for Nursing Classification and Clinical Effectiveness, processes requests for permissions to use the Classification. See the inside front cover for directions on whom to contact for permission to use or licensing.

When we first began working on the NIC classification, we had little idea of the magnitude of the work or its current widespread use, and we did not know that it would be followed by NOC. We were looking for a way to get the work in print and disseminated quickly. As academics, we were familiar with the book publishing world, and, after some very serious review of alternative mechanisms and talks with other publishers, we selected Mosby as the publisher. Publication with Mosby has several advantages. First, they have the resources and the contacts to produce a book, to market it, and to sell it. In addition, Mosby has the legal staff and resources to process requests for permission and protect the copyright. This is especially important with standardized language, where alteration of terms will impede the goal of communication among nurses across specialties and between delivery sites. We continue to have a good relationship with Mosby, which involves frequent and active participation in permissions requests. We view our relationship as a partnership.

Copyright does *not* restrict fair use. According to guidelines by the American Library Association, fair use allows materials to be copied if: (1) the portion copied is selective and sparing in comparison to the whole work; (2) the materials are not used repeatedly; (3) no more than one copy is made for each person; (4) the source and copyright notice are included on each copy; and (5) persons are not assessed a fee for the copy beyond the actual cost of reproduction. The determination of the amount that can be copied under fair use policies has to do with the effect of the copying on sales of the original material. The American Library Association says that no more than 10% of a work should be copied.

When someone puts NIC on an information system that will be used by multiple users, copyright is violated (a book is now being "copied" for use by hundreds of nurses) and so a licensing agreement is needed. Also, when someone uses large amounts of NIC in a book or software product that is then sold and makes money for that individual, then a permissions fee is necessary. Schools of nursing and health care agencies that want to use NIC in their own organizations and have no intention of selling a resulting product are free to do so. Fair use policies exist, however. For example, NIC and NOC should not be photocopied and used in syllabi semester after semester—the Classification books should be adopted for use. Similarly, health care agencies should purchase a reasonable number of books (say, one per unit) rather than copy the interventions and place them in some procedure manual.

Requests for use of NIC and NOC should be sent to the permissions department of Mosby. Many requests for permission to use material do not violate copyright, and permission is given with no fee. Fees for use in a book depend on the amount of material used. Fees for use in information systems depend on the number of users and average about $5.00 per user per year. There is a flat fee for incorporating NIC into a vendor's database and then a sublicense fee for each sublicense undertaken based on the number of users. The fees are reasonable, and a substantial portion of the fees is forwarded to the Center for Nursing Classification and Clinical Effectiveness to help support the ongoing development and use of NIC.

14. How do I explain to the administrator at my institution that a license is needed? First of all, we want to repeat that only use in an information system requires a license and a fee; if you want to use NIC manually or for a particular project that does not violate copyright, please go ahead. In our experience, it is nurses and not health care administrators who are unfamiliar with licenses and fees. Most other health care classifications are copyrighted, and fees are required for use. For example, the *Current Procedural Terminology* (*CPT*) is copyrighted by the American Medical Association, the *Diagnostic and Statistical Manual of Mental Disorders* (*DSM*) is copyrighted by the American Psychiatric Association, and SNOMED is copyrighted by the College of American Pathologists. Health care institutions regularly pay license fees now, but most nurses are not aware of these. At one Midwestern tertiary care hospital, 97 vendor software products are installed, and more than $1,220,000 is spent annually on software license fees.

License fees are often included as part of the software costs. NIC can be licensed from Mosby (use of the language) for incorporation in an existing information system or purchased from a vendor with software (the vendor has purchased the license from Mosby, and the software price includes the cost of the license). As more nurses understand the advantages of using standardized language and desire this in purchases of new information systems, more vendors will include NIC in their products.

In nursing, none of the professional organizations have the resources to maintain NIC, so another avenue was needed. We have been told by those in the medical field that having the Classification housed in a university setting has advantages over the professional organizational model, in which politics (what is in and what is out) may play a part. Ongoing development and maintenance, however, require resources. Classifications and other works in the public domain are often those for which there will be no upkeep—you can use what is there but do not expect it to be kept current. We have attempted to make NIC as accessible as possible but also to collect fees so that we can have a revenue stream to finance the maintenance work that must continue.

15. Should we use a nursing classification when most of health care is being delivered by interdisciplinary teams? Occasionally we hear something like, "We can't use anything that is labeled *nursing* and comes from nursing when everything is now going to be interdisciplinary." We hear this, by the way, from nurses rather than from physicians or other power holders in the interdisciplinary arena. At the same time, it is assumed that using medical language does not violate this artificial interdisciplinary principle. We believe that nurses who are members of an interdisciplinary team addressing the development and implementation of a computerized integrated patient care record should be, in fact, must be, the spokespersons for use of NIC and NOC. Yes, these have the *nursing* word in their titles because they were developed inductively through research based on the work of nurses by nurses. Taken as a whole, they reflect the discipline of nursing, but any one individual intervention may be done by other types of providers and any one outcome may be influenced by the treatments of other providers or by many other factors. This is a situation in which nursing has something of value that the other providers, for the most part, do not, and which documents the contributions of nurses and can be used or adapted and used by others if they wish. Nurses should not shrink from talking about these nursing initiatives; rather, they should stand tall and offer them as a nursing contribution to the interdisciplinary goal of a computerized patient record that can cross settings and specialties.

This is *not* inconsistent with being a good team member in an interdisciplinary environment. For successful outcomes to be achieved by interdisciplinary teams, it is essential that nurse members communicate their unique perspective and knowledge. What makes a good team member? There are three essential qualities: (1) the person has something that contributes to the overall functioning of the team, (2) the person is good at what he or she does, and (3) others understand what the person can do. Would a baseball team welcome a member who could not play any position and was a poor batter? Definitely not. Would the team welcome someone who was eager to help but unable to say how he or she could help? Maybe, but this person would end up being water boy or girl rather than playing a position. Being a good team member means that the person has something to contribute and communicates ideas. Baseball teams emphasize the importance of specific and different roles and skills of members. No one suggests that because a team member is called a pitcher or a shortstop, he or she is not a team player. Players are not told that they are not good team members if they sharpen their individual knowledge and skills and are acknowledged for individual performance. A baseball team, or any team for that matter, improves effectiveness by maximizing and integrating the contributions of individual members. Baseball managers would undoubtedly get a good laugh from the notion that they should conceal and minimize the contributions of individual team members to increase the effectiveness of the team.

We have heard a few individuals say that there should be only one language that is shared by all health disciplines. If this is possible, we believe that the one language should develop inductively through the sharing and adding on to the current languages that exist. Perhaps, over time, we will build one large common language in which some intervention and outcome terms are shared by many providers. But even if we can build one large common language, it will always be used in parts because the whole is too great to learn, communicate, and study and because all interventions and outcomes are not the business of every discipline. The one very large language will be broken down and used in parts for the same reasons that there are disciplines—the whole is too large and complex to be mastered by any one individual. Hence, different disciplines represent different specialized perspectives.

16. I want to implement NIC in our agency/facility. What is the best way to go about this? Other related questions include: **Should I implement NIC and NOC together? Should I implement NIC at the same time I orient nurses to a new computer system? Should we do this on just a pilot unit first or put this up "live" for everyone at the same time?** This is what Chapter 3 is all about. In particular, see the Steps for Implementation in Box 3-2 for practice agencies and Box 3-9 for educational facilities. There are also other helpful materials in Chapter 3, such as a list of helpful readings related to change and evaluation, as well as many examples of implementation forms used by practice agencies that have implemented NIC. As for the questions related to how much to do at one time, there is no one right way; it truly does depend on the situation and the amount and nature of the changes, the resources and support available, and the time constraints. The companion NOC book has many helpful suggestions about implementation of NOC. We would caution not to make too many changes at once, for this is often more than most can handle. On the other hand, don't drag a change out in small pieces for a long time. Duplicate charting (recording the same thing in more than one place) is a no-no. Piloting a change to work the bugs out (say, starting on one unit where the nurse manager and staff are supportive) is always a good idea. Providing time for training and having support staff available when the change is first made are important. The Center for Nursing Classification and Clinical Effectiveness has available a 4-hour web course on the basics of standardized language and NIC and NOC, as well as a film made by the National League for Nursing on the development and purpose of NIC, which are helpful teaching aides. It is important in the beginning to think about the uses of the data in the future, beyond the initial care planning or documentation purposes. Chapter 3 also covers the idea of setting up a comprehensive database for effectiveness research in the future.

17. How does NIC compare with other classifications? Usually this question has a specific "other" in the question, most often the International Classification of Nursing Practice (ICNP) or the Omaha System, but sometimes the Home Health Care Classification, the Perioperative Data Set, or the Patient Care Data Set. We include brief information about these here to help the reader make a comparison.

International Classification of Nursing Practice. The need for language to facilitate communication by and among nurses is a worldwide concern. In 1996, the International Council of Nurses (ICN) published the Alpha Version of the ICNP[9] and, in 1999, the Beta 1 Version.[10] The initial intent was to construct an organizing structure for existing classifications, but under the direction of Randi Mortensen and Gunnar Nielsen of Denmark, the ICNP developed into a separate classification. The Beta Version has three components: nursing phenomena, nursing outcomes, and nursing actions. Each component consists of axes; for example, the nursing phenomena classification axes are focus of practice, judgment, frequency, duration, body site, topology, likelihood, and distribution. The outcomes classification is simply the status of a nursing diagnosis at some point in time after a nursing intervention. The nursing actions classification consists of action type, target, means, time, location, topology, route, and beneficiary. While each of the axes has a definition, there are no standardized lists of terms for each of the axes. The development and testing of the ICNP has raised awareness of the need for nursing terminology around the globe, but the Classification itself is difficult to use clinically. In our opinion, the components are most useful for the development of a reference information model (see question 19) that can assist with the transfer of languages across differing computer systems. Information can be found at the International Council of Nurses' web site: http://www.icn.ch/icnp.htm.

Omaha System. The Omaha System is the oldest of the nursing classifications and was developed in the 1970s by Karen Martin and colleagues for use in community health.[15,23] It consists of three parts: problems, interventions, and outcomes. The Problem Classification Scheme consists of four domains (Environmental, Psychosocial, Physiological, and Health Related Behaviors) that include 40 problems or diagnoses. Modifiers for the diagnoses identify the problem as either an individual or family problem and as a health promotion, potential, or actual problem. There are also signs and symptoms specific to each problem. The Intervention Scheme is composed of four categories (Health Teaching, Guidance and Counseling; Treatments and Procedures; Case Management; and Surveillance) that include 62 targets defined as objects of health-related interventions or activities. The third part is the Problem Rating Scale for Outcomes, a simple five-point, ordinal scale composed of Knowledge, Behavior, and Status subscales. Each of the three concepts is rated for degree of response. Ratings are done at appropriate intervals and when the patient is discharged from service. The three parts of the system are not linked to each other; a nurse makes an independent selection in each of the parts.

The Omaha System is used in numerous community health settings and in some educational settings. In 1994 a software program called *the Nightingale Tracker*, was developed based on the Omaha System and funded by the Helene Fuld Health Trust. An article by the development team overviews the software and some of the issues in its development.[17] The Classification has been translated into Danish and Japanese and the problem scheme has been linked to both NIC[11] and NOC by the Iowa researchers with a review by Karen Martin. While the Omaha System has received widespread recognition in multiple arenas, it has not changed substantially since the original work.[15] The Winter 1999 issue of *On-line Journal of Nursing Informatics* contains a series of articles about the system.

Home Health Care Classification (HHCC). The Home Health Care Classification (HHCC), developed by Virginia Saba at Georgetown University in the late 1980s for use in home health care, consists of two vocabularies for diagnoses and interventions.[21,22] The diagnoses vocabulary consists of 50 major categories and 95 subcategories; the interventions vocabulary consists of 60 major categories and 100 subcategories. Each vocabulary uses modifiers to expand the codes. The diagnoses can be modified by the terms *improved, stabilized*, and *deteriorated* to indicate the expected or actual outcomes of care. The interventions can be modified by the terms *assess, care, teach*, and *manage* to indicate the type of nursing action. The two vocabularies are organized by 20 care components, similar to the classes of NIC and NOC, and include a coding scheme. The Classification has been widely disseminated, but the extent of use is unclear. More information can be found at the web site: http://www.dml.georgetown.edu/research/hhcc. An article comparing the first edition of NIC with the intervention schemes of the Omaha System and the HHCC was published in the *Journal of Nursing Administration* in 1993.[16] To our knowledge, the HHCC has not been updated since the original publication.

Perioperative Data Set. This was developed by the Association of periOperative Registered Nurses (AORN) in the early 1990s. It contains diagnoses, interventions, and outcomes identified for the specialty of perioperative nursing. The interventions in it are at the discrete activity level of NIC. In an article in *Nursing Diagnosis* in 2001,[2] Suzanne Beyea, then the Director of Research for the Association who spearheaded the development of the data set, explains the reasons for development of the specialty data set and then puts forth the case that, since the development of the comprehensive classifications of NIC and NOC, specialty organizations should *not* develop their own vocabularies and data sets but should use and help refine existing classifications.

Patient Care Data Set. The Patient Care Data Set was developed by Judy Ozbolt at the University of Virginia and then underwent substantial revisions at Vanderbilt University Medical Center. It began in 1994 as a comprehensive catalog of terms used in patient care records of nine hospitals to name the phenomenon of care: problems, actions, and goals.[20] In 1998 version 4 consisted of a data dictionary and 363 terms for problems, 311 terms for goals, and 1357 terms for patient care orders organized into 22 components modified from those identified by Virginia Saba. These terms are now being parsed into atomic-level elements, and rules are being established for combining these into more complex concepts. For example, the elements proposed for the problem concepts are subject, object, likelihood, status, degree, duration, value, frequency, body site, and laterality. The Patient Care Data Set is different from the other classifications that have been previously described. It is not in a clinically usable form but, rather, may prove to be a helpful model for the development of a behind-the-scenes information model that can facilitate the translation of one vocabulary to another. In June of 1999, Ozbolt organized an invitational conference on nursing vocabularies with the goal of developing a reference information model.[19] The idea is similar to what she is attempting to develop with the Patient Care Data Set—the identification of components of diagnoses, interventions, and outcomes so that standardized language concepts in any of the classifications can be parsed behind the scenes to facilitate transfer and comparison among different computer systems. Representatives of each of the nursing classifications, as well as representatives from standards organizations, were at the conference. A similar conference has been held yearly since 1999 to continue the dialogue.

In summary then, compared with other classifications, NIC is the most comprehensive for interventions. Of all the classifications, only NANDA, NIC, and NOC are comprehensive and have ongoing research efforts to keep them current. The relationships that link these classifications[13] and the proposal for a common organizing structure[8] present users with a comprehensive classification system that can be used to document care across settings and specialties.

18. In a care plan, what's the structure for NIC and NOC? What do you choose and think about first? The answer to this reflects the clinical decision making of the provider planning and delivering the care. Individuals have different approaches to this, reflecting how they learned to do this in school, refined by what they find works best for them and their typical patient population. As a general approach, we suggest first making the diagnosis or diagnoses, then selecting outcomes and indicators, rating the patient on these, then selecting the interventions and appropriate activities, implementing these, and then rating the outcomes again. If you want to set goals, these can be derived from the NOC outcomes; for example, the patient is at 2 on X outcome and by discharge he should be at a level of 4. In some situations, this process is not possible or even desirable, and you would want to use a different order. For example, in a crisis you would move immediately to the implementation of the intervention and leave the diagnosis and identification of the outcome for later. The advantage of the standardized classifications is that they provide the language for the knowledge base of nursing. Educators and others can now focus on teaching and practice of skills in clinical decision making; researchers can focus on examining the effects of interventions on patient outcomes in real practice situations. See the model in Chapter 3 that shows how standardized language can be used at the individual level, the unit/organizational level, and the network/state/country level.

19. What is a reference terminology model? Why are these being developed? Will they make classifications such as NIC obsolete? A reference terminology (RT) model identifies the parts of a concept (i.e., the parts of any diagnosis or any intervention) that can be used "behind the screens" in computer systems to help these systems "talk with each other." For example, an intervention might consist of an action, a recipient, and a route. When we went to high school in the 1960s, we were asked to diagram sentences in order to learn the parts of speech (e.g., the noun, verb, adverb); an RT model is used to help represent concepts in a similar way. Theoretically, an RT model enables different vocabularies (e.g., NIC and the Omaha System) to be mapped to one model and thus compared with each other. We say "theoretically" because this approach has not yet been tested in practice. In 1999, Judy Ozbolt organized the Nursing Vocabulary Summit Conference, which has been held yearly at Vanderbilt University, with the identified need to develop and test a reference terminology model.[19] In the late 1990s and early 2000s, terminology models mushroomed; examples include HL7 (in the United States for all of health care), CEN (in Europe for all of health care), SNOMED (for use in the United States and Great Britain), and ISO-Nursing (for nursing internationally). As we stated earlier, we consider the ICNP in the Beta version with its axes a reference terminology model that is more helpful "behind the screens" than useful for practicing nurses as a "front-end terminology." A reference terminology model is sometimes called a *reference information model*; although those in the informatics standards area say that there are differences between the two, it is hard to distinguish the differences.

A second part of this question is whether the creation of a reference terminology model will make classifications such as NIC obsolete. No, NIC is a "front-end" language designed for communication among nurses and between nurses and other providers. We want nurses to be able to write and talk NIC. On the other hand, reference terminology models are for use "behind the screens": if they do succeed, they will help vendors to build computer systems that can use and compare different front-end languages. Reference terminology models are pretty hard to understand and not clinically useful. Even if they allow the user to document care in his or her own words (versus standardized language), this is not desirable (except in a free text notes section that supplements and elaborates on the standardized language) for the profession because we would still have the problem of lack of communication among ourselves and others as to what we do. We do not want to leave the impression that you need a reference terminology model in order to have a computer system; you don't. You can put the clinical classifications in certain fields and use the identified linkages to help users access these. But we will always need a common language to communicate the work of nursing—NIC is intended to be just that.

20. Is there commercial software available with NIC in it? Are there vendors that have clinical nursing software with NIC? Yes. This is a growing area. First, when a licensing agreement for NIC is made with Mosby, the user is sent a CD-ROM to make it easier to transfer the language to a computer system. Available from Mosby in 2003, NANDA, NIC, and NOC are linked in care planning software ("NANDA, NOC, and NIC: Electronic Linkages") based on the linkage book.[13] A growing number of vendors are including NIC in their information systems. In 2003 the vendors who have signed licensing agreements to use NIC are **Ergo**, Lake Quivira, Kansas [http://www.ergopartners.com]; **Nurse's Aide** (for school nurses), Keller, Texas [http://www.nursesaide.net]; **McKesson**, Alpharetta, Georgia [http://www.mckesson.com]; **Tech Time**, Billings, Montana [http://www.techtimeinc.com]; **DXR Development Group**,

Carbondale, Illinois [http://www.dxrgroup.com]; **Purkinje**, Montreal, Quebec, Canada [http://www.purkinje.com]; and **Dairyland Healthcare Solutions,** Glenwood, Montana [http://www.dhsnet.com]. Additional licensing agreements are in process. We do not endorse any particular product; prospective users should contact the vendors directly for review of their products. Other software has been developed for specific purposes and is not available commercially, at least not at this date. For example, the government of Iceland has mandated the use of NANDA, NIC, and NOC in all of their facilities and has built software (eMR) (A. Thoroddsen, personal communication, November 14, 2002) to document care and collect data. Another example is the software built for research data collection by Gail Keenan and her colleagues in Michigan.[14] We believe that the inclusion of NIC in SNOMED will facilitate and encourage the incorporation of NIC in vendor products. If your vendor does not include NIC, ask about future plans at their user meetings. Vendors will build their products according to user demand. Nurses need to speak up and ask for standardized language to be included in clinical information systems.

CENTER FOR NURSING CLASSIFICATION AND CLINICAL EFFECTIVENESS (CNC)

Because we have made reference to the Center several times in this chapter, it seems advisable to provide a bit more detail about the Center located at the College of Nursing, the University of Iowa. The Center was approved by the Iowa Board of Regents (the governing body that oversees the state's three public universities) in 1995 with the name of "Center for Nursing Classification." In 2001 the name was expanded to the Center for Nursing Classification and Clinical Effectiveness. The purpose of the Center is to facilitate the continued development and use of NIC and NOC. The Center conducts the review processes and procedures for updating the classifications, disseminates materials related to the classifications, provides office support to assist faculty investigators in obtaining funds, and offers research and education opportunities for students and visiting fellows. The Center provides a structure for the continued upkeep of the classifications and for communication with the many nurses and others in education and health care facilities who are putting the languages in their curricula and documentation systems. The Center is physically located in three rooms on the fourth floor of the College of Nursing. One of the rooms is a conference room with a small library. Currently (2003), Joanne Dochterman is the director and Sharon Sweeney is the coordinator. They are assisted in their decision making by an executive board composed of the editors of the NIC and NOC books, as well as a few others. The "fellows" (see pp. xvii-xviii) assist with the work of the Center. Financial support for the Center comes from a variety of sources, including university and college funds; licensing, permission, and product revenue from NIC and NOC; and related publications, grants, and income from Center courses. The Center is under a mandate to be self-supporting in 2004 and towards that end has been raising funds, with the assistance of the Fundraising Advisory Board and the University of Iowa Foundation, for a $1 million endowment. In fall 2002, the money raised for the endowment was just over $600,000. The endowment is needed to provide some permanent long-range security for the work of the Center.

The Center publishes *The NIC/NOC Letter* twice a year, as well as its annual report. These publications and other information about the Center and products and happenings can be found on the web site: http://www.nursing.uiowa.edu/cnc. The Center receives visitors who come for a short period of study, as well as national and international scholars who come for an extended period to work on a project. The Center cosponsors the Institute for Informatics and Classification, held at the University of Iowa annually since 1998. This institute for a small number (50 or less) of individuals provides an intensive experience in current information about the classifications and their use, as well as cutting-edge issues in informatics. In the future it is likely to be held every other year opposite the NNN conference, which is also cosponsored by the Center. One web course on the basics of standardized language and NANDA, NIC, and NOC is offered through the Center, and one more on implementation in education is underway.

SUMMARY

This chapter provides an overview of NIC and the Center for Nursing Classification and Clinical Effectiveness at the College of Nursing, the University of Iowa, where the Classification is maintained. A brief overview of four related projects—NOC, NDEC, the NNN Alliance, and the NMMDS—is also included. A series of frequently asked questions about NIC is presented and answered. The chapter provides a convenient way to quickly become familiar with NIC, but serious users will also want to read other publications that provide more detail about many of the topics covered here. In Appendix E, we have included a fairly complete bibliography on writings about NIC prepared by authors from the University of Iowa and others.

References

1. Alternative Link Systems, Inc. (2001). *The CAM and nursing coding manual*. Albany, NY: Delmar.
2. Beyea, S. (2001). Nursing specialties: Structured vocabularies, synergy of efforts—a win-win for nursing. *Nursing Diagnosis, 12*, 63-65.
3. Center for Nursing Classification. (Cox, R., Preparer). (2000). *Standardized nursing language in long term care*. Iowa City: Author.
4. Center for Nursing Classification. (2000). *NIC interventions and NOC outcomes linked to the OASIS Information Set*. Iowa City: Author.
5. Craft-Rosenberg, M., Delaney, C., Denehy, J., & NDEC Research Team. (1999). Nursing Diagnosis Extension Classification (NDEC): History, methods, completed work, and future directions. In M. Rantz & P. LiMone (Eds.), *Classification of Nursing Diagnoses: Proceedings of the Thirteenth Conference* (pp. 71-218). Glendale, CA: Cinahl Information Systems.
6. Delaney, C., & Huber, D. (1996). *A Nursing Management Minimum Data Set (NMMDS): Report of an invitational conference*. Chicago: American Organization of Nurse Executives.
7. Dochterman, J. M., & Jones, D. (2001). *Collaboration in nursing classification: A conference*. National Library of Medicine Conference Grant Proposal, R13 LM07243.
8. Dochterman, J. M., & Jones, D. (Eds.). (2003). *Unifying nursing languages: The harmonization of NANDA, NIC, and NOC*. Washington, DC: American Nurses Association.
9. International Council of Nurses. (1996). *The International Classification of Nursing Practice (ICNP): A unifying framework—alpha version*. Geneva, Switzerland: Author.
10. International Council of Nurses. (1999). *International Classification for Nursing Practice (ICNP): ICNP update—beta 1 version*. Geneva, Switzerland: Author.
11. Iowa Intervention Project. (1996). *NIC interventions linked to Omaha System problems*. Iowa City: Center for Nursing Classification.
12. Johnson, M., Maas, M. L., & Moorhead S. (Eds.). (2000). *Nursing Outcomes Classification (NOC)* (2nd ed.). St. Louis, MO: Mosby.
13. Johnson, M., Bulechek, G., Dochterman, J. Maas, M., & Moorhead, S. (2001). *Nursing diagnoses, outcomes, interventions: NANDA, NOC, and NIC linkages*. St. Louis, MO: Mosby.
14. Keenan, G. M., Stocker, J. R., Geo-Thomas, A. T., Soparkar, N. R., Barkauskas, V. J., & Lee, J. L. (2002). The HANDS project: Studying and refining the automated collection of a cross-setting clinical data set. *Computers in Nursing, 20*, 89-100.
15. Martin, K.S., & Scheet, N. J. (1992). *The Omaha System: Applications for community health nursing*. Philadelphia: W. B. Saunders.
16. Moorhead, S. A., McCloskey, J. C., & Bulechek, G. M. (1993). Nursing interventions classification: A comparison with the Omaha system and the home healthcare classification. *The Journal of Nursing Administration, 23*, 23-29.
17. The Nightingale Tracker Field Test Nurse Team. (1999). Designing an information technology application for use in community-focused nursing education. *Computers in Nursing, 17*, 73-81.
18. North American Nursing Diagnosis Association (NANDA). (1999). *Nursing diagnoses: Definitions & classification, 1999-2000*. Philadelphia: Author.
19. Ozbolt, J. (2000). Terminology standards for nursing: Collaboration at the summit. *Journal of the American Informatics Association: JAMIA 7*, 517-522.
20. Ozbolt, J., Fruchtnicht, J. N., & Hayden, J. R. (1994). Toward data standards for clinical nursing information. *Journal of the American Informatics Association: JAMIA, 1*, 175-185.
21. Saba, V. K. (1992). The classification of home health care nursing: Diagnoses and interventions. *Caring Magazine, 11*, 50-57.

22. Saba, V. K. (2002). Nursing classifications: Home Health Care Classification system (HHCC): An overview. *Online Journal of Issues in Nursing, 7,* Article 3. Retrieved August 2000, from http://nursing world.org/ojin/tpc/tpc 7.htm

23. Visiting Nurse Association of Omaha. (1986). *Client management information system for community health nursing agencies* (Publication No. HRP-0907023). Washington, DC: U.S. Government Printing Office.

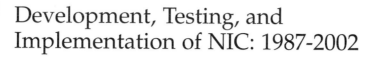

CHAPTER TWO

Development, Testing, and Implementation of NIC: 1987-2002

THE BEGINNING

We are sometimes asked how this all began. In 1987 Joanne McCloskey and Gloria Bulechek established a research team to develop a classification of nursing interventions parallel to the North American Nursing Diagnosis Association (NANDA) classification of nursing diagnoses. We had been teaching a master's adult health course on concepts for several years, which evolved into nursing diagnoses and then into diagnoses and interventions. We had done some conceptual work for a book on independent nursing interventions.[9] After attending the NANDA conference in St. Louis, Missouri, in 1986, we realized that the profession needed an intervention classification because once you have made a diagnosis, you have an obligation to do something about it. We had the background, motivation, and interest to begin such a task. We had no idea at the time how we would go about doing this, and, if we had known all that would be involved, we probably would not have begun this exciting but all-consuming journey.

We began by inviting eight others (all colleagues at the University of Iowa College of Nursing) to a 2-hour brainstorming meeting to discuss the idea of developing a classification of interventions. Each of the eight was selected for some specific expertise; together the 10 of us represented the whole of nursing. Some individuals were experts in pediatrics and some in gerontology; some had clinical backgrounds; some had administrative backgrounds; some were qualitative researchers, some quantitative. At the end of the first meeting, nothing was resolved, but the idea had been presented and discussed. The group was then asked to commit to three more meetings in the next few months. At the end of those three meetings, they were all asked to commit to 1 year as members of a research team. During the course of the first year of work, when we were sorting out the conceptual issues, we came up with the idea that we should build on the extensive care planning and documentation data sources in nursing. This led us to investigate possible sources of data in information systems. We knew that a large database of nursing orders was used by our university hospital, and we requested the use of this as an initial data source. As a condition for use of the data set, the director of nursing requested that two of her staff be included on the research team. This addition of two members from the clinical area was important and helped to broaden the perspective of the team. As others in the college and hospital learned about the team, they asked to join. Over the 15 years since the beginning of the project, we have had approximately 80 individuals actively participating in the teamwork. These individuals represent many diverse academic and clinical settings and multiple specialty areas. Many of the individuals have been on the research team for several years; many of the original 12 individuals are still with the project. In 1995 the Center for Nursing Classification was founded at the College of Nursing, the University of Iowa (see Chapter 1) to assist with the ongoing development of Nursing Interventions Classification (NIC) and Nursing Outcomes Classification (NOC); in 2002 the name was expanded to the Center for Nursing Classification and Clinical Effectiveness. In 2002, with the ongoing work being mostly upkeep of the Classifications, implementation, and effectiveness research based on use in practice, the research teams of both NIC and NOC became "fellows" appointed for 3 years to the Center for Nursing Classification and Clinical Effectiveness.

BEFORE NIC: REASONS TO DEVELOP NIC

Classifications have existed since early times. For example, in the eleventh century, a monk named Guido d'Arezzo invented a musical scale (Guido's scale) whereby a musician of any land can today read or play any composition from any part of the world.[57] Other examples include the symbols of chemical elements and the categories in biology (i.e., phylum, class, order, family, genus, species, and variety) that arrange living organisms into related groups. Classifications bring order to our environment and help us to communicate with each other. A small terrier with floppy ears in the natural state, but often with cropped ears for show, that likes to pull on a leash is a miniature schnauzer (this description may fit other dogs as well). A rather formal looking chair with a high winged back, often found in living rooms, which is comfortably upholstered is a Queen Anne chair. Classifications help to advance the knowledge base of a field through the organization of the knowledge and the discovery of the principles governing what is known. They also identify gaps in knowledge that can then be addressed by research. In addition, classifications facilitate understanding. For example, when nurses use a common language to communicate their treatment plans, then communication among nurses is enhanced and the patient benefits from greater continuity of care, from shift to shift and setting to setting. NIC was developed for several reasons.

Reason One: Standardization of the Nomenclature of Nursing Treatments

The phenomenon of concern with nursing interventions is nurse behavior or nurse activity, that is, those things that nurses do to assist patient status or patient behavior to move toward a desired outcome. This phenomenon differs from nursing diagnoses or patient outcomes sensitive to nursing care in which the phenomenon of concern is patient behavior or patient status. A classification of nursing interventions was needed to standardize the language that nurses use to describe their specific behaviors when delivering nursing treatments. Before NIC, multiple terms were used for the intervention step of the nursing process (e.g., *action, activity, intervention, treatment, therapeutics, order,* and *implementation*); and there was confusion among intervention, assessment, and evaluation activities and a lack of conceptualization as to what constitutes an intervention. Interventions were described at a very discrete level of detail, for example:

> Position the limb with sandbags.
> Raise the head of the bed 30 degrees.
> Explore with the patient her need for attention.
> Observe for coughing.
> Inspect the nails for abnormalities.
> Monitor respiratory pattern.

There was little conceptualization of how these actions fit together to form interventions. The result was long, wordy care plans that were seldom used and nursing information systems that contained thousands of nursing actions, although nurses generally selected a much smaller number. Nursing textbooks also addressed nursing interventions at the most discrete level. Typically, textbooks included long lists of nursing actions for each type of patient; the list in one book was not the same as the list in another, even though the same type of patient was discussed. Lists would change with each new edition.

In contrast, the NIC labels are concepts that are implemented by a set of nursing activities (actions) directed toward the resolution of patients' actual or potential health care problems. A nurse can describe the care given to any one patient using only a few labels.

At the opposite end of the discrete actions, there were also some beginning classification schemes for nursing interventions such as the following: Henderson's components of basic nursing,[31] Verran's taxonomy of ambulatory care nursing,[70] Benner's eight domains of nursing,[8] the Omaha classification scheme for interventions,[42,71] the National Council of State Boards of Nursing's categories of nurse activities,[41] Sigma Theta Tau's International Classification of Nursing Knowledge,[64]

Bulechek and McCloskey's beginning taxonomy of nursing interventions,[10] the minimum data set intervention lists,[72] and Saba and colleagues' Home Health Care Classification.[62,63] Most of these schemes contained only broad categories that are not clinically useful. (See a more detailed review and listing of these schemes in either of two previous publications.[46,47]) Those schemes that did contain clinically useful interventions (the Omaha System and the classifications of Sigma Theta Tau, Bulechek & McCloskey, and Saba) were incomplete. (An article comparing NIC with Omaha and Saba classifications was published in the *Journal of Nursing Administration* in 1993.[54])

In summary, before NIC, nursing interventions were viewed either as lengthy lists of discrete actions or as large categories. What was needed was a clinically useful language between these two extremes.

Reason Two: Expansion of Nursing Knowledge about the Links between Diagnoses, Interventions, and Outcomes

The widespread use of NANDA's nursing diagnosis language had increased awareness of the need for similar standardized classifications in the areas of interventions and outcomes. The impetus for guideline development by the Agency for Health Care Policy and Research[1] further clarified the need. Guidelines were proposed to assist practitioners in determining which of several courses of action has the highest probability of producing effective outcomes, given a particular set of circumstances surrounding the patient's condition—in other words—which interventions are known to be most effective for patients with a particular diagnosis or set of diagnoses. Medicine has used standardized databases to routinely collect massive amounts of computerized clinical data and from the data has begun to explore outcomes as a function of medical interventions. In contrast, nursing's knowledge about the effectiveness of nursing care is limited. Standardized terminologies in the areas of diagnoses, interventions, and outcomes were needed to build large databases that will help determine the linkages among these variables. When nurses systematically document the diagnoses of their patients, the treatments they perform, and the resulting patient outcomes using a common standardized language, then we will be able to determine which nursing interventions work best for a given diagnosis or population. Not only will the nursing care to that population be improved, but nursing as a profession will gain recognition for that demonstrated contribution to desirable patient outcomes.

Reason Three: Development of Nursing and Health Care Information Systems

The documentation of nursing care is increasingly being computerized. But, until NIC was developed, there was no standardized system for describing the treatments that nurses perform. Individual agencies developed their own sets of nursing orders or actions by copying ideas from one another, using lists of orders that had been generated from care plans used at the institution, or brainstorming. Because nursing interventions had traditionally been considered a series of discrete actions, a computer list of these to which NIC has not been applied results in many thousands of items, and the nursing care plan for a patient may have 75 "interventions." Although a particular agency's list of "standardized" interventions may be agreed upon and useful to those in the agency, it is very unlikely that this list is the same as another agency's list. This inconsistency results in the inability to collect comparable data from multiple agencies or even within agencies from one unit to the next. The NIC, in conjunction with NANDA and NOC, provides the discipline of nursing with the clinical data elements for an automated patient record.

Reason Four: Teaching Decision Making to Nursing Students

Nursing diagnoses have been included in most of the major care planning textbooks since the 1980s, but there was no systematic approach to the teaching of interventions before NIC. Students practice technical skills in a lab before performing them with patients, but there has been little opportunity to practice the more difficult decision-making skills. Eventually, nursing diagnosis, intervention, and outcome textbooks based on tested theory will replace the more medically oriented medical-surgical, pediatric, mental health, and other textbooks. Additionally, there will be more films and audiocassettes demonstrating independent nursing interventions. We envision that the analysis of actual client data will assist in the instruction of clinical decision making. For example, a database on the diagnosis of Body Image Disturbance can be accessed, and the student can study the associated etiologies, interventions, and outcomes to determine for which populations certain interventions are most effective for this diagnosis. The relationships of the nursing diagnoses and interventions with the patient's signs and symptoms, demographic characteristics, and medical diagnoses and therapies can also be determined. Defining and classifying nursing interventions will help in the important process of teaching beginning nurses how to determine a patient's needs and respond appropriately. In addition, a classification of nursing interventions makes it easier to identify nursing interventions requiring higher knowledge and skill levels that should be taught in a graduate program.

Reason Five: Determination of the Costs of Services Provided by Nurses

In the 1980s, multiple efforts were reported in the literature to "cost out" nursing services. Most of the studies had small sample sizes, were conducted in one institution, and used patient classification systems without much regard to their validity and reliability.[44,51] The wide variety of nonstandardized patient classification systems was a key reason for the difficulty of obtaining large data sets for comparison of nursing costs. The determination of nursing costs based on interventions performed would be a great improvement but would require a standardized list of interventions. NIC provides the language for interventions delivered to patients that can be the basis for determining costs of services.

Physicians bill for their services based on the codes in the *Physicians' Current Procedural Terminology* (*CPT*) manual published by the American Medical Association.[3] Hurdis Griffith and colleagues[28,29] demonstrated that nurses often perform some of the procedures for which physicians are paid. The *CPT*, however, includes only a few of the interventions that nurses perform and thus is inadequate as a means to reimburse nurses. More recently, a new multidisciplinary classification, the ABC Codes by Alternative Link,[2] has been developed for reimbursement for alternative providers. NIC interventions are a part of the ABC coding system. Alternative Link is seeking recognition from the U.S. federal government as a code set that can be used for Medicare reimbursement, and some states are currently using the ABC codes in the Medicaid programs.

Reason Six: Planning for Resources Needed in Nursing Practice Settings

Ultimately, identification of costs for specific nursing interventions will allow evaluation of the cost-effectiveness of nursing care. Knowing the cost and the effectiveness of specific interventions allows the reduction of costs through elimination or substitution of services and helps in the determination of whether present costs will prevent or reduce future costs.[43] The first step in this important process is the identification of the interventions that nurses perform. Then, the time for delivery, the cost, and the effectiveness of these interventions can be studied. This information will help nursing administrators to plan more effectively for staff and equipment needed to deliver the interventions. In the past, resource use has been based on tradition; the identification of nursing interventions is the first step toward more effective planning and use of resources in the future.

Reason Seven: Language to Communicate the Unique Function of Nursing

In the first of a three-part series in the *Journal of the American Medical Association* in December 1990, the journal's staff asked, "How can such a pervasive element of health care be so invisible?"[4] They continued on to identify the core dilemma: "What does a nurse do that is unique?" Similarly, in a series of examples, Gebbie[27] outlined the invisibility of the profession. According to Gebbie, others increasingly acknowledge the importance of the care component of health care in affecting the outcomes achieved, yet nursing is not recognized as an important contributor.

"There is no indication of an understanding of the complete domain of nursing and how the nursing profession might add to the entire discussion [of health care effectiveness]" (p. 5). What Gebbie and many others within the nursing profession have recognized is that we need to systematically describe what it is that nurses do, so that nursing's contribution to health care can be understood. A classification of nursing interventions assists in nursing's efforts to describe its uniqueness, as well as its similarities to other health professions.

Reason Eight: Articulation with the Classification Systems of Other Health Care Providers

For purposes of reimbursement and research, the federal government, insurance companies, and the medical community have been collecting standardized health information for several years. Several Uniform Minimum Health Data Sets (UMHDS) have been developed under the auspices of the National Committee on Vital and Health Statistics. The Uniform Hospital Discharge Data Set (UHDDS) is incorporated into uniform hospital billing requirements. Fourteen items are included: patient identification, date of birth, sex, race and ethnic group, residence, hospital identification, admission and discharge dates, primary medical diagnoses, secondary diagnoses, procedures, disposition of the patient, expected principal source of payment, and physician identification. The Ambulatory Medical Care Minimum Data Set is similar to the UHDDS but is based on an encounter in which the patient is neither hospitalized nor institutionalized. The Long-term Health Care Minimum Data Set is used in long-term care, defined broadly to cover ambulatory, domiciliary, and institutional services in a wide range of settings. This data set is longer than the previous two and covers basic activities of daily living, mobility, behavior problems, vision, hearing, and other functional capabilities.[56]

For every item or variable defined for a data set, a classification for the variable's terms is needed. For example, each of the nursing variables of diagnoses, interventions, and outcomes requires a classification. The major classifications of physician terms are the International Classification of Diseases (ICD and ICD-CM),[58,59,75] Current Procedural Terminology (CPT),[3] Diagnostic and Statistical Manual of Mental Disorders (DSM),[6] the Systematized Nomenclature of Medicine (SNOMED),[20,65] and the Health Care Financing Administration's Common Procedural Coding System (HCPCS).[30] For a comparison of these classifications with NIC, see Chapter 2 of the second edition of this book.

These data sets and medical classification systems do not include nursing care. As a result, nursing's impact on patient care quality and health care costs is unknown and invisible. Harriet Werley and colleagues have published extensively on the need for a uniform Nursing Minimum Data Set (NMDS) that would be collected systematically in all agencies.[72-74] The nursing care variables identified for inclusion in the NMDS are nursing diagnoses, nursing interventions, patient outcomes, and intensity of nursing care. NIC is intended as the classification of nursing interventions that can be used to implement the NMDS.

DEVELOPMENT OF NIC

So, with these reasons in mind, the work to develop NIC began in 1987, and as indicated in Chapter 1, the research has progressed through four phases, each with some overlap in time:

Phase I: Construction of the Classification (1987-1992)
Phase II: Construction of the Taxonomy (1990-1995)
Phase III: Clinical Testing and Refinement (1993-1997)
Phase IV: Use and Maintenance (1996-ongoing)

The development research received 7 years of funding from the National Institutes of Health, National Institute of Nursing (1991-1998); and most recently, funding for effectiveness research has been received from the National Institute of Nursing Research (NINR) and the Agency for Healthcare

Research and Quality (AHRQ). The remainder of this chapter is an overview of the work of each of the phases. Although the early years of development can now be viewed historically, an overview of them is included here so that those who are new to the classification will understand the origins.

Phase I: Construction of the Classification (1987-1992)

In phase I, nursing activities were identified, grouped together, and given a conceptual intervention label. Three steps were used to construct the classification: identification and resolution of the conceptual and methodological issues, generation of an initial list of interventions, and refinement of the intervention list and activities. Each of these is discussed below, but the reader is referred to the first edition of this book,[45] where this phase of the research is explained in more detail.

Step 1: Identification and resolution of the conceptual and methodological issues

During the first step of the research, several methodological and conceptual issues were evident and eventually resolved. For example, a major methodological issue was whether we should use an inductive or deductive approach. A deductive approach, whereby interventions could be identified and placed within some existing conceptual framework, was ruled out after systematic review of existing intervention classification schemes.[46] An inductive approach, beginning with the activities that nurses in practice were using to plan and document care, was chosen. A major conceptual issue was the question of what sorts of nursing behaviors should be included in an intervention taxonomy. For the purpose of answering the question, nurse behaviors, which capture all assessment, intervention, and evaluation activities that nurses do to benefit patients, were identified. Nurses perform, for patient benefit, the following types of behaviors:

1. Assessment behaviors to make a nursing diagnosis.
2. Assessment behaviors to gather information for a physician to make a medical diagnosis.
3. Nurse-initiated treatment behaviors in response to nursing diagnoses.
4. Physician-initiated treatment behaviors in response to medical diagnoses.
5. Behaviors to evaluate the effects of nursing and medical treatments. These are also assessment behaviors, but they are done for purposes of evaluation, not diagnosis.
6. Administrative and indirect care behaviors that support interventions.

To be useful for multiple purposes, a classification of nursing interventions must include all types of treatments that nurses perform. The core of nursing interventions should be the nurse-initiated treatments (number 3 in the list), but any listing of nursing interventions (e.g., for a computerized care planning system) must also include physician-initiated treatments (number 4). Nurse-initiated treatment behaviors in response to nursing diagnoses also include those nursing treatments that result from the client's response to medical interventions. If a medical intervention caused a patient problem amenable to nursing treatment, then the nurse would make a diagnosis and treat it. For example, some medical treatments might render a patient unable to perform his or her own daily hygiene activities. A nurse observing this situation would make a nursing diagnosis of Bathing/Hygiene Self-Care Deficit and perform the required interventions of Bathing and Hair Care. Categories 3 and 4 in the preceding list include the monitoring and assessment activities of nurses, when these are done as treatments. Unfortunately, the words *monitoring* and *assessment* are used in many ways to mean different things in nursing. When they are used to refer to only data gathering behaviors, they would be included in categories 1, 2, and 5.

The behaviors in categories 1 and 2 are assessment (before diagnosis), not intervention (after diagnosis), functions. Category 5 focuses on evaluation and is included in the classification of patient outcomes. Category 6, administrative and indirect care behaviors, involves the supporting activities related to staff development, record-keeping, staffing, scheduling, and so on. These were not initially targeted for inclusion in this classification; however, because of feedback from nurses and because of their importance, the second edition of this book included many indirect care interventions and subsequent editions have added additional ones. An indirect care intervention is a treatment performed away from the patient but on behalf of a patient or group of patients. Examples include Controlled Substance Checking, Critical Path Development, and Emergency Cart Checking. Indirect care interventions support the effectiveness of direct care interventions. NIC does not include administrative interventions that are performed by a nurse manager rather than a nurse clinician, although some of the indirect care interventions in NIC (e.g., Cost Containment, Delegation, and Staff Supervision) performed by a nurse manager would then be administrative interventions.

Step 2: Generation of an initial list of interventions

Nursing activities, or those things a nurse does as the implementation step of the nursing process, were readily available in nursing textbooks, nursing care planning guides, and information systems. In all of these sources, before NIC, an intervention was viewed as a discrete action or a list of discrete activities with little conceptualization of how these fit together. For example, the following were typical of "interventions" listed in pre-NIC nursing textbooks: "Auscultate breath sounds before and after suctioning," "Monitor level of consciousness," and "Cut food in small pieces." Typically, textbooks include several hundred of these "interventions," with the list for any one patient or diagnosis numbering several dozen. More often than not, these actions were a mixture of assessment and treatment activities, as well as a mixture of nurse-initiated and physician-initiated activities. A list of nursing interventions for a particular condition in one book was not the same as the list in another book for the same condition. For example, if we compare the suggested nursing interventions for the nursing diagnosis of Activity Intolerance in several books, we find huge differences. For treatment of Activity Intolerance, Moorhouse, Geissler, and Doenges[55] listed six independent interventions (e.g., "Check vital signs before and immediately after activity") and one collaborative intervention ("Follow graded cardiac rehabilitation and activity program"); McFarland and McFarlane[52] listed three goals with 24 interventions (e.g., "Assess the patient's past and present activity pattern" and "Engage immobile patient in passive exercise regimen"); and Carpenito[13] listed eight major categories of interventions and 46 discrete activities (e.g., "Instruct person to practice controlled coughing four times a day" and "Discuss the need for annual immunizations [against flu, bacteria]"). Despite the mix of actions and enormous differences in approach, it seemed to us that we could begin the task of intervention classification construction by grouping the available data. Thus an inductive approach that made use of these rich data was a logical choice.

The investigators designed a data source rating form and used it to review and rate data sources from a variety of specialty areas. (See the first edition of this book for a copy of the rating form, a listing of all of the sources that were reviewed, and an overview of the process used.[45]) The criteria used to select the sources were (1) presents clear, discrete nursing actions; (2) includes a comprehensive list of actions; and (3) represents current practice.

Forty-five sources from a variety of specialty areas were reviewed. Every attempt was made to be comprehensive in the selection of sources; the main idea was to "get started," to generate an initial list of interventions. The review of care planning books included those published in the 5 years prior (1983-1988); the review of information systems was limited to three in the state of Iowa for which access was available and a fourth whose handbook was published and available. It was decided to include some information systems as sources because the intervention lists in these systems added an additional practice dimension.

Fourteen of the highest rated sources were then used in eight content analysis exercises to create an initial list of intervention labels. The first couple of exercises used more general sources (medical-surgical), two exercises used computerized lists, and three exercises used specialty books in areas that may not have been well captured by the general or information system sources. The exact description of the exercise sources, the numbers of activities used in each exercise, and the methods used to select activities are included in Box 3-3 in the first edition of this book.[45]

Before the preparation of each exercise, the research team reviewed the label/activity progress to date and selected from the highly rated sources those that were judged most likely to produce new intervention labels. Once the sources for the next exercise were determined, they were reviewed by the principal investigators and the method of activity selection was determined. For nearly all sources, the activities were chosen by systematic random selection, but the frequency of selection (e.g., select every fifth item or every second item) varied by the number of activities listed in the source. Also, some books were organized by nursing diagnosis and required the selection of specific nursing diagnoses to identify intervention activities. Content analysis was used to categorize the selected nursing activities. Each of the exercises was done as follows:

1. Approximately 250 concrete nursing activities from two related sources were randomly selected and entered into a computer file.
2. Each activity was printed on a separate slip of paper, and the slips were distributed to all members of the research team.
3. Each team member independently categorized the activities and gave each category an intervention label.

In the beginning, each label had to be generated by the team members based on their knowledge and experience. Beginning with the third exercise, members selected a label already identified or added a new label if an appropriate one was not on the list. Approximately 250 activities were used in each exercise because the team found that this was a manageable number of activities that also produced a good yield of labels. These exercises were very labor-intensive, each requiring 4 to 6 hours per researcher to complete and many more hours per exercise to enter the results on the computer. Some of the strategies used by group members and the team leaders to accomplish this stage of the research are discussed in a 1991 article[19] and on pages 37 to 39 of the first edition of this book.[45]

Because the seventh and eighth exercises produced only a few new labels and the research team agreed that these exercises were duplications of earlier ones, it was determined that an initial list of intervention labels had been generated and that it was time to proceed to the next step of refinement. We did not believe that all the intervention labels for the taxonomy had been generated, but we thought that the vast majority had been determined and that the exercises no longer represented the most helpful method of refining and expanding the list.

Step 3: Refinement of the intervention list and activities

Following the content analysis exercises, each intervention label had one to several hundred associated activities. Many of these activities were redundant because different sources proposed the same activity but with different wording. The task was to refine the labels and activities to move toward face and content validity. Two refinement methods were used: expert survey and focus group.

For the expert surveys, a two-round Delphi questionnaire process was used. National samples of certified master's prepared nurses received questionnaires composed of interventions relating to their specialty areas. The first-round questionnaire was developed from the label/activity lists generated from the exercises. In addition, clinical nursing and research literature was reviewed by a team investigator who refined the activities and added any missing labels and activities. The investigator also wrote a definition of the intervention that was included in one or both survey rounds. The process, then, was that groups of related intervention labels were selected; lists of their accompanying activities were generated by the computer; and, after refinement by a team investigator based on the literature, a questionnaire was constructed. Participants were asked to rate each activity according to the extent to which it is characteristic of the label. Fehring's methodology[24,25] for content validation of nursing diagnoses was adapted for use with interventions and yielded Intervention Content Validity (ICV) scores with critical and supporting activities.

Fehring's method, which was adapted for intervention labels, consisted of the following steps:

1. Nurse experts rated the activities for each intervention on a Likert-like scale of 1 (activity is not at all characteristic of intervention) to 5 (activity is very characteristic). They were also asked to suggest any activities that were missing and to comment on the definition.

2. The Delphi technique was used to enhance consensus among experts. Two rounds of questionnaires were used. The second round presented a refinement of the first list of activities and interventions based on responses by the nurses to round one.
3. Weighted ratios were calculated for each activity. These were obtained by summing the weights assigned to each response and then dividing by the total number of responses. The weights established by Fehring were used: $5 = 1, 4 = 0.75, 3 = 0.50, 2 = 0.25$, and $1 = 0$.
4. Activities with ratios equal to or greater than 0.80 were labeled critical activities. Activities with ratios less than 0.50 were discarded. These cutoffs, set by Fehring, are established conventions based on accepted standards for establishing reliability.
5. The total ICV score was obtained for each intervention by summing the individual activity ratings and averaging the results.

Over a 2-year period (June 1989 to June 1991), 14 surveys were completed, and 138 interventions were validated. The process and results of 12 of the surveys are reported in a symposium in *Nursing Clinics of North America*.[11] These surveys include the topics of Circulatory Care, Compliance, Family Interventions, Fluids and Electrolytes, Maternal-Infant Attachment, Activity and Movement, Neurologic Care, Pain, Patient Teaching, Respiratory Care, Safety, and Surveillance. In addition, one of the early surveys on labels related to skin care was published in *Nursing Diagnosis*.[69] In these publications, the ICV score for each intervention and ratio scores for each activity are reported.

The second method, focus group work, was instituted when it became apparent that the survey process was very time-consuming, costly, and not appropriate for all labels. For the focus group validation method, a team member prepared a draft of the label definition and activities for initial review by a small core group of team members, which was followed by a review by the entire team. Sets of related labels were often developed and reviewed as a cluster because this helped to clarify the similarities and differences among labels. Typically, each label was reviewed three times, twice by the core group and once by the entire team. For each review, 5 to 20 people provided input. Each successive review led to further refinement of the label, definition, and activities. Sometimes the review of one intervention led to repeated review and revision of an intervention developed previously.

The focus group method did not result in ICV scores or the grouping of categories by major and supporting activities. It did, however, result in well-defined interventions with well-edited and complete activity lists. The results were 198 interventions validated by focus group.

In summary, the result of phase I work was 336 interventions, each with a label, a definition, a set of related activities that describe the behaviors of the nurse who implements the intervention, and a short list of background readings. At this point in the research, we submitted the manuscript for the first edition of this book, which was published in May of 1992.[45] Although we knew that the work was just a beginning, we believed it was necessary to publish so the project would be known and others could use the interventions and provide feedback. We did, however, continue the work, and in the second edition[48] we added new interventions and grouped the interventions into a taxonomy with numerical codes.

Phase II: Construction of the Taxonomy (1990-1995)

In phase II, construction of the taxonomy, the interventions were clustered together in related groups and organized at three levels of abstraction. Two additional steps were used to generate a taxonomy.

Step 4: Arrangement of the Intervention list in an initial taxonomic structure
Once the interventions had been defined, an organizing structure was needed. It was necessary that the structure be easy to use and clinically meaningful. Similarity ratings and hierarchical clustering techniques were used to guide the development of the taxonomy. Hierarchical cluster analysis helped us group similar interventions into clusters of related interventions, and the clusters in turn were grouped into "super clusters" on the basis of their similarities.[23,32] The methods for the development of the taxonomy are explained in detail in an article published in *Image* in the fall of 1993.[33] Only a brief overview is given here, and the reader is referred to the article for more information.

Seventeen nurse members of the intervention research team were given the intervention labels and definitions on separate cards to generate the similarity ratings. Each person sorted the interventions into related groups. They were instructed to use an inductive process and to let the categories emerge from the data (interventions and their definitions). They were also asked to put a name on each resulting group if they wanted to, but this was not necessary. They were restricted to 25 total groups because it was believed that more than this would not be useful clinically. An extra piece of paper was provided on which they were asked to write their comments about the strategies and guidelines they used for grouping.

The data from the group placements were then entered into the computer, and hierarchical clustering was used to analyze the number of raters who put every two interventions in the same group. A "proximity" score for each pair of interventions, for example, "Blood Products Administration" and "Intravenous (IV) Therapy," was computed. Proximity was determined by how many raters placed these two intervention labels in the same group. Proximity for each pair was expressed as the proportion of the maximum number of points possible. If everyone put a particular pair of interventions in the same category, then that pair had a proximity of 1. Conversely, a pair of interventions, for example, "Intravenous (IV) Therapy" and "Animal-Assisted Therapy," that never appeared together for any rater, received a proximity of 0. A total of 57,970 pairs of interventions were rated, and therefore 57,970 proximities were to be computed.

Complete linkage analysis was chosen as the best cluster analysis technique for this exercise, and printouts of five different clusterings of the data were reviewed by the team members for clinical consistency and usefulness. The team believed that 20 to 30 groups defined clusters that were most clinically useful and initially chose 27 clusters that appeared to group the data well. These were referred to as *classes* of interventions. Names were assigned to each by using the suggestions made by team members during the exercise.

Each class was systematically reviewed by a select group of four to six team members. Distinguishing characteristics of each class were identified, and a definition for each class was written. Some revisions were made, and then each team member reviewed, as a whole, the revised classes and their definitions. Additional small modifications were made, and one class was eliminated. The group believed that there was consensus about the remaining 26 classes, their names and definitions, and the interventions that each contained. They did not believe, however, that this was the "top" of the taxonomy. A decision was made to try the same exercise with sorting of the classes.

Thus the 26 classes, each with their definitions and interventions, were printed on cards, and team members sorted the classes into related groups. They were again instructed to use an inductive process and let the groups emerge from the data. They were asked to suggest names for each group and to record comments on the decision-making process they engaged in while sorting. This time they were restricted to seven groups because it was believed that the top level of the taxonomy would be unwieldy with more.

Hierarchical cluster analysis of 26 classes resulted in six "super clusters." The team members reviewed these and determined that they represented clinical practice and decided to call them *domains*. Domain labels and definitions were developed. The entire taxonomic structure, consisting of domains, classes, and interventions, was printed and distributed to all team members. A discussion was held, and each team member was invited to submit written comments.

At this point, we had a three-tiered taxonomic structure composed of 6 domains, 26 classes, and 357 interventions (the original 336 plus others that had been developed since the publication).[32] The taxonomy was printed in a booklet, which was available at cost to interested individuals. Following a validation study (see next step, validation survey 4), the taxonomy was revised to include the 6 domains and 27 classes published in the second edition.

Step 5: Validation of the intervention labels, defining activities, and taxonomy
Now that we had the interventions developed and organized, we wanted to make sure that our work was useful to the nurse in practice. Four validation surveys were administered.

Validation survey 1: Use survey to specialty organizations. A three-part questionnaire was distributed in 1992 to heads of 32 clinical practice organizations who were members of the American Nurses Association's National Organization Liaison Forum (NOLF). In the first part of the questionnaire, the label and definition for each of the 336 interventions were listed. Similar interventions were placed together into the taxonomy's 26 interventions. The organizational representatives were asked to rate how often their members performed each intervention. The five-point rating scale consisted of several times a day; about once a day; about once a week; about once a month; and rarely, if at all. In the second part of the questionnaire, respondents were asked to identify any interventions they believed were missing from the list and interventions that are core to the specialty. *Core* was defined as "if someone read the list, they would know the nature of the specialty." Part three of the questionnaire collected demographic information.

Each organizational head determined how to provide the requested information. Some had a practice committee complete the questionnaire, and others designated one organization official to provide the data. Twenty-eight usable questionnaires were returned to the research team. The NOLF respondents estimated that 84% of their 264,493 total members are employed; that 43% have 10 or more years experience in the specialty; that 41% hold a baccalaureate degree and 27% have a graduate degree; that 37% hold certification for specialty practice; and that 46% of the members use nursing diagnoses.

The survey results are partially reported in four articles.[7,12,66,67] The results demonstrate that NIC does include interventions appropriate to all specialties and also provide beginning data on the types of use of different interventions. Thirty-six interventions were reported to be used several times a day by 50% of the specialty organizations. The six most frequently used interventions (used by 75% of the organizations several times a day) were Active Listening, Emotional Support, Infection Control, Vital Signs Monitoring, Infection Protection, and Medication Management. This survey demonstrated that NIC is helpful in defining the nature of specialty nursing practice, and it provided the basis for a follow-up survey in 1995 related to defining of core interventions (see next section).

Validation survey 2: Use survey to individual nurses. The use survey to specialty organizations was modified and sent to individual nurses from a variety of specialty areas who were actively engaged in clinical practice.[12] The names were obtained from a list of respondents who had served as expert raters in prior NIC work. The respondents were asked to duplicate and pass on the questionnaire to other expert nurses. A total of 442 questionnaires were mailed, and 277 usable surveys were received. The respondents were experienced, highly educated practitioners: 90% reported more than 6 years of experience, with the median being 17 years; 77% had a baccalaureate or a higher degree, with 55% holding a master's degree. They lived in all regions of the country, with the majority in the north central states. The majority were employed in hospitals, with 91% working in communities with more than 30,000 people.

This survey also demonstrated that all interventions in NIC are used by nurses in clinical practice. The use ratings provided by the individual nurses were analyzed by work setting and specialty. There were 219 (79%) nurses employed in hospitals and 58 (21%) practicing in nonhospital settings. There were 111 (40%) working in intensive care and 166 (60%) practicing in other specialties. The results were analyzed to determine which interventions were used most frequently by work setting and specialty. Of the 336 interventions rated, 159 interventions were used significantly more frequently by hospital nurses than by nurses in other settings. Interventions such as Acid-Base Management, Bleeding Precautions, Electrolyte Management, and Fluid Management, which support homeostatic regulation, were very evident. Nurses who did not practice in hospitals identified 52 interventions that they used more frequently than hospital nurses. These included Abuse Protection, Anticipatory Guidance, Attachment Promotion, Reminiscence Therapy, and Therapy Group. These interventions support the family unit and facilitate lifestyle changes. There were 185 interventions used more frequently by intensive care nurses, including the interventions that support homeostatic regulation, for example, Artificial Airway Management, Bleeding Precautions, Cardiac Care, and Code Management, as well as interventions for self-care assistance, for example, Bathing, Bed Rest Care, Bowel Incontinence Care, and Eye Care. There were 65 interventions used more frequently by nonintensive care nurses, including a number of interventions that support the family unit, for example, Abuse Protection, Anticipatory Guidance, Attachment Promotion, and Family Integrity Promotion: Childbearing Family, and those that facilitate lifestyle changes, for example, Coping Enhancement, Counseling, Learning Facilitation, and Memory Training. Other interventions were used equally by all groups. (See Box 2-4 on pp. 27-30 in the second edition of NIC[48] for the complete results.) Although the survey represented only beginning data about interventions used by nurses, it demonstrated that NIC is useful to describe the work of the practicing nurse in a variety of settings and in different specialty areas.

Validation survey 3: Use of indirect care interventions. In each of the previous two surveys, respondents were asked to identify any interventions that they believed were missing from NIC. Many of the suggestions for additional interventions were in the area of indirect care: treatments performed away from the patient but important for the effectiveness of the direct care interventions. Examples include Controlled Substance Checking, Critical Path Development, Emergency Cart Checking, Environmental Management, and Supply Management. The input from the survey participants confirmed for the team members that it was important to develop more of the indirect care interventions. According to Prescott and colleagues,[60] one half of a nurse's time is spent in indirect and unit management activities, compared with only one third of the nurse's time spent in direct care activities (estimates vary some by study; remaining percent of time is in category of personnel). Defining indirect care interventions is becoming more important as case management and the use of unlicensed assistive personnel increase. Defining both direct and indirect care interventions is necessary in order to decide what to delegate to others. The research team had several discussions about the nature of nursing interventions and decided that it was time to expand NIC to include both direct and indirect care treatments. The definition of a nursing intervention was revised to include indirect care interventions. A validation survey of some of the indirect care interventions was undertaken when we had a sufficient number developed. The following four purposes were outlined for the survey:

1. To determine the use rate (validity) of the indirect care interventions
2. To assist in the identification of missing indirect care interventions
3. To determine time estimates for interventions
4. To determine level of provider preparation needed to perform interventions

Purposes 3 and 4 were included as pilot work for future study.

A questionnaire asking about use of 26 indirect care interventions was developed and sent to 500 members of the Academy of Medical Surgical Nursing. This group was chosen because it was believed these generalist nurses would perform most of the indirect care interventions. One hundred seventy-one usable surveys were returned. Results show that all of the 26 interventions are used in practice, which supports the validity of including these in the Classification. The interventions used several times a day by 50% or more of the respondents were Documentation (97%), Delegation (80%), Order Transcription (77%), Environmental Management (70%), and Technology Management (62%). Several interventions were also used several times a day by 40% or more of the respondents: Controlled Substance Checking (49%), Telephone Consultation (48%), Shift Report (45%), Specimen Management (45%), Visitation Facilitation (43%), and Transport (42%). Those used rarely or only monthly were Triage (83% rarely, 9% monthly), Code Management (61% rarely, 32% monthly), Product Evaluation (56% rarely, 33% monthly), and Preceptor: Employee (rarely 43%, monthly 40%). Details about the results of this survey, including information on times to perform the interventions and decisions to delegate, are available in an article.[50]

Validation survey 4: Taxonomy validation. The fourth validation survey was a question-naire developed to assess the meaningfulness of the classes and domains. It was distributed in May 1993 to a sample of nurses expert in theory development who were members of the Midwest Nursing Research Society (MNRS).[34] One hundred sixty-one MNRS members from the interest groups of theory development, qualitative methods, and nursing diagnosis were sent question-naires; and 121 usable surveys were analyzed. The participants were, on average, 47 years of age, with a mean of 24 years of experience in nursing. Twenty (16%) had a master's degree and the remaining 101 subjects (83%) had a doctorate.

The participants were each supplied with a copy of the draft taxonomy and a questionnaire survey. Each participant was asked to rate each domain and each class as to how character-istic (1, not at all characteristic, to 5, very characteristic) it is according to the following five criteria:

- Clarity: The class label and definition are stated in clear understandable terms.
- Homogeneity: All interventions are variations of the same class.
- Inclusiveness: The class includes every possible intervention.
- Mutual exclusiveness: The class excludes interventions that do not belong.
- Theory neutral: The class can be used by any institution, nursing specialty, or care delivery model regardless of philosophical orientation.

Analysis of the results indicated that the taxonomy was well developed. Specifically, 77% of the respondents rated the domains as either quite characteristic or very characteristic according to all criteria, and 88% of the respondents rated the classes as either quite characteristic or very characteristic according to all criteria. The criteria of theory neutral and mutual exclusiveness received the highest ratings; the criterion of inclusiveness received the lowest ratings. The Physiological: Complex domain received the highest ratings, and the Health System domain received the lowest ratings. The Health System domain received low ratings chiefly because respondents did not believe it included all of the interventions in this area. Because this is the domain in which most of the indirect care interventions are located, the need for development of more indirect care interventions was validated.

Based on both the quantitative and qualitative results, revisions were made in the taxonomy. Changes occurred mostly in definitions. Three class names were modified and one new class (Information Management) was created. In addition, a few interventions moved classes and some cross-referencing was added or omitted. All in all, the review demonstrated the validity of the taxonomy; the changes that were made were done to enhance clarity. Also at this time, all new interventions that had been developed since the publication of the NIC book in 1992 were placed in the taxonomy. Most of the interventions were easy to place and needed very little discussion. At this time, each intervention was also given a unique number. The validated taxonomy with 6 domains, 27 classes, and 443 coded interventions was published in the second edition of NIC in 1996.[48]

Phase III: Clinical Testing and Refinement (1993-1997)

In Phase III, clinical testing and refinement, the interventions were field tested in five clinical facilities, and guidelines were developed to assist others with implementation. Feedback from nurses in the field sites and other users was received, and the system for refinement of interven-tions was developed. Core interventions were also identified for 39 nursing specialties.

Field testing

A major strength of NIC is its comprehensiveness. NIC includes all interventions that nurses do on behalf of patients. It is useful to nurses in all specialties and in all settings. In phase III we worked with five field sites to implement NIC on their nursing information systems and to establish mechanisms to help others with implementation. The participating sites and a brief description of their computer systems at the time of testing (1993-1997) follows:

- Genesis Medical Center in Davenport, Iowa, following a consolidation of two community hospitals in 1994, was a 500-bed community hospital with approximately 680 registered nurses physically located on two sites, the east and west campuses. Nursing diagnosis had served as the focus for planning patient care in the west campus site since 1982. A mainframe Spectra 2000 computerized nursing information system based on the NANDA list of diagnoses was used to generate and document patient care plans in this site since 1984. The east campus used manual care planning.
- The University of Iowa Hospitals and Clinics in Iowa City, Iowa, in 1994 was an 820-bed teaching hospital and a regional tertiary care center with a staff of 1500 registered nurses. The hospital has been computerized since the early 1970s with an IBM mainframe system. The nursing information system called *INFORMM* was designed in house and implemented for care planning in 1988. On-line documentation of nursing orders was being piloted in 1994 in one unit.
- Oaknoll Retirement Residence is an independent living complex and long-term care facility located in Iowa City. In 1994, it had 133 apartments for elderly persons able to live independently and a 48-bed long-term care facility (32 skilled and 16 intermediate). The nursing department employed 16 registered nurses. The nursing information system, newly purchased in 1993, was an IBM-compatible personal computer and used a MED-COM medical records software program.
- Dartmouth-Hitchcock Medical Center, in 1994, was a 435-bed teaching hospital and tertiary care center with a staff of more than 650 registered nurses located in Lebanon, New Hampshire. The hospital was working with Cerner Corporation of Kansas City to develop a nursing information system. The Cerner applications run on digital hardware and represent a strongly integrated system based on a relational database.
- Loyola University Medical Center's Mulcahy Outpatient Center in Chicago, Illinois, is a multispecialty ambulatory care facility with an associated community nursing service, a hospice program, and a nurse managed center. In 1994 the ambulatory programs provided 226,126 patient visits and employed 223 registered nurses. The medical center hospital used a Technicon (TDS) medical information system called *LUCI*. The system was installed in the outpatient center, but the care planning and documentation functions were not on-line.

Field implementation had different levels of success in each agency (see the previous edition for more information). Despite the tremendous challenges to implementation during a time of down-sizing and fiscal constraints, NIC was implemented in some way in all the agencies, and we learned from their attempts. Representatives from each of the five field sites collaborated on an article describing the implementation of NIC in the sites and the associated issues.[21] Although the challenges related to computerization of NIC differed some by type of facility, whether the facility already had a nursing information system, and sophistication of the staff, several issues were common to all. Based on the field site work, we wrote "Steps for Implementation of NIC in a Clinical Practice Agency" and "Implementation Rules of Thumb for Using NIC on a Nursing Information System" (see Chapter 3, Box 3-2 and Box 3-5) to help others who were beginning to implement NIC. In addition, "Steps for Implementation of NIC in an Educational Setting" (see Box 3-9) was also written to assist educators in implementing NIC.

We constructed a scale to measure the extent of implementation and asked representatives of each agency to compete the scale in 1997. This scale attempts to measure the "dose" of NIC as the independent variable. The scale was derived from two sources: (1) a degree of implementation scale obtained from Joyce Verran and colleagues, who had developed indexes to measure the strength of concepts that were a part of a differentiated group practice model (we heard about these at a national presentation and obtained samples from Dr. Verran; the scale has since been published[53]); and (2) the Iowa Steps for Implementation of NIC in a Practice Setting and Steps for

Implementation of NIC in an Educational Setting. The scale is consistent with Rogers' model of the innovation-decision process,[61] which consists of five stages: (1) knowledge, (2) persuasion, (3) decision, (4) implementation, and (5) confirmation. The scale was pilot tested in June 1995 at 106 agencies whose representatives had previously contacted us for information about NIC and was revised slightly based on their answers. Figure 2-1 contains the scale for measuring the degree of use of NIC in practice or education facilities with the 1997 responses from each of our previous field sites. One can see from the ratings of each of the previous five field sites that all of them implemented NIC in some degree. The scale was included in an implementation manual[35] that was produced to assist other agencies in implementing NIC.

To monitor the implementation of NIC closely and to learn from the field sites what would assist others with implementation, we encouraged and worked with a doctoral student who conducted a qualitative study of the implementation of NIC in the five field sites. The investigation used a prospective design to (1) determine the strategies used to introduce the Classification, (2) identify issues that emerged, and (3) provide guidelines facilitating smooth implementation in other agencies.[14] Rogers' model of diffusion of innovations in organizations[61] provided the conceptual framework for conducting the study. Data collection included recording participant interviews at each site, recording group meetings, and analyzing electronic data transactions on a NIC message board. Key individuals in each site were interviewed three times during the first year of implementation: at the start of the implementation process, midway through the study, and immediately before the study was completed. These key individuals included (1) the decision maker for adopting NIC, (2) the on-site coordinator, (3) the research team's liaison, and (4) four staff nurses. Ethnograph, a computer program for the analysis of text-based data, was used for coding and organizing the data. Interrater reliability was established by having two persons review 10% of the interview and meeting transcriptions. The 86 interviews provided code words, which were collapsed into 11 categories: decision to adopt, efficiency of nursing work, enhancing

No
Use: _____   There is no current activity or planned activity related to use

Use: For each item give a number
    0 = Not at all
    1 = Somewhat
    2 = A moderate amount
    3 = A good deal or item has been completed

Dartmouth	Genesis	Loyola	Oaknoll	UIHC	
3	3	3	3	3	The idea of NIC use is being explored.
1	3	3	2	3	An expressed commitment to use is made by key persons in the agency.
3	3	3	2	3	An implementation task force is established and discussions regarding NIC use are taking place.
0	3	3	1	3	A written plan for implementation is made and distributed.
3	3	3	2	3	NIC is implemented in pilot units or a few courses.
1	3	1-2	2	3	NIC is integrated into agency forms (e.g., philosophy, policies, standards/objectives, syllabi).
1	3	1	2	3	Implementation of NIC is achieved "house-wide" (i.e., majority of staff/faculty/students know about and use NIC).
0	3	1	2	3	NIC is an integral aspect of agency functioning.
0	3	1	2	3	Information regarding use of NIC is used for ongoing strategy formulation (e.g., the database of interventions chosen by the staff or students for a particular population of patients is analyzed and used for staff or faculty development).

Fig. 2-1 Scale to measure the degree of use of NIC in practice or education facilities.

the work of nursing, planning strategies, interactive strategies, positive reaction, negative reaction, changing practice, documentation, information dissemination, and environmental influences. The findings demonstrated that the communications channels used to process information and the leadership were key for successful implementation. The derived benefits of using NIC showed a change (negative to positive) as nurses started using NIC. Two major themes emerged, showing that the use of NIC increased efficiency and demonstrated effectiveness of nursing care. Documentation was a dominant issue for users. The guidelines (Steps for Implementation of NIC in a Clinical Setting, see Box 3-2) developed by the principal investigators of the Iowa Intervention Project research team were corroborated by this study.

In addition to our five "official" field sites, numerous other agencies began to implement NIC during this time. In 1997 we estimated that approximately 200 clinical practice agencies and more than 100 educational facilities were beginning to use NIC in some way; in 2002 clinical practice agencies and an increasing number of vendors were signing licenses to put NIC into their computerized information systems. To provide some assistance to others who were not a part of our grant-funded field site effort, we began in October 1993 *The NIC Letter*, which in March 1997 became *The NIC/NOC Letter*. In 1998, the mailing list for this newsletter, produced three times a year, included more than 1200 individuals; in 2001, the *Letter* was published only two times a year because of the cost of increased subscribers, numbering over 1600. A LISTSERV discussion list, which was begun to assist with communication among personnel at the field sites, was opened up to anyone interested and now has more than 300 active participants from several countries. The video made by the National League for Nursing *(Meet NIC: The Nursing Interventions Classification System)* is also a good means of introducing both staff nurses and students to NIC. We produced an anthology of our publications from the first in 1990 through June 1996[16]; it is available from the Center for Nursing Classification and Clinical Effectiveness and is a good resource for those interested in the early development of NIC. The anthology is a convenient way to obtain all of the early relevant readings and is especially helpful to those who are just discovering standardized language and NIC and those in other countries who have difficulty accessing some of the U.S. journals.

Core interventions
As we observed the nurses in particular units discuss how best to implement NIC, we saw that an early step was their struggle to determine which of the interventions were most related to their patient population and should be targeted first for implementation. At the same time, educators were asking for directions on which interventions related to which courses. To assist in the identification of interventions that are core to specialty areas of practice, we mailed a questionnaire to 49 clinical specialty organizations in June 1995. Each organizational representative was to identify, on behalf of the organization, those NIC interventions that are core to their specialty. Core interventions were defined as a "limited, central set of interventions that define the nature of the specialty. A person reading the list of core interventions would be able to determine the area of specialty practice. The core set of interventions does not include all the interventions used by nurses in the specialty but rather includes those interventions used most often by nurses in the specialty or used predominately by nurses in the specialty." Instructions in the survey urged the respondents to keep the list of core interventions short, preferably less than 30 interventions. A list of all 433 interventions and their definitions was attached to the questionnaire. Because the survey required a response that represents the nature of the specialty, the organizational representatives requested input from others in the organization to verify their answers. Thirty-nine organizations responded to the survey. The core interventions of each of the 39 specialty organizations were first reported in a monograph published by the Center and then in the third edition of NIC in Part Five. An article reporting on the initial survey was published in *Nursing Outlook* in 1998.[49] For this edition, the initial survey was updated by using a focus group approach, and core interventions were identified for four new specialties. This work is published in Part Five (see pp. 903-932).

Phase IV: Use and Maintenance (1996-Ongoing)

Classification systems are not useful if they do not reflect current practice. The current work relates to the ongoing development and use of NIC. Topics discussed in this section include updating NIC through feedback from users, development of community interventions, establishment of linkages with other languages, ongoing work through the Center for Nursing Classification and Clinical Effectiveness, and work with other organizations.

Development and use of a feedback and review process

In earlier editions of NIC, a review form was included, which allowed users to make suggestions for new interventions and revision of existing interventions (see Appendix B for guidelines for submission). Each submission is sent through a review process.

Between the publications of the first and second editions, approximately a dozen submissions for new or revised interventions were received. Most of these came from members of one of the field sites or from students working with a member of the research team. Since the publication of the second edition, the number of submissions has increased, with input coming from a broader user base. Some of the submissions have been based on validation studies, and changes have been suggested based on the study. Others have been made based on clinician use, and suggestions for change have been based on changes in practice. Some of the new interventions in this edition, as well as some of the changes in existing interventions, have resulted from submissions to the research team. We have been told that a strength of NIC is the consistent format. Individuals who submit suggestions for changes should be familiar with the Principles for Intervention Development and Refinement (see Appendix B). They should also be familiar with the structure and content of the Classification to be sure that their idea is unique and is presented well. All submitters whose suggestions have been used in NIC are acknowledged in the next edition.

From the beginning, we have kept an "Interventions Under Consideration" list of ideas for new interventions that may be needed in NIC. Sometimes, when an idea is further explored and work is begun on it for a new intervention, it is discovered that NIC already includes the intervention (just called something else). For the purpose of keeping NIC current with practice changes, there will always be a list of suggestions for new interventions. (This "Interventions Under Consideration" list is not published in NIC because it is constantly changing, but it is available upon request from the Center for Nursing Classification and Clinical Effectiveness.)

In preparation for the publication of this edition, we placed all of the new interventions in the appropriate class and domain of the taxonomy. This was very easy to do and no new classes or domains were added. As we explained in Chapter 1, we also placed all interventions in the NNN Taxonomy of Nursing Practice (see Appendix D) in order to work toward the goal of a common organizing structure for NANDA diagnoses, NIC interventions, and NOC outcomes.

Community interventions

Although the second edition of NIC did include some interventions (e.g., Environmental Management: Community, Health Education, Health Screening, Immunization/Vaccination Administration, Risk Identification, and Smoking Cessation Assistance) that can be used with communities (aggregates), the number of these interventions was small and not visible in NIC. The entire research team decided to study this area, and over the course of a year or more before the publication of the third edition of NIC in 2000, read and discussed multiple writings related to the nature of community practice. This area of intervention was acknowledged as especially important in third-world countries where nursing action is often aimed at the entire community. It is also an area of growing importance in the United States as health care becomes more prevention and community focused. According to Deal, "As the devastating impact of public health problems such as AIDS, infant mortality, adolescent pregnancy, child abuse, and domestic violence become more evident nationwide, a clear need exists for effective population-based health programs . . . it is imperative that community health nurses define their services and provide evidence supporting the effectiveness of interventions they offer" (p. 315).[22] The American Nurses Association Division on Community Health Nursing[5] defines community health nursing as a synthesis of nursing practice and public health practice applied to promoting and preserving the health of populations, with the dominant responsibility to the population as a whole. A *population* is a collection of individuals who have one or more personal (e.g., sex, age) or environmental (e.g., country, work site) characteristics in common. After reading and discussion, we defined a community health intervention as follows: "A community (or public health) intervention is targeted to promote and preserve the health of populations. Community interventions emphasize health promotion, health maintenance, and disease prevention of populations and include strategies to address the social and political climate in which the population resides."

Following this period of study, several of the newer members of the research team who had expertise in community health (Mary Tarbox, Mary Aquilino, Eleanor McClelland, and Barbara Head) took the lead for the development of several new community interventions. After review and discussion by the entire research team, the new domain of *community* was created and added to the NIC taxonomy in the third edition. We believe that this gives this important area of nursing appropriate recognition and will encourage the identification and articulation of the unique interventions in this area.

Linkages with NANDA, the Omaha System, NOC, Resident Assessment Protocols (RAP), and Outcome and Assessment Information Set (OASIS)

A major effort during the past several years has been directed toward the development of linkages. This began during the field testing of NIC, when the nurses in the clinical agencies noted linkages with nursing diagnoses. One of the team members who was also director of nursing at one of the field sites (Jeanette Daly), assisted by other team members, undertook a series of steps in 1992 to link NIC interventions to NANDA nursing diagnoses. These initial linkages were printed in a monograph in 1993, and an expanded and updated linkage list was published in the second edition of NIC.[48] For both the third edition and this edition, we updated the linkages of NIC interventions to NANDA diagnoses (see Part Four). As can be seen, NIC interventions are provided for each NANDA diagnosis in two sections: suggested interventions and additional optional interventions. The most obvious of the suggested interventions are also indicated. The format provides guidance for the nurse but requires that clinical reasoning be used for the selection of the appropriate interventions.

NIC has also been linked with other classifications. In 1996 we published in monograph form *NIC Interventions Linked to Omaha System Problems.*[36] This linkage list (providing linkages between the Omaha System 1992 list of problems and the NIC 1996 list of interventions) was completed as a result of requests from nurses in community settings who were using Omaha System problems but wished for the more comprehensive set of interventions that NIC provides. The format for this publication, available from the Center for Nursing Classification and Clinical Effectiveness, is similar to that of NIC linkages with NANDA diagnoses.

In 1998, we completed linkages with the NOC outcomes[40] and also published these in monograph form.[37] For each of the 190 outcomes in the 1997 NOC book, we provided interventions from the NIC 1996 book in the same categories as those in the linkages with diagnoses. In 2001 the principal investigators of NIC and NOC, under the leadership of Marion Johnson, linked NOC outcomes and NIC interventions to NANDA diagnoses and published these in a book.[39] The format is that for each NANDA diagnosis, the key outcomes are identified and then the appropriate interventions are identified in relationship to the outcome and in consideration of the diagnosis. There is a web site, accessible with a pass code that comes with the purchase of the book, that includes a care plan constructor that uses the linkages related to a specific patient condition (e.g., alcoholism, burns, chest pain, chicken pox, peptic ulcer). A software program based on this care planning book is also now available.

In the past few years, linkages between NIC and NOC and two other classifications (Resident Assessment Protocols [RAP] for use in long-term care facilities and Outcome and Assessment Information Set [OASIS] for use in skilled home care) have been completed and are available as monographs [15,18] from the Center for Nursing Classification and Clinical Effectiveness. Each of these linkages is designed to assist in use of NIC and NOC with federally mandated assessment instruments required for reimbursement in these settings.

We are told that these linkages are very helpful in constructing computer information systems. Although the linkages to date are based on expert opinion, in the future they will be able to be validated through study of actual use in practice. The work is time-consuming, especially when new updates must be produced, but the result is helpful to nurses in making clinical decisions and useful for teaching students how to reason.

Implementation help and effectiveness research
Since the publication of the last edition of NIC, we have also produced a number of other works that assist in implementation.

Estimated time and educational requirements for NIC interventions. This was first published as a monograph[17] and is included in this edition as Part Six. We have estimated the time to perform and type of personnel to deliver each of the 513 interventions in this book. The reader is referred to an article titled "Determining Cost of Nursing Interventions: A Beginning"[38] for information about how the information in Part Six can be used to determine nursing cost and nursing charges for care delivered. The introduction to Part Six explains the method and rationale for the ratings. The section also includes some summary tables that might assist educators or managers in deciding at what level to teach the interventions or what type of staff are needed to perform the interventions.

Curriculum guide for implementation of NANDA, NIC, and NOC into an undergraduate curriculum. This is available as a monograph[26] from the Center for Nursing Classification and Clinical Effectiveness. This work can be used to assist faculty in education programs in implementing standardized languages in their curricula and courses. Authors Cynthia Finesilver and Debbie Metzler, faculty members at Bellin College in Green Bay, Wisconsin, with their colleagues and some of their students, have written about the process and course assignments they use to integrate nursing standardized language in 12 nursing courses in their curriculum. Actual completed student assignments are included for each course. As far as we know, this is the first publication demonstrating use of standardized language across an entire undergraduate curriculum. We thank the authors for taking the time to write and organize the material. The authors of this publication are now designing a web course to assist others in the teaching of standardized language; we hope that this course will be available through the Center beginning in 2004.

NIC and NOC 101: The basics. This 4-hour web course examines the importance of using standardized language for patient care and for the discipline of nursing and focuses on documentation of nursing interventions and nursing-sensitive patient outcomes. The course begins with an overview of standardized language then presents basic information about the development of NANDA and its association with the Iowa research team of NDEC (Nursing Diagnosis Extension Classification). An overview of the development and current information about the two standardized languages developed at Iowa, NIC and NOC, are the main focus of the course. Information about the Center for Nursing Classification and Clinical Effectiveness at the College of Nursing that facilitates the ongoing work is included. Participating faculty are Joanne McCloskey Dochterman, Marion Johnson, and Martha Craft-Rosenberg. For more information go to http://ceu.nursing.uiowa.edu/nicnoc101.

Methods to conduct effectiveness research. Once standardized language is implemented and used to document nursing care, effectiveness research is possible (see the next chapter). In 2001 we had a 4-year grant funded by NINR and AHRQ (Marita Titler and Joanne Dochterman, co-principal investigators), *Nursing Interventions & Outcomes in 3 Older Populations.*[68] The research uses existing clinical and operational data that reside in electronic data repositories in one tertiary care setting to determine the impact of nursing interventions on patient outcomes for three elderly populations: those with heart failure and shock, those with hip fractures, and those who receive the intervention of fall prevention. This is one of the first nursing effectiveness studies in which a large database is used, made possible by the use of standardized nursing language for documentation. The study's four aims are the following:

1. To identify frequently used nursing diagnoses, nursing interventions, pharmacological treatments, and medical treatments for hospitalized elderly with diagnosis-related group (DRG) 127 or 209 and for those who receive the Fall Prevention nursing intervention
2. To describe the relationships among patient characteristics, patient clinical conditions (nursing diagnoses, medical diagnoses, severity of illness), treatments (nursing interventions, medical treatments, pharmacological treatments), characteristics of nursing units, and outcomes of hospitalized elderly patients (DRG 127; DRG 209, Fall Prevention) by using a cross-sectional, retrospective design
3. To compare the cost of acute care for patients (a) who *receive* the nursing intervention Fall Prevention with those who do not receive this nursing intervention, (b) who receive the most frequently used nursing treatment for heart failure (DRG 127) with those who do not receive this intervention, and (c) who receive the most frequently used nursing treatment for hip fracture (DRG 209) with those who do not receive this intervention
4. To develop a guideline for construction and use of a nursing effectiveness research database built from electronic data repositories

Working with other organizations
Over the years, we have worked with multiple groups and organizations to implement NIC. Recently, we have worked with national health care standards organizations to include NIC and NOC. For example, in 1998 we submitted information about NIC and NOC to the American National Standards Institute (ANSI) Health Informatics Standards Board (HISB) to be included in the Inventory of Clinical Information Standards Report, which was presented to the Department of Health and Human Services. Also, since June 1998, we have been working with individuals from Alternative Link, a company located in Las Cruces, New Mexico, to incorporate NIC interventions into the ABC Codes[2] they are developing for reimbursement for alternative providers. Alternative Link has applied to Centers for Medicare and Medicaid Services (CMS) (formerly the Health Care Financing Administration [HCFA]) to be recognized as a reimbursement system. In 2001, NIC was submitted and registered in HL7 (Health Level 7), the U. S. standards organization for health care. In 2002, NIC was licensed for inclusion in SNOMED (Systematized Nomenclature of Medicine), which is under development by the College of American Pathologists in Chicago, Illinois, and aims to be the comprehensive reference terminology for the computerized patient record. During 2003 and 2004, we will be reviewing this work with the SNOMED developers.

We are also consulting, as requested, with authors and vendors who are incorporating NIC in their books and information systems. A growing number of nursing information system vendors are putting NIC and NOC into their systems, and more are demonstrating interest as a result of frequent user requests. We continue to receive many requests for presentations about NIC and NOC; with the availability of web conferencing technology, this is becoming easier. In Appendix C, we have included a timeline and highlights of the major events related to the development and implementation of NIC over the years.

SUMMARY

A large research team has been working since 1987 to construct, validate, and implement a standardized language for nursing treatments. This chapter first describes how the work began and the reasons for development of NIC. The development of NIC is then described in four phases: construction of the Classification, construction of the taxonomy, clinical testing and refinement, and use and maintenance. We have given a comprehensive, although not detailed, overview of the development of NIC in this book so that those who are new to the Classification can understand its history. A variety of qualitative and quantitative methods have been used to construct NIC, including content analysis, survey to experts, focus group review, similarity ratings, hierarchical analysis, and multidimensional scaling. Since the 2000 edition of the book, 29 new interventions have been developed and 93 revised. The major achievement of the past years has been the recognition of the usefulness of NIC and its implementation in growing numbers of practice agencies and educational programs. The next chapter focuses on the use of NIC and includes many examples from agencies that have adopted NIC for a variety of purposes.

References

1. Agency for Health Care Policy and Research. (1990, August). *AHCPR program note*. Rockville, MD: U. S. Department of Health and Human Services, Public Health Service.
2. Alternative Link Systems, Inc. (2001). *The CAM and nursing coding manual*. Albany, NY: Delmar.
3. American Medical Association. (1986). *Physicians' current procedural terminology* (4th ed.). Chicago: Author.
4. American Medical Association. (1990). Troubled past of "invisible" profession. *JAMA: The Journal of the American Medical Association, 264*, 2851-2857.
5. American Nurses Association. (1980). *A conceptual model of community health nursing practice*. Kansas City, KS: Author.
6. American Psychiatric Association. (1992). *Diagnostic and statistical manual of mental disorders* (3rd ed.). Washington, DC: Author.
7. Barry-Walker, J., Bulechek, G. M., & McCloskey, J. C. (1994). A description of medical-surgical nursing. *Medical Surgical Journal, 3*, 261-268.
8. Benner, P. (1984). *From novice to expert*. Menlo Park, CA: Addison-Wesley.
9. Bulechek, G. M., & McCloskey, J. C. (Eds.). (1985). *Nursing interventions: Treatments for nursing diagnoses*. Philadelphia: W. B. Saunders.
10. Bulechek, G. M., & McCloskey, J. C. (1987). Nursing interventions: What they are and how to choose them. *Holistic Nursing Practice, 1*, 36-44.
11. Bulechek, G. M., & McCloskey, J. C. (Eds.). (1992). *Symposium on nursing interventions: Nursing Clinics of North America*. Philadelphia: W. B. Saunders.
12. Bulechek, G. M., McCloskey, J. C., Titler, M. G., & Denehy, J. A. (1994). Report on the NIC project: Interventions used in practice. *The American Journal of Nursing, 49*, 59-64, 66.
13. Carpenito, L. J. (1989). *Nursing diagnoses: Application to clinical practice* (3rd ed.). Philadelphia: JB Lippincott.
14. Carter, J. (1995). *Implementation of the Nursing Interventions Classification (NIC) in five clinical sites*. Unpublished doctoral dissertation, University of Iowa, Iowa City.
15. Center for Nursing Classification (1996). *Nursing Interventions Classification (NIC) Publications: An anthology*. Iowa City, IA: Author.
16. Center for Nursing Classification. (2000). *NIC interventions and NOC outcomes linked to the OASIS Information Set*. Iowa City, IA: Author.
17. Center for Nursing Classification. (2001). *Estimated time and educational requirements to perform 486 nursing interventions*. Iowa City, IA: Author.
18. Center for Nursing Classification. (Cox, R., Preparer). (2000). *Standardized nursing language in long term care*. Iowa City, IA: Author.
19. Cohen, M. Z., Kruckeberg, T., McCloskey, J. C., Bulechek, G., Craft, M. J., Crossley, J. D., et al. (1992). A taxonomy of nursing interventions: Inductive methodology with a research team and a large data set. *Nursing Outlook, 39*, 162-165.
20. Cote, R. A., Rothwell, D. J., Palotay, J. L., Beckett, R. S., Brochy L. (1993). *SNOMED international*. Northfield, IL: College of American Pathologists.
21. Daly, J. M., Button, P., Prophet, C., Clarke, M. Androwich, I. (1997). Nursing Interventions Classification implementation issues in five test sites. *Computers in Nursing, 15*, 23-29.

22. Deal, L. W. (1994). The effectiveness of community health nursing interventions: A literature review. *Public Health Nursing, 11,* 315-323.
23. Everitt, B. (1974). *Cluster analysis.* London: Heinemann.
24. Fehring, R. J. (1986). Validating diagnostic labels: Standardized methodology. In M. E. Hurley (Ed.), *Classification of nursing diagnoses: Proceedings of the Sixth Conference.* St. Louis, MO: Mosby.
25. Fehring, R. J. (1987). Methods to validate nursing diagnoses. *Heart & Lung: The Journal of Critical Care, 16,* 625-629.
26. Finesilver, C., & Metzler, D. (Eds.). (2002). *Curriculum guide for implementation of NANDA, NIC, and NOC into an undergraduate nursing curriculum.* Iowa City: Center for Nursing Classification, the University of Iowa College of Nursing.
27. Gebbie, K. M. (1990, Fall). Distinguished scholar address highlight of convention luncheon. *SCAN—News of the American Nursing Foundation,* 4-6.
28. Griffith, H. M., & Robinson, K. R. (1993). Current Procedural Terminology (CPT) coded services provided by nurse specialists. *Image, 25,* 178-186.
29. Griffith, H. M., Thomas, N., Griffith, L. (1991). MDs bill for these routine nursing tasks. *The American Journal of Nursing, 91,* 22-25.
30. Health Care Financing Administration. (1992). *HCFA Common Procedure Coding System (HCPCS).* Washington, DC: U. S. Department of Health and Human Services, U. S. Government Printing Office.
31. Henderson, V. (1961). *Basic principles of nursing care.* London: ICN House.
32. Iowa Intervention Project. (1992). *Nursing Interventions Classification (NIC): Taxonomy of nursing interventions.* Iowa City: University of Iowa College of Nursing. (Out of Print).
33. Iowa Intervention Project. (1993). The NIC taxonomy structure. *Image, 25,* 187-192.
34. Iowa Intervention Project. (1995). Validation and coding of the NIC taxonomy structure. *Image, 27,* 43-49.
35. Iowa Intervention Project. (1996). *NIC implementation manual.* Iowa City: The University of Iowa College of Nursing, Center for Nursing Classification. (Out of Print).
36. Iowa Intervention Project. (1996). *NIC interventions linked to Omaha System problems.* Iowa City: The University of Iowa College of Nursing, Center for Nursing Classification.
37. Iowa Intervention Project. (1998). *NIC interventions linked to NOC outcomes.* Iowa City: The University of Iowa College of Nursing, Center for Nursing Classification.
38. Iowa Intervention Project. (2001). Determining cost of nursing interventions: A beginning. *Nursing Economics, 19,* 146-160.
39. Johnson, M., Bulechek, G., Dochterman, J., Maas, M., & Moorhead, S. (2001). *Nursing diagnoses, outcomes, interventions: NANDA, NOC, and NIC linkages.* St. Louis, MO: Mosby.
40. Johnson, M., Maas, M. (Eds.). (1999). *Nursing outcomes classification (NOC).* St. Louis, MO: Mosby.
41. Kane, M., Kingsbury, C., Colton, D., Estes, C. (1986). *A study of nursing practice and role delineation and job analysis of entry-level performance of registered nurses.* Chicago: National Council of State Boards of Nursing.
42. Martin, K. S., & Scheet, N. J. (1992). *The Omaha System: Applications for community health nursing.* Philadelphia: W. B. Saunders.
43. McCarty, P. (1989). Nurses see new horizons for organized nursing. *The American Nurse, 1,* 10-11.
44. McCloskey, J. C. (1989). Implications of costing out nursing services for reimbursement. *Nursing Management, 20,* 44-49.
45. McCloskey, J. C., & Bulechek, G. M. (Eds.). (1992). *Nursing Interventions Classification (NIC).* St. Louis, MO: Mosby.
46. McCloskey, J. C., & Bulechek, G. M. (1993). Defining and classifying nursing interventions. In P. Moritz (Ed.), *Patient outcomes research: Examining the effectiveness of nursing practice* (Publication No. 93-3411). Washington, DC: U. S. Government Printing Office.
47. McCloskey, J. C., & Bulechek, G. M. (1993). Nursing intervention schemes. In *Papers from the Nursing Minimum Data Set Conference.* Ottawa, Ontario, Canada: Canadian Nurses Association.
48. McCloskey, J. C., & Bulechek, G. M. (Eds.) (1996). *Nursing Interventions Classification (NIC)* (2nd ed.). St. Louis, MO: Mosby.
49. McCloskey, J. C., Bulechek, G. M., & Donahue, W. (1998). Nursing interventions core to specialty practice. *Nursing Outlook, 46,* 67-76.
50. McCloskey, J. C., Bulechek, G. M., Moorhead, S., & Daly, J. (1996). Nurses' use and delegation of indirect care interventions. *Nursing Economic$, 14,* 22-23.
51. McCloskey, J. C., Gardner, D. L., & Johnson, M. (1987). Costing out nursing services: An annotated bibliography. *Nursing Economic$, 5,* 245-253.
52. McFarland, G. K., & McFarlane, E. (1989). *Nursing diagnosis and intervention.* St. Louis, MO: Mosby.
53. Milton, D. A., Verran, J. A., Gerber, R. M., Fleury, J. (1995). Tools to evaluate reengineering progress. In S. S. Blancett & L. Flarey (Eds.), *Reengineering nursing and health care.* Gaithersburg, MD: Aspen.
54. Moorhead, S. A., McCloskey, J. C., & Bulechek, G. M. (1993). Nursing interventions classification: A comparison with the Omaha System and the Home Healthcare Classification. *The Journal of Nursing Administration, 23,* 23-29.

55. Moorhouse, M. F., Geissler, A. C., & Doenges, M. E. (1987). *Critical care plans: Guidelines for patient care.* Philadelphia: F. A. Davis.

56. Pearce, N. D. (1988). Uniform minimum health data sets: Concept, development, testing, recognition for federal health use, and current status. In H. H. Werley & N. M. Lang (Eds.), *Identification of the nursing minimum data set.* New York: Springer.

57. Pei, M. (1964). *The story of language.* Philadelphia: J. B. Lippincott.

58. Practice Management Information Corporation. (1992). *HCPCS: National level II Medicare codes—HCFA common procedure coding system.* Los Angeles: Author.

59. Practice Management Information Corporation. (1989). *ICD-9-CM International classification of diseases* (9th rev., 3rd ed., clinical modification). Los Angeles: Author.

60. Prescott, P. A., Phillips, C. Y., Ryan, J. W., & Thompson, K. O. (1991). Changing how nurses spend their time. *Image, 23,* 23-28.

61. Rogers, F. (1995). *Diffusion of innovations* (4th ed.). New York: Free Press.

62. Saba, V. K. (1992.) The classification of home health care nursing: Diagnoses and interventions. *Caring Magazine, 11,* 50 57.

63. Saba, V. K., O'Hare, P. A., Zuckerman, A. E., Boondas, J., Levine, E., & Oatway, D. M. (1991). A Nursing intervention Taxonomy for home health care. *Nursing & Health Care, 12,* 296-299.

64. Sigma Theta Tau International Honor Society of Nursing. (1987). *Introduction to the international classification of nursing knowledge.* Indianapolis, IN: Author.

65. Systematized Nomenclature of Medicine (SNOMED). Web site: http://www.snomed.org

66. Steelman, V., Bulechek, G. M., & McCloskey, J. C. (1994). Toward a standardized language to describe perioperative nursing. *AORN Journal, 60,* 786-795.

67. Titler, M., Bulechek, G. M., & McCloskey, J. C. (1996). Use of the Nursing Interventions Classification by critical care nurses. *Critical Care Nursing, 16,* 38-54.

68. Titler, M., & Dochterman, J. (Co-PIs). Nursing Interventions & Outcomes in 3 Older Populations, 5 R01 NR05331-02, National Institute of Nursing Research & the Agency for Healthcare Research and Quality. Funded grant proposal, 07/01/2001–03/31/2005.

69. Titler, M., Pettit, D., Bulechek, G. M., McCloskey, J. C., Craft, M. J., Cohen, M. Z., et al. (1991). Classification of nursing interventions for care of the integument. *Nursing Diagnosis, 2,* 45-56.

70. Verran, J. (1981). Delineation of ambulatory care nursing practice. *The Journal of Ambulatory Care Management, 4,* 1-13.

71. Visiting Nurse Association of Omaha. (1986). *Client management information system for community health nursing agencies* (Publication No. HRP-0907023). Washington, DC: U. S. Government Printing Office.

72. Werley, H. H., & Devine, E. C. (1987). The Nursing Minimum Data Set: Status and implications. In K. J. Hannah, M. Reimer, W. C. Mills, S. Letourneau (Eds.), *Clinical judgment and decision making: The future with nursing diagnosis.* New York: John Wiley and Sons.

73. Werley, H. H., & Lang, N. M. (Eds.). (1988). *Identification of the Nursing Minimum Data Set.* New York: Springer.

74. Werley, H. H., Lang, N. M., & Westlake, S. K. (1986) The Nursing Minimum Data Set Conference: Executive summary. *Journal of Professional Nursing, 2,* 217-224.

75. World Health Organization. (1992). *International statistical classification of diseases and related health problems* (10th rev.). Geneva: Author.

CHAPTER THREE

Use of NIC

The Nursing Interventions Classification (NIC) should be used to communicate the interventions that nurses use with patients. When NIC is used to document practice, then we have the beginning of a mechanism to determine the impact of nursing care on patient outcomes. This chapter has four parts and an appendix. Part One identifies and discusses six factors that should be considered when a nurse selects an intervention for a particular patient. Part Two discusses the implementation of NIC in a clinical practice agency. Several useful guidelines for implementation are included; and computerization, the potential uses of the computerized data, and construction of a useful database are addressed. Part Three addresses use in education. Part Four is an overview of a model illustrating how nursing practice data (diagnoses, interventions, and outcomes) can be used at three levels. Following the overview, there is a discussion of some of the advantages of use of standardized language. An appendix to the chapter includes examples of use of NIC in both practice and education. These examples should be helpful to others who are considering implementation. Nearly all of the examples included here are new to this edition. The previous edition of NIC also includes examples and the majority of those are still in use and relevant.

SELECTING AN INTERVENTION

The selection of a nursing intervention for a particular patient is part of the clinical decision making of the nurse. Six factors should be considered when choosing an intervention: desired patient outcomes, characteristics of the nursing diagnosis, research base for the intervention, feasibility for doing the intervention, acceptability to the patient, and capability of the nurse. These are outlined here briefly; for more detail, consult Bulechek and McCloskey's text.[3,4]

Desired Patient Outcomes

Patient outcomes should be specified before an intervention is chosen. They serve as the criteria against which to judge the success of a nursing intervention. Outcomes describe behaviors, responses, and feelings of the patient in response to the care provided. Many variables influence outcomes, including the clinical problem; interventions prescribed by the health care providers; health care providers themselves; environment in which care is received; patient's own motivation, genetic structure, and pathophysiology; and patient's significant others. There are probably more intervening or mediating variables in each situation, making it difficult to establish a causal relationship between nursing interventions and patient outcomes in some instances. The nurse must identify for each patient the outcomes that can be reasonably expected and can be attained as the result of nursing care. Pinkley[13] urges us to choose the outcomes for a patient in the context of all the nursing diagnoses, not just those aimed at the alleviation of the etiology of one diagnosis. According to Pinkley, the choosing of outcomes should be directed at optimizing health, as well as alleviating problems.

An excellent way to specify outcomes is by use of the Nursing Outcomes Classification (NOC).[11] As indicated in a previous chapter, NOC contains outcomes for individual patients and family caregivers that are representative for all settings and clinical specialties. NOC describes patient states at a conceptual level with indicators expected to be responsive to nursing intervention. This allows measurement of the outcomes at any point on a continuum from most negative to most positive at different points in time. NOC outcomes can be used to monitor the extent of progress, or lack of progress, throughout an episode of care and across different care settings. The NOC outcome of Anxiety Self-Control is displayed in Box 3-1 to show the label, definition, indicators, and measuring scale. NOC outcomes have been linked to North American Nursing Diagnosis Association (NANDA) diagnoses, and these linkages appear in the back of the NOC book. NIC interventions have also been linked to NOC outcomes, and to NANDA diagnoses, and those linkages are available in a book entitled *Nursing Diagnoses, Outcomes, Interventions: NANDA, NOC and NIC Linkages*.[10]

Characteristics of the Nursing Diagnosis

Outcomes and interventions are selected in relationship to particular nursing diagnoses. The intervention is directed toward altering the etiological factors (in NANDA's taxonomy, the *related factors*) associated with the diagnosis. If the intervention is successful in altering the etiology, the patient's status can be expected to improve. According to Bulechek and McCloskey,[3,4] it is not always possible to change the etiological factors; when this is the case, it is necessary to treat the signs and symptoms (in NANDA's taxonomy, the *defining characteristics*). For potential or high-risk diagnoses, the intervention is aimed at altering or eliminating the risk factors for the diagnosis.

Research Base for the Intervention

The nurse who uses an intervention should be familiar with its research base. The research will indicate the effectiveness of using the intervention with certain types of patients. Some interventions have been widely tested for specific populations, whereas others are still in the concept development phase and have had little or no empirical testing. Nurses know about the research related to particular interventions through their education programs and by keeping their knowledge current. If there is no research base for an intervention to assist a nurse in the choosing of an intervention, then the nurse may use scientific principles (e.g., infection transmission) or consult an expert about the specific populations for which the intervention might work.[14]

Feasibility for Performing the Intervention

Feasibility concerns include the ways in which the particular intervention interacts with other interventions, both those of the nurse and those of other health care providers. It is important that the nurse be involved in the total plan of care for the patient. Other feasibility concerns, critical in today's health care environment, are the cost of the intervention and time for implementation. The nurse needs to consider the interventions of other providers, the cost of the intervention, and the time it takes to choose an intervention.

Acceptability to the Patient

An intervention must be acceptable to the patient and family. The nurse is frequently able to recommend a choice of interventions to assist in reaching a particular outcome. For each intervention, to facilitate an informed choice, the patient should be given information about how he or she is expected to participate. The patient's values, beliefs, and culture must all be considered in the choice of an intervention.

Capability of the Nurse

The nurse must be able to carry out the particular intervention. Bulechek and McCloskey[3,4] outline three areas in which the nurse must be competent; the nurse must (1) have knowledge of the scientific rationale for the intervention, (2) possess the necessary psychomotor and interpersonal skills, and (3) be able to function within the particular setting to effectively use health care resources. It is clear from just glancing at the total list of interventions that no one nurse has the

Box 3-1

One Example of a NOC (Nursing Outcomes Classification) Outcome
Anxiety Self-Control (1402)

Domain—Psychosocial Health (III)

Class—Self Control (O)

Scale(s)—Never demonstrated to Consistently demonstrated (m)

Care Recipient:

Data Source

Definition: Personal actions to eliminate or reduce feelings of apprehension, tension, or uneasiness from an unidentifiable source

OUTCOME TARGET RATING: Maintain at _____   Increase to _____

Anxiety Self-Control Overall Rating	Never demon- strated 1	Rarely demon- strated 2	Sometimes demon- strated 3	Often demon- strated 4	Consistently demon- strated 5	
Indicators:						
140201 Monitors intensity of anxiety	1	2	3	4	5	NA
140202 Eliminates precursors of anxiety	1	2	3	4	5	NA
140203 Decreases environmental stimuli when anxious	1	2	3	4	5	NA
140204 Seeks information to reduce anxiety	1	2	3	4	5	NA
140205 Plans coping strategies for stressful situations	1	2	3	4	5	NA
140206 Uses effective coping strategies	1	2	3	4	5	NA
140207 Uses relaxation techniques to reduce anxiety	1	2	3	4	5	NA
140208 Monitors duration of episodes	1	2	3	4	5	NA
140209 Monitors length of time between episodes	1	2	3	4	5	NA
140210 Maintains role performance	1	2	3	4	5	NA
140211 Maintains social relationships	1	2	3	4	5	NA
140212 Maintains concentration	1	2	3	4	5	NA
140213 Monitors sensory perceptual distortions	1	2	3	4	5	NA
140214 Maintains adequate sleep	1	2	3	4	5	NA
140215 Monitors physical manifestations of anxiety	1	2	3	4	5	NA
140216 Monitors behavioral manifestations of anxiety	1	2	3	4	5	NA
140217 Controls anxiety response	1	2	3	4	5	NA

First edition 1997, revised second edition, revised third edition (formerly Anxiety Control).

Outcome Content References:

Hudson, W.W. (1992). The WALMYR assessment scales scoring manual. Tempe, AZ: WALMYR Publishing Co.

Laraia, M.T., Stuart, G.W., & Best, C.L. (1989). Behavioral treatment of panic-related disorders: A review. *Archives of Psychiatric Nursing, 3*(3), 125-133.

Moorhead, S.A., & Brighton, V.A. (2001). Anxiety and fear. In M. Maas, K. Buckwalter, M. Hardy, T. Tripp-Reimer, M. Titler, & J. Specht (Eds.), *Nursing care of older adults: Diagnoses, outcomes & interventions* (pp. 571-592). St. Louis, MO: Mosby.

Stuart, G. W., & Laraia, M.T. (2001). *Principles and practice of psychiatric nursing* (7th ed.). St. Louis, MO: Mosby.

Tucker, S., Moore, W., & Luedtke, C. (2000). Outcomes of a brief inpatient treatment program for mood and anxiety disorders. *Outcomes Management for Nursing Practice, 4*(3), 117-123.

Waddell, K.L., & Demi, A.S. (1993). Effectiveness of an intensive partial hospitalization program for treatment of anxiety disorders. *Archives of Psychiatric Nursing, 7*(1), 2-10.

Source: Moorhead, S., Johnson, M., & Maas, M. (Eds.). (2004). *Nursing outcomes classification (NOC)* (3rd ed.). St. Louis, MO: Mosby.

capability to perform all of the interventions. Nursing, like other health disciplines, is specialized, and individual nurses perform within their specialty and refer or collaborate when other skills are needed.

After considering each of the these factors for a particular patient, the nurse selects the intervention(s). This is not as time-consuming as it sounds when elaborated in writing. As Benner[1] has demonstrated, the student and beginning nurse should examine these things systematically, but with experience, the nurse synthesizes this information and is able to recognize patterns rapidly. One advantage of the Classification is that it facilitates the teaching and learning of decision making for the novice nurse. Using standardized language to communicate the nature of our interventions does not mean that we stop delivering individualized care. Interventions are tailored to individuals by selection of the activities and by modification of the activities as appropriate for the patient's age and the patient's and family's physical, emotional, and spiritual status. These modifications are made by the nurse, using sound clinical judgment.

In the taxonomy (see pp. 109-125) similar interventions are grouped together. The domains and classes of the taxonomy help clinicians locate and select interventions most appropriate for patients. The domain level helps a clinician to make an initial sort, then the classes provide more focus. For example, to locate interventions for a patient having trouble breathing, the nurse should review the class on Respiratory Management; to locate teaching interventions, the nurse should review the class on Patient Education. The interventions in classes can be grouped together on an information system. Another way to locate an intervention is to use the linkages with NANDA interventions provided in this book or the linkages with NANDA diagnoses and NOC outcomes provided in the linkage book.[10] Over time, as we determine which interventions are frequently used together for best success with a particular patient, these population clusters can also be grouped. We have also included, for the first time in this edition, the location of interventions in a second taxonomic structure (see Appendix D). As explained in the introduction to this structure, this was developed in the hope that with time, we can evolve to one common structure for NANDA, NIC, and NOC. This structure is untested to date, however, so, in this edition, we have provided placement of interventions in both our own structure and the proposed common structure.

IMPLEMENTING NIC IN A CLINICAL PRACTICE AGENCY

The time and cost for implementation of NIC into a nursing information system in a clinical practice agency depends on the agency's selection and use of a nursing information system, the computer competency of nurses, and nurses' previous use and understanding of standardized nursing language. The change to the use of a nursing standardized language with a computer represents, for many, a major change in the way in which nurses have traditionally documented, and effective change strategies need to be used. Complete implementation of NIC throughout an agency may take months to several years; the agency should allocate resources for computer programming, education, and training. As major vendors complete clinical nursing information systems that include NIC, implementation will be easier. In this section we include tools for implementation.

Box 3-2 provides steps for implementation. Although not all of the steps must be done in every institution, the list is helpful in planning for implementation. We have found that successful implementation of the steps requires knowledge about change and nursing information systems. In addition, it is a good idea to have an evaluation process established. Box 3-3 is an annotated list of readings in the areas of change, evaluation, and nursing information systems that we have found helpful in assisting others to implement NIC. Also included are other readings about NIC and NOC that may be helpful for implementation. Those who are in charge of the implementation effort would be wise to read many of the readings, and some of these might be selected as helpful resources for administrators and practicing nurses. Another way to get basic information about NIC and NOC and an overview of standardized language is to take the 4-hour web course available from the Center for Nursing Classification and Clinical Effectiveness (see Box 3-4).

NIC can be used as either a manual or computerized system. Use of NIC in a computerized system facilitates data aggregation and analysis. Box 3-5 includes "rules of thumb" for using NIC on an information system. Following these will help ensure that data are captured in a consistent

---

Box 3-2

Steps for Implementation of NIC in a Clinical Practice Agency

A. Establish Organizational Commitment to NIC

- Identify the key person responsible for implementation (e.g., person in charge of nursing informatics).
- Create an implementation task force with representatives from key areas.
- Provide NIC materials to all members of the task force.
- Invite a member of the NIC project team to do a presentation to the staff and to meet with the task force.
- Purchase copies of the NIC book, circulate readings about NIC and *The NIC/NOC Letter* to units.
- Show the NIC video.
- Have members of the task force begin to use the NIC language in everyday discussion.
- Have key individuals from the task force sign onto the Center for Nursing Classification and Clinical Effectiveness LISTSERV.

B. Prepare an Implementation Plan

- Write the specific goals to be accomplished.
- Do a force field analysis to determine driving and restraining forces.
- Determine whether an in-house evaluation will be done and the nature of the evaluation effort.
- Identify which NIC interventions are most appropriate for the agency or unit.
- Determine the extent to which NIC is to be implemented; for example, in standards, care planning, documentation, discharge summary, performance evaluation.
- Prioritize the implementation efforts.
- Choose 1 to 3 pilot units. Get members from these units involved in the planning.
- Develop a written timeline for implementation.
- Review current system and determine the logical sequence of actions for integration of NIC.
- Create work groups of expert clinical users to review NIC interventions and activities, determine how these will be used in agency, and develop needed forms.
- Distribute the work of the expert clinicians to other users for evaluation and feedback before implementation.
- Encourage the development of a *NIC champion* in each of the units.
- Keep other key decision makers in agency informed.
- Determine the nature of the total nursing data set. Work to ensure that all units are collecting data on all variables in a uniform manner so that future research can be done.
- Make plans to ensure that all nursing data are retrievable.
- Identify learning needs of staff and plan ways to address these.

C. Carry Out the Implementation Plan

- Develop the screens/forms for implementation. Review each NIC intervention and decide whether all parts (e.g., label, definition, activities, reference) are to be used. Determine which are critical activities to document and whether further details are desired.
- Provide training time for staff.
- Implement NIC in the pilot unit(s) and obtain regular feedback.
- Update content or create new computer functions as needed.
- Use focus groups to clarify issues and address concerns/questions.
- Use data on positive aspects of implementation in house-wide presentations.
- Implement NIC house-wide.
- Collect postimplementation evaluation data and make changes as needed.
- Identify key markers to use for ongoing evaluation and continue to monitor and maintain the system.
- Provide feedback to the Center for Nursing Classification and Clinical Effectiveness.

Box 3-3

Annotated List of Helpful Readings Related to Implementation

Change

Berwick, D. (1997). Spreading innovation. **Quality Connection, 6,** *1-3.*

Health care is burgeoning with innovations, but spreading them is frustratingly slow. Berwick gives seven rules a leader can use to spread innovation based on E. Rogers' summary of empirical work published in *The Diffusion of Innovations* (see reference below).

Brennan, P. F. (1999). Harnessing innovative technologies: What can you do with a shoe? **Nursing Outlook, 47,** *128-131.*

Emerging computer and information system technologies portend great benefit to enable nursing to fulfill its social contract. It is the prerogative and responsibility of nursing to design, develop, or evaluate emerging technologies; to re-engineer practice to capitalize on them; and to reconceptualize education to prepare nurses to use them.

Clark, P. C., & Hall,, H. S. (1990). Innovations probability chart. A valuable tool for change. **Nursing Management, 21,** *128v-128x.*

Contains an easy-to-use tool that can be used to determine the factors within the organization that may facilitate or hinder the change process.

Hersey, P., Blanchard, K., Johnson, D. E. (2001). Planning and implementing change. In **Management of organizational behavior** *(8th ed, pp. 376-398). Upper Saddle River, NJ: Prentice-Hall, Inc.*

Overviews the processes of planned versus directive change. Describes how to do a force field analysis to determine the driving and restraining forces for the change.

Ingersoll, G. L., Brooks, A. M., Fischer, M. S., Hoftere, D. A., Lodge, R. H., Janken J. K., et al. (1995). Professional practice model: Research collaboration: Issues in longitudinal, multisite design. **Journal of Nursing Administration, 25,** *39-46.*

The article is a result of the authors' experience of implementing an enhanced professional practice model in five general medical surgical units. Nineteen recommendations for others who might undertake similar projects are discussed according to three phases of the project—the "buying on" phase, the "sustaining momentum" phase, and the "moving on" phase. The recommendations make good administrative sense, and attention to these will facilitate the success of any change process.

Katzenbach, J. R., & Smith, D. K. (1993). **The wisdom of teams.** *Boston: Harvard Business School Press. (Book summary by Soundview Executive Book Summaries, Bristol, VT).*

Defines teams and types of teams. Discusses resistance to teams and strategies to use to get teams unstuck.

Rogers, E. (1995). **Diffusion of innovation** *(4th ed.). New York: The Free Press.*

A classic. Book is helpful but NOT an easy read. The first edition, published in 1962, was recognized as a landmark work in the field and became established as the standard introduction to diffusion studies. This fourth edition synthesizes 4000 publications on diffusion research. Rogers' model of the innovation-decision process consists of five stages: (1) knowledge, (2) persuasion, (3) decision, (4) implementation, and (5) confirmation.

Keep in mind that an innovation, to be accepted:
• needs to be an improvement over what previously existed
• should not eliminate or interfere with other things valued
• needs to enhance prestige of individuals who adopt it
• must be supported by high-prestige individuals
• should involve those who will use it in the implementation
• should be able to be modified to accommodate valued traditional practices
(Lundsgaarde, Fisher, & Steele, 1981—see evaluation section).

Evaluation

Aaronson, L. S., & Burman, M. E. (1994). Focus on psychometrics. Use of health records in research: Reliability and validity issues. **Research in Nursing and Health, 17,** *67-73.*

Not an easy read but is a good overview of the issues related to reliability and validity that need to be addressed when data obtained from health records are used.

Continued

Annotated List of Helpful Readings Related to Implementation—cont'd

Lundsgaarde, H., Fischer, P., & Steele, D. (1981). Human problems in computerized medicine. **Anthropology, 13,** *197-204.*
Provides a comprehensive evaluation of the process of implementing a computerized system. The article overviews a study in a medical unit at a 750-bed hospital to evaluate physician attitudes towards the Problem-Oriented Medical Information System (PROMIS).

McCloskey, J. C., Maas, M., Gardner-Huber, D., Kasparek, A., Specht, J., Ramler, C., Watson, C., et al. (1994). Nursing management innovations: A need for systematic evaluation. **Nursing Economic$, 12,** *35-45.*
Introduces the idea of nursing management innovations, summarizes the research related to four such innovations, and then proposes a method for more systematic evaluation of nursing innovations. The four innovations that are reviewed are (1) use of nurse extenders, (2) hospital-based case management, (3) nursing shared governance, and (4) product line management.

Meisenhelder, J. B. (1993). Health care reform: Opportunity for evaluation research. **Nursing Scan in Research Application for Clinical Practice, 6,** *1-3.*
Identifies the key points in development of the evaluation plan for a new system: write measurable objectives, make a plan that is cost-effective, and evaluate the major goals. Short but to-the-point piece.

Nursing Information Systems

Burkes, M. (1991). Identifying and relating nurses' attitudes toward computer use. **Computers in Nursing, 9,** *190-201.*
Describes a study to measure nurses' attitudes toward computer use. Includes description of an investigator-designed survey to measure knowledge, satisfaction, and motivation about computer use. A beliefs part consists of the questionnaire of Stronge (Stronge & Brodt, 1985).

Stronge, J. H., & Brodt, A. (1985). Assessment of nurses' attitudes toward computerization. **Computers in Nursing, 3,** *154-158.*
Reports on the development and availability of a questionnaire designed to measure nurses' attitudes toward computerization. The tool has been widely used.

Turley, J. P. (1992). A framework for the transition from nursing records to a nursing information system. **Nursing Outlook, 40,** *177-181.*
Urges nurses to reevaluate their current modes of record keeping. Says that we need links between the professional knowledge structure and the record of transactions (care given) but that these links cannot be too tight. Computer jargon makes it hard to understand in some places.

Other Helpful Readings about NIC

Iowa Intervention Project. (2001). Determining cost of nursing interventions: A beginning. **Nursing Economic$, 19,** *146-160.*
Determination of cost of nursing services has long been a concern for nurse executives and others. A key component of nursing cost is the interventions delivered. An essential step for determining cost of interventions is the determination of the time to deliver the intervention and the type of provider who can do the intervention. This manuscript reports time estimates and provider education required for interventions listed in the second edition of NIC based on expert judgment. In addition to being useful for contracting for nursing services and for evolving reimbursement mechanisms, the knowledge is helpful for planning for staffing and other resource use.

Iowa Intervention Project. (1997). Proposal to bring nursing into the information age. **Image—Journal of Nursing Scholarship, 29,** *275-281.*
Addresses issues related to documentation of nursing care and proposes a model that illustrates how nursing practice data, collected through use of standardized languages, are useful to staff nurses, nurse administrators, researchers, and policy makers. Concludes that there are three main challenges: (1) the level of detail to document, (2) the inclusion of nursing language in critical paths, and (3) the need for articulation among different nursing classifications.

McCloskey, J. C., Bulechek, G. M. & Donahue, W. (1998). Nursing interventions core to specialty practice. **Nursing Outlook, 46,** *67-76.*
Reports on a survey mailed to 39 specialty practice organizations in 1995. Ninety-six percent of the 433 NIC interventions were identified as core by at least one specialty; 82 interventions were listed as core for six or more specialties. Discusses how the lists of core interventions can be used in practice, education, and research. The core interventions in this book are an expansion of this early work.

Box 3-3

Annotated List of Helpful Readings Related to Implementation—cont'd

McCloskey, J. C., & Bulechek, G. M. (1994). Standardizing the language for nursing treatments: An overview of the issues. **Nursing Outlook, 42,** *56-63.*

Overviews the issues involved in using standardized language. Argues that proper use will assist nurses in making good judgments, will help make nursing services visible to others, and will facilitate research related to the effectiveness of nursing care. Although this publication is a decade old, it is still helpful to those who are new to standardized language.

McCloskey, J. C., & Maas, M. L. (1998). Interdisciplinary team: The nursing perspective is essential. **Nursing Outlook, 46,** *157-163.*

Discusses the trend toward interdisciplinarity in health care and its tendency to conceal the identity and contributions of nursing professionals. Authors urge nurses to maintain a nursing perspective while participating collaboratively on interdisciplinary teams. The value of nurses' knowledge of NIC ad NOC is highlighted because these languages are among the most well-developed standardized languages in health care and are potentially useful for the development of standardized languages for other disciplines.

Box 3-4

Web Course on the Basics of NIC and NOC

Check out the course overview at http://www.ceu.nursing.uiowa.edu/nicnoc101/. This web course examines the importance of using standardized language for patient care and for the discipline of nursing, focusing on documentation of nursing interventions and nursing-sensitive patient outcomes. The course begins with an overview of standardized language, then presents basic information about the development of NANDA (North American Nursing Diagnosis Association) and its association with the Iowa research team of NDEC (Nursing Diagnosis Extension Classification). An overview of the development and current information about the two standardized languages developed at the University of Iowa, the Nursing Interventions Classification (NIC) and the Nursing Outcomes Classification (NOC), are the main foci of the course. Information about the Center for Nursing Classification and Clinical Effectiveness at the College of Nursing that facilitates the ongoing work is included. The course consists of approximately 4 hours of lecture content with PowerPoint slides and related handouts. Faculty for the course are Joanne McCloskey Dochterman, Director, Center for Nursing Classification and Clinical Effectiveness and principal investigator of NIC; Marion Johnson, principal investigator of NOC; and Martha Craft-Rosenberg, principal investigator of NDEC and President-Elect of NANDA.

The course may be taken for Continuing Education Units (.4) or a certificate. Cost in 2002 was $75. (Group rates, e.g., for a course requirement may be negotiated.)

Required software and bandwidth: Internet Explorer 5.0 or higher, Netscape 6.0 or higher, RealOne Player; 56K modem connection or faster (your actual connection speed *must be above 43 Kbps* to receive the content). All of this software is free for download from web sites.

manner. In some computer systems, because of space restrictions, there is a need to shorten some of the NIC activities. While this is becoming less of a necessity as computer space for nursing expands, Box 3-6 provides guidelines for shortening NIC activities to fit in a computer system with two examples.

Most institutions that adopt NIC do so because of the need for data about the use and effectiveness of clinical interventions. To have good data that can be used for a variety of analyses, it is necessary to also collect, in a systematic way, other information that can be used in conjunction with the NIC data about interventions to address a variety of questions. Early in the process of implementation, an institution should identify key research questions to be addressed with data

---

Box 3-5

Implementation RULES OF THUMB for Using NIC on a Nursing Information System

1. The information system should clearly indicate that NIC is being used.
2. NIC intervention labels and definitions should appear in whole and should be clearly labeled as interventions and definitions.
3. Activities are not interventions and should not be labeled as such on the screens.
4. Documentation that the intervention was planned or delivered should be captured at the intervention label level. In addition, an agency may choose to have nurses identify specific activities within the intervention for patient care planning and documentation.
5. The number of activities required in an information system should be kept as few as possible for each intervention so as not to overburden the provider.
6. If activities are included on the information system, they should be written to the extent possible (given the constraints of the data structure) as they appear in NIC. Activities that must be rewritten to fit short field constraints should reflect the intended meaning.
7. All additional or modified activities should be consistent with the definition of the intervention.
8. Modification of NIC activities should be done sparingly and only as needed in the practice situation.
9. NIC interventions should be a permanent part of the patient's record with capability to retrieve this information.

Box 3-6

Guidelines for Shortening NIC Activities to Fit in a Computer System

Introduction: While things are changing, some computer systems still restrict space, thereby not allowing for the number of characters necessary for including the entire length of the NIC activities. If this is the case, we would advise requesting more space. However, if for whatever reason, this is not possible, the following guidelines should be used to decrease the length of the activities. If these guidelines are followed, all activities should be less than 125 characters.

Guidelines
1. Eliminate all "as appropriate" and "as needed" found after a comma at the end of some activities.
2. Remove all e.g.'s found inside of parentheses.
3. Delete words or dependent clauses that describe other parts of an activity.
4. Use the abbreviation pt for patient and nse for nurse.
5. Do NOT create new language and do not replace words.
(Note: We have decided not to suggest word abbreviations in addition to what is already in NIC because most agencies have an agreed-upon list of abbreviations that they are required to use; these lists are not uniform across agencies, and creating yet another list may lead to further confusion.)

Examples:
Perform and document the patient's health history and physical assessment ~~evaluating preexisting conditions, allergies, and contraindications for specific anesthetic agents or techniques~~.
Deliver anesthetic consistent with ~~each~~ patient's physiological needs, clinical judgment, ~~patient's requests,~~ and Standards ~~for Nurse Anesthesia Practice~~.
Obtain ordered specimen for laboratory analysis of acid-base balance ~~(e.g. ABC, urine, and serum levels), as appropriate~~.
Screen for symptoms of a history of domestic abuse. ~~(e.g., numerous accidental injuries, multiple somatic symptoms, chronic abdominal pain, chronic headaches, pelvic pain, anxiety, depression, post traumatic stress syndrome, and other psychiatric disorders.)~~

collected through documentation. After the research questions are identified, the variables needed to address the questions and whether the data are currently collected or should be collected in the new system can be determined. The data that will be obtained from the identified variables must be linked with each other at the individual patient level. Addressing these concerns when setting up a nursing information system will prevent problems later.

The analysis of data collected through documentation of practice is sometimes referred to as *effectiveness research*. Documentation of practice through the use of standardized language opens up many exciting possibilities for nursing in effectiveness research. The identification of research questions to be addressed is referred to by two health policy authors at Harvard Medical School as the "effectiveness space."[8] That is, as nurses we must identify the variables (e.g., interventions, outcomes, specific patient characteristics, specific provider characteristics, specific treatment setting characteristics) and their measures necessary to evaluate effectiveness.

For example, an agency wishes to have data that can answer the following three research questions: What interventions typically occur together? Which nurses use which interventions? What are the related diagnoses and outcomes for particular interventions? The rationale for desiring data related to these questions is as follows:

- *What interventions typically occur together?* When information is systematically collected about the treatments nurses perform, clusters of interventions that typically occur together for certain types of patients can be identified. We need to identify interventions that are frequently used together for certain types of patients so we can study their interactive effects. This information will also be useful in the construction of critical paths, in determining costs of services, and in planning for resource allocation.
- *Which nurses use which interventions?* Systematic documentation of intervention use will allow us to study and compare the use rate of particular interventions by type of unit and facility. Implementation of NIC will allow us to learn which interventions are used by which nursing specialties. Determining the interventions used most frequently in a specific type of unit or in a certain type of agency will help to determine which interventions should be in that unit's or agency's nursing information system. It will also help in the selection of personnel to staff that unit and in the structuring of the continuing education provided to the personnel in the unit.
- *What are the related diagnoses and outcomes for particular interventions?* Knowing which interventions work best for specific diagnoses and lead to certain outcomes can assist nurses in making better clinical decisions. In addition, this information can help us to design treatment plans for patients that have the best chances of success.

The recommended data elements to address these questions are listed in Box 3-7 and include both definitions and the proposed measurements. Consistent definition and measurement are necessary to aggregate and compare data from different units in different settings. These variables and their measures have been discussed with representatives from several types of agencies and care settings in an attempt to make them meaningful in all settings; wherever possible, we have made our definitions and measurement indicators consistent with those of the Nursing Minimum Data Set (NMDS)[15] and the other health care uniform data sets, such as the Uniform Hospital Discharge Data Set (UHDDS).[12] As can be seen from the list, more than clinical nursing data is needed. The patient's identity number is needed to link information; age, sex, and race/ethnicity are included to provide some demographic information on the patient population; the physician's diagnoses and interventions; medications; and the work unit's type, staff mix, average patient acuity, and workload are included for controls. That is, for some analyses we may need to control for one or more of these effects to determine whether the nursing intervention was the cause of the effect on the patient outcome.

Our work with these variables demonstrates that the profession must still grapple with several issues related to the collection of standardized data. For example, the collection and coding

Box 3-7

Data Elements for Effectiveness Research in Nursing
Definitions and Measurement

FACILITY

1. Facility identification number

Definition: a number that identifies the organization where the patient/client was provided nursing care
Measurement: use Medicare identification number

ADMISSION DATA

2. Patient identification number

Definition: the unique number, assigned to each patient/client within a health care facility, that distinguishes and separates one patient record from another in that facility
Measurement: use the facility's record number

3. Date of birth

Definition: the day of the patient's birth
Measurement: month, day, and year of birth

4. Gender

Definition: the patient's sex
Measurement: male, female, unknown

5. Race

Definition: a class or kind of people unified by community of interests, habits, or characteristics
Measurement: use Uniform Hospital Discharge Data Set (UHDDS) codes: 1. American Indian or Alaska Native; 2. Asian/Pacific Islander; 3. black, not Hispanic; 4. Hispanic; 5. white, not Hispanic; 6. other (please specify); 7. unknown

6. Marital status

Definition: legally recognized union of man and woman
Measurement: 1. married, 2. widowed, 3. divorced, 4. separated, 5. never married, 6. unknown

7. Admission date

Definition: date of initiation of care
Measurement: month, day, year

MEDICATIONS

8. Medications

Definition: medicinal substances used to cure disease or relieve symptoms
Measurement: 1. name of drug; 2. route of administration (1. PO, 2. IM/SC, 3. IV, 4. aerosol, 5. rectal, 6. eye drops, 7. other); 3. dose (amount of drug prescribed); 4. frequency (number times given per day); 5. start date (date drug first used in this episode of care: month, day, year); 6. stop date (date drug discontinued in this episode of care: month, day, year)

PHYSICIAN DATA

9. Physician identification number

Definition: a number across settings that identifies the physician who is primarily responsible for the medical care of the patient /client during the care episode
Measurement: unique number used by provider to bill for services (UHDDS uses attending and operating)

10. Medical diagnosis

Definition: the medical conditions that coexist at the time of admission, that develop subsequently, or that affect the treatment received and/or the length of stay; all diagnoses that affect the current episode of care

Box 3-7

Data Elements for Effectiveness Research in Nursing
Definitions and Measurement—cont'd

Measurement: names of medical diagnoses as listed on the patient's bill using *International Classification of Diseases, Ninth Revision, Clinical Modification (ICD-9-CM)* codes

11. Diagnosis-related group (DRG)

Definition: The U.S. prospective payment system used for reimbursement of Medicare patients; categorizes discharged patients into approximately 500 groups based on medical diagnosis, age, treatment procedure, discharge status, and sex.
Measurement: the 3-digit number and name of the DRG that this patient was assigned

12. Medical intervention

Definition: a treatment prescribed by a physician; any significant procedure for the current episode of care
Measurement: 1. names of physician procedures listed on the patient bill using *Current Procedural Terminology (CPT)* codes; 2. start date (date procedure began this episode of care: month, day, year); 3. stop date (date procedure discontinued this episode of care: month, day, year)

NURSING DATA

13. Nurse identification number

Definition: a number across settings that identifies the nurse who is primarily responsible for the nursing care of the patient or client during the care episode
Measurement: Does not exist at this time; make own codes

14. Nursing diagnosis

Definition: a clinical judgment made by a nurse about the patient's response to an actual or potential health problem or life process during this episode of care, which affects the treatments received and/or the length of stay
Measurement: names of nursing diagnoses using NANDA terms and codes

15. Nursing intervention

Definition: a treatment performed by a nurse
Measurement: 1. names of treatments delivered to patient during episode of care using NIC terms and codes; 2. start date (date intervention began this episode of care: month, day, year); 3. stop date (date intervention discontinued this episode of care: month, day, year)

OUTCOMES

16. Patient outcome

Definition: an aspect of patient/client health status that is influenced by nursing intervention during this episode of care
Measurement: 1. names of outcomes using NOC terms, 2. date identified, 3. date outcome is stopped, 4. status of outcome at beginning and end of episode of care (use NOC scale)

17. Discharge date

Definition: date of termination of an episode of care
Measurement: month, day, and year

18. Disposition

Definition: plan for continuing health care made on discharge
Measurement: use NMDS with modification: 1. discharged to home or self-care (routine discharge); 2. discharged to home with referral to organized community nursing service; 3. discharged to home with arrangements to see nurse in ambulatory care setting; 4. transfer to a short-term care hospital; 5. transfer to a long-term care institution; 6. died; 7. left against medical advice; 8. still a patient; 9. other

Continued

Box 3-7

Data Elements for Effectiveness Research in Nursing
Definitions and Measurement—cont'd

19. Cost of care

Definition: provider's charges for the services rendered to the client incurred during the episode of care
Measurement: total charges billed for episode of care (from patient's bill)

UNIT DATA

20. Unit type

Definition: name of type of unit or specialty area that best characterizes where majority of patient care is delivered
Measurement: all units answer both parts a and b:
A. Where is the location of nursing care? (Check only one site.)
____Ambulatory care/outpatient
____Community
____Home
____Hospital
____Long-term care setting/nursing home
____Occupational health
____Rehabilitation agency
____School
____Other: Please describe_____
B. What is the specialty that best characterizes the type of care being delivered? (Choose only one.)
____General medical
____General surgical
____General medical surgical
____Geriatric
____Intensive or emergency care (e.g., CCU, MICU, PICU, SICU, ER, OR, RR)
____Maternal-child
____Psychiatric (adult or child, including substance abuse)
____Specialty medicine (e.g., bone marrow, cardiology, dermatology, hematology, hemodialysis, neurology, oncology, pulmonary, radiology)
____Specialty surgery (e.g., EENT, neurosurgery, orthopedics, urology)
____Other (Please describe):_____

21. Staff mix

Definition: ratio of professional to nonprofessional nursing care providers in the unit/clinic/group where care is being provided
Measurement: number of RNs to nonprofessional staff who *worked* in unit/clinic/group each day of patient's stay (Collect daily for patient's length/episode of care—if cannot get daily, take weekly average. Allocate 12-hour shifts or other irregular shifts to times actually worked, i.e., a person who works 12 hours 7:30 am to 7:30 pm is allocated 8 hours [1 FTE] on days and 4 hours [.5 FTE] on evenings. Count only actual direct care hours, i.e., remove the head nurse and charge nurse unless they are providing direct care, remove the unit secretary and do not include nonproductive hours [such as orientation, continuing education])
   No. of FTE RNs days_____
   No. of FTE RNs evenings_____
   No. of FTE RNs nights _____
   No. of FTE LPN/LVNs days_____
   No. of FTE LPN/LVNs nights_____
   No. of FTE LPN/LVNs evenings_____
   No. of FTE aides days _____
   No. of FTE aides evenings_____
   No. of FTE aides nights_____
   No. of others days (please identify) _____
   No. of others evenings (please identify) _____
   No. of others nights (please identify) _____

Box 3-7

Data Elements for Effectiveness Research in Nursing Definitions and Measurement—cont'd

22. Hours of nursing care

Definition: hours of nursing care administered per patient day in unit/clinic/group where care is delivered

Measurement: hours of care (actual staffing) by RNs, LPNs, and aides

Days: RN hours _____LPN hours_____aide hours _____others hours _____
Evenings: RN hours _____LPN hours_____aide hours _____others hours _____
Nights: RN hours _____LPN hours_____aide hours _____others hours _____
NOTE: These are the same people as in number 21.

23. Patient acuity

Definition: average illness level of patients cared for in the unit

Measurement: patient is rated on agreed-upon patient acuity scale (for example, see Box 3-8)

24. Workload

Definition: the amount of nursing service provided in a unit

Measurement: the average patient acuity (number 23) times the number of occupied beds per day (or number of patients seen in ambulatory care) divided by the number of RNs working or number of total nursing personnel working (number 21)

_____midnight census or number of patients encountered per day

of medications (number 8) in an easily retrievable form is not yet available in many facilities. Although nursing effectiveness research can be done without the knowledge of medications, many of the outcomes that are achieved by nurses are also influenced by certain drugs, and so the control for medication effect is desirable. At present, there is no unique number that identifies the primary nurse (number 13). Consequently, it is not currently possible to attribute clinical interventions or outcomes to particular nurses based on documentation data. Additionally, health care facilities do not collect the unit data (numbers 20 through 24) in a standardized way. Thus if one wished to compare these data across facilities, the data would need to be translated facility by facility to common measures such as those proposed in Box 3-7.

Item 23 proposes use of a patient acuity scale that can be used to compare data across institutions. Many agencies have their own patient classification scale or use one from the literature; however, these are typically not usable across different settings. To fill this void, we have constructed, with help from individuals in different settings, an easy-to-use prototype patient acuity scale that can be used across settings (Box 3-8). Although testing of the scale has been limited, its usefulness in all settings has been demonstrated.

An additional challenge is having a measure of the "dose" of the intervention. Maintaining the integrity of the intervention across participants and settings is important in effectiveness research because inconsistent intervention delivery may result in variability in the outcomes achieved.[2,5] When NIC is used, this means that a substantial number of the activities listed for a particular intervention should be done and that all activities that are done should be consistent with the definition of the intervention. It is important that the activities be tailored for individual care, but they must not vary so much that the intervention is no longer the same. In experimental research when a particular intervention is studied under controlled conditions (called *efficacy research*), the consistent delivery of the intervention is possible. These ideal conditions rarely happen in actual practice, so effectiveness research (what actually happens in practice) is imperative. At present, there is no solution to the issue of "dose" of the intervention. A proxy measure, such as the amount of time a practitioner uses when doing the intervention, is helpful and may suffice as a measure of "dose" in some studies. But the best solution is to know the number and extent of

Box 3-8

NIC Patient Acuity Scale

Instructions: Rate each patient on this scale once a day (or as appropriate in your practice).

Acuity Level of Patient (Circle One):

1. A self-care patient who is primarily in contact with the health care system for assistance with health promotion activities. The patient may require some assistance to cope with the effects of disease or injury but the amount of treatment provided is not more than that which could be provided on a brief outpatient visit. *The patient in this category is often seeking routine health screening tests, such as mammograms, Pap smears, parenting instructions, weight loss and blood pressure checks, sports physicals, and well-baby check-ups. The teaching aspects of care are usually brief and often limited to take-home written instructions.*

2. A patient who is relatively independent as a self-care agent but may have some limitations in total self-care. The patient requires periodic nursing assessment and interventions for needs that may be simple or complex. Teaching activities form a good part of the care delivered and health care requirements include the need for education about prevention. *Examples of patients who may fit in this category include women at high risk for a complicated pregnancy, individuals with hard-to-control diabetes or newly diagnosed diabetes, individuals who have a stable psychiatric illness, a family with a child with attention deficit disorder, and cardiac patients in the rehabilitation stage.*

3. A patient who is unable to find enough resources or energies to meet his or her own needs and is dependent on others for self-care requirements. This person requires continuing nursing intervention but the care is predictable and not in the nature of an emergency. *Examples of patients who fit this category are someone with an unstable or energy-draining chronic illness, a woman in active labor, a long-term care patient, a hospice patient, a depressed psychiatric patient, and a stabilized postoperative patient.*

4. A patient who is acutely ill and dependent on others for self-care requirements with needs that may change quickly. The patient requires continuing nursing assessment, and intervention and care requirements are not predictable. *Examples of patients in this category are a postoperative patient recovering from major surgery during the first 24 to 36 hours, someone experiencing an acute psychiatric episode, and a woman in a high-risk pregnancy category in active labor.*

5. A patient who is critically ill and requires life-saving measures to maintain life. The patient has no ability to act as his or her own self-care agent and requires constant assessment and nursing intervention to maintain an existence. *Examples of patients in this category are patients in intensive care receiving full life support, psychiatric patients in intensive care; low birth weight preemies; head injury accident victims; and, in general, those individuals with multisystem failures.*

the specific activities that are done. Some of the databases being developed by individual agencies and vendors include this information, but others do not have the memory storage capacity required for large data sets and the agencies have chosen not to document this level of detail. Although the documentation of the intervention label is most important for comparison of data across sites, it is also important to have a way to ascertain the consistent implementation of the intervention. This can be done by an agency's adoption of a standard protocol for the delivery of the intervention, by the collection of the time spent for intervention delivery, or by documentation of the activities related to the intervention.

More refinement must be done on all of these measures; the beginning drafts included here illustrate the challenges that face us as we move forward to conduct effectiveness research. Despite the challenges, we must continue making progress. Individuals who are considering implementing NIC must not get overwhelmed by the challenges; rather, they should join in the excitement about the capability to generate data to demonstrate the worth of nursing care. In this chapter's appendix, we include several examples submitted by those in practice who have implemented NIC.

USE IN EDUCATION

It is our experience that changes in education are slower to develop than those in practice and only take place if educators view the practice changes as somewhat lasting. Nursing diagnoses have been included in most of the major care planning textbooks since the 1980s; in the past few years, many authors of nursing care planning books and textbooks have included NIC. Educators still typically use books and journal articles for teaching, rather than computer software programs. Although this is beginning to change, there are few computer software programs for teaching care planning and documentation. We hope that the software based on our linkage book[10] will be useful for teaching standardized nursing language and clinical decision making to students. In this section we include guidelines for use by faculty members to implement NIC in the curriculum, and in this chapter's appendix there are some examples of forms used by faculty members who are using NIC to facilitate the teaching of care planning and clinical decision making. Another useful resource to assist faculty in implementing standardized language in an undergraduate curriculum is a monograph written by Cynthia Finesilver and Debbie Metzler and their colleagues and students at Bellin College in Green Bay, Wisconsin, which is available from the Center for Nursing Classification and Clinical Effectiveness at the University of Iowa.[7]

Implementation of NIC in an educational setting is easier than implementation in a practice setting because fewer individuals are involved and there are usually no issues related to use in an information system. Nevertheless, this is a big change, and some guidelines for making the change are useful (see readings listed in Box 3-3). Box 3-9 lists Steps for Implementation of NIC in an Educational Setting. These are similar to Steps for Implementation of NIC in a Practice Agency (see Box 3-2), but the specific actions relate to the academic setting and course development. The central decision that must be made is that faculty adopt a nursing philosophical orientation and focus, rather than the more traditional medical orientation with nursing implications added on. If the faculty members are not familiar with NIC and NOC, the 4-hour web course offered by the Center for Nursing Classification and Clinical Effectiveness may be an easy way to quickly gain an understanding of the basics (see Box 3-4).

Not all interventions can or should be addressed at the undergraduate level; faculty must decide which interventions should be learned by all undergraduate students and which require advanced education and should be learned in a master's program. Some interventions are unique to specialty areas and perhaps are best taught only in specialty elective courses. Connie Delaney, a professor at the University of Iowa, has elaborated the steps for identifying which interventions are taught in what courses. In an e-mail communication, Delaney recommends the following steps, which we have expanded:

1. Identify the NIC interventions that are never taught in the curriculum (e.g., associate, baccalaureate, master's) and eliminate these from further action.
2. Using the remaining interventions, have each course group identify the interventions that are taught in their course or area of teaching responsibility. That is, identify what is currently taught with the NIC intervention terms.
3. Compile this information into a master grid (interventions on one axis and each course on the other axis) and distribute it to all faculty members.
4. Have a faculty discussion, noting the interventions that are unique to certain courses and those that are taught in more than one course. Clearly articulate the unique perspective offered by each course for each intervention that is taught in more than one place (e.g., Is the intervention being delivered to a different population?). Should both courses continue to include the intervention or should content be deleted from one course? Review interventions that are not located in any courses but that faculty believe should be taught at this level. Should content be added?
5. Affirm consensus of the faculty on what interventions are taught where.

The same process can, of course, be done with nursing diagnoses (by using NANDA) and with patient outcomes (by using NOC). Many educational programs already use NANDA diagnoses and can implement NIC by reviewing the NANDA to NIC linkages and determining the interventions that might be taught in relationship with NANDA diagnoses.

Box 3-9

Steps for Implementation of NIC in an Educational Setting

A. Establish organizational commitment to NIC
- Identify the key person responsible for implementation (e.g., head of curriculum committee).
- Create an implementation task force with representatives from key areas.
- Provide NIC materials to all members of the task force.
- Invite a member of the NIC project team to do a presentation to the faculty and to meet with the task force.
- Purchase and distribute copies of the NIC book.
- Circulate readings about NIC and copies of *The NIC/NOC Letter* to faculty. Show the NIC video at a faculty meeting.
- Examine the philosophical issues regarding the centrality of nursing interventions in nursing.
- Have members of the task force and other key individuals begin to use the NIC language in everyday discussion.
- Have key individuals from the task force sign onto the Center for Nursing Classification and Clinical Effectiveness LISTSERV.

B. Prepare an implementation plan
- Write specific goals to be accomplished.
- Do a force field analysis to determine driving and restraining forces.
- Determine whether an in-house evaluation will be done and the nature of the evaluation.
- Determine the extent to which NIC is to be implemented; for example, in graduate, as well as undergraduate programs; in philosophy statements; in process recordings, care plans, case studies; in orientation for new faculty.
- Prioritize the implementation efforts.
- Develop a written timeline for implementation.
- Create work groups of faculty and perhaps students to review NIC interventions and activities, determine where these will be taught in the curriculum and how they relate to current materials, and develop or redesign any needed forms.
- Identify which NIC interventions should be taught at the graduate level and which at the undergraduate level. Identify which interventions should be taught in which courses.
- Distribute the drafts of decisions to other faculty for evaluation and feedback.
- Encourage the development of a *NIC champion* in each department or course group.
- Keep other key decision makers informed of your plans.
- Identify learning needs of faculty and plan ways to address these.

C. Carry out the implementation plan
- Revise the syllabi; order the NIC books; ask library to order books.
- Provide time for discussion and feedback in course groups.
- Implement NIC one course at a time and obtain feedback from both faculty and students.
- Update course content as needed.
- Determine impact on and implications for supporting courses and prerequisites and restructure these as needed.
- Report progress on implementation regularly at faculty meetings.
- Collect postimplementation evaluation data and make changes in curriculum as needed.
- Identify key markers to use for ongoing evaluation and continue to monitor and maintain the system.
- Provide feedback to the Center for Nursing Classification and Clinical Effectiveness.

Inclusion of standardized nursing language in a curriculum focuses the teaching on clinical decision making (the selection of the appropriate nursing diagnoses, outcomes, and interventions for a particular patient/client). Two helpful books for the teaching of clinical decision making to new students are listed in Box 3-10, as well as one instrument that could be used to measure the development of critical thinking. As more educational programs teach standardized nursing language as the knowledge base of nursing, these resources will expand.

USE OF A STANDARDIZED LANGUAGE MODEL

This chapter concludes with explanation of a model (Figure 3-1) that indicates the relationship of use of standardized language for documentation of actual care delivered by the nurse at the bedside

Box 3-10

Helpful Resources for Teaching Clinical Decision Making in Nursing

Two introductory texts that incorporate NIC:
Pesut, D. J., & Herman, J. (1999). *Clinical reasoning: The art and science of critical and creative thinking.* Albany, NY: Delmar Publishers.
Rubenfeld, M. G., & Scheffer, B. K. (1999). *Critical thinking in nursing: An interactive approach* (2nd ed.). Philadelphia: Lippincott.

Instrument to measure critical thinking:
Facione, P. A., Facione, N. C., & Giancarlo, C. A. (1998). *The California Critical Thinking Disposition Inventory.* Millbrae, CA: California Academic Press.
    Measures seven mental attributes of critical thinkers: truth-seeking, open-mindedness, analyticity, systematicity, self-confidence, inquisitiveness, and maturity. Consists of 75 items rated with a 6-point Likert scale.

to the generation of data for decision making about cost and quality issues in the agency and for inclusion in databases used for health policy making. The three-level model indicates that use of standardized language for documentation of patient care not only assists the practicing nurse in communicating with others but also leads to several other important uses.

At the *individual level,* each nurse uses standardized language in the areas of diagnoses, interventions, and outcomes to communicate patient care plans and to document care delivered. We recommend the use of NANDA, NIC, and NOC as the classifications in the areas of diagnoses, interventions, and outcomes. Each of these classifications is comprehensive across specialties and practice settings, and each has ongoing research efforts to maintain the currency of the classifications. An individual nurse working with a patient or group of patients/clients asks himself or herself several questions according to the steps of the nursing process. What are the patient's nursing diagnoses? What are the patient outcomes that I am trying to achieve? What interventions do I use to achieve these outcomes? The identified diagnoses, outcomes, and interventions are then documented by using the standardized language in these areas. A nurse working with an information system that contains the Classification will document care by choosing the concept label for the intervention. Not all of the activities will be done for every patient. To indicate which activities have been done, the nurse can either highlight those done or simply document the exceptions, depending on the existing documentation system. A nurse working with a manual information system will write in the chosen NIC intervention labels as care planning and documentation are done. The activities can also be specified depending on the agency's documentation system. Although the activities may be important in communicating the care of an individual patient, the intervention label is the place to begin when planning care.

This part of the model can be thought of as documentation of the key decision points of the nursing process with standardized language. It makes apparent the importance of nurses' skills in clinical decision making. We have found that even though NIC requires nurses to learn a new language and a different way to conceptualize what they do (naming the intervention concept rather than listing a series of discrete behaviors), they quickly adapt and in fact become the driving force to implement the language. With or without computerization, the adoption of NIC makes it easier for nurses to communicate what they do—with each other and with other providers. Care plans are much shorter, and interventions can be linked to diagnoses and outcomes. Because an individual nurse's decisions about diagnoses, interventions, and outcomes are collected in a uniform way, the information can be aggregated to the level of the unit or organization.

At the *unit/organizational level,* the information about individual patients is aggregated for all the patients in the unit (or other group) and, in turn, in the entire facility. This aggregated nursing practice data can then be linked to information contained in the nursing management database.

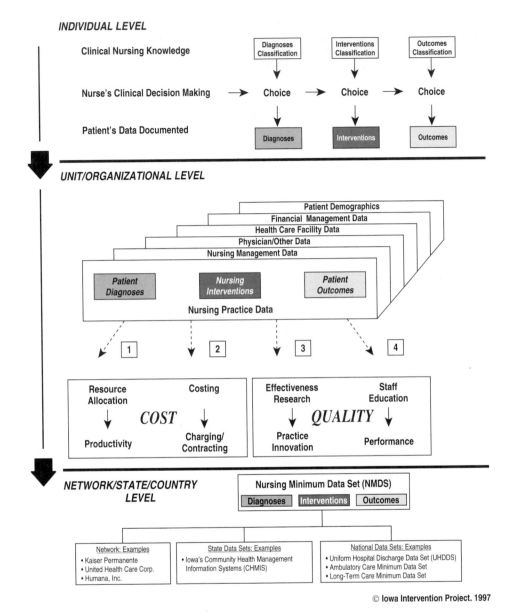

INDIVIDUAL LEVEL

Clinical Nursing Knowledge — Diagnoses Classification / Interventions Classification / Outcomes Classification

Nurse's Clinical Decision Making → Choice → Choice → Choice

Patient's Data Documented — Diagnoses / Interventions / Outcomes

UNIT/ORGANIZATIONAL LEVEL

Patient Demographics
Financial Management Data
Health Care Facility Data
Physician/Other Data
Nursing Management Data

Patient Diagnoses — Nursing Interventions — Patient Outcomes

Nursing Practice Data

1   2   3   4

Resource Allocation   Costing
COST
Productivity   Charging/Contracting

Effectiveness Research   Staff Education
QUALITY
Practice Innovation   Performance

NETWORK/STATE/COUNTRY LEVEL

Nursing Minimum Data Set (NMDS)
Diagnoses   Interventions   Outcomes

Network: Examples
• Kaiser Permanente
• United Health Care Corp.
• Humana, Inc.

State Data Sets: Examples
• Iowa's Community Health Management Information Systems (CHMIS)

National Data Sets: Examples
• Uniform Hospital Discharge Data Set (UHDDS)
• Ambulatory Care Minimum Data Set
• Long-Term Care Minimum Data Set

© Iowa Intervention Project, 1997

Fig. 3-1 Nursing Pactice Data: Three Levels.

The management database includes data about the nurses and others who provide care and the means of care delivery. This is another area in which standardization is needed. To that end, Delancy and Huber[6] have proposed the collection of a nursing management minimum data set that includes standardized measures for a host of management information, including method of care delivery, staff mix, facility vacancy rate, and unit size and type. These two databases (nursing practice and nursing management) comprise the nursing information system. In turn, the nursing practice and management data can be linked with data about the treatments done by physicians and other providers, facility information, patient information, and financial data. Most of these data, with the exception of data about treatments done by providers other than physicians, are already collected in a uniform way and are available for use.

The model illustrates how the clinical practice data linked with other data in the agency's information system can be used to determine both cost and quality of nursing care. The cost side of the model addresses resource allocation and costing out of nursing services; the quality side of the model addresses effectiveness research and staff education. The use of standardized language to plan and document care does not automatically result in knowledge about cost and quality but provides the potential for data collection for decision making in these areas. The steps to accomplish these four purposes are briefly outlined below. Explanation of some managerial and financial terms is provided in parentheses for those not familiar with these areas.

Cost

Resource allocation—the distribution of staff and supplies
- Determine the interventions and related outcomes per type of population.
- Determine and apply the rules for staffing mix (ratio of professional to nonprofessional nursing care providers) per type of population.
- Allocate other resources (supplies and equipment) accordingly.
- Determine productivity (ratio of output to input or the ratio of work produced to people and supplies needed to produce the work) of the staff.

Costing—determining the cost of nursing services rendered to the patient
- Identify the interventions delivered to the patient.
- Affix a price per intervention, taking into account the level of provider and time spent.
- Determine an overhead charge (amount billed for business expenses that are not chargeable to a particular service but are essential to the production of services such as heat, light, building, and repairs); allocate evenly to all patients and be able to provide justification.
- Determine the cost of care delivery per patient (direct care interventions plus overhead).
- Determine the charge per patient or use the information to contract for nursing services (establishing a business arrangement for the delivery of nursing services at a fixed price).

Quality

Effectiveness research—research to determine effects or outcomes of nursing interventions
- Identify the research questions (e.g., what combination of interventions results in the best outcomes for a particular type of patient?).
- Select the outcomes to be measured.
- Identify and collect the intervening variables (e.g., patient characteristics, physician treatments, staff mix, workload).
- Analyze the data.
- Make recommendations for practice innovations.

Staff education—providing education for staff to ensure competency to deliver the needed interventions
- Determine the level of competence of the nurses related to particular interventions.
- Provide education as needed and remeasure competence.
- Determine the nurse's level of accountability for the interventions and whether the intervention or part of the intervention is delegated.
- Provide education as needed related to decision making, delegation, and team building.
- Evaluate performance in terms of achievement of patient outcomes.
- Use information in nurse's performance evaluation, taking into consideration ability to competently perform the intervention and overall level of professional accountability.

The two sides of the model are interactive. Cost and quality should always be considered hand in hand. In addition, the four paths do not mean to imply that these are mutually exclusive. Research can be conducted on the cost side, and costs can be determined for research and education. The four distinct paths, however, are helpful to indicate the main areas of use of these data at an organizational level.

The *network/state/country level* involves the "sending forward" of nursing data (NMDS) to be included in large databases that are used for bench marking for determination of quality and for health policy making. Werley and colleagues[15] have identified 16 variables that should be included in large policy-making databases. These include the three clinical variables of diagnoses, interventions, and outcomes; nursing intensity (defined as staff mix and hours of care), which will be collected in the nursing management database; and 12 other variables such as patient's age, sex, and race and the expected payer of the bill (which are available from other parts of the clinical record). The model indicates that the nursing data on diagnoses, interventions, and outcomes are aggregated by facility and then included in the larger regional and national databases. Examples of two national databases and one state database are listed on the model. A growing number of networks of care providers (the model lists three) are also constructing databases. According to Jacox,[9] nursing has remained essentially invisible in these clinical and administrative databases. She lists the following ramifications of the invisibility of nursing and nursing care in the databases:

- We cannot describe the nursing care received by patients in most health care settings.
- Much of nursing practice is described as the practice of others, especially physicians.
- We cannot describe the effects of nursing practice on patient outcomes.
- We often cannot describe nursing care within a single setting, let alone across settings.
- We cannot identify what nurses do so that they may be reimbursed for it.
- We cannot tell the difference in patient care and costs when care is delivered by physicians as contrasted with nurses.
- This invisibility perpetuates the view of nursing as part of medicine that does not need to be separately identified.

Advantages of the Use of Standardized Data

The use of standardized language to document practice provides a way to overcome the invisibility described by Jacox[9]; it brings the vision of the NMDS to reality. Systematic collection of clinical practice data helps every segment of nursing. We believe that if nurses working in all settings systematically document their care using standardized language, the benefits of the model can be realized.

Our patients will benefit from the systematic collection and use of nursing information because their continuity of care will be enhanced. As they move from one health care setting to another, there will be a standardized way to communicate the care plan and the outcomes remaining to be achieved. As nurses become more familiar with the standardized language contained in the classifications, they can more precisely communicate what has been done and what still must be done for each patient. We will also have better terminology to describe our services to patients so they might be more active partners in their health care. Patients in the future will benefit from the research that will be conducted on the standardized databases.

The staff nurse or care provider will also find many advantages. Level one of the model provides a systematic, efficient way for nursing care to be documented. As computer systems become more available, the burden of paper work and multiple recordings should be eased. The use of standardized language will help the nurse to concentrate on the clinical judgment portion of the nursing process rather than on the description of phenomena. Communication with other nurses and other providers at the time of patient transfer or discharge will be much easier.

The nurse manager/administrator will have richer data for use in planning the allocation of resources. Level two of the model will provide information on the most frequently occurring patient diagnoses within the unit or the organization and the frequency of the nursing interventions that are delivered. Planning for staff selection and staff development activities can be based on patient data. There will be a better rationale for staff mix and the determination of activities to be delegated to unlicensed assistants. Level two will provide the nurse manager with the information to balance the cost and quality components of care. Cost is currently receiving a great deal of attention, but cost concerns must be balanced by concerns for quality. The implementation of this model allows us to do both.

The benefits to nurse researchers (and ultimately to patients) are numerous. Databases for nursing practice information obtained from care actually delivered will become available. Questions concerning which interventions work best for which patients at what cost can readily be studied from the existing sources of data. Nursing will be able to participate in bench marking types of research to evaluate care from one region of the country to another. When new technologies are introduced, the databases will contain baseline information for comparison of effectiveness. The progress of nursing science should move more quickly when existing data can be used, rather than making it necessary for each researcher to collect new data each time a research question or hypothesis is proposed.

Nursing educators will find many benefits in the model. Curricula will emphasize two major foci: the information contained in the classifications and the process of making clinical decisions or deciding how to apply the content knowledge of each of the classifications to an individual patient. We should see more commonalties evolve in curricula across the country so that there is more consensus about the preparation of a professional nurse. The standardized languages will be adopted in nursing textbooks (this is already happening) so that students will see more consistency as they progress through their programs of study.

Our professional associations will benefit greatly from the information that will be collected at level three of the model. They can use this information to better articulate the contributions of nurses at state and national levels. Information from the databases can be used when decisions are made about which health policies to develop and support. Legislation that will benefit our consumers can be developed based on actual patient data. The manpower needs for the profession can be more adequately estimated.

SUMMARY

This chapter is an overview of the potential uses of NIC, and the appendix includes several new examples of use in practice and education. Since the first edition of NIC was published in 1992, there has been rapid movement in both settings to incorporate use. We recognize that implementation of NIC is not without difficulties and that work to continuously improve the Classification and links with other classifications should be ongoing. We welcome and look forward to your feedback and suggestions for improvement.

References

1. Benner, P. (1994). *From novice to expert*. Menlo Park, CA: Addison-Wesley.
2. Braden, S., & Braden, C. J. (1998). *Evaluating nursing interventions: A theory driven approach.* Thousand Oaks, CA: Sage.
3. Bulechek, G. M., McCloskey, J. C. (Eds.). (1992). *Nursing interventions: Essential nursing treatments* (2nd ed.). Philadelphia: W. B. Saunders.
4. Bulechek, G. M., & McCloskey, J. C. (Eds.). (2000). *Nursing interventions: Effective nursing treatments* (3rd ed.). Philadelphia: W. B. Saunders.
5. Carter, J. J., Moorhead, S. A., McCloskey, J. C., & Bulechek G. M. (1995). Using the Nursing Interventions Classification to implement Agency for Health Care Policy and Research guidelines. *Journal of Nursing Care Quality, 9,* 76-86.
6. Delaney, C., & Huber, D. (Eds.). (1996). *Nursing Management Minimum Data Set (NMMDS).* Chicago: American Organization of Nurse Executives.
7. Finesilver, C., & Metzler, D. (Eds.). (2002). *Curriculum guide for implementation of NANDA, NIC and NOC in an undergraduate curriculum,* Iowa City, IA: Center for Nursing Classification and Clinical Effectiveness.

8. Guadagnoli, E., & McNeil, B. J. (1994). Outcomes research: Hope for the future or the latest rage? *Inquiry 31*, 14-24.
9. Jacox, A. (1995). Practice and policy implications of clinical and administrative databases. In N. M. Lang (Ed.), *Nursing data systems: The emerging framework*. Washington, DC: American Nurses Association.
10. Johnson, M., Bulechek, G., Dochterman, J., Maas, M., & Moorhead, S. (2001). *Nursing diagnoses, outcomes, interventions: NANDA, NOC and NIC linkages*. St. Louis, MO: Mosby.
11. Johnson, M., Maas, M., & Moorhead, M. (Eds.). (2000). *Nursing Outcomes Classification (NOC)* (2nd ed.). St. Louis, MO: Mosby.
12. National Committee on Vital and Health Statistics. (1980). *Uniform hospital discharge data: Minimum data set* (Publication No. PHS 80-1157). Hyattsville, MD: U. S. Department of Health, Education, and Welfare, National Center for Health Statistics.
13. Pinkley, C. L. (1991). Exploring NANDA's definition of nursing diagnosis: linking diagnostic judgments with the selection of outcomes and interventions. *Nursing Diagnosis, 2*, 26-32.
14. Titler, M. G. (1994). Infusing research into practice to promote quality care. *Nursing Research, 4*, 306-313.
15. Werley, H. H., & Lang, N. M. (Eds.). (1988). *Identification of the nursing minimum data set*. New York: Springer.

Examples of Use in Practice and Education

In this section we have included some examples of forms, computer screens, class assignments, and so on that demonstrate the use of NIC in practice and education. We are not advocating any of the forms; rather, they are included here as examples of how NIC is being used. We thank the contributors who have submitted materials. Requests for more information about these materials should be addressed to the identified person or institution. Please note that copyright for each of the items is held by the person/organization that submitted it, and an item cannot be reprinted or used without permission from the copyright holder.

ElderCARE ♥
1324 North Sheridan Road, Waukegan, IL 60085   ~   (847) 360-4004

CARE RECEIVER:		AGE:	DOB:		TODAY'S DATE:

PAST MEDICAL HISTORY   ○ NONE   CANCER (LOCATION) _____

○ CVA	○ HYPO / HYPERTENSION	○ SLEEP APNEA	○ BOWEL DISORDERS	HOSPITALIZATIONS/SURGERIES _____
○ HEAD INJURY	○ MI / ANGINA	○ DIABETES	○ HEPATITIS/JAUNDICE	_____
○ MS	○ PACEMAKER	○ IMMUNE DISORDER	○ ULCERS	_____
○ OBS / DEMENTIA	○ ANEMIA	○ THYROID PROBLEM	○ ARTHRITIS	_____
○ SEIZURES	○ SICKLE CELL	○ KIDNEY DISEASE	○ BACK INJURY	ANESTHESIA COMPLICATIONS _____
○ ARRHYTHMIA	○ ASTHMA / COPD	○ STD	○ JOINT REPLACEMENT	_____
○ CABG/ANGIOPLASTY	○ CHF	○ SKIN DISORDER	○ OTHER:	

NURSING OUTCOME COMPREHENSION SCALE: 1 = NONE   2 = LIMITED   3 = MODERATE   4 = SUBSTANTIAL   5 = EXTENSIVE

1. BASIC PHYSIOLOGY	NURSING DIAGNOSIS	NURSING INTERVENTIONS	NURSING OUTCOME	SCALE
A. ACTIVITY AND EXERCISE ○ DENIES PROBLEM ○ STIFFNESS	○ ACTIVITY INTOLERANCE	○ ACTIVITY THERAPY: (FOCUS ON WHAT PATIENT CAN DO RATHER THAN DEFICITS. IDENTIFY PREFERENCES FOR ACTIVITY. ENCOURAGE ALTERNATIVE ACTIVITY AND REST.)	○ ENDURANCE	
○ WEAKNESS ○ HISTORY OF FALLS	○ FATIGUE ○ RISK FOR INJURY	○ ENERGY MANAGEMENT ○ FALL PREVENTION	○ ENERGY CONSERVATION ○ SAFETY: FALL PREVENTION	
C. IMMOBILITY MANAGEMENT **ASSISTIVE DEVICES:** ○ DENIES PROBLEM ○ CANE ○ WALKER ○ BRACE ○ CRUTCHES ○ WHEELCHAIR	○ IMPAIRED PHYSICAL MOBILITY	○ EXERCISE PROMOTION ○ BODY MECHANICS PROMOTION	○ MOBILITY ○ KNOWLEDGE OF IMMOBILITY CONSEQUENCES	
E. PHYSICAL COMFORT ○ DENIES PROBLEM ○ PAIN _____ LOCATION _____ INTENSITY	○ PAIN ○ SLEEP DISTURBANCE	○ PAIN MANAGEMENT ○ SLEEP MANAGEMENT	○ COMFORT ○ ENVIRONMENTAL MANAGEMENT ○ REST	
F. SELF CARE ABILITY (0 = INDEPENDENT 1 = ASSISTIVE DEVICE 2 ASSISTANCE FROM OTHERS 3 ASSISTANCE FROM PERSONS & DEVICES 4 = DEPENDENT)				
○ DENIES PROBLEM ___ AMBULATION ___ EATING/DRINKING ___ BATHING ___ DRESSING/GROOMING ___ TOILETING ___ SHOPPING ___ FOOD PREPARATION ___ HOME MAINTENANCE/ HOUSEKEEPING ___ STAIR CLIMBING ___ BED MOBILITY ___ TRANSFERRING ___ TELEPHONE ABILITY ___ LAUNDRY ___ TRANSPORTATION ___ FINANCES	○ SELF-CARE DEFICIT	○ SELF-CARE ASSISTANCE (MONITOR CLIENT'S NEED FOR ADAPTIVE DEVICES) (ASSIST CLIENT IN ACCEPTING DEPENDENCY NEEDS) (TEACH CAREGIVERS TO ENCOURAGE INDEPENDENCE) (ESTABLISH ROUTINE FOR SELF-CARE ACTIVITIES)	○ MOBILITY ○ ANXIETY CONTROL ○ COMFORT LEVEL ○ COGNITIVE ABILITY ○ ENDURANCE ○ ENERGY CONSERVATION ○ TRANSFER PERFORMANCE ○ MOOD EQUILIBRIUM ○ ROLE PERFORMANCE	

HEALTH ASSESSMENT   © VICTORY MEMORIAL HOSPITAL 1998

Fig. 3A-1 Health Assessment/Wellness Plan—Vista ElderCARE, Victory Memorial Hospital, Waukegan, IL.
Three pages of a six-page plan developed as part of a hospital-based community outreach program to low-income, underserved, homebound elders age 65 and older. Volunteer registered nurses, through interview and noninvasive techniques, complete the in-home assessment to identify actual or potential health problems and to provide health education and referral. (*Submitted by Carole E. Johnson, RN, BSN, [847-615-8424 or email: carolejohnson3@msn.com] Former Geriatric Care Manager at Vista Health. Used with permission.*)

ElderCARE ♥
1324 North Sheridan Road, Waukegan, IL 60085   ~   (847) 360-4004

3. BEHAVIORAL	NURSING DIAGNOSIS	NURSING INTERVENTIONS	NURSING OUTCOME	SCALE

P. COGNITIVE:
MENTAL STATUS
○ ALERT
○ ORIENTED
○ CONFUSED:
  ○ ACUTE ○ CHRONIC
○ COMBATIVE
○ UNRESPONSIVE
○ IMPAIRED MEMORY
○ IMPAIRED
  COMPREHENSION
	○ ALTERED THOUGHT
	PROCESSES
	
	○ MEMORY IMPAIRED
		○ DELUSION MANAGEMENT:
		SAFE & THERAPEUTIC
		ENVIRONMENT
		○ DEMENTIA MANAGEMENT
		MODIFIED ENVIRONMENT
		○ COGNITIVE STIMULATION
		(USE MEMORY AIDS, A
		CALENDAR, TALK ABOUT
		NON-THREATENING NEWS
		EVENTS, USE RADIO,
		MUSIC, TV AS STIMULATION)
		○ REMINISCENSE THERAPY
		(RECALL PAST EVENTS TO
		FACILITATE ADAPTATION
		TO PRESENT)
			○ SAFETY - PHYSICAL
			ENVIRONMENT
			○ COGNITIVE
			ORIENTATION	

Q. COMMUNICATION:
HEARING: _____ RIGHT
○ WNL   _____ LEFT
○ IMPAIRED
○ HEARING AID
○ DEAF
VISION: _____ RIGHT
○ WNL   _____ LEFT
○ IMPAIRED
○ EYE GLASSES
○ CONTACT LENS
SPEECH:
○ WNL
○ SLURRED
○ EXPRESSIVE APHASIA
INTERPRETER: _____
LANGUAGE
SPOKEN: _____
	○ SENSORY/PERCEPTUAL
	ALTERATION:
	  ○ HEARING
	  ○ VISION
	
	○ IMPAIRED VERBAL
	COMMUNICATION
		○ COMMUNICATION
		ENHANCEMENT
		(HEARING DEFICIT)
		(SPEECH DEFICIT)
		
		○ ENVIRONMENTAL
		MANAGEMENT
		
		○ ACTIVE LISTENING
			○ COMMUNICATION
			ABILITY
			
			○ SAFETY - PHYSICAL
			ENVIRONMENT	

R. COPING: ○ EFFECTIVE
MAJOR CONCERNS _____ _____ MAJOR LOSS/CHANGE _____
 	
○ MUSIC/TV
○ DISTRACTION
○ READING
○ PRAYER
○ PHYSICAL ACTIVITY
○ ALCOHOL/DRUGS
○ MEDICATION
○ TALK ON TELEPHONE
○ CRYING
○ FRIENDS
○ _____
Y N **SPIRITUAL ASSESSMENT:**
○○ BELIEVE IN HIGHER
  POWER
○○ LIFE HAS MEANING &
  PURPOSE
○○ HAVE SENSE OF HOPE
○○ FEEL SENSE OF
  CONNECTEDNESS/
  HARMONY
RITUALS: _____
PRACTICE _____
	○ ALTERED HEALTH
	MAINTENANCE
	○ DENIAL
	○ ANXIETY
	○ DECISIONAL CONFLICT
	○ SEXUAL DYSFUNCTION
	○ GRIEVING
	○ IMPAIRED ADJUSTMENT
	○ HOPELESSNESS,
	POWERLESSNESS*
	○ *BECK DEPRESSION
	INVENTORY COMPLETED
	
	○ SPIRITUAL DISTRESS
	○ QUESTION MEANING OF
	EXISTENCE
	○ QUESTION MEANING OF
	SUFFERING
	○ ANGER TOWARD GOD
		○ HEALTH EDUCATION
		
		○ ANXIETY REDUCTION
		○ DECISION MAKING
		SUPPORT
		○ SEXUAL COUNSELING
		
		○ GRIEF WORK FACILITATION
		○ COPING ENHANCEMENT
		○ HOPE INSTILLATION
		○ SELF ESTEEM
		ENHANCEMENT
		○ SPIRITUAL SUPPORT
		(ENCOURAGE USE OF
		SPIRITUAL REFERRAL
		RESOURCES)
		○ LISTENING
		○ PRESENCE (DEMONSTRATE
		ACCEPTING ATTITUDE,
		COMMUNICATE EMPATHY,
		BE SENSITVE TO
		PATIENT'S TRADITIONS &
		BELIEFS)
		○ BIBLIOTHERAPY
		(SCRIPTURE READINGS)
			○ HEALTH PROMOTING
			BEHAVIOR
			
			○ ANXIETY CONTROL
			○ DECISION MAKING
			
			○ KNOWLEDGE:
			SEXUALITY
			○ GRIEF RESOLUTION
			○ COPING
			○ ACCEPTANCE
			○ SELF ESTEEM
			
			○ SPIRITUAL WELL BEING
			○ HOPE	

HEALTH ASSESSMENT
ⓒ VICTORY MEMORIAL HOSPITAL 1998

Fig. 3A-1, cont'd

Continued

ElderCARE ♥
1324 North Sheridan Road, Waukegan, IL 60085   ~   (847) 360-4004

5. FAMILY:	NURSING DIAGNOSIS	NURSING INTERVENTIONS	NURSING OUTCOME	SCALE
X. LIFESPAN CARE: ◯ DENIES PROBLEM ◯ EXPRESSED NEED FOR CAREGIVER SUPPORT LEVEL OF FAMILY INVOLVEMENT: ◯ ADEQUATE ◯ LIMITED ◯ NONE	◯ CAREGIVER ROLE STRAIN ◯ ALTERED FAMILY PROCESSES ALTERED ROLE PERFORMANCE ◯ CAREGIVER ◯ SPOUSE ◯ FAMILY	◯ CAREGIVER SUPPORT: (EXPLORE STRENGTHS & WEAKNESSES) (ENCOURAGE CAREGIVER SUPPORT GROUP & SPIRITUAL RESOURCES) (IDENTIFY SOURCES OF RESPITE CARE) ◯ FAMILY INVOLVEMENT: (FACILITATE FAMILY UNDERSTANDING OF MEDICAL ASPECTS OF ILLNESS) (IDENTIFY & RESPECT FAMILY'S COPING MECHANISMS) (DISCUSS OPTIONS FOR CARE i.e. GROUP LIVING, RESIDENTIAL CARE, RESPITE CARE) ◯ FAMILY INTEGRITY PROMOTION ◯ ROLE ENHANCEMENT	◯ CAREGIVER EMOTIONAL HEALTH & WELL-BEING ◯ INFORMATION PROCESSING (HEALTH SYSTEM GUIDANCE) ◯ ROLE ENHANCEMENT	
6. HEALTH SYSTEM	NURSING DIAGNOSIS	NURSING INTERVENTIONS	NURSING OUTCOME	SCALE
Y.a. HEALTH SYSTEM MEDIATION ◯ N/A ◯ INFORMATION REQUESTED ADVANCE DIRECTIVES IN PLACE: ◯ Y ◯ N LIVING WILL ◯ Y ◯ N POA HEALTHCARE ◯ Y ◯ N FINANCIAL POA HEALTH SYSTEMS KNOWLEDGE ◯ ADEQUATE ◯ REQUESTS INFORMATION	◯ DECISIONAL CONFLICT ◯ KNOWLEDGE DEFICIT	◯ DECISION MAKING SUPPORT: (INFORM PATIENT & FAMILY OF ALTERNATIVES) ◯ HEALTH SYSTEM GUIDANCE (HEALTHCARE PROVIDERS HEALTHCARE FACILITIES EMERGENCY SERVICES SECOND OPINION COORDINATE REFERRALS ENCOURAGE FAMILY TO ASK QUESTIONS ABOUT SERVICES & CHARGES)	◯ DECISION MAKING ◯ KNOWLEDGE: HEALTH RESOURCES	

ASSESSMENT SUMMARY

1. BASIC PHYSIOLOGY 2. COMPLEX PHYSIOLOGY 3. BEHAVIORAL 4. SAFETY 5. FAMILY 6. HEALTH SYSTEM

A _____	H _____	O _____	U _____	X _____	Y.a. _____
C _____	K _____	P _____	V _____		
E _____	L _____	Q _____			
F _____	M _____	R _____			
D _____	N _____	T _____			
B _____		S _____			

REFERRAL: ◯ CLERGY
◯ PHYSICIAN
◯ ELDERCARE
  ◯ CASE MANAGER
    ◯ MEALS ON WHEELS
    ◯ CATHOLIC CHARITIES
    ◯ SUPPORT GROUP
◯ VOLUNTEER REQUEST

REVISIT:
◯ _____ WK

TELEPHONE:
◯ _____ WK

R.N. SIGNATURE:

HEALTH ASSESSMENT

© VICTORY MEMORIAL HOSPITAL 1998

Fig. 3A-1, cont'd

CLAXTON-HEPBURN MEDICAL CENTER
JOB DESCRIPTION/PERFORMANCE APPRAISAL

Position: RN – Medical/Surgical

Employee: _____

Review Date: _____

Type of Review: ☐ Self ☐ 90 Day ☐ Annual

Position Summary: Provides general and specialized nursing care to patients of all ages in a medical-surgical setting that includes pediatric, elderly and oncologic patients.

Qualifications: Valid and current registration on N.Y.S. RN license. Successful completion of a Pediatric Advance Life Support class within two years of hire. Knowledge of growth & development across the life span and the ability to use that knowledge to individualize the plan and delivery of care.

Strengths:
_____
_____

Areas for Improvement:
_____
_____

Plans for Development:
_____
_____

Employee Comments:
_____
_____

Evaluator _____ Date _____   Employee _____ Date _____

Fig. 3A-2 Job Description/Performance Appraisal—Claxton-Hepburn Medical Center, Ogdensburg, NY.
Two pages of an eight-page document that uses NIC interventions as the basis of performance appraisal. The interventions are viewed as competencies and those that are included for this position related to the care of medical-surgical patients are based on the specialty core interventions identified in NIC for medical-surgical nursing. NIC is also used in the agency as the documentation structure so there is consistency in the job description, patient care documentation, and assessment of performance. (*Submitted by Sharon LaDuke, BS, RN, Patient Documentation Analyst. Used with permission.*)

Continued

III. MEDICAL/SURGICAL DEPARTMENT RESPONSIBILITIES	COMPETENCIES	Does Not Yet Meet	Meets
A. Provides individualized, age-specific care that supports physical functioning	1. Enteral Tube Feeding - Delivers nutrients and water through a gastrointestinal tube	☐	☐
	2. Gastrointestinal Intubation - Inserts a tube in the gastrointestinal tract	☐	☐
	3. Nutrition Management - Assists with or provides a balanced dietary intake of foods and fluids	☐	☐
	4. Tube Care: Gastrointestinal - Manages a patient with a gastrointestinal tube	☐	☐
B. Provides age-specific, individualized care that supports homeostatic regulation	1. Acid-Base Management - Promotes acid-base balance and prevents complications resulting from imbalance	☐	☐
	2. Airway Management - Facilitates patency of air passages	☐	☐
	3. Blood Products Administration - Administers blood or blood products and monitors patient response	☐	☐
	4. Dysrhythmia Management - Prevents, recognizes and facilitates treatment of abnormal cardiac rhythms	☐	☐
	5. Electrolyte Management - Promotes electrolyte balance and prevents complications resulting from abnormal or undesired serum electrolyte levels	☐	☐
	6. Fluid Management - Promotes fluid balance and prevents complications resulting from abnormal or undesired fluid levels	☐	☐
	7. Incision Site Care - Cleans, monitors and promotes healing in the wound that is closed with sutures, clips or staples	☐	☐
	8. Intravenous Insertion - Inserts a needle into a peripheral vein for the purpose of administering fluids, blood or medications	☐	☐
	9. Intravenous Therapy - Administers and monitors intravenous fluids and medications	☐	☐
	10. Medication Administration - Prepares, gives and evaluates the effectiveness of prescription and nonprescription drugs	☐	☐

Fig. 3A-2, cont'd

INITIATE APPROPRIATE PROBLEMS

Surgical Plan of Care

Date	Initials	Nursing Diagnosis	Patient Outcomes — For specific indicators see NOC book.*	***NOTIFY PHYSICIAN IF ANY CHANGES IN PATIENT CONDITION — Activities listed under NIC interventions are clinical guidelines only and do not replace nursing clinical judgment. For other activities see NIC book.	Start date	Stop Date
		Pain	1=Severe ② 2=Substantial ③ 3=Moderate ④ 4=Slight 5= None ⑤ Pain Level 2102 **Score Outcome Definition:** Amount of reported or demonstrated pain ON INITIATION 1 2 3 4 5 PATIENT GOAL 1 2 3 4 5 AT RESOLUTION/DISCHARGE 1 2 3 4 5 If Discharge Outcome at 3 or less, select all that apply. ☐ Chronic condition ☐ DC with services ☐ Compliance issues ☐ Transfer to other hosp ☐ Transfer to ECF ☐ AMA ☐ Expired ☐ Learning Barrier ☐ Physical Limitations ☐ Pt/Family Discussions ☐ If none apply, make a note	**Pain Management: Pain Assessment** 1 Instruct pt to rate pain using 1 to 10 scale and determine realistic pain goals. 2 Assess pain level and document pain location, type, and intensity q 2-4h and PRN or per protocol 3 Intervene at onset of pain providing appropriate analgesic care 4 Assess VS prior to and after administration of medication 5 Monitor effectiveness of medication 20–30 min after administration or per protocol 6 Select and implement a variety of measures to facilitate pain relief, as appropriate **Analgesic Administration–Intraspinal** 1 Check patency/function of catheter, port, or pump. 2 Monitor and record VS per protocol. 3 Monitor for adverse reactions: resp depression, urinary retention, undue somnolence, itching, seizures, nausea, and vomiting 4 Remove catheter according to agency protocol **Medication Management: SAM Kit** 1 Determine patient's ability to self-medicate 2 Teach pt and/or family expected action, side effecs, administration method, interactions, as appropriate 3 Monitor for effectiveness, side effects, toxicity **Patient-Controlled Analgesia (PCA) Assistance** 1 Teach pt and family how to use the PCA device 2 Teach patent/family the action and side effects of pain-relieving agents 3 Monitor and document effectiveness, side effects of medication *Document care where you currently document i.e. flowsheet		
		Impaired Skin Integrity	1=None ② 2=Slight ③ 3=Moderate ④ 4=Substantial 5=Complete ⑤ Wound Healing: Primary Intention 1102 **Score Outcome Definition:** The extent to which cells and tissues have regenerated following intentional closure ON INITIATION 1 2 3 4 5 PATIENT GOAL 1 2 3 4 5 AT RESOLUTION/DISCHARGE 1 2 3 4 5 If Discharge Outcome at 3 or less, select all that apply. ☐ Chronic condition ☐ DC with services ☐ Compliance issues ☐ Transfer to other hosp ☐ Transfer to ECF ☐ AMA ☐ Expired ☐ Learning Barrier ☐ Physical Limitations ☐ Pt/Family Discussions ☐ If none apply, make a note	**Incision Site Care** 1. Inspect incision for redness, swelling, or signs of dehiscence or evisceration 2. Note characteristics of any drainage 3. Monitor healing 4. Change or remove dressing as appropriate 5. Instruct patient/family in care of incis on **Tube Care** 1. Maintain patency of tube, monitoring drainage 2. Instruct patient/family in tube purpose and care 3. Administer skin/tube care as appropriate		
		Initials	Signature	Addressograph		

*Moorhead, S., Johnson, M., & Maas, M. (2004). Nursing outcomes classification (NOC) (3rd ed.). St. Louis: Mosby

Fig. 3A-3 Surgical Plan of Care—Good Samaritan Hospital in Puyallup, WA.
Plan of care for surgical patients using seven NANDA diagnoses with related NOC outcomes and NIC interventions with activities. *(Developed by Good Samaritan Hospital, Puyallup, WA, with special thanks to Rosalind Willis, RN, Joyce Mitchell, RN, Julie Clobes, RN, Kari Newman, RN, Karen Graybeal, RN, and PCS Core Team. Used with permission.)*

Continued

INITIATE APPROPRIATE PROBLEMS

Date	Initials	Nursing Diagnosis	SURGICAL PLAN OF CARE		**NOTIFY PHYSICIAN IF ANY CHANGES IN PATIENT CONDITION Activities listed under NIC interventions are clinical guidelines only and do not replace nursing clinical judgment. See NIC book for other activities.	Start date	Stop Date
			Patient Outcomes For specific indicators see NOC book*				
		ineffective airway clearance	1=Extremely Compromised ☺ 2=Substantially compromised 3=Moderately compromised ☺ 4=Mildly compromised ☺ 5= Not compromised ☺				
			Respiratory Status: Ventilation 0403 **Score Outcome** **Definition**	Definition: Movement of air in and out of lungs	**Respiratory Monitoring: Respiratory Assessment** 1. Assess resp. status q 4 h and PRN 2. Turn, cough and deep breath q2h and PRN 3. Obtain baseline O2 sat ____% 4. Administer O2 if sat 92% on RA or per MD order		
			ON INITIATION	1 2 3 4 5			
					Ventilation Assistance: IS 1. Instruct and assist with IS as appropriate 2. Encourage TCDB q2h and PRN 3. Administer appropriate pain meds to prevent hypoventilation 4. Teach breathing techniques as appropriate 5. Administer O2 as appropriate		
			PATIENT GOAL	1 2 3 4 5	If Discharge Outcome at 3 or less, select all that apply. ☐ Chronic condition ☐ DC with services ☐ Compliance issues ☐ Transfer to other hosp ☐ Transfer to ECF ☐ AMA ☐ Expired ☐ Learning Barrier ☐ Physical Limitations ☐ Pt/Family Discussions ☐ If none apply, make a note		
			AT RESOLUTION/ DISCHARGE	1 2 3 4 5			
		Impaired Physical Mobility	1=Severe ☺ 2=Substantial 3=Moderate ☺ 4=Slight 5=None ☺				
			Immobility Consequences: Physiological **Score Outcome** **Definition**	Definition: Compromise in physiological functioning due to impaired physical mobility	**Exercise Therapy: Ambulation** 1. Encourage to dangle or up in chair as tolerated 2. Instruct and assist in transfer techniques as needed 3. Encourage independent ambulation within safe limits 4. Encourage to be up ad lib if appropriate 5. Assess activity pattern daily _ Obtain Physical therapy consult if requires max assist of 2 6. Consider OT consult **Positioning:** 1. Position of comfort with proper body alignment if immobile 2. Position to promote ventilation/perfusion 3. Turn per schedule while in bed		
			ON INITIATION	1 2 3 4 5	If Discharge Outcome at 3 or less, select all that apply. ☐ Chronic condition ☐ DC with services ☐ Compliance issues ☐ Transfer to other hosp ☐ Transfer to ECF ☐ AMA ☐ Expired ☐ Learning Barrier ☐ Physical Limitations ☐ Pt/Family Discussions ☐ If none apply, make a note		
			PATIENT GOAL	1 2 3 4 5			
			AT RESOLUTION/ DISCHARGE	1 2 3 4 5			
		Risk of con-stipation	1=Extremely compromised ☺ 2=Substantially compromised 3=Moderately compromised ☺ 4=Mildly compromised 5=Not compromised ☺				
			Bowel Elimination 0501 **Score Outcome** **Definition**	Definition Ability of the GI tract to form and evacuate effectively	**Bowel Management:** 1. Note date of last bowel movement 2. Monitor bowel movements including frequency, consistency, color 3. Assess and record bowel sounds 4. Monitor for S/S of diarrhea, constipation, and impaction 5. Teach patient a high fiber diet as appropriate 6. Evaluate medications for GI side effects 7. Administer bowel meds as appropriate and as ordered		
			ON INITIATION	1 2 3 4 5	If Discharge Outcome at 3 or less, select all that apply. ☐ Chronic condition ☐ DC with services ☐ Compliance issues ☐ Transfer to other hosp ☐ Transfer to ECF ☐ AMA ☐ Expired ☐ Learning Barrier ☐ Physical Limitations ☐ Pt/Family Discussions ☐ If none apply, make a note		
			PATIENT GOAL	1 2 3 4 5			
			AT RESOLUTION/ DISCHARGE	1 2 3 4 5			

*Moorhead, S., Johnson, M., & Maas, M. (2004). Nursing outcomes classification (NOC) (3rd ed.). St. Louis: Mosby

Fig. 3A-3, cont'd

INITIATE APPROPRIATE PROBLEMS

SURGICAL PLAN OF CARE

Date	Initials	Nursing Diagnosis	Patient Outcomes (For specific indicators see NOC book*)		**NOTIFY PHYSICIAN IF ANY CHANGES IN PATIENT CONDITION** Activities listed under NIC interventions are clinical guidelines only and do not replace nursing clinical judgment.	Start date	Stop Date
		Anxiety	1=Never demonstrated ☺ 2=Rarely Demonstrated 3=Sometimes demonstrated ☺ 4=Often demonstrated 5=Consistently demonstrated ☺				
			Anxiety control 1402 **Score Outcome Definition**: Ability to eliminate or reduce feelings of apprehension and tension from an unidentifiable source	If Discharge Outcome at 3 or less, select all that apply. ☐ Chronic condition ☐ DC with services ☐ Compliance issues ☐ Transfer to other hosp ☐ Transfer to ECF ☐ AMA ☐ Expired ☐ Learning Barrier ☐ Physical Limitations ☐ Pt/Family Discussions ☐ If none apply, make a note	Anxiety Reduction: Encourage verbalization of feelings 1. Use a calm, reassuring approach 2. Explain all procedures 3. Listen attentively 4. Support the use of appropriate defense mechanisms 5. Instruct patient on the use of relaxation techniques 6. Administer medications as appropriate		
			ON INITIATION 1 2 3 4 5				
			PATIENT GOAL 1 2 3 4 5				
			AT RESOLUTION/ DISCHARGE 1 2 3 4 5				
		Knowledge deficit	1=None ☺ 2=Limited 3=Moderate ☺ 4=Moderate ☺ 5=Extensive ☺				
			Knowledge: Illness Care 1824 **Score Outcome Definition**: Extent of understanding of illness-related information needed to achieve and maintain optimal health	If Discharge Outcome at 3 or less, select all that apply. ☐ Chronic condition ☐ DC with services ☐ Compliance issues ☐ Transfer to other hosp ☐ Transfer to ECF ☐ AMA ☐ Expired ☐ Learning Barrier ☐ Physical Limitations ☐ Pt/Family Discussions ☐ If none apply, make a note	Teaching: Disease Process 1. Evaluate patient understanding of disease process 2. Describe disease process 3. Provide information Video Handout Community Resources Verbal 4. Provide information re: patient; progress 5. Refer to community agencies/support groups as indicated 6. Instruct on measures to prevent complications 7. Consider pharmacy consult for ≥ 5 discharge meds		
			ON INITIATION 1 2 3 4 5				
			PATIENT GOAL 1 2 3 4 5				
			AT RESOLUTION/ DISCHARGE 1 2 3 4 5				

*Moorhead, S., Johnson, M., & Maas, M. (2004). Nursing outcomes classification (NOC) (3rd ed.). St. Louis Mosby

Fig. 3A-3, cont'd

Sample
Parish Nursing Services
Brief Client Interaction Form—Spiritual

Client Name:_____

DOB:_____   Age/Age Range _____   Date: _____

Gender M F   Marital Status _____   Time:_____

Address :_____

_____

Phone:_____

Ethnic Heritage[1](circle):   C   A   H   OA   NA   ME   FE   MC   U   O

Congregational Status (circle):   Parishioner   Non-Parishioner

Referral Source[2] (circle):   S   P   NP   PS   MD   HCP   M   O   PN   FAM

Location[3]: C   PNO   V   H   HV   NH   P   PA   M   Other

Progress Note:

_____

_____

_____

_____

_____

_____

_____

_____

_____

_____

_____

                          Parish Nurse X_____

                          Congregation_____

❑ Has screening documentation

---

[1] C=Caucasian; A=African American/Black; H=Hispanic; OA=Oriental/Asian; NA=Native American; ME=Middle Eastern; FE=Far Eastern; MC=Multi-Cultural; U=Unknown; O=Other
[2] S=Self; P=Parishioner; NP=Non-Parishioner; PS=Pastoral Staff; MD=Physician; HCP=Other Health Care Professional; M=Media; O=Other; PN=Parish Nurse; FAM=Family
[3] C=Church; PNO=Parish nurse office; V=Visit to HCP; H=Hospital; NH=Nursing Home; P=Phone; PA=Pantry; M=Mail; Other=Other

©This form cannot be modified or used without written permission, 1/02

Fig. 3A-4 Brief Client Interaction Form—
    The two-sided template is designed for one-time or short-term interactions. The parish nurse checks off labels that are appropriate for the interaction. If the intervention label is checked, the information need not be documented in the narrative note unless additional detail is required. This minimizes the time spent in record-ing information. *(Submitted by Lisa Burkhart, MPH, PhD, RN, Assistant Professor, Marcella Niehoff School of Nursing, Loyola University, Chicago. Used with permission.)*

Sample

Parish Nursing Services

Brief Client Interaction Form—Spiritual

Client Name: _____

NURSING DIAGNOSIS[1]

Life Principles

- ☐ Spiritual Distress
- ☐ Readiness for Enhanced Spiritual Well-Being
- ☐ Decisional Conflict

Health Promotion

- ☐ Ineffective Health Maintenance

Activity/Rest

- ☐ Disturbed Sleep Pattern

Cognitive/Perceptual

- ☐ Disturbed Thought Process

Self-Perception

- ☐ Powerlessness
- ☐ Hopelessness
- ☐ Situational Low Self-Esteem
- ☐ Chronic Low Self-Esteem

Role/Relationship

- ☐ Interrupted Family Processes
- ☐ Impaired Social Interaction

Comfort

- ☐ Chronic Pain
- ☐ Acute Pain
- ☐ Social Isolation

Coping/Stress Tolerance

- ☐ Anxiety
- ☐ Fear
- ☐ Ineffective Coping
- ☐ Compromised Family Coping
- ☐ Disabled Family Coping
- ☐ Readiness for Enhanced Family Coping

Safety/Protection

- ☐ Risk for Self-mutilation
- ☐ Risk for Injury

NURSING INTERVENTIONS[2]

Physiological Basic

- ☐ Pain Management
- ☐ Progressive Muscle Relaxation
- ☐ Sleep Enhancement
- ☐ Transport

Behavioral/Cognitive Therapy

- ☐ Bibliotherapy
- ☐ Music Therapy
- ☐ Mutual Goal Setting
- ☐ Patient Contracting

Communication Enhancement

- ☐ Active Listening
- ☐ Complex Relationship Building
- ☐ Conflict Mediation
- ☐ Meditation
- ☐ Socialization Enhancement

Coping/Spiritual/Religious

- ☐ Anticipatory Guidance
- ☐ Body Image Enhancement
- ☐ Coping Enhancement
- ☐ Counseling
- ☐ Crisis Intervention
- ☐ Decision-Making Support
- ☐ Dying Care
- ☐ Emotional Support
- ☐ Forgiveness Facilitation
- ☐ Grief Work Facilitation
- ☐ Hope Instillation
- ☐ Humor
- ☐ Mood Management
- ☐ Presence
- ☐ Recreational Therapy
- ☐ Religious Ritual Enhancement

Coping/Spiritual/Religious (cont.)

- ☐ Role Enhancement
- ☐ Security Enhancement
- ☐ Self-awareness Enhancement
- ☐ Spiritual Growth Facilitation
- ☐ Spiritual Support
- ☐ Support System Enhancement
- ☐ Touch
- ☐ Values Clarification

Psychological Comfort Promotion

- ☐ Anxiety Reduction
- ☐ Calming Technique
- ☐ Simple Guided Imagery
- ☐ Simple Relaxation Therapy

[1] Diagnosis Labels reprinted with permission from NANDA.

[2] NIC labels reprinted with permission from Mosby.

©This form cannot be modified or used without written permission, 1/02

Fig. 3A-4, cont'd

Parish Nursing Services
Client Interaction Form

Client Name:_____

DOB:_____   Age/ Age Range _____   Date: _____

Gender M F   Marital Status _____   Time:_____

Address :_____   _____

_____

Phone:_____

Ethnic Heritage[1] (circle):   C   A   H   OA   NA   ME   FE   MC   U   O

Congregational Status (circle):   Parishioner   Non-Parishioner

Referral Source[2] (circle):   S   P   NP   PS   MD   HCP   M   O   PN   FAM

Contact Person: _____   Phone: _____

Advanced Directives: Y N   Living Will Y N   Durable Power of Attorney for Health Care Y N

Primary Health Care Professional: _____   _____

Address: _____   Phone: _____

Pertinent Medical History (circle):   DM   HTN   Cardiovascular   Pulmonary

        Cancer   Glaucoma   Urinary   Other: _____

Pertinent Medication History: _____

_____

Comments/ Additional Information:

_____

_____

_____

_____

_____

_____

❏   Has BP screening form   Parish Nurse X_____

                            Congregation_____

_____

[1] C=Caucasian; A=African American/Black; H=Hispanic; OA=Oriental/Asian; NA=Native American; ME=Middle
Eastern; FE=Far Eastern; MC=Multi-Cultural; U=Unknown; O=Other
[2] S=Self; P=Parishioner; NP=Non-Parishioner; PS=Pastoral Staff; MD=Physician; HCP=Other Health Care Professional;
M=Media; O=Other; PN=Parish Nurse; FAM=Family

©This form cannot be modified or used without written permission, 1/02

Fig. 3A-5 Long-term Interaction Template—
    This template is used with clients that are seen regularly over an extended period. The NANDA, NIC, and NOC labels are listed on separate flow sheets, which are dated and initialed. Each health record includes one demographic form, a series of progress notes, a nursing diagnosis flow sheet, and a NIC flow sheet. This is an example of the first page of a NIC flow sheet. (*Submitted by Lisa Burkhart, MPH, PhD, RN, Assistant Professor, Marcella Niehoff School of Nursing, Loyola University, Chicago. Used with permission.*)

Sample
Parish Nursing Services
Nursing Intervention List: Chronic Care/Caregiver/   CLIENT NAME: _____

Grief/Loss/Aging

Interventions:	Inits Date	Inits Date	Inits Date	Inits Date	Inits Date	Inits Date	Inits Date	Inits Date	Inits Date	Inits Date	Inits Date	Inits Date	Inits Date	Inits Date	Inits Date	Inits Date	Inits Date
Physiological Basic																	
1. Bed Rest Care																	
2. Bowel Management																	
3. Eating Disorders Management																	
4. Exercise Promotion																	
5. Exercise Promotion: Stretching																	
6. Exercise Therapy: Joint Mob.																	
7. Nutritional Counseling																	
8. Nutritional Monitoring																	
9. Pain Management																	
10. Progressive Muscle Relaxation																	
11. Self-Care Assistance: Toileting																	
12. Sleep Enhancement																	
13. Therapeutic Touch																	
14. Transport																	
15. Urinary Elimination Management																	
16. Urinary Incontinence Care																	
17. Urinary Inc. Care: Enuresis																	
18. Weight Management																	
19. Weight Reduction Assistance																	
Physiological: Complex																	
20. Cardiac Care																	
21. Circulatory Precautions																	
22. Fluid Management																	
23. Skin Surveillance																	
24. Unilateral Neglect Management																	

Parish Nurse Signature/Initials: _____

©This form cannot be modified or used without written permission. 1/02

Fig. 3A-5, cont'd

University of New Mexico Health Sciences Center
2211 Lomas Blvd NE
Albuquerque, NM, 87106

Medication Refill Note (Pediatric Cardiology)

Last, First, MR# **4XXXXXX**

Date of Birth: 05/05/xxxx

Dictation Date and Time: Jan. 4th, 200x at xx00

Date Refilled: Jan. 4th, 200x

Pharmacy Name and Phone Number: XXXXX Pharmacy, xxx-xxxx

Medication(s):

XXXXXXXX 2 mg/mL, 1.5 ml = 3 mg PO twice daily -- refills X 2

Comments:

I reviewed the current note by Dr. ZZZZs on XXXXXX's dosage and his next planned adjustment for weight change. I then called the pharmacy to authorize two refills, which should cover the patient until he visits our clinic again.

Total time spent: 10 minutes

NIC # 2380 – Medication Management

_____

Signature

Fig. 3A-6 Dictation forms—University of New Mexico Health Sciences Center, Albuquerque, NM.
   Two forms for use with a dictation charting system for nurses, viewable by any user through Cerner Powerchart. The first is a medication refill note and the second is a nurse visit note. The forms track the time the nurse spends with the patient/family and are potentially billable (NIC codes would need to be matched to *CPT* for billing under current system). *(Submitted by Scott Chisholm Lamont, BSN, RN, CCRN, CFRN, ENC(C), Specialty Nurse III, Pediatric Pain Team and Children's Heart Center. Used with permission.)*

University of New Mexico Health Sciences Center
2211 Lomas Blvd NE
Albuquerque, NM, 87106
Xxxxxxx, Xxxx, MR# xxxxxxx

Date of Birth: 08/15/xxxx

Assessment Data:

Reason for visit, physical exam, psychosocial & family systems assessment, history and current medications and treatments.

Primary Nursing Diagnosis: Acute Pain (00132)

Additional Nursing Diagnoses: none

Desired Outcome (NOC): Pain Control (1605)

> **Selected Indicators:** 04 (score: 3, goal: 5); 05 (score: 4, goal: 5); 07 (score: 4, goal: 5); 11 (score: 2, goal: 4)

Desired Outcome (NOC): Pain: Disruptive Effects (2101)

> **Selected Indicators:** 03 (score: 2, goal: 5); 13 (score: 3, goal: 5)

Dictation Date and Time: 02/01/2002 @ 1700

Total Time Spent: 60 minutes

Nursing Note:

I saw Xxxx in clinic today as a nurse visit, due to hxx complaint of ongoing leg pain, which has been worsening over time, limiting hxx mobility ......

Intervention(s) Implemented or Utilized (NIC):

1. Pain Management (1400)
2. Heat/Cold Application (1380)
3. Teaching: Prescribed Activity/Exercise (5612)
4. Teaching: Prescribed Medication (5616)
5. Exercise Promotion: Stretching (0202)
6. Exercise Therapy: Ambulation (0221)
7. Telephone Follow Up (8190)

Actual Outcome (NOC): Pain Control (1605)

> **Selected Indicators:** No changes expected or observed at this point, will follow-up with family by phone Monday to determine outcome scores

Actual Outcome (NOC): Pain: Disruptive Effects (2101)

> **Selected Indicators:** No changes expected or observed at this point, will follow-up with family by phone Monday to determine outcome scores

---

Signature

Fig. 3A-6, cont'd

Exhibit 1

```
NURSING – ADD/UPDATE ORDERS                         PAGE   001
87-00001-8    XXXXX, XXXX X.                    F      90 YRS
Place an 'X' before the desired group(s).  6JCE  CEREBRAL VASC. ACCIDENT
= = = = = = = = = = = = = = = = = = = = = = = = = = = = = = = = = = = = = = = = =

    (    ) CEREBRAL EDEMA MANAGEMENT                  | NIC
    (    ) CEREBRAL PERFUSION PROMOTION               | NIC
    (    ) DISCHARGE PLANNING                         | NIC
    (    ) ENTERAL TUBE FEEDING: ADULT                | NIC+
    (    ) EXERCISE THERAPY: JOINT MOBILITY           | NIC
    ( X  ) FALL PREVENTION                            | NIC
    (    ) HYPERGLYCEMIA MANAGEMENT                   | NIC
    (    ) INTRAVENOUS (IV) THERAPY                   | NIC
    (    ) INVASIVE HEMODYNAMIC MONITORING            | NIC
    (    ) MEDICAL IMMOBILIZATION                     | NIC+
    (    ) NEUROLOGIC MONITORING                      | NIC
    (    ) OXYGEN THERAPY                             | NIC
    (    ) ROUTINE CARE                               | DEPT
    (    ) SURVEILLANCE: ADULT, ACUTE                 | NIC+
    (    ) TEACHING: NEUROSCIENCE                     | NIC+
    (    ) TEACHING: PROCEDURE/TREATMENT              | NIC
    (    ) TUBE CARE: URINARY                         | NIC
    (    ) VITAL SIGNS MONITORING                     | NIC


Selection ==> (    )              RETURN=R
- - - - - - - - - - - - - - - - - - - - - - - - - - - - - - - (Nurse's signature) - - - - - - - - - -

        HELP=PF1                        MASTER=PF10     SIGNOFF=PF11
```

Fig. 3A-7 Selected computer screens from the Information Network for Online Retrieval & Medical Management (INFORMM) System at the University of Iowa Hospital and Clinics, Iowa City, IA.
The screens are from the hospital's nursing information system, available in all general inpatient care and selected ambulatory care units. NIC interventions may be selected by users in multiple online pathways: via patient population (shown in the first screen), nursing diagnosis, defining characteristic, etiology, NIC taxonomy, care plan category, and alphabetical list. NIC+ are those interventions modified by the agency for use with a specific population. When a NIC intervention is selected, the user may individualize the associated patient care orders (see third screen). NIC is used in the facility for both care planning and documentation. The data are stored and can be retrieved and analyzed for quality improvement and research. *(Submitted by Gloria Dorr, MA, RN, Advance Practice Nurse, Nursing Informatics. Used with permission.)*

Exhibit 5

NURSING - ADD/UPDATE/ORDERS
   87-00004-7 xxxxx, xxxx x.   F   90 YRS
==

PHYSIOLOGICAL DOMAIN: BASIC	PHYSIOLOGICAL DOMAIN: COMPLEX
10 ACTIVITY/EXERCISE MANAGEMENT	23 DRUG MANAGEMENT
11 ELIMINATION MANAGEMENT	24 ELECTROLYTE & ACID-BASE MANAGEMENT
12 IMMOBILITY MANAGEMENT	25 NEUROLOGICAL MANAGEMENT
13 NUTRITION SUPPORT	26 PERIOPERATIVE CARE
14 PHYSICAL COMFORT PROMOTION	27 RESPIRATORY MANAGEMENT
15 SELF-CARE FACILITATION	28 SKIN/WOUND MANAGEMENT
FAMILY DOMAIN	29 THERMOREGULATION
16 CHILDBEARING CARE	30 TISSUE PERFUSION MANAGEMENT
17 LIFESPAN CARE	BEHAVIORAL DOMAIN
SAFETY DOMAIN	31 BEHAVIOR THERAPY
18 CRISIS MANAGEMENT	32 COGNITIVE THERAPY
19 RISK MANAGEMENT	33 COMMUNICATION ENHANCEMENT
HEALTH SYSTEM DOMAIN	34 COPING ASSISTANCE
20 HEALTH SYSTEM MANAGEMENT	35 PATIENT EDUCATION
21 HEALTH SYSTEM MEDIATION	36 PSYCHOLOGICAL COMFORT PROMOTION
22 INFORMATION MANAGEMENT	

Selection ==> (   )   RETURN=R   NIC ALPHA=A
- (Nurse's Signature) - - - - - - - - - - - - - - - -

         HELP=PF1   MASTER=PF10   SIGNOFF=PF11

Exhibit 9

   NURSING - DISPLAY ORDER DATABASE   PAGE 001

   Place an 'X' before the desired orders from the order group
   FALL PREVENTION | NIC   ***MAINTAINED GROUP***
== =

   (   ) BP, PULSE/ORTHOSTATIC –ONCE
   (   ) RISK POTENTIAL/FALLS –ONCE   REQ
   (   ) PRECAUTIONS: FALL, SIDERAILS UP - 4, BED   REQ
   (   )   LOW/LOCKED, NIGHTLIGHT –CNSTNT
   (   ) VOIDS: TIMED W/ASSISTANCE, STAY WITH PATIENT -q2H
   (   )   WA
   (   ) AMBULATION: NON-SLIP SHOES, ASSISTANCE 1 PERSON
   (   )   -PRN
   (   ) ORIENTATION: ENVIRONMENT –PRN
   (   ) CALL LIGHT WITHIN REACH -CNSTNT
   (   ) COMMUNICATION MODE: HEARING AID/GLASSES –PRN
   (   ) INSTRUCTION; FALL PRECAUTIONS, PATIENT/FAMILY   REQ
   (   )   -ONCE +PRN
   (   ) REFERRAL: PHYSICAL THERAPY –PRN   REQ

   Selection ==> (   )   RETURN=R   ALL OF GROUP=A
- (Nurse's Signature) - - - - - - - - - - - - - - - - - -

         HELP=PF1   MASTER=PF10   SIGNOFF=PF11

Fig. 3A-7, cont'd

Costing Out An Indirect NIC Paper

Student Name_____

Overall Expectations: Student will provide evidence of understanding costing out an indirect nursing intervention as a basis for budgeting and staffing in a 3-5 page paper.

Steps:
1. Describe fully and "ideally" an invented case scenario based on the use of an indirect NIC. Select from the list of NIC activities those that fit best with the case scenario. Include NIC activities that require resources.

2. Using cost-effectiveness analysis (CEA) techniques (see references) and the NIC case scenario, compute a cost effectiveness (C/E) ratio.

    a. Use relevant resources consumed components in the **numerator** and
    b. Use savings in clinical or quality outcomes/health of staff or organization effectiveness components in the **denominator.**
    c. Define each component in measurable dollar terms. Identify total costs and savings in a ratio.
    d. State if cost-effective. Cost will include all direct and indirect care resources used: personnel, supplies/equipment, time. Effectiveness will include savings to the patient, payer, or institution.

3. Identify and justify the one perspective selected and used in the C/E ratio: community/society OR payer OR consumer OR institution/provider.

4. List all assumptions made in constructing the C/E ratio.

Grading Checklist:		Possible Points	Points Earned
1.	Case	40:	_____
2.	C/E Ratio	20:	_____
3.	Perspective	10:	_____
4.	Assumptions	15:	_____
5.	APA/writing	15:	_____
		Total Points	_____

Fig. 3A-8 Costing Out an Indirect NIC Paper—University of Michigan, Flint, MI.
This contains the instructions for a paper assignment for determining cost of an indirect NIC intervention in a course taught at University of Michigan, Flint, by Mary Killen, as well as one paper written to meet the assignment written by Gabrielle Tysar. The assignment helps undergraduate students to understand the basis of budgeting and staffing. *(Submitted by Mary Killeen, PhD, RNC, CNAA, Associate Professor. Used with permission.)*

Grading Criteria
Costing Out Indirect NIC Paper

Costing Paper Grading Elements/ Possible Points	D: does not meet expectations	C: meets minimal expectations	B: fully meets expectations	A: exceeds expectations
Case /40 points	Poor case: unclear and resources not identified and not relevant **(24 or fewer points)**	Partial case: unclear or resources not identified. Questionable relevance **(28-31)**	Full description of case, i.e., clear story with resources identified. Somewhat relevant. **(32-35)**	In addition, story is totally relevant to NIC definition and most of the activities **(36-40)**
C/E Ratio/20 points	C/E ratio computed w/ missing components; Components not completely defined and $ attached AND Total costs & savings missing **(13 or fewer points)**	C/E ratio computed w/ missing components; Components not completely defined and $ attached OR Total costs & savings missing **(14-16)**	C/E ratio computed w/ all components; Components not completely defined and $ attached OR Total costs & savings missing. **(16-17)**	C/E ratio computed w/ all components; Components completely defined and $ attached AND Total costs & savings present **(18-20)**
Perspective/10 points	Not identified or justified **(6 or fewer points)**	Either identified or justified **(7-8)**	Identified and partially justified **(8-9)**	Completely identified and justified. **(9-10)**
Assumptions/15 points	No assumptions apparent **(10 or fewer points)**	Assumptions unclear AND incomplete **(10.5-12)**	Assumptions unclear OR incomplete **(12-13.5)**	Assumptions clear, complete and consistent with case and C/E ratio **(13.5-15)**
APA/Writing/15 points	**(10 or fewer points)**	**(10.5-12)**	**(12-13.5)**	**(13.5-15)**

Fig. 3A-8, cont'd

Continued

Outline
Costing Out an Indirect NIC Paper
Title of the Costing Assignment (Use Level 1 APA Heading for Title)

Introduction
The Case Scenario (Use Level 3 APA Headings)
- Order of events using resources (people, equipment, time, supplies) using the selected indirect intervention activities
- In the scenario, include the results (nursing outcomes).

C/E (Cost/Effectiveness) Ratio:
Benefits (Outcomes-Denominator)
- Level of health benefits to the patient or institution or society from the use of the intervention
- Immediate and long-term benefits = outcomes
- Use the perspective that has been identified. For example, if institution perspective for Orientation NIC: outcome is "90% competent staff will result in what benefits to the patient? Faster discharge, less complications, etc." Must express all outcomes in $.

Resource Costs (Activities in the NIC - Numerator) List all resources consumed.
- Direct Costs: changes in resource used due to the NIC. (These vary with patient numbers [census] & acuity)
- Indirect Costs: fixed or overhead; productivity gains or losses; time costs; psychic costs; costs to family
  (try for these two types of costs to get extra points):
    1. Opportunity Costs: use market prices, i.e. salaries, office visit, travel cost
    2. Marginal Costs see ex. In Stone, 1998, p. 231 under Analysis
- Display Formula: (Note: Benefits denominator must be larger than Cost numerator to be cost effective)

Resource Cost A + Resource Cost B + Resource Cost C, etc. = Total Resource Costs
Benefit A + Benefit B + Benefit C, etc   = Total Benefit Cost
=C/E ratio (e.g. 1:4) and $ cost per unit of outcome (for every dollar spent, x dollars of benefits

---

Perspective
Who is receiving the intervention? (Be unambiguous and make one choice)
Assumptions
Take nothing for granted - the assumptions underpinning the case are important, e.g., the organization will save money by employing BSN prepared RNs to ___
Conclusion

References

Allred, C. A., Arford, P.H., Mauldin, P.D., & Goodwin, L. K. (1998). Cost-effectiveness analysis in the nursing literature, 1992-1996. *Image: Journal of Nursing Scholarship, 30* (3), 235-242.

McCloskey, J.C., & Bulechek, G.M. (Eds.). (2000). *Nursing Interventions Classification (NIC)* (3rd ed.). St. Louis: Mosby.

Stone, P.W. (1998). Methods for conducting and reporting cost-effectveness analysis in nursing. *Image: Journal of Nursing Scholarship, 30* (3), 229-234.

Fig. 3A-8, cont'd

Multidisciplinary Care Conference

Gabrielle C. Tysar

University of Michigan - Flint

References

An extensive search of the literature produced three articles that could be added to the existing citations referenced for the NIC label Multidisciplinary Care Conference. An article by Coopman (2001) covered benefits of the multidisciplinary team (MDT) that included increased quality of patient care and improved performance of the team members through collaborative decision-making. The article goes on to state that greater equality in decision-making in health care teams generally leads to healthy relationships among team members, producing better patient care. The second article, by Schofield and Amodeo (1999), is a research study discussing the need for interdisciplinary cooperation in patient care. Through progressive communication and utilizing the broad spectrum of knowledge, the MDT can provide comprehensive care to individuals with multiple problems. Moreover, the article cites improved access to care, reduction in length of stay, and patient efficacy in self-care behaviors as added patient benefits of the multidisciplinary team. The same article shows that healthcare providers also benefit from these teams. For the staff, the burden of treatment is relieved and team members share the facilitation of difficult patients. The last article, by Van Ess Coeling and Cukr (2000), presents evidence that collaboration between nurses and doctors is significantly and positively associated with desired patient outcomes and that predicted risk of negative outcomes decreased in collaborative situations. This article also discussed that health team collaboration is related to decreased resource use and cost of care. With these findings, it is obvious that multidisciplinary teams are not only beneficial, but also necessary in many settings.

Since there are only two references, Mariano (1989) and Richardson (1986), listed under the multidisciplinary care conference intervention in the Nursing Interventions Classification

Fig. 3A-8, cont'd

Continued

(Bulechek & McCloskey, 2000), it was assumed that there would be no difficulty in finding additional references to add to the list. However, a preliminary keyword search through the library databases proved otherwise. Several days of searching, over a period of three weeks, produced no acceptable results. This student got frustrated and consulted colleagues in an attempt to learn what types of searches had provided adequate results for their labels. One kind student provided direction toward the Cumulative Index of Nursing and Allied Health Literature (CINAHL) books in the library to look up the label. This exercise was fruitful in generating seven possible keyword phrases that would be useful when searching the computerized databases. The course instructor was also helpful in suggesting multiple search engines and criteria to obtain the desired results. Given that this was such a lengthy process, only the searches producing the articles used for this paper will be detailed.

The search to extend the short list of sources already published for the NIC intervention, and notated by an asterisk on the reference page, began at home, on-line, via Internet Explorer to the university databases. Once at the library homepage, "Periodicals: Indexes & Full Texts" was selected to conduct the search. Utilizing the "FirstSearch (OCLC)" engine, the CINAHL database and full text articles were chosen to narrow the search results. Many keyword phrases using "and" as the Boolean operator were input for the search criteria. These keyword phrases included: multidisciplinary care conference, professional-ancillary services, health care team, interdisciplinary health team, medical care team, patient care team, multidisciplinary research, and multidisciplinary health team. The results for this search were minimal (under ten articles) and the articles had nothing to do with the intervention or the activities that help define it. It was on to the "ProQuest Direct" engine for another try.

Fig. 3A-8, cont'd

Again the index for full text periodicals was chosen and ProQuest was selected. Under collections, "ProQuest Nursing Journals" was elected to help narrow the search. To further narrow the results, the guided search method was used. The keyword phrase "interdisciplinary health team" using "and" as the Boolean operator was the criteria. Instructions for this paper specifically stated that the new articles that would be added to the previous citations needed to be from 1998 to the current year, so the date range was limited to 1999-2003. In addition to the date limitation, only English language periodicals were searched. All article types were searched at this time. Of the 16 articles matching the search, only the Schofield (1999) article was chosen because it met the requirements for this paper.

To find additional articles, the same engine, database, and limitations were used, except the last keyword of the search criteria was changed to "care." This search produced 38 articles and only the one by Van Ess Coeling (2000) fit the paper's criteria. The last search was conducted through ProQuest's general database. The limitations remained the same, but the criteria were returned to "interdisciplinary health team." Twenty-one articles matched the search and the Coopman (2001) article was chosen as part of the research base.

The Multidisciplinary Care Conference Scenario

After attending a hospital board meeting on patient care quality and cost containment through early discharge, the director of the brain rehabilitation unit, Beth, agreed it was time to make some changes. The board had gone into detail about their plans to initiate multidisciplinary teams to manage the care of patients and hopefully reduce costs at the same time. Beth had volunteered to do the 60-day trial run on brain rehabilitation because it was a small unit of 12 beds and the staff already worked well as a team. After an extensive search and study of the literature on such teams, Beth found that all the current articles showed evidence

Fig. 3A-8, cont'd

Continued

that multidisciplinary teams benefited the staff as well as the patients. The staff would have more people to help with the difficult cases while the patients would get more comprehensive care. Both benefits would save the hospital money. It sounded like everybody would win by implementing the conferences. Impressed by what she read, Beth reviewed the definition and activities listed under the multidisciplinary care conference label in the Nursing Interventions Classification (Bulechek & McCloskey, 2000). She found that numerous caregivers performed many of the activities that were listed and often the discharge paperwork was delayed or lost when it came time for the patients to leave. Beth believed the conferences would be the perfect solution to the problem.

Family conferences were already taking place on the unit, but they only involved the discharge planner, the nurse, and a physical therapist. This conference was used to teach the family what to expect when the patient was at home and to discuss patient needs. The new conferences would be held in the unit conference room for one hour every Tuesday morning. A physician, the primary nurse, discharge planner, physical therapist, occupational therapist, and other pertinent staff would be obligated to attend as mandated by the hospital board.

After weeks of planning, Beth was ready for the first conference. By typing up an agenda for the conferences, Beth had prepared her staff and the doctors for what they could expect. The conferences would be used to plan and evaluate patient care with the professional disciplines previously noted. They would focus on the health status data pertinent to planning patient care. They would also discuss and establish mutually agreeable goals and the patient's progress toward those goals. Each team member would be asked for his/her evaluation of the patient in order to make adequate adjustments to their plan of care so that necessary referrals could be made. When all of the disciplines are in agreement, a projected date of patient

Fig. 3A-8, cont'd

discharge will be set. The result of these conferences will be a multidisciplinary team that provides the patient with quality care in one setting by collaborating on a plan of care that effectively meets the patient's needs in the least amount of steps. In so doing, the workload of the team is shared and confusion is eliminated. The board would be evaluating the success of the multidisciplinary conferences after sixty days to study the cost benefits. After making necessary changes or improvements, the board will be implementing the practice hospital within thirty days.

Cost/Effectiveness Ratio

To determine whether or not the intervention is cost effective, the following cost analysis will provide figures to do so. Costs will be based on a one-hour multidisciplinary care conference.

Resource Costs

1. Beth's time (indirect): $39.00/hr = $30.00/hr wage + 30% ($9) for benefits = $39.00.

2. Physician's time (indirect): $117.00/hr = $90.00/hr + 30% ($27) for benefits = $117.00.

3. Discharge planner (indirect): $36.40/hr = $28.00/hr + 30% ($8.40) for benefits = $36.40.

4. Physical therapist (indirect): $32.50/hr = $25.00/hr + 30% ($7.50) for benefits = $32.50.

5. Occupational therapist (indirect): $32.50/hr = $25.00/hr + 30% ($7.50) for benefits = $32.50.

6. Primary nurse (indirect): $35.10/hr = $27.00/hr + 30% ($8.10) for benefits = $35.10.

7. Unit clerk (indirect): $18.20/hr = $14.00/hr + 30% ($4.20) for benefits = $18.20.

8. Cost to print patient list and agenda for meeting: 15 copies x 2 pages @ .7 cents per copy = $2.10.

Fig. 3A-8, cont'd

Continued

Total resource costs for the one hour conference = 1+2+3+4+5+6+7+8= $312.80. Projected cost for one full year of conferences is $312.80 x 4 weeks = $1251.20 x 12 months = $15, 014.40.

The cost for the conference seems extremely low, but the benefits do not stop at the patients and staff. The hospital and insurance companies will experience immediate and long-term savings from this simple intervention. If each of the twelve possible patients on the unit went home one day sooner than the projected discharge date, an estimated savings to the hospital could be calculated something like this:

Average cost for each hospital day per patient is $700 x 12 = $8,400.00

If the average length of stay on the unit is 21 days per patient, that is an average of 17 patients per month and 204 patients per year. If each of those 204 patients were discharged just one day early, the total savings would be $700 x 204 = $142,800.00 annually. The ratio of costs ($15,014.40) to benefits ($142,800.00) = 0.11 or 1 to 10.

Another way to estimate possible benefits would be to look at the savings from pain medications the patient did not need due to early discharge.

1. One IM shot of Demerol q 4/hr per patient = $20.00 x 6 doses/d = $120.00/day.

    $120.00 x 12 patients = $1,440.00/day.

    $120.00/day x 204 patients annually = $24,480.00 annually.

2. Syringes with needles @ 6 per patient per day = $5.00 x 6 = $30.00/day.

    $30.00/day x 12 patients = $360.00/day.

    $30.00/day x 204 patients annually = $6,120.00 annually.

3. Alcohol swabs @ 6 per patient per day = $.50 x 6 = $3.00/day.

    $3.00/day x 12 patients = $36.00/day.

    $3.00/day x 204 patients annually = $612.00 annually.

Fig. 3A-8, cont'd

Total single patient cost for one day of IM Demerol is 1+2+3 = $153.00, $153.00 x 12 patients = $1,836.00/day, and 204 patients annually = $31,212.00. The cost ($31,212.00) to benefit ($142,800.) ratio is 0.22 or 1 to 5.

Perspective

This cost analysis is taken from the perspective of the hospital. It is obvious by the dollar amounts that the benefits of the multidisciplinary care conference far outweigh the costs to the hospital. However, the marginal costs of one more unit of activity could be calculated. For instance, if the institution wanted to implement an additional trial on another unit. In calculating the cost, it would be essential not to compare apples to oranges. A 12-bed unit as compared to one with 30 beds will have dramatically lower costs. So, one would need to consider if the unit's staffing is larger, if the unit had its own conference room, the total number of patients housed on the unit, and number of members from all disciplines required to attend the conference. There would also be increased printing charges for copies of the agenda and protocol for the conference.

However, the opportunity cost could be looked at in many different ways. The one hour time allotment for the conference could be the highest value of the benefits not realized. For instance, if the conference takes too many staff members away from their duties, thus endangering the patients' well-being, then the benefit is not cost effective since the resources used to pay the healthcare staff would have been spent more effectively on patient care.

Assumptions

There are several basic assumptions in this analysis. The first assumption is that the hospital board made implementing multidisciplinary care conferences mandatory to increase the quality of patient care and in effect reduce patient care costs. The second assumption is that all

Fig. 3A-8, cont'd

Continued

patients on the brain rehabilitation unit would require, and receive, multiple daily doses of Demerol for pain. The third assumption is that patients would be discharged at least one day early without regard to possible complications in their recovery or difficulty in placing them after discharge. The fourth assumption is that the brain unit had its own conference room on the floor. The final assumption is that all other disciplines would be agreeable to participating in multidisciplinary conferences.

References

McCloskey, J. & Bulechek, G. (2000). *Nursing interventions classification (NIC)* (3rd ed.). St. Louis: Mosby.

Coopman, S. (2001, July). Democracy, performance, and outcomes in interdisciplinary health care teams. *The Journal of Business Communication, 38*(3), 261-284.

*Mariano, C. (1989). The case of interdisciplinary collaboration. *Nursing Outlook, 37*(6), 285-288.

*Richardson, A. T. (1986). Nurses interfacing with other members of the team. In D. A. England (Ed.), *Collaboration in Nursing* (pp. 163-185). Rockville, MD: Aspen.

Schofield, R., & Amodeo, M. (1999, August). Interdisciplinary teams in health care and human services settings: Are they effective? *Health & Social Work, 24*(3), 210-219.

Stone, P. (1998, Third Quarter). Methods for conducting and reporting cost-effectiveness analysis in nursing. *Image: Journal of Nursing Scholarship, 30*(3), 229-234.

Van Ess Coeling, H., & Cukr, P. (2000, January). Communication styles that promote perceptions of collaboration, quality, and nurse satisfaction. *Journal of Nursing Care Quality, 14*(2), 63-74.

* Denotes references already cited under the NIC label.

Fig. 3A-8, cont'd

University of Pittsburgh School of Nursing
NURSING PLAN OF CARE - Individualized

Name: _____

Patient Initials: _____
Date: _____

Nursing Diagnosis: Pain

Definition: An unpleasant sensory and emotional experience arising from actual or potential tissue damage or described in terms of such damage (International Association for the Study of Pain); sudden or slow onset of any intensity from mild to severe with an anticipated or predictable end and a duration of less than 6 months.

NIC		NOC		Indicators
a) Label	**Pain Management**	**a) Label**	Pain Level	**a1)** Reported Pain
	Activities (Individualized and Prioritized)			
	a1) Perform a comprehensive assessment of pain to include location, characteristics, onset/duration, frequency, quality, intensity or severity of pain, and precipitating factors.			**a2)** Frequency of Pain
	a2) Observe for non-verbal cues of discomfort, especially in those unable to communicate effectively.	NOC #	2102	
NIC #	1400	*Definition:*	Severity of reported or demonstrated pain.	
Definition:	Alleviation of pain or a reduction in pain to a level of comfort that is acceptable to the patient.			
	a3) Reduce or eliminate factors that precipitate or increase the pain experience (e.g., fear, fatigue, monotony, and lack of knowledge).	Scale	Severe to None	
	a4) Select and implement a variety of measures (e.g., pharmacologic, nonpharmacologic, interpersonal) to facilitate pain relief, as appropriate.			
	a5) Collaborate with the patient, significant other, and other health professionals to select and implement nonpharmacologic pain relief measures, as appropriate.			
b) Label	**Analgesic Administration**	**b) Label**	Pain Control	**b1)** Uses preventive measures.
	b1) Determine pain location, characteristics, quality, and severity before medicating patient.	NOC #	1605	**b2)** Uses analgesics appropriately.
NIC #	2210			
	b2) Attend to comfort needs and other activities that assist relaxation to facilitate response to analgesia.			

Fig. 3A-9 Nursing Plan of Care for Pain—University of Pittsburgh School of Nursing, Pittsburgh, PA.
The nursing plan of care for pain was done as part of an independent study in the nursing informatics graduate program. The current plan of care in use by the school of nursing (which already contained NANDA) was revised to incorporate NIC and NOC. The purpose was to expose faculty to the NIC and NOC vocabulary and demonstrate how they could be used in conjunction with NANDA for student care plans. (*Submitted by Dariada Sutton, Director of Nursing Informatics, University of Pittsburgh Medical Center [UPMC] Health System. Used with permission.*)

Continued

University of Pittsburgh School of Nursing
NURSING PLAN OF CARE - Individualized

Patient Initials: _____   Name: _____
Date: _____

Nursing Diagnosis: Pain
Definition: An unpleasant sensory and emotional experience arising from actual or potential tissue damage or described in terms of such damage (International Association for the Study of Pain); sudden or slow onset of any intensity from mild to severe with an anticipated or predictable end and a duration of less than 6 months.

NIC	Activities (Individualized and Prioritized)	NOC	Indicators
Definition: Use of pharmacologic agents to reduce or eliminate pain.	**b3)** Evaluate the effectiveness of analgesic at regular frequent intervals after each administration, but especially after the initial doses, also observing for any signs and symptoms of untoward effects (e.g., respiratory depression, nausea and vomiting, dry mouth, and constipation).	*Definition:* Personal actions to control pain.	**b3)** Reports symptoms to health care professional. **b4)** Reports pain controlled.
	b4) Document response to analgesic and any untoward effects.	Scale Never demonstrated to	Consistently demonstrated.
	b5) Teach about the use of analgesics, strategies to decrease side effects, and expectations for involvement in decisions about pain relief.		
c) Label Simple Massage	**c1)** Massage, using continuous, even, and rhythmical movements.		
NIC # 1480	**c2)** Massage the hands or feet, if other areas are inconvenient, or if more comfortable for the patient.		
Definition: Stimulation of the skin and underlying tissues with varying degrees of hand pressure to decrease pain, produce relaxation, and/or improve circulation.	**c3)** Establish a period of time for massage that achieves the desired response.		

Fig. 3A-9, cont'd

University of Pittsburgh School of Nursing
NURSING PLAN OF CARE - Individualized

Name: _____

Patient Initials: _____
Date: _____

Nursing Diagnosis:
Definition: Pain

An unpleasant sensory and emotional experience arising from actual or potential tissue damage or described in terms of such damage (International Association for the Study of Pain); sudden or slow onset of any intensity from mild to severe with an anticipated or predictable end and a duration of less than 6 months.

NIC	Activities (Individualized and Prioritized)	NOC	Indicators
	c4) Avoid lengthy conversations during the massage, unless it is used as a distraction technique.		
	c5) Avoid massaging over areas of open lesion or tender skin areas.		

d) Label Humor

NIC # 5320

Definition: Facilitating the patient to perceive, appreciate, and express what is funny, amusing, or ludicrous in order to establish relationships, relieve tension, release anger, facilitate learning, or cope with painful feelings.

d1) Determine the types of humor appreciated by the patient.

d2) Determine the patient's typical response to humor (e.g., laughter or smiles)

d3) Determine the time of day that patient is most receptive.

d4) Make available a selection of humorous games, cartoons, jokes, videos, tapes, books, etc.

d5) Monitor patient response and discontinue humor strategy, if ineffective.

d6) Respond positively to humor attempts made by the patient

Fig. 3A-9, cont'd

Welcome to the
Wayne State University
Clinical Log

An academic and clinical exercise in standardized language that describes what nursing students do in the field.

Introduction

The Wayne State University Clinical Log is a web-accessible database designed for students to keep track of clinical information generated during their undergraduate and graduate educational programs. FOR INFORMATION REGARDING THE UNDERGRADUATE VERSION, SEND AN EMAIL INQUIRY. This introduction will focus on Advanced Practice Field Experiences.

This database has been designed using MS Access 2000 to provide for optimal, seamless integration into the Office 2000 suite. It is accessed via the Internet anytime using Netscape or Internet Explore browsers. Students enter their data that are coded for School, Program, Course, and Semester. For example, the Wayne State University, Adult NP Program, Clinical Decision Making Course NUR 7160, given in Fall, 2001 is attached to all the data generated during that student's practicum for that course.

Fig. 3A-10 Clinical Log web site—Wayne State University, Detroit, MI.
The Wayne State University Clinical Log is a web-accessible database designed for students to keep track of clinical information generated during their undergraduate and graduate educational programs. The clinical log incorporates several standardized languages including NIC and NOC. Schools may subscribe to the services—both instructors and students have access to the data generated. The web site address is http://www.apnlog.wayne.edu. *(Submitted by Michael Morgan, MPH, PhD, APRN, Assistant Professor. Used with permission.)*

Patients/Clients are not identified by name, medical record number, or social security number. Students have immediate access to their data and have the capability for copying their data in MS Excel for making graphs and tables.

Instructors have access to all the data their students generate. Should the Program elect, additional data regarding Preceptor and Clinical Site These data can be helpful in making decisions regarding preceptor characteristics (e.g., amount of independence for students) and site characteristics (e.g. patient mix, acuity).

In addition to drop-down boxes (for short list variables, hyperlinks contain specific information regarding coding and choices for many of the more complex variables. They are able to edit and view their own data. Instructors are able to view all the data generated by their students.

The Clinical Log incorporates several standardized languages, including NURSING languages in addition to ICD, CPT, and others. This not only provides the students an opportunity to use the languages but encourages cross-comparison among the different taxonomies.

Advantages

The Wayne State Clinical Log has some advantages, which make it quite attractive to students and program faculty.

1) Data collection is uniform through out the database . This means data entered and updated in this database have same pattern and scalability so that students will never have any problem accessing it.

2) The format of the database is designed so that the Schools participating in this log will have all of their data in a well-defined form which can be customized to reflect the data fields each college requires.

3) There is 24/7 access for the student. Students can go online anytime to access the database and can have their data all the time.

4) The report generation system in this database can be customized for every program or every college. Reports has been generated in MS Excel and customized according to the need of the program and then sent to the recipient appropriately.

5) The Clinical Log format is updated on a regular basis. We do all the work so you don't have to hire your own database manager.

6) Commonly available software is incorporated throughout the Log. The database was made by using MS Access 2000, which is the most common database engine in any Windows machine. Reports are formatted for MS Excel which has easy-to-use chart and graph functions.

7) Commonly used standardized languages (nursing, pharmacy, medicine) are used—students SEE how taxonomies unfold. Students develop expertise in the ICD-9 (for medical diagnoses),

Fig. 3A-10, cont'd

Continued

CPT (for medical procedures), DSM (for psychiatric diagnoses) NANDA/NIC/NOC (for standardized nursing language), American Hospital Formulary System (for medications), and the Evaluation and Management (E/M) codes (for ambulatory care visits).

Disadvantages

1) Data cannot be traced back to individual patients, so if a student sees that same patient twice, the encounter is a NEW entry. No tracking of individual patients is possible.

2) While there is no charge for use of this service, a cost-recovery mechanism is being developed. Charges will be minimal—around $5/student per semester.

Data fields

Not all students have to fill out all the data fields, depending on the requirements of the School the student attends. Current data fields include:

Patient demographics: E/M age codes; ethnicity; sex; payor status
Clinical Information: ICD-9, CPT-4 (plus measure of student involvement); DSM-
                                        IV (5 axis capability);
                                      NANDA (Taxonomy II) codes;
                                      NIC (Nursing Interventions Classification) codes;
                                      NOC (Nursing Outcomes Classification) code and score; Visit time (minutes face to face);
                                      Student involvement in visit;
                                      Level of Service (E/M codes);
                                      labs;
                                      Medications prescribed (AHFS codes);
Program information: Preceptor; site; number of hours in field/week

We are open to designing an interface that is friendly to YOUR students.

Copyright

Copyright permission has been secured from Elsevier for use of NIC and NOC.

McCloskey, J.C. & G.M. Bulechek (Eds.), (2000). *Nursing Interventions Classification* (3rd ed.). St. Louis: Mosby

Johnson, M., M. Maas, & S. Moorhead, (Eds.), (2000). *Nursing Outcomes Classification* (2nd ed.). St. Louis: Mosby.

Johnson, M., G. Bulechek, J.M. Dochterman, M. Maas, & S. Moorhead (Eds.), (2001). *Nursing Diagnoses, Outcomes, & Interventions: NANDA, NOC, and NIC Linkages*. St. Louis: Mosby

Fig. 3A-10, cont'd

In addition:

> "*AHFS* Pharmacologic-Therapeutic Classification used with permission (c) 2001 American Society of Health-System Pharmacists. The Classification is part of the *AHFS Drug Information*; the Society is not responsible for the accuracy of transpositions from the original context."

For further information

If you would like further information regarding this project, please send email to:

Michael J. Morgan, MPH, PhD, APRN
Wayne State University College of Nursing

Below is copy of what the data entry interface looks like.

Case ID		Date of Service		Course	
Site ID		Preceptor ID		Age Code	
Ethnicity Code		Sex Code		Payer Code	

NANDA # 1		NIC # 1		ICD # 1	
NANDA # 2		NIC # 2		ICD # 2	
NANDA # 3		NIC # 3		ICD # 3	
More than 3 NANDA	☐	More than 3 NIC	☐	More than 3 ICD	☐

Fig. 3A-10, cont'd

Continued

MED Code # 1		CPT Code		# Interp Today	
MED Code # 2		Procedure Involvement		# Labs Rx'd	
MED Code # 3		Multiple Procedure	☐	# X-rays Rx'd	
More than 3 MED	☐				
Visit Involvement		Level of Service		Time Spent	

NOC # 1		NOC # 2		NOC # 3	
Indicator A		Indicator A		Indicator A	
Rating A		Rating A		Rating A	
Indicator B		Indicator B		Indicator B	
Rating B		Rating B		Rating B	
Indicator C		Indicator C		Indicator C	
Rating C		Rating C		Rating C	
Indicator D		Indicator D		Indicator D	
Rating D		Rating D		Rating D	
NOC 1 Score		NOC 2 Score		NOC 3 Score	

Fig. 3A-10, cont'd

Foundations of Nursing
NU152C

STUDENT OBJECTIVES	SUBJECT MATTER	STUDENT ACTIVITIES	TEACHING AIDS
57. Describe the purpose of documentation.	C. Documentation 1. Purpose	Potter and Perry; CH 7	
58. Identify types of information found in various parts of the medical record.	2. Parts of medical record	NIC: **Documentation p. 260**	
59. Describe types of documentation.	3. Common abbreviations 4. Types of documentation	NIC: **Incident Reporting p. 395**	
60. Describe legal guidelines for documentation.	5. Legal guidelines		
61. Define and describe the techniques utilized by the nurse when performing an assessment.	6. Special types of documentation a. computerized charting b. Nursing Minimum Data Set c. incident/variance reports		
62. Describe various positions used during a physical exam.	IV. Assessment of the Client A. Assessment techniques	Potter and Perry; CH 12	VHS # 602 Vital signs
63. Define terms used to describe vital signs.	1. inspection 2. palpation 3. auscultation	Vital signs lab NIC: **Examination Assistance p.315**	
64. Explain physiologic basis for vital signs.	4. percussion		
65. Identify normal ranges for vital signs throughout the life span.	B. Positioning for assessment C. Assessment of vital signs	Potter and Perry; CH 11 Handouts Castillo p 3-17 & 37-41	
66. Select appropriate equipment to use when taking vital signs.	1. physiologic basis for vital signs 2. parameters assessed a. temperature b. pulse		
67. Demonstrate correct technique for measuring vital signs.	c. respirations d. blood pressure 3. normal ranges for vital signs 4. appropriate equipment	NIC: **Vital Signs Monitoring p. 700**	
68. Describe routine assessments performed at the beginning of a shift.	D. Assessment of the hospitalized client 1. admission/transfer/discharge 2. shift assessment	NIC: **Specimen Management p. 605**	
69. Describe the role of the LPN in the admission/transfer/discharge process.	3. role of the LPN	NIC: **Visitation Facilitation p. 698**	

Fig. 3A-11 Selected pages from syllabi—Iowa Lakes Community College, Emmetsburg, IA.
Selected pages from syllabi of three courses (Foundations of Nursing [NU152C], Foundations of Nursing Skills Lab [NU158C], and Adult Health Nursing II [NU213C]), which demonstrate where specific NIC interventions and NANDA diagnoses are taught. In parentheses after some NICs, *I* means taught for the first time and *R* means taught as a review. (*Submitted by Judith Donahue, RN, MSN, Director of Nursing Education. Used with permission.*)

Continued

Foundations of Nursing Skills Lab
NU158C

STUDENT OBJECTIVES	SUBJECT MATTER	STUDENT ACTIVITIES	TEACHING AIDS
1. Describe basic mechanisms of ventilation, circulation, and oxygenation	I. Nursing Care of Client Needs A. Promoting optimal oxygenation 1. Review normal oxygenation function	Potter & Perry; CH 27 Handouts	
2. Identify effect of hyperventilation, hypoventilation and hypoxia on oxygenation.	2. Factors affecting oxygenation a. hyperventilation b. hypoventilation c. hypoxia		
3. Identify subjective and objective data used to assess oxygenation status.	3. Assessment of oxygenation a. respiratory monitoring 1) subjective data	NIC: **Respiratory Monitoring p. 559**	
4. Describe techniques used to monitor respiratory functioning.	a) dyspnea b) cough		
5. State client outcomes to meet oxygenation needs.	2) objective data a) lung sounds b) pulse oximetry	**Ineffective Airway Clearance**	
6. Identify nursing diagnoses/outcomes related to oxygenation needs.	4. Nursing diagnoses	NIC: **Airway Management p. 132** NIC: **Aspiration Precautions p. 151**	
7. Identify nursing interventions related to airway management and promotion of optimal oxygenation.	5. Planning a. outcomes related to oxygenation needs	NIC: **Respiratory Monitoring p. 559**	
8. Identify principles of oxygen therapy including safety measures.	6. Implementation a. airway management		
9. Describe correct techniques in oxygen administration.	b. positioning c. incentive spirometry	**Impaired Gas Exchange**	
10. Demonstrate accurate documentation of assessment and interventions for the client with an oxygenation need.	d. oxygen therapy e. pulse oximetry f. gerontological nursing practice	NIC: **Oxygen Therapy p. 484**	
11. Evaluate effectiveness of nursing interventions in maintenance of oxygenation.	g. documentation 7. Evaluation		

Fig. 3A-11, cont'd

Continued

Foundations of Nursing Skills Lab
NU158C

STUDENT OBJECTIVES	SUBJECT MATTER	STUDENT ACTIVITIES	TEACHING AIDS

40. Discuss proper methods of foot and nail care.	d. oral care
	  1) conscious
	  2) unconscious
	e. positioning
	f. bedmaking
	  1) unoccupied
		Bathing/Hygiene
		Self Care Deficit
		NIC: **Bathing p. 157**
		NIC: **Perineal Care**
		  p. 500
		NIC: **Foot Care p. 354**	

41. Describe nursing interventions that promote a client's personal hygiene.
42. Demonstrate accurate documentation of assessment and interventions for the client with hygiene needs.
43. Describe methods to evaluate interventions designed to promote hygiene.
	g. maintaining comfortable room environment
	h. gerontological nursing practice
	i. documentation
	6. Evaluation of nursing interventions
		NIC: **Self-Care**
		  Assistance: Bathing/
		  Hygiene p. 576
		NIC: **Contact Lens**
		  Care p. 232
		NIC: **Hair care p. 361**
		Impaired Dentition
		NIC: **Oral Health**
		  Maintenance p. 478
		NIC: **Oral Health**
		  Restoration p. 480	

44. List the basic motor skills used in daily living.
45. Discuss the physiologic effects of exercise.
46. Discuss benefits and hazards of bedrest.
47. Discuss physiologic changes associated with immobility.
48. Explain principles of body mechanics nurses use to prevent injury to self and clients.
	E. Promoting exercise and activity
	1. Principles of mobility
	  a. normal motor function skills
	  b. factors that interfere with motor function
	  c. benefits of exercise
	  d. problems related to immobility
	  e. principles of body mechanics
	2. Assessment
	  a. motor function skills
	  b. complications of bedrest
		Potter and Perry;
		  CH 24, 33
		
		Handouts
		Castillo p. 21
		Risk for Impaired Skin
		Integrity
		NIC: **Pressure Ulcer**
		  Prevention p. 535
		NIC: **Pressure**
		  Management p. 533
			VHS # 645
			Body
			Mechanics

Fig. 3A-11, cont'd

Adult Health Nursing II
NU 213 C

STUDENT OBJECTIVES	SUBJECT MATTER	STUDENT ACTIVITIES	TEACHING AIDS
19. Describe guidelines for planning and implementing nursing care incorporating setting of priorities.			
20. Discuss evaluation of the nursing process.			
21. Describe ways of communicating the nursing process.			
22. Describe the interaction between components of the nursing process.			
23. Discuss the purposes of client teaching/ learning in health care delivery.	D. Client Teaching	LC & H Ch 6	VHS: The Nurse As Teacher
24. Identify factors contributing to successful learning for the adult client.	1. Purpose	**Knowledge Deficit**	
25. Identify principles of effective teaching.	2. Method of knowing/Sources of knowledge	NIC: Teaching; Individual p. 643	
26. Discuss types of teaching strategies that can be used to teach adult clients.	3. Assessment of the learner	NIC: Learning Facilitation p. 423	
27. Identify health problems related to various cultures that impact patient education.	4. Principles of effective teaching	NIC: Learning Readiness Enhancement p. 425	
	5. Teaching strategies	NIC: Teaching; Disease Process p. 640	
		NIC: Teaching; Procedure/Treatment p. 652	
		NIC: Teaching; Group p. 641	
28. Discuss the importance of health promotion.	E. Health Promotion	**Health-Seeking Behaviors**	
29. Identify a model of health promotion.	1. Model of health promotion	NIC: Health Education p. 365	
30. Discuss sociocultural perspectives of health promotion.	2. Health assessment	NIC: Self-modification assistance p. 581	
31. Discuss health promotion strategies utilized with adult clients.	3. Promoting self care and health promotion	NIC: Exercise Promotion p. 316	
		Potential for Enhanced Spiritual Well-Being	
		NIC: Self-awareness Enhancement p. 574	

Fig. 3A-11, cont'd

Adult Health Nursing II
NU 213 C

STUDENT OBJECTIVES	SUBJECT MATTER	STUDENT ACTIVITIES	TEACHING AIDS
32. Define how the body maintains biological homeostasis.	II. Concepts and Challenges Encountered in Adult Health Nursing	**NIC: Spiritual Support p. 607** **NIC: Bibliotherapy p. 169**	
33. List factors that affect the body's ability to maintain homeostasis.	A. Homeostasis/Stress 1. Mechanisms for maintaining homeostasis	LC&H Ch 7 Stress Study Guide Ch 7 Short answers & case study	VHS: Conquering Stress in Changing Times
34. Describe the stages of Selye's general adaptation syndrome.	2. Adaptation factors		
35. Identify and explain the physiologic and psychologic signs and symptoms of stress.	3. Stress theory 4. Cell adaptation to injury	LC&H Ch 11 Inflammation Study Guide Ch 11	
36. Discuss the relationship between stress, adaptation and homeostasis and their impact on the immune system.	5. Systemic response to injury	**NIC: Risk Identification p 565 (I)** **NIC: Calming Technique p. 194 (R)**	
37. Describe the causes and mechanisms of cellular injury, ischemia and necrosis.		**NIC: Coping Enhancement p. 234 (R)**	
38. Explain components of the inflammatory response.		**NIC: Anxiety Reduction p. 146 (R)** **NIC: Presence p. 532 (R)**	
39. Explain the response of the adrenal medulla and cortex to injury.		**Decisional Conflict (I)**	
40. Identify and discuss nursing diagnoses commonly applied to client with disruption in homeostasis.		**NIC: Support System Enhancement p. 624 (R)** **NIC: Humor p. 380 (I)**	
41. Identify NIC interventions utilized when caring for the client with disruption in homeostasis.		**NIC: Simple Relaxation Therapy p. 598 (R)** **NIC: Progressive Muscle Relaxation p. 539 (I)** **NIC: Simple Guided Imagery p. 595 (I)** **NIC: Cutaneous Simulation p. 242**	

Fig. 3A-11, cont'd

PART TWO

Taxonomy of Nursing Interventions

Overview of the NIC Taxonomy

The 514 interventions in the *Nursing Interventions Classifications (NIC)* fourth edition have been organized, as in the last edition, into 7 domains and 30 classes. This three-level taxonomic structure is included on the following pages. At the top, most abstract level are 7 *domains* (numbered 1 to 7). Each domain includes *classes* (assigned alphabetical letters) or groups of related interventions (each with a unique code of four numbers) that are at the third level of the taxonomy. Only intervention label names are used in the taxonomy. Refer to the alphabetical listing in the book for the definition and defining activities for each intervention. The taxonomy was constructed using the methods of similarity analysis, hierarchical clustering, clinical judgment, and expert review. Refer to Chapter 2 for more details on the construction, validation, and coding of the taxonomy.

The taxonomy clusters related interventions for ease of use. The groupings represent all areas of nursing practice. Nurses in any specialty should remember that they should use the whole taxonomy with a particular patient, not just interventions from one class or domain. The taxonomy is theory neutral; the interventions can be used with any nursing theory and in any of the various nursing settings and health care delivery systems. The interventions can also be used with various diagnostic classifications, including NANDA (North American Nursing Diagnosis Association), ICD (International Classification of Diseases), DSM (Diagnostic & Statistical Manual of Mental Disorders), and Omaha.

Each of the interventions has been assigned a unique number to facilitate computerization. If one wishes to identify the class and domain of the intervention, one would use six digits (e.g., 1A-0140 is Body Mechanics Promotion and is located in the Activity and Exercise Management class in the Physiological: Basic domain). Activity codes are not included in this book as we did not wish the classification to be dominated by numbers. If one wishes to assign codes, then each intervention's activities can be numbered using two spaces after a decimal (e.g., 1A-0140.01). Given the sheer number of activities and the amount of resources that would be needed to keep track of them and the changes in activities over time, there has been no attempt to assign unique codes to activities. If activities are coded in a particular facility, they need to be used together with the related intervention code.

Some interventions have been included in two classes but are coded according to the primary class. We have attempted to keep cross-referencing to a minimum because the taxonomy could easily become long and unwieldy. Interventions are listed in another class only if they were judged to be sufficiently related to the interventions in that class. No intervention is listed in more than two classes. Interventions that are more concrete (i.e., those with colons in the title) have been coded at the fourth digit (e.g., Exercise Therapy: Ambulation is coded 0221). Occasionally an intervention is located in only one class but has a code that is assigned to another class (e.g., Nutritional Counseling is located in class D, Nutrition Support, but is coded 5246 to indicate that it is a counseling intervention). The interventions in each class are listed alphabetically, but the numbers may not be sequential because of additions and deletions. In the class of Elimination Management the interventions related to the bowel are first listed alphabetically and then those related to the bladder are listed. The last two classes in the domain Health System (Health System Management, coded a, and Information Management, coded b) contain many of the indirect care interventions (those that would be included in overhead costs). The taxonomy first appeared in the second edition of NIC in 1996 with 6 domains and 27 classes. The third edition, published in 2000, included one new domain (Community) and three new classes: Childrearing Care (coded Z) in the Family domain and Community Health Promotion and Community Risk Management in the Community domain (c and d). In this edition, no new domains or classes were added; the 28 new interventions were easily placed in the existing classes.

The coding guidelines used for this and previous editions are summarized as follows:

- Each intervention is assigned a unique four-digit code, which belongs to the intervention as long as the intervention exists, regardless of whether it should change class in some future edition.
- Codes are retired when interventions are deleted; no code is used more than once. Interventions that have a modification in label name only that does not change the nature of the intervention will keep the same code number. In this case the label name change does not affect the intervention, but the change was needed for a compelling reason (e.g., Abuse Protection was changed to Abuse Protection Support in edition 3 to distinguish the intervention from an outcome in NOC that had the same name; Conscious Sedation was changed in this edition to Sedation Management to better reflect current practice).
- Interventions that have a modification in label name only that *does* change the nature of the intervention are assigned a new code, and the previous code is retired (e.g., in edition 3 Triage became Triage: Disaster, indicating the more discrete nature of this intervention and distinguishing it from the new interventions of Triage: Emergency Center and Triage: Telephone.)
- Cross-referencing is avoided if possible, and no intervention is cross-referenced in more than two classes; the number assigned is selected from the primary class.
- Interventions that are most concrete are coded using the fourth digit.
- Interventions are listed alphabetically within each class; the code numbers may not be sequential because of changes, additions, and deletions.
- Although the codes originally begun in the second edition were assigned logically and this logical order is being continued when possible, *codes are context free* and should not be interpreted to have any meaning except as a four-digit number.
- Activities are not coded, but if one desires to do this, use two (or more if indicated in your computer system) spaces to the right of a decimal and number the activities as they appear in each intervention (e.g., 0140.01, 0140.02).

NIC TAXONOMY

	Domain 1	Domain 2	Domain 3
Level 1 Domains	**1. Physiological: Basic** Care that supports physical functioning	**2. Physiological: Complex** Care that supports homeostatic regulation	**3. Behavioral** Care that supports psychosocial functioning and facilitates lifestyle changes
Level 2 Classes	**A Activity and Exercise Management:** Interventions to organize or assist with physical activity and energy conservation and expenditure	**G Electrolyte and Acid-Base Management:** Interventions to regulate electrolyte/acid base balance and prevent complications	**O Behavior Therapy:** Interventions to reinforce or promote desirable behaviors or alter undesirable behaviors
	B Elimination Management: Interventions to establish and maintain regular bowel and urinary elimination patterns and manage complications due to altered patterns	**H Drug Management:** Interventions to facilitate desired effects of pharmacologic agents	**P Cognitive Therapy:** Interventions to reinforce or promote desirable cognitive functioning or alter undesirable cognitive functioning
	C Immobility Management: Interventions to manage restricted body movement and the sequelae	**I Neurologic Management:** Interventions to optimize neurologic function	**Q Communication Enhancement:** Interventions to facilitate delivering and receiving verbal and nonverbal messages
	D Nutrition Support: Interventions to modify or maintain nutritional status	**J Perioperative Care:** Interventions to provide care prior to, during, and immediately after surgery	**R Coping Assistance:** Interventions to assist another to build on own strengths, to adapt to a change in function, or achieve a higher level of function
	E Physical Comfort Promotion: Interventions to promote comfort using physical techniques	**K Respiratory Management:** Interventions to promote airway patency and gas exchange	**S Patient Education:** Interventions to facilitate learning
	F Self-Care Facilitation: Interventions to provide or assist with routine activities of daily living	**L Skin/Wound Management:** Interventions to maintain or restore tissue integrity	**T Psychological Comfort Promotion:** Interventions to promote comfort using psychological techniques
		M Thermoregulation: Interventions to maintain body temperature within a normal range	
		N Tissue Perfusion Management: Interventions to optimize circulation of blood and fluids to the tissue	

Domain 4	Domain 5	Domain 6	Domain 7
4. Safety Care that supports protection against harm	**5. Family** Care that supports the family	**6. Health System** Care that supports effective use of the health care delivery system	**7. Community** Care that supports the health of the community
U Crisis Management: Interventions to provide immediate short-term help in both psychological and physiological crises	**W Childbearing Care:** Interventions to assist in the preparation for childbirth and management of the psychological and physiological changes before, during, and immediately following childbirth	**Y Health System Mediation:** Interventions to facilitate the interface between patient/family and the health care system	**c Community Health Promotion:** Interventions that promote the health of the whole community
V Risk Management: Interventions to initiate risk reduction activities and continue monitoring risks over time	**Z Childrearing Care:** Interventions to assist in raising children	**a Health System Management:** Interventions to provide and enhance support services for the delivery of care	**d Community Risk Management:** Interventions that assist in detecting or preventing health risks to the whole community
	X Lifespan Care: Interventions to facilitate family unit functioning and promote the health and welfare of family members throughout the lifespan	**b Information Management:** Interventions to facilitate communication about health care	

Level 1 Domains	1. PHYSIOLOGICAL: BASIC — Care That Supports Physical Functioning		
Level 2 Classes	**A Activity and Exercise Management** Interventions to organize or assist with physical activity and energy conservation and expenditure	**B Elimination Management** Interventions to establish and maintain regular bowel and urinary elimination patterns and manage complications resulting from altered patterns	**C Immobility Management** Interventions to manage restricted body movement and the sequelae
Level 3 Interventions	0140 Body Mechanics Promotion 0180 Energy Management 0200 Exercise Promotion 0201 Exercise Promotion: Strength Training 0202 Exercise Promotion: Stretching 0221 Exercise Therapy: Ambulation 0222 Exercise Therapy: Balance 0224 Exercise Therapy: Joint Mobility 0226 Exercise Therapy: Muscle Control 5612 Teaching: Prescribed Activity/Exercise **S***	0410 Bowel Incontinence Care 0412 Bowel Incontinence Care: Encopresis **Z** 0420 Bowel Irrigation 0430 Bowel Management 0440 Bowel Training 0450 Constipation/Impaction Management 0460 Diarrhea Management 0470 Flatulence Reduction 0480 Ostomy Care **L** 0490 Rectal Prolapse Management 0550 Bladder Irrigation 0560 Pelvic Muscle Exercise 0630 Pessary Management 0640 Prompted Voiding 1876 Tube Care: Urinary 0570 Urinary Bladder Training 0580 Urinary Catheterization 0582 Urinary Catheterization: Intermittent 0590 Urinary Elimination Management 0600 Urinary Habit Training 0610 Urinary Incontinence Care 0612 Urinary Incontinence Care: Enuresis **Z** 0620 Urinary Retention Care 1804 Self-Care Assistance: Toileting **F**	0740 Bed Rest Care 0762 Cast Care: Maintenance 0764 Cast Care: Wet 6580 Physical Restraint **V** 0840 Positioning 0846 Positioning: Wheelchair 1806 Self-Care Assistance: Transfer **F** 0910 Splinting 0940 Traction/Immobilization Care 0960 Transport
	0100 to 0399	**0400 to 0699**	**0700 to 0999**

*Letter indicates another class where the intervention is also included.

D Nutrition Support
Interventions to modify or maintain nutritional status

1020 Diet Staging
1030 Eating Disorders Management
1050 Feeding **F**
1056 Enteral Tube Feeding
1080 Gastrointestinal Intubation
1100 Nutrition Management
1120 Nutrition Therapy
5246 Nutritional Counseling
1160 Nutritional Monitoring
1803 Self-Care Assistance: Feeding **F**
1860 Swallowing Therapy **F**
5614 Teaching: Prescribed Diet **S**
1200 Total Parenteral Nutrition (TPN) Administration **G**
1874 Tube Care: Gastrointestinal
1240 Weight Gain Assistance
1260 Weight Management
1280 Weight Reduction Assistance

1000 to 1299

E Physical Comfort Promotion
Interventions to promote comfort using physical techniques

1320 Acupressure
1330 Aromatherapy
1340 Cutaneous Stimulation
6482 Environmental Management: Comfort
1380 Heat/Cold Application
1450 Nausea Management
1400 Pain Management
1440 Premenstrual Syndrome Management
1460 Progressive Muscle Relaxation
3550 Pruritus Management **L**
1480 Simple Massage
5465 Therapeutic Touch
1540 Transcutaneous Electrical Nerve Stimulation (TENS)
1570 Vomiting Management

1300 to 1599

F Self-Care Facilitation
Interventions to provide or assist with routine activities of daily living

1610 Bathing
1620 Contact Lens Care
6462 Dementia Management: Bathing **V**
1630 Dressing
1640 Ear Care
1650 Eye Care
1050 Feeding **D**
1660 Foot Care
1670 Hair Care
1680 Nail Care
1710 Oral Health Maintenance
1720 Oral Health Promotion
1730 Oral Health Restoration
1750 Perineal Care
1770 Postmortem Care
1780 Prosthesis Care
1800 Self-Care Assistance
1801 Self-Care Assistance: Bathing/Hygiene
1802 Self-Care Assistance: Dressing/Grooming
1803 Self-Care Assistance: Feeding **D**
1805 Self-Care Assistance: IADL
1804 Self-Care Assistance: Toileting **B**
1806 Self-Care Assistance: Transfer **C**
1850 Sleep Enhancement
5603 Teaching: Foot Care **S**
1860 Swallowing Therapy **D**
1870 Tube Care

1600 to 1899

**Level 1
Domains**

**Level 2
Classes**

**Level 3
Interventions**

2. PHYSIOLOGICAL: COMPLEX
Care That Supports Homeostatic Regulation

G   Electrolyte and Acid-Base Management
Interventions to regulate electrolyte/acid
base balance and prevent complications

1910 Acid-Base Management
1911 Acid-Base Management: Metabolic Acidosis
1912 Acid-Base Management: Metabolic Alkalosis
1913 Acid-Base Management: Respiratory
        Acidosis **K***
1914 Acid-Base Management: Respiratory
        Alkalosis **K**
1920 Acid-Base Monitoring
2000 Electrolyte Management
2001 Electrolyte Management: Hypercalcemia
2002 Electrolyte Management: Hyperkalemia
2003 Electrolyte Management: Hypermagnesemia
2004 Electrolyte Management: Hypernatremia
2005 Electrolyte Management: Hyperphos-
        phatemia
2006 Electrolyte Management: Hypocalcemia
2007 Electrolyte Management: Hypokalemia
2008 Electrolyte Management: Hypomagnesemia
2009 Electrolyte Management: Hyponatremia
2010 Electrolyte Management:
        Hypophosphatemia
2020 Electrolyte Monitoring
2080 Fluid/Electrolyte Management **N**
2100 Hemodialysis Therapy
2110 Hemofiltration Therapy
2120 Hyperglycemia Management
2130 Hypoglycemia Management
2150 Peritoneal Dialysis Therapy
4232 Phlebotomy: Arterial Blood Sample **N**
1200 Total Parenteral Nutrition (TPN)
        Administration **D**

H   Drug Management
Interventions to facilitate desired effects of
pharmacological agents

2210 Analgesic Administration
2214 Analgesic Administration Intraspinal
2840 Anesthesia Administration **J**
6430 Chemical Restraint **V**
2240 Chemotherapy Management **S**
2280 Hormone Replacement Therapy
2300 Medication Administration
2308 Medication Administration: Ear
2301 Medication Administration: Enteral
2310 Medication Administration: Eye
2311 Medication Administration: Inhalation
2302 Medication Administration: Interpleural
2312 Medication Administration: Intradermal
2313 Medication Administration: Intramuscular
2303 Medication Administration: Intraosseous
2319 Medication Administration: Intraspinal
2314 Medication Administration: Intravenous
2320 Medication Administration: Nasal
2304 Medication Administration: Oral
2315 Medication Administration: Rectal
2316 Medication Administration: Skin
2317 Medication Administration: Subcutaneous
2318 Medication Administration: Vaginal
2307 Medication Administration: Ventricular
        Reservoir
2380 Medication Management
2390 Medication Prescribing
2400 Patient Controlled Analgesia (PCA) Assistance
2260 Sedation Management
5616 Teaching: Prescribed Medication **S**
2440 Venous Access Devices (VAD) Maintenance **N**

1900 to 2199   **2200 to 2499**

*Letter indicates another class where the intervention is also included.

I	**Neurologic Management**	**J**	**Perioperative Care**

I   Neurologic Management
Interventions to optimize neurologic function

2540 Cerebral Edema Management
2550 Cerebral Profusion Promotion
2560 Dysreflexia Management
2570 Electroconvulsive Therapy Management
2590 Intracranial Pressure (ICP) Monitoring
2620 Neurologic Monitoring
2660 Peripheral Sensation Management
0844 Positioning: Neurologic
2680 Seizure Management **V**
2690 Seizure Precautions
2720 Subarachnoid Hemorrhage Precautions
1878 Tube Care: Ventriculostomy/Lumbar Drain
2760 Unilateral Neglect Management

J   Perioperative Care
Interventions to provide care before, during, and immediately after surgery

2840 Anesthesia Administration **H**
2860 Autotransfusion **N**
3000 Circumcision Care **W**
6545 Infection Control: Intraoperative
0842 Positioning: Intraoperative
2870 Postanesthesia Care
2880 Preoperative Coordination **Y**
3582 Skin Care: Donor Site **L**
3583 Skin Care: Graft Site **L**
2900 Surgical Assistance
2920 Surgical Precautions **V**
2930 Surgical Preparation
5610 Teaching: Preoperative **S**
3902 Temperature Regulation: Intraoperative **M**

Continued

Level 1 *Domains*	**2. PHYSIOLOGICAL: COMPLEX—cont'd** **Care That Supports Homeostic Regulation**

Level 2
Classes

K Respiratory Management	**L Skin/Wound Management**
Interventions to promote airway patency and gas exchange	Interventions to maintain or restore tissue integrity

Level 3
Interventions

K Respiratory Management	L Skin/Wound Management
1913 Acid-Base Management: Respiratory Acidosis **G**	3420 Amputation Care
1914 Acid-Base Management: Respiratory Alkalosis **G**	3440 Incision Site Care
3120 Airway Insertion and Stabilization	3460 Leech Therapy
3140 Airway Management	3480 Lower Extremity Monitoring
3160 Airway Suctioning	0480 Ostomy Care **B**
6412 Anaphylaxis Management **V**	3500 Pressure Management
3180 Artificial Airway Management	3520 Pressure Ulcer Care
3200 Aspiration Precautions **V**	3540 Pressure Ulcer Prevention **V**
3210 Asthma Management	3550 Pruritus Management **E**
3230 Chest Physiotherapy	3582 Skin Care: Donor Site **J**
3250 Cough Enhancement	3583 Skin Care: Graft Site **J**
4106 Embolus Care: Pulmonary **N**	3584 Skin Care: Topical Treatments
3270 Endotracheal Extubation	3590 Skin Surveillance
3300 Mechanical Ventilation	3620 Suturing
3310 Mechanical Ventilatory Weaning	3660 Wound Care
3320 Oxygen Therapy	3662 Wound Care: Closed Drainage
3350 Respiratory Monitoring	3680 Wound Irrigation
1872 Tube Care: Chest	
3390 Ventilation Assistance	

3100 to 3399	**3400 too 3699**

M Thermoregulation
Interventions to maintain body temperature within a normal range

3740 Fever Treatment
3780 Heat Exposure Treatment
3800 Hypothermia Treatment
3840 Malignant Hyperthermia Precautions **U**
3900 Temperature Regulation
3902 Temperature Regulation: Intraoperative **J**

N Tissue Perfusion Management
Interventions to optimize circulation of blood and fluids to the tissue

2860 Autotransfusion **J**
4010 Bleeding Precautions
4020 Bleeding Reduction
4021 Bleeding Reduction: Antepartum Uterus **W**
4022 Bleeding Reduction: Gastrointestinal
4024 Bleeding Reduction: Nasal
4026 Bleeding Reduction: Postpartum Uterus **W**
4028 Bleeding Reduction: Wound
4030 Blood Products Administration
4035 Capillary Blood Sample
4040 Cardiac Care
4044 Cardiac Care: Acute
4046 Cardiac Care: Rehabilitative
4050 Cardiac Precautions
4062 Circulatory Care: Arterial Insufficiency
4066 Circulatory Care: Venous Insufficiency
4064 Circulatory Care: Mechanical Assist Device
4066 Circulatory Care: Venous Insufficiency
4070 Circulatory Precautions
4240 Dialysis Access Maintenance
4090 Dysrhythmia Management
4104 Embolus Care: Peripheral
4106 Embolus Care: Pulmonary **K**
4110 Embolus Precautions
2080 Fluid/Electrolyte Management **G**
4120 Fluid Management
4130 Fluid Monitoring
4140 Fluid Resuscitation
4150 Hemodynamic Regulation
4160 Hemorrhage Control
4170 Hypervolemia Management
4180 Hypovolemia Management
4190 Intravenous (IV) Insertion
4200 Intravenous (IV) Therapy
4210 Invasive Hemodynamic Monitoring
4220 Peripherally Inserted Central (PIC) Catheter Care
4232 Phlebotomy: Arterial Blood Sample **G**
4234 Phlebotomy: Blood Unit Acquisition
4235 Phlebotomy: Cannulated Vessel
4238 Phlebotomy: Venous Blood Sample
4250 Shock Management
4254 Shock Management: Cardiac
4256 Shock Management: Vasogenic
4258 Shock Management: Volume
4260 Shock Prevention
4092 Temporary Pacemaker Management
2440 Venous Access Devices (VAD) Maintenance **H**

Level 1 Domains	**3. BEHAVIORAL** Care That Supports Psychosocial Functioning and Facilitates Lifestyle Changes		
Level 2 Classes	**O Behavior Therapy** Interventions to reinforce or promote desirable behaviors or alter undesirable behaviors	**P Cognitive Therapy** Interventions to reinforce or promote desirable cognitive functioning or alter undesirable cognitive functioning	**Q Communication Enhancement** Interventions to facilitate delivering and receiving verbal and nonverbal messages
Level 3 Interventions	4310 Activity Therapy 4320 Animal-Assisted Therapy **Q*** 4330 Art Therapy **Q** 4340 Assertiveness Training 4350 Behavior Management 4352 Behavior Management: Overactivity/Inattention 4354 Behavior Management: Self-Harm 4356 Behavior Management: Sexual 4360 Behavior Modification 4362 Behavior Modification: Social Skills 4370 Impulse Control Training 4380 Limit Setting 4390 Milieu Therapy 4400 Music Therapy **Q** 4410 Mutual Goal Setting 4420 Patient Contracting 6926 Phototherapy: Mood/Sleep Regulation 4470 Self-Modification Assistance 4480 Self-Responsibility Facilitation 4490 Smoking Cessation Assistance 4500 Substance Use Prevention 4510 Substance Use Treatment 4512 Substance Use Treatment: Alcohol Withdrawal 4514 Substance Use Treatment: Drug Withdrawal 4516 Substance Use Treatment: Overdose 4439 Therapeutic Play **Q**	4640 Anger Control Assistance 4680 Bibliotherapy 4700 Cognitive Restructuring 4720 Cognitive Stimulation 5520 Learning Facilitation **S** 5540 Learning Readiness Enhancement **S** 4760 Memory Training 4820 Reality Orientation 4860 Reminiscence Therapy	4920 Active Listening 4320 Animal-Assisted Therapy **O** 4330 Art Therapy **O** 4974 Communication Enhancement: Hearing Deficit 4976 Communication Enhancement: Speech Deficit 4978 Communication Enhancement: Visual Deficit 5000 Complex Relationship Building 5020 Conflict Mediation 4400 Music Therapy **O** 5100 Socialization Enhancement 4430 Therapeutic Play **O**
	4300 to 4599	**4600 to 4899**	**4900 to 5199**

*Letter indicates another class where the intervention is also included.

R Coping Assistance Interventions to assist another to build on own strengths, to adapt to a change in function, or achieve a higher level of function	**S Patient Education** Interventions to facilitate learning	**T Psychological Comfort Promotion** Interventions to promote comfort using psychological techniques
5210 Anticipatory Guidance Z 5220 Body Image Enhancement 5230 Coping Enhancement 5240 Counseling 5242 Genetic Counseling W 5248 Sexual Counseling 6160 Crisis Intervention U 5250 Decision-Making Support Y 5260 Dying Care 5270 Emotional Support 5280 Forgiveness Facilitation 5290 Grief Work Facilitation 5294 Grief Work Facilitation: Perinatal Death W 5300 Guilt Work Facilitation 5310 Hope Instillation 5320 Humor 5330 Mood Management 5340 Presence 5360 Recreation Therapy 5422 Religious Addiction Prevention 5424 Religious Ritual Enhancement 5350 Relocation Stress Reduction 5370 Role Enhancement X 5380 Security Enhancement 5390 Self-Awareness Enhancement 5400 Self-Esteem Enhancement 5426 Spiritual Growth Facilitation 5420 Spiritual Support 5430 Support Group 5440 Support System Enhancement 5450 Therapy Group 5410 Trauma Therapy: Child 5440 Touch 5470 Truth Telling 5480 Values Clarification	2240 Chemotherapy Management H 6784 Family Planning: Contraception W 5510 Health Education c 5520 Learning Facilitation P 5540 Learning Readiness Enhancement P 5562 Parent Education: Adolescent Z 5566 Parent Education: Childrearing Family Z 5568 Parent Education: Infant Z 5580 Preparatory Sensory Information 5602 Teaching: Disease Process 5603 Teaching: Foot Care F 5604 Teaching: Group 5606 Teaching: Individual 5626 Teaching: Infant Nutrition Z 5628 Teaching: Infant Safety Z 5605 Teaching: Infant Stimulation Z 5610 Teaching: Preoperative J 5612 Teaching: Prescribed Activity/Exercise A 5614 Teaching: Prescribed Diet D 5616 Teaching: Prescribed Medication H 5618 Teaching: Procedure/Treatment 5620 Teaching: Psychomotor Skill 5622 Teaching: Safe Sex 5624 Teaching: Sexuality 5630 Teaching: Toddler Nutrition Z 5632 Teaching: Toddler Safety Z 5634 Teaching: Toilet Training Z	5820 Anxiety Reduction 5840 Autogenic Training 5860 Biofeedback 5880 Calming Technique 5900 Distraction 5920 Hypnosis 5960 Meditation Facilitation 5922 Self-Hypnosis Facilitation 6000 Simple Guided Imagery 6040 Simple Relaxation Therapy

5200 to 5499   **5500 to 5799**   **5800 to 6099**

Level 1 Domains	**4. SAFETY** Care That Supports Protection Against Harm	
Level 2 Classes	**U Crisis Management** Interventions to provide immediate short-term help in both psychological and physiological crises	**V Risk Management** Interventions to initiate risk reduction activities and continue monitoring risks over time
Level 3 Interventions	6140 Code Management 6160 Crisis Intervention **R*** 6200 Emergency Care 7170 Family Presence Facilitation **X** 6240 First Aid 3840 Malignant Hyperthermia Precautions **M** 6260 Organ Procurement 6300 Rape-Trauma Treatment 6320 Resuscitation 6340 Suicide Prevention **V** 6362 Triage: Disaster 6364 Triage: Emergency Center 6366 Triage: Telephone	6400 Abuse Protection Support 6402 Abuse Protection Support: Child **Z** 6403 Abuse Protection Support: Domestic Partner 6404 Abuse Protection Support: Elder 6408 Abuse Protection Support: Religious 6410 Allergy Management 6412 Anaphylaxis Management **K** 6420 Area Restriction 3200 Aspiration Precautions **K** 6522 Breast Examination 6430 Chemical Restraint **H** 6440 Delirium Management 6450 Delusion Management 6460 Dementia Management 6462 Dementia Management: Bathing **F** 6470 Elopement Precautions 6480 Environmental Management 6486 Environmental Management: Safety 6487 Environmental Management: Violence Prevention 6490 Fall Prevention 6500 Fire Setting Precautions 6510 Hallucination Management 6520 Health Screening **d** 6530 Immunization/Vaccination Management **c** 6540 Infection Control 6550 Infection Protection 6560 Laser Precautions 6570 Latex Precautions 6580 Physical Restraint **C** 6590 Pneumatic Tourniquet Precautions 3540 Pressure Ulcer Prevention **L** 6600 Radiation Therapy Management 6610 Risk Identification **d** 6630 Seclusion 2680 Seizure Management **I** 6648 Sports-Injury Prevention: Youth **Z** 6340 Suicide Prevention **U** 2920 Surgical Precautions **J** 6650 Surveillance 6654 Surveillance: Safety 9050 Vehicle Safety Promotion **d** 6680 Vital Signs Monitoring
	6100 to 6399	**6400 to 6699**

*Letter indicates another class where the intervention is also included.

Level 1 Domains	**5. FAMILY** Care That Supports the Family		
Level 2 Classes	**W Childbearing Care** Interventions to assist in the preparation for childbirth and management of the psychological and physiological changes before, during, and immediately following childbirth	**Z Childrearing Care** Interventions to assist in raising children	**X Lifespan Care** Interventions to facilitate family unit functioning and promote the health and welfare of family members throughout the lifespan
Level 3 Interventions	6700 Amnioinfusion 6720 Birthing 4021 Bleeding Reduction: Antepartum Uterus **N*** 4026 Bleeding Reduction: Postpartum Uterus **N** 1054 Breastfeeding Assistance 6750 Cesarean Section Care 6760 Childbirth Preparation 3000 Circumcision Care **J** 6771 Electronic Fetal Monitoring: Antepartum 6772 Electronic Fetal Monitoring: Intrapartum 6481 Environmental Management: Attachment Process 7104 Family Integrity Promotion: Childbearing Family 6784 Family Planning: Contraception **S** 6786 Family Planning: Infertility 6788 Family Planning: Unplanned Pregnancy 7160 Fertility Preservation 5242 Genetic Counseling **R** 5294 Grief Work Facilitation: Perinatal Death **R** 6800 High-Risk Pregnancy Care 6830 Intrapartal Care 6834 Intrapartal Care: High-Risk Delivery 6840 Kangaroo Care 6850 Labor Induction 6860 Labor Suppression 6870 Lactation Suppression 6880 Newborn Care 6890 Newborn Monitoring 6900 Nonnutritive Sucking 6924 Phototherapy: Neonate 6930 Postpartal Care 5247 Preconception Counseling 6950 Pregnancy Termination Care 6960 Prenatal Care 7886 Reproductive Technology Management 6972 Resuscitation: Fetus 6974 Resuscitation: Neonate 6612 Risk Identification: Childbearing Family 6656 Surveillance: Late Pregnancy 1875 Tube Care: Umbilical Line 6982 Ultrasonography: Limited Obstetric	6402 Abuse Protection Support: Child **V** 5210 Anticipatory Guidance **R** 6710 Attachment Promotion 1052 Bottle Feeding 0412 Bowel Incontinence Care: Encopresis **B** 8250 Developmental Care 8272 Developmental Enhancement: Adolescent 8274 Developmental Enhancement: Child 6820 Infant Care 5244 Lactation Counseling 7200 Normalization Promotion 5562 Parent Education: Adolescent **S** 5566 Parent Education: Childrearing Family **S** 5568 Parent Education: Infant **S** 8300 Parenting Promotion 8340 Resiliency Promotion 7280 Sibling Support 6648 Sports Injury Prevention: Youth **V** 5626 Teaching: Infant Nutrition **S** 5628 Teaching: Infant Safety **S** 5605 Teaching: Infant Stimulation **S** 5630 Teaching: Toddler Nutrition **S** 5632 Teaching: Toddler Safety **S** 5634 Teaching: Toilet Training **S** 0612 Urinary Incontinence Care: Enuresis **Z**	7040 Caregiver Support 7100 Family Integrity Promotion 7110 Family Involvement Promotion 7120 Family Mobilization 7170 Family Presence Facilitation **U** 7130 Family Process Maintenance 7140 Family Support 7150 Family Therapy 7180 Home Maintenance Assistance 7260 Respite Care 6614 Risk Identification: Genetic 5370 Role Enhancement **R**
	6700 to 6999	**8200 to 8499**	**7000 to 7299**

*Letter indicates another class where the intervention is also included.

Level 1 Domains	**6. HEALTH SYSTEM** Care That Supports Effective Use of the Health Care Delivery System		
Level 2 Classes	**Y Health System Mediation** Interventions to facilitate the interface between patient/family and the health care system	**a Health System Management** Interventions to provide and enhance support services for the delivery of care	**b Information Management** Interventions to facilitate communication about health care
Level 3 Interventions	7310 Admission Care 7320 Case Management **c*** 7330 Culture Brokerage 5250 Decision-Making Support **R** 7370 Discharge Planning 6485 Environmental Management: Home Preparation 7380 Financial Resource Assistance 7400 Health System Guidance 7410 Insurance Authorization 7440 Pass Facilitation 7460 Patient Rights Protection 2880 Preoperative Coordination **J** 7500 Sustenance Support 7560 Visitation Facilitation	7610 Bedside Laboratory Testing 7620 Controlled Substance Checking 7630 Cost Containment 7640 Critical Path Development 7650 Delegation 7660 Emergency Cart Checking 7680 Examination Assistance 8550 Fiscal Resource Management **c** 7690 Laboratory Data Interpretation 7700 Peer Review 7710 Physician Support 7722 Preceptor: Employee 7726 Preceptor: Student 7760 Product Evaluation 7800 Quality Monitoring 7820 Specimen Management 7850 Staff Development 7830 Staff Supervision 7840 Supply Management 7880 Technology Management	7910 Consultation 7930 Deposition/Testimony 7920 Documentation 7960 Health Care Information Exchange 7970 Health Policy Monitoring **c** 7980 Incident Reporting 8020 Multidisciplinary Care Conference 8060 Order Transcription 8100 Referral 8120 Research Data Collection 8140 Shift Report 6658 Surveillance: Remote Electronic 8180 Telephone Consultation 8190 Telephone Follow-up
	7300 to 7599	**7600 to 7899**	**7900 to 8199**

*Letter indicates another class where the intervention is also included.

Level 1 *Domains*	**7. COMMUNITY** **Care That Supports the Health of the Community**

Level 2 *Classes*	**c Community Health Promotion** Interventions that promote the health of the whole community	**d Community Risk Management** Interventions that assist in detecting or preventing health risks to the whole community

Level 3 *Interventions*	7320 Case Management **Y*** 8500 Community Health Development 8550 Fiscal Resource Management **a** 5510 Health Education **S** 7970 Health Policy Monitoring **b** 6530 Immunization/Vaccination Management **V** 8700 Program Development	8810 Bioterrorism Preparedness 8820 Communicable Disease Management 8840 Community Disaster Preparedness 6484 Environmental Management: Community 6489 Environmental Management: Worker Safety 8880 Environmental Risk Protection 6520 Health Screening **V** 6610 Risk Identification **V** 6652 Surveillance: Community 9050 Vehicle Safety Promotion **V**

8500 to 8799   **8800 to 9099**

*Letter indicates another class where the intervention is also included.

PART THREE

The
Classification

Abuse Protection Support   6400

Definition: Identification of high-risk dependent relationships and actions to prevent further infliction of physical or emotional harm

Activities:

Identify adult(s) with a history of unhappy childhoods associated with abuse, rejection, excessive criticism, or feelings of being worthless and unloved as children

Identify adult(s) who have difficulty trusting others or feel disliked by others

Identify whether individual feels asking for help is an indication of personal incompetence

Identify level of social isolation present in family situation

Determine whether family needs periodic relief from care responsibilities

Identify whether adult at risk has close friends or family available to help with children when needed

Determine relationship between husband and wife

Determine whether adults are able to take over for each other when one is too tense, tired, or angry to deal with a dependent family member

Determine whether child/dependent adult is viewed differently by an adult based on sex, appearance, or behavior

Identify crisis situations that may trigger abuse, such as poverty, unemployment, divorce, or death of a loved one

Monitor for signs of neglect in high-risk families

Observe a sick or injured child/dependent adult for signs of abuse

Listen to the explanation of how the illness or injury happened

Identify when the explanation of the cause of the injury is inconsistent between those involved

Encourage admission of child/dependent adult for further observation and investigation, as appropriate

Record times and durations of visits during hospitalization

Monitor parent-child interactions and record observations, as appropriate

Monitor for underreactions or overreactions on the part of an adult

Monitor child/dependent adult for extreme compliance, such as passive submission to hospital procedures

Monitor child for role reversal, such as comforting the parent or overactive or aggressive behavior

Listen attentively to adult who begins to talk about own problems

Listen to a pregnant woman's feelings about pregnancy and expectations about the unborn child

Monitor new parent's reactions to infant, observing for feelings of disgust, fear, or unrealistic expectations

Monitor for a parent who holds newborn at arm's length, handles him/her awkwardly, or asks for excessive assistance

Monitor for repeated visits to a clinic, emergency room, or physician's office for minor problems

Monitor for a progressive deterioration in the physical and emotional care provided to a child/dependent adult in the family

Monitor child for signs of failure to thrive, depression, apathy, developmental delay, or malnutrition

Determine expectations adult has for child to determine if expected behaviors are realistic

Instruct parents on realistic expectations of child based on developmental level

Establish rapport with families with a history of abuse for long-term evaluation and support

Help families identify coping strategies for stressful situations

Continued

A

Activities:—cont'd

Instruct adult family members on signs of abuse

Refer adult(s) at risk to appropriate specialists

Inform the physician of observations indicative of abuse

Report any situations where abuse is suspected to the proper authorities

Refer adult(s) to shelters for abused spouses, as appropriate

Refer parents to Parents Anonymous for group support, as appropriate

Encourage patient to contact police when physical safety is threatened

Inform patient of laws and services relevant to abuse

Background Readings:

Bohn, D.K. (1990). Domestic violence and pregnancy: Implications for practice. Journal of Nurse-Midwifery, 35(2), 86-98.

Lancaster, J., & Kerschner, D. (1992). Violence and human abuse. In M. Stanhope & J. Lancaster (Eds.), Community health nursing (3rd ed.) (pp. 411-427). St. Louis: Mosby–Year Book.

Roberts, C., & Quillan, J. (1992). Preventing violence through primary care intervention. Nurse Practitioner, 17(8), 62-70.

Vickrey, P.G. (2001). Protecting the older adult. Nursing Management, 30(7), 34-38.

Abuse Protection Support: Child   6402

Definition: Identification of high-risk, dependent child relationships and actions to prevent possible or further infliction of physical, sexual, or emotional harm or neglect of basic necessities of life

Activities:

Identify mothers who have a history of late (4 months or later) or no prenatal care

Identify parents who have had another child removed from the home or have placed previous children with relatives for extended periods

Identify parents who have a history of substance abuse, depression, or major psychiatric illness

Identify parents who demonstrate an increased need for parent education (e.g., parents with learning problems, parents who verbalize feelings of inadequacy, parents of a first child, teen parents)

Identify parents with a history of domestic violence or a mother who has a history of numerous "accidental" injuries

Identify parents with a history of unhappy childhoods associated with abuse, rejection, excessive criticism, or feelings of being worthless and unloved

Identify crisis situations that may trigger abuse (e.g., poverty, unemployment, divorce, homelessness, and domestic violence)

Determine whether the family has an intact social support network to assist with family problems, respite child care, and crisis child care

Identify infants/children with high-care needs (e.g., prematurity, low birth weight, colic, feeding intolerances, major health problems in the first year of life, developmental disabilities, hyperactivity, and attention deficit disorders)

Identify caretaker explanations of child's injuries that are improbable or inconsistent, allege self-injury, blame other children, or demonstrate a delay in seeking treatment

Determine whether a child demonstrates signs of physical abuse, including numerous injuries in various stages of healing; unexplained bruises and welts; unexplained pattern, immersion, and friction burns; facial, spiral, shaft, or multiple fractures; unexplained facial lacerations and abrasions; human bite marks; intracranial, subdural, intraventricular, and intraoccular hemorrhaging; whiplash shaken infant syndrome; and diseases that are resistant to treatment and/or have changing signs and symptoms

Determine whether the child demonstrates signs of neglect, including poor or inconsistent growth patterns, failure to thrive, wasting of subcutaneous tissue, consistent hunger, poor hygiene, constant fatigue and listlessness, bald patches on scalp or other skin afflictions, apathy, unyielding body posture, and inappropriate dress for weather conditions

Determine whether the child demonstrates signs of sexual abuse, including difficulty walking or sitting; torn, stained, or bloody underclothing; reddened or traumatized genitals; vaginal or anal lacerations; recurrent urinary tract infections; poor sphincter tone; acquired sexually transmitted diseases; pregnancy; promiscuous behavior or prostitution; a history of running away, sudden massive weight loss or weight gain, aggression against self, or dramatic behavioral or health changes of undetermined etiology

Determine whether the child demonstrates signs of emotional abuse, including lags in physical development, habit disorders, conduct learning disorders, neurotic traits/psychoneurotic reactions, behavioral extremes, cognitive developmental lags, and attempted suicide

Encourage admission of child for further observation and investigation, as appropriate

Record times and durations of visits during hospitalizations

Monitor parent-child interactions and record observations

Determine whether acute symptoms in child abate when child is separated from family

Continued

A

Activities:—cont'd

Determine whether parents have unrealistic expectations for child's behavior or whether they have negative attributions for their child's behavior

Monitor child for extreme compliance, such as passive submission to invasive procedures

Monitor child for role reversal, such as comforting the parent, or overactive or aggressive behavior

Listen to pregnant woman's feelings about pregnancy and expectations about the unborn child

Monitor new parents' reactions to their infant, observing for feelings of disgust, fear, or disappointment in gender

Monitor for a parent who holds newborn at arm's length, handles newborn awkwardly, asks for excessive assistance, and verbalizes or demonstrates discomfort in caring for the child

Monitor for repeated visits to clinics, emergency rooms, or physicians' offices for minor problems

Establish a system to flag the records of children who are suspected victims of child abuse or neglect

Monitor for a progressive deterioration in the physical and emotional state of the infant/child

Determine parent's knowledge of infant/child basic care needs and provide appropriate child care information as indicated

Instruct parents on problem solving, decision making, and childrearing and parenting skills, or refer parents to programs where these skills can be learned

Help families identify coping strategies for stressful situations

Provide parents with information on how to cope with protracted infant crying, emphasizing that they should not shake the baby

Provide the parents with noncorporal punishment methods for disciplining children

Provide pregnant women and their families with information on the effects of smoking, poor nutrition, and substance abuse on the baby's and their health

Engage parents and child in attachment-building exercises

Provide parents and their adolescents with information on decision making and communication skills and refer to youth services counseling, as appropriate

Provide older children with concrete information on how to provide for the basic care needs of their younger siblings

Provide children with positive affirmations of their worth, nurturing care, therapeutic communication, and developmental stimulation

Provide children who have been sexually abused with reassurance that the abuse was not their fault and allow them to express their concerns through play therapy appropriate for age

Refer at-risk pregnant women and parents of newborns to nurse home visitation services

Provide at-risk families with a Public Health Nurse referral to ensure that the home environment is monitored, that siblings are assessed, and that families receive continued assistance

Refer families to human services and counseling professionals, as needed

Provide parents with community resource information that includes addresses and phone numbers of agencies that provide respite care, emergency child care, housing assistance, substance abuse treatment, sliding-fee counseling services, food pantries, clothing distribution centers, health care, human services, hot lines, and domestic abuse shelters

Inform physician of observations indicative of abuse or neglect

Report suspected abuse or neglect to proper authorities

Refer a parent who is being battered and at-risk children to a domestic violence shelter

Refer parents to Parents Anonymous for group support, as appropriate

A

Background Readings:

Campbell, J., & Humphreys, J. (1993) Nursing care of survivors of family violence (2nd ed.). St. Louis: Mosby.

Campbell, J., & Humphreys, J. (1984). Nursing care of victims of family violence. Reston, VA: Reston Publishing.

Cicchetti, D., & Carlson, V. (Eds.). (1990). Child maltreatment: Theory and research on the causes and consequences of child abuse and neglect. New York: Cambridge University Press.

Cowen, P.S. (1994). Child abuse—What's nursing's role? In J.C. McCloskey & H.K. Grace (Eds.), Current issues in nursing (4th ed.) (pp. 731-741). St. Louis: Mosby.

Cowen, P.S., & Van Hoozer, H. (1993). Family violence computer assisted instruction programs. Chapel Hill: Health Sciences Consortium.

Dove, A., & Kobryn, M. (1991). Computer detection of child abuse. Nursing Standard, 6(10), 38-39.

Dykes, L.J. (1986). The whiplash shaken infant syndrome: What has been learned? Child Abuse & Neglect, 10, 211-221.

Rosenberg, D.A. (1987). Web of deceit: A literature review of Munchausen syndrome by proxy. Child Abuse & Neglect, 11(4), 547-563.

A

Abuse Protection Support: Domestic Partner 6403

Definition: Identification of high-risk, dependent domestic relationships and actions to prevent possible or further infliction of physical, sexual, or emotional harm or exploitation of a domestic partner

Activities:

Screen for risk factors associated with domestic abuse (e.g., history of domestic violence, abuse, rejection, excessive criticism, or feelings of being worthless and unloved; difficulty trusting others or feeling disliked by others; feeling that asking for help is an indication of personal incompetence; high physical care needs; intense family care responsibilities; substance abuse; depression; major psychiatric illness; social isolation; poor relationships between domestic partners; multiple marriages; pregnancy; poverty; unemployment; financial dependence; homelessness; infidelity; divorce; or death of a loved one)

Screen for symptoms of a history of domestic abuse (e.g., numerous accidental injuries, multiple somatic symptoms, chronic abdominal pain, chronic headaches, pelvic pain, anxiety, depression, post-traumatic stress syndrome, and other psychiatric disorders)

Monitor for signs and symptoms of physical abuse (e.g., numerous injuries in various stages of healing; unexplained lacerations, bruises, or welts of the face [particularly periorbital], mouth, torso, back, buttocks, or upper extremities; unexplained fractures of the skull, nose, ribs, or hips; patches of missing hair or tender scalp; bruises, chafing, or excoriation of the wrists or ankles or other restraining marks; "defensive" bruises on forearms; and human bite marks)

Monitor for signs and symptoms of sexual abuse (e.g., presence of semen or dried blood; injury to external genital, vaginal, anal, or penile areas; request to check fetal heart sounds; acquired sexually transmitted diseases; or dramatic behavioral or health changes of an undetermined etiology)

Monitor for signs and symptoms of emotional abuse (e.g., low self-esteem, depression, humiliation and defeat; overly cautious behavior around partner; aggression against self or suicide gestures)

Monitor for signs and symptoms of exploitation (e.g., inadequate provision for basic needs when adequate resources are available; deprivation of personal possessions; unexplained loss of social support checks; evidence that personal assets are taken without consent or approval or through the use of undue influence; or lack of knowledge of personal finances or legal matters)

Document evidence of physical or sexual abuse using standardized assessment tools and photographs

Listen attentively to individual who begins to talk about own problems

Identify inconsistencies in explanation of cause of injury(ies)

Determine congruence between the type of injury and the description of cause

Interview patient and/or knowledgeable other about suspected abuse in the absence of partner

Encourage admission to a hospital for further observation and investigation, as appropriate

Monitor partner interactions and record observations, as appropriate (e.g., record times and durations of partner visits during hospitalization, underreactions or overreactions by partner)

Monitor the individual for extreme compliance, such as passive submission to hospital procedures

Monitor for progressive deterioration in the physical and/or emotional state of individuals

Monitor for repeated visits to a clinic, emergency room, or physician's office for minor problems

Establish a system to flag individual records where there is suspicion of abuse

Provide positive affirmation of worth

Encourage expression of concerns and feelings, which may include fear, guilt, embarrassment, and self-blame

Provide support to empower victims to take action and make changes to prevent further victimization

Assist individuals and families in developing coping strategies for stressful situations

Assist individuals and families to objectively evaluate strengths and weaknesses of relationships

Refer individuals at risk for abuse or who have suffered abuse to appropriate specialists and services (e.g., public health nurse, human services, counseling, legal assistance)

Refer abusive partner to appropriate specialists and services

Provide confidential information regarding domestic violence shelters, as appropriate

Initiate development of a safety plan for use in the event that violence escalates

Report any situations in which abuse is suspected in compliance with mandatory reporting laws

Initiate community education programs designed to decrease violence

Monitor use of community resources

Background Readings:

Alpert, E. (1995). Violence in intimate relationships and the practicing internist: New "disease" or new agenda. Annals of Internal Medicine, 123(10), 774-781.

Campbell, J., Harris, M., & Lee, R. (1995). Violence research: An overview. Scholarly Inquiry for Nursing Practice: An International Journal, 9(2), 105-126.

Campbell, J., & Humphreys, J. (1993). Nursing care of survivors of family violence. St. Louis: Mosby.

Erickson, R., & Hart, S. (1998). Domestic violence: Legal, practice, and educational issues. Med Surg Nursing 7(3), 142-147, 164.

McFarlane, J., Christoffel, K., Bateman, L., Miller, V., & Bullock, L. (1991). Assessing for abuse: Self-report versus nurse interview. Public Health Nursing, 8(4), 245-250.

Parker, B., & McFarlane, J. (1991). Identifying and helping battered pregnant women. Maternal-Child Nursing, 16, 161-164.

Roberts, C., & Quillan, J. (1992). Preventing violence through primary care intervention. Nurse Practitioner, 17(8), 62-70.

A

Abuse Protection Support: Elder 6404

Definition: Identification of high-risk, dependent elder relationships and actions to prevent possible or further infliction of physical, sexual, or emotional harm; neglect of basic necessities of life; or exploitation

Activities:

Identify elder patients who perceive themselves to be dependent on caretakers due to impaired health status; functional impairment; limited economic resources; depression; substance abuse; or lack of knowledge of available resources and alternatives for care

Identify care arrangements that were made or continue under duress with only minimal consideration of the elder's care needs; the caregivers' abilities, characteristics, and competing responsibilities; need for environmental accommodations; and the history and quality of the relationships between the elder and the caregivers

Identify family crisis situations that may trigger abuse, such as poverty, unemployment, divorce, homelessness, or death of a loved one

Determine whether the elder patients and their caretakers have a functional social support network to assist the patient in performing activities of daily living and in obtaining health care, transportation, therapy, medications, community resource information, financial advice, and assistance with personal problems

Identify elder patients who rely on a single caretaker or family unit to provide extensive physical care assistance and monitoring

Identify caretakers who demonstrate impaired physical or mental health; substance abuse; depression; fatigue; financial problems or dependency; injuries that were inflicted by patient; failure to understand patient's condition or needs; intolerant or hypercritical attitudes towards patient; caregiver burnout; back injuries due to unassisted lifting or caretakers who threaten patient with abandonment, hospitalization, institutionalization, or painful procedures

Identify family caretakers who have a history of being abused or neglected in childhood

Identify caretaker explanations of patient's injuries that are improbable, inconsistent, allege self-injury, blame others, include activities beyond elder's physical abilities, or demonstrate a delay in seeking treatment

Determine whether elder patient demonstrates signs of physical abuse including numerous injuries in various stages of healing; unexplained lacerations, abrasions, bruises, or burns; unexplained fractures, blunt trauma, patches of missing hair or a tender scalp; and human bite marks

Determine whether the elder patient demonstrates signs of neglect including poor hygiene; inadequate or inappropriate (torn, dirty) clothing or deprivation of warm clothing or footwear; untreated skin lesions; contractures, impaired skin integrity, and decubiti; malnutrition or lack of adherence to prescribed diet; deprivation or inadequate aids to mobility and perception (canes, glasses, hearing aids); no dentures or decayed fractured teeth; perineal excoriation and skin breakdown; untreated health problems or repeated admissions due to inadequate health care surveillance; vermin infestation; medication deprivation or oversedation; and deprivation of social contacts

Determine whether the elder patient demonstrates signs of sexual abuse including presence of semen or dried blood; injury to external genital, vaginal, anal, or penile areas; acquired sexually transmitted diseases; or dramatic behavioral or health changes of undetermined etiology

Determine whether the elder patient demonstrates signs of emotional abuse including fear, anger, confusion, withdrawal, low self esteem, depression, humiliation and defeat; overly cautious behavior around caretaker; aggression against self or suicide gestures

Determine whether the elder patient demonstrates signs of exploitation including inadequate provision for basic needs when adequate resources are available; deprivation of personal possessions; unexplained loss of Social Security or pension checks; evidence that personal assets are taken without consent or approval or through the use of undue influence; or a lack of knowledge of personal finances or legal matters including guardianships and power of attorney

Encourage admission of patient for further observation and investigation, as appropriate

Monitor patient-caretaker interactions and record observations

Determine whether acute symptoms in patients abate when they are separated from caretakers

Determine whether caretakers have unrealistic expectations for patient's behavior or if they have negative attributions for the behavior

Monitor for extreme compliance with caretakers' demands or passive submission to invasive procedures

Monitor for repeated visits to clinics, emergency rooms, or physicians' offices for injuries, inadequate health care monitoring, inadequate surveillance, or inadequate environmental adaptations

Provide patients with positive affirmation of their worth and allow them to express their concerns and feelings, which may include fear, guilt, embarrassment, and self-blame

Assist caretakers to explore their feelings about relatives or patients in their care and to identify factors that are disturbing and appear to contribute to abusive and neglectful behaviors

Assist patients in identifying inadequate and harmful care arrangements and help them and their family members identify mechanisms for addressing these problems

Discuss concerns about observations of at-risk indicators separately with the elder patient and the caretaker

Determine the patient's and caretaker's knowledge and ability to meet the patient's care and safety needs and provide appropriate teaching

Help patients and their families identify coping strategies for stressful situations including the difficult decision to discontinue home care

Determine deviations from normal aging and note early signs and symptoms of ill health through routine health screenings

Promote maximum independence and self-care through innovative teaching strategies and the use of repetition, practice, reinforcement, and individualized pacing

Provide environmental assessment and recommendations for adapting the home to promote physical self-reliance or refer to appropriate agencies for assistance

Assist with restoration of full range of activities of daily living as possible

Instruct on the benefits of a routine regimen of physical activity, provide tailored exercise regimens, and refer to physical therapy or exercise programs as appropriate in order to prevent dependency

Implement strategies to enhance critical thinking, decision making, and remembering

Provide a Public Health Nurse referral to ensure that the home environment is monitored and that patient receives continued assistance

Provide referrals for patients and their families to human services and counseling professionals

Provide community resource information to elder patients and their caretakers that includes addresses and phone numbers of agencies that provide senior service assistance; home health care; residential care, respite care, emergency care, housing assistance, transportation; substance abuse treatment, sliding-fee counseling services, health care, and human services; food pantries and Meals on Wheels; clothing distribution centers; and hot lines

Caution patients to have their Social Security or pension checks directly deposited, not to accept personal care in return for transfer of assets, and not to sign documents or make financial arrangements before seeking legal advice

Encourage patients and their families to plan in advance for care needs, including who will assume responsibility if the patient becomes incapacitated and how to explore abilities, preferences, and options for care

Consult with community resources for information

Inform physician of observations indicative of abuse or neglect

Report suspected abuse or neglect to proper authorities

Continued

A

Background Readings:

Fulmer, T., Paveza, G., Abraham, I., Fairchild, S. (2000). Elder neglect assessment in the emergency department. Journal of Emergency Nursing 26(5), 436-443.

Klienschnmidt, K.C. (1997). Elder abuse: A review. Annals of Emergency Medicine, 30(4), 463-472.

White, S.W. (2000). Elder abuse: Critical care nurse role in detection. Critical Care Nurse Quarterly, 23(2), 20-25.

Abuse Protection Support: Religious   6408

Definition: Identification of high-risk, controlling religious relationships and actions to prevent infliction of physical, sexual, or emotional harm and/or exploitation.

Activities:

Identify individuals who are dependent on the religious "leader" due to impaired or altered religious development, mental or emotional impairment, depression, substance abuse, lack of social resources or financial issues

Identify patterns of behavior, thinking, and feeling in which a person experiences "control over" his/her religious journey by another

Identify church/family history for religious and/or ritual abuse, problem-solving and coping methods, emotional stability, degree of persuasive and manipulative techniques used and religious addiction

Determine whether the individual demonstrates signs of physical abuse, emotional abuse, exploitation, or religious addiction

Monitor individual and "leader" interactions, noting level of obedience demanded, tolerance for differences, persuasive and manipulation techniques employed, maturationally appropriate methods, content, and sense of "love" principle/life force/deity

Determine whether individual has a religious functional network to assist in meeting needs for belonging, care, and transcendence in a healthy manner

Offer prayer and healing services for the person and for past generational healing of the family/congregation

Help identify resources to meet the religious "safety" and support of the individual and group

Provide interpersonal support on a regular basis as needed

Refer for appropriate religious counseling

Refer to professional specialist if occult and/or satanic ritual abuse is suspected

Report suspected abuse to proper church and/or legal authorities

Background Readings:

Linn, M., Linn, S.F., & Linn, D. (1994). Healing spiritual abuse and religious addiction. New York: Paulist Press.
Linn, M., Linn, D., & Fabricant, S. (1985). Healing the greatest hurt. New York: Paulist Press.
McAll, K. (1982). Healing the family tree. London: Sheldon Press.
MacNutt, F. (1995). Deliverance from evil spirits: A practical manual. Grand Rapids, MI: Baker Book House Company.

A

Acid-Base Management   1910

Definition: Promotion of acid-base balance and prevention of complications resulting from acid-base imbalance

Activities:

Maintain patent IV access

Maintain a patent airway

Monitor arterial blood gases (ABGs) and serum and urine electrolyte levels, as appropriate

Monitor hemodynamic status, including CVP, MAP, PAP, and PCWP levels, if available

Monitor for loss of acid (e.g., vomiting, nasogastric output, diarrhea, and diuresis), as appropriate

Monitor for loss of bicarbonate (e.g., fistula drainage and diarrhea), as appropriate

Position to facilitate adequate ventilation (e.g., open airway and elevate head of bed)

Monitor for symptoms of respiratory failure (e.g., low PaO_2 and elevated $PaCO_2$ levels and respiratory muscle fatigue)

Monitor respiratory pattern

Monitor determinants of tissue oxygen delivery (e.g., PaO_2, SaO_2, and hemoglobin levels and cardiac output), if available

Provide oxygen therapy, if necessary

Provide mechanical ventilatory support, if necessary

Monitor determination of oxygen consumption (e.g., SvO_2 and $avDO_2$ levels), if available

Obtain ordered specimen for laboratory analysis of acid-base balance (e.g., ABG, urine, and serum levels), as appropriate

Monitor for worsening electrolyte imbalance with correction of the acid-base imbalance

Reduce oxygen consumption (e.g., promote comfort, control fever, and reduce anxiety), as appropriate

Monitor neurological status (e.g., level of consciousness and confusion)

Administer prescribed alkaline medications (e.g., sodium bicarbonate) as appropriate, based on ABG results

Provide frequent oral hygiene

Instruct the patient and/or family on actions instituted to treat the acid-base imbalance

Promote orientation

Background Readings:

American Association of Critical-Care Nurses. (1998). Core curriculum for critical care nursing (5th ed.). Philadelphia: WB Saunders.

Baer, C.L. (1993). Acid-base balance. In M.R. Kinney, D.R. Packa, & S.B. Dunbar (Eds.), AACN's clinical reference for critical-care nursing (pp. 209-216). St. Louis: Mosby.

Shapiro, B., Peruzzi, W.T., Kozelowski-Templin, R. (1994). Clinical application of blood gases (5th ed.). St. Louis: Mosby.

Kraut, J.A., & Madeas, N.E. (2001). Approach to patients with acid-base disorders. Respiratory Care, 46(4), 392-402.

Tasota, F.J., & Wesmiller, S.W. (1998). Keeping blood pH in equilibrium. Nursing 98, December, 35-40.

Acid-Base Management: Metabolic Acidosis   1911

A

Definition: Promotion of acid-base balance and prevention of complications resulting from serum HCO_3 levels lower than desired

Activities:

Obtain ordered specimen for laboratory analysis of acid-base balance (e.g., ABG, urine, and serum levels), as appropriate

Monitor ABG levels for decreasing pH level, as appropriate

Maintain patent IV access

Monitor intake and output

Position patient to facilitate ventilation

Monitor determinants of tissue oxygen delivery (e.g., PaO_2, SaO_2, and hemoglobin levels and cardiac output), if available

Monitor for electrolyte imbalances associated with metabolic acidosis (e.g., hyponatremia, hyperkalemia or hypokalemia, hypocalcemia, hypophosphatemia, and hypomagnesemia), as appropriate

Reduce oxygen consumption (e.g., promote comfort, control fever, and reduce anxiety), as appropriate

Monitor loss of bicarbonate through the GI tract (e.g., diarrhea, pancreatic fistula, small bowel fistula, and ileal conduit), as appropriate

Monitor for decreasing bicarbonate from excessive nonvolatile acids (e.g., renal failure, diabetic ketoacidosis, tissue hypoxia, and starvation), as appropriate

Administer prescribed alkaline medications (e.g., sodium bicarbonate) as appropriate, based on ABG results

Avoid administration of medications resulting in lowered HCO_3 level (e.g., chloride-containing solutions and anion exchange resins), as appropriate

Prevent complications from excessive $NaHCO_3$ administration (e.g., metabolic alkalosis, hypernatremia, volume overload, decreased oxygen delivery, decreased cardiac contractility, and enhanced lactic acid production)

Administer fluids as prescribed

Administer insulin and fluid hydration (isotonic and hypotonic) for diabetic ketoacidosis, causing metabolic acidosis, as appropriate

Prepare patient for dialysis (e.g., assist with catheter placement for dialysis), as appropriate

Assist with dialysis (e.g., hemodialysis or peritoneal dialysis), as appropriate

Institute seizure precautions

Provide frequent oral hygiene

Maintain bed rest, as indicated

Monitor for CNS manifestations of metabolic acidosis (e.g., headache, drowsiness, decreased mentation, seizures, and coma), as appropriate

Monitor for cardiopulmonary manifestations of metabolic acidosis (e.g., hypotension, hypoxia, arrhythmias, and Kussmaul respiration), as appropriate

Monitor for GI manifestations of metabolic acidosis (e.g., anorexia, nausea, and vomiting), as appropriate

Provide comfort measures to deal with the GI effects of metabolic acidosis

Encourage diet low in carbohydrate to decrease CO_2 production (e.g., administration of hyperalimentation and total parenteral nutrition), as appropriate

Instruct the patient and/or family on actions instituted to treat the metabolic acidosis

Continued

A

Background Readings:

Baer, C.L. (1993). Acid-base balance. In M.R. Kinney, D.R. Packa, & S.B. Dunbar (Eds.), AACN's clinical reference for critical-care nursing (pp. 209-216). St. Louis: Mosby.

Shapiro, B., Peruzzi, W.T., Kozelowski-Templin, R. (1994). Clinical application of blood gases (5th ed.). St. Louis: Mosby.

Speakman, E. (2001). Fluid, electrolyte, and acid-base balances, In Potter, P.A., & Perry A. (Eds.), Fundamental of Nursing (5th ed.). St Louis: Mosby.

Tasota, F.J., & Wesmiller, S.W. (1998). Keeping blood pH in equilibrium. Nursing 98, December, 35-40.

Acid-Base Management: Metabolic Alkalosis   1912

Definition: Promotion of acid-base balance and prevention of complications resulting from serum HCO_3 levels higher than desired

Activities:

Obtain ordered specimen for laboratory analysis of acid-base balance (e.g., ABG, urine, and serum levels), as appropriate

Monitor ABG levels for increased pH level

Maintain patent IV access, as appropriate

Monitor intake and output

Monitor determinants of tissue oxygen delivery (e.g., PaO_2, SaO_2, and hemoglobin levels and cardiac output), if available

Avoid administration of alkaline substances (e.g., IV sodium bicarbonate and PO or NG antacids), as appropriate

Monitor for electrolyte imbalances associated with metabolic alkalosis (e.g., hypokalemia, hypercalcemia, and hypochloremia), as appropriate

Monitor for associated excesses of bicarbonate (e.g., hyperaldosteronism, glucocorticoid excess, and licorice abuse), as appropriate

Monitor for renal loss of acid (e.g., diuretic therapy), as appropriate

Monitor for GI loss of acid (e.g., vomiting, NG tube suctioning and high chloride content diarrhea), as appropriate

Administer dilute acid (isotonic hydrochloride) or arginine monohydrochloride, as appropriate

Administer H_2-receptor antagonist (e.g., ranitidine or cimetidine) to block hydrochloride secretion from the stomach, as appropriate

Administer carbonic anhydrase–inhibiting diuretics (e.g., acetazolamide and methazolamide) to increase excretion of bicarbonate, as appropriate

Administer chloride to replace deficient anion (e.g., ammonium chloride or arginine hydrochloride, normal saline), as appropriate

Administer prescribed IV potassium chloride until underlying hypokalemia is corrected

Administer potassium-sparing diuretics (e.g., Spironolactone/Aldactone and Triamterene/Dyrenium), as appropriate

Administer antiemetics to reduce loss of HCl in emesis, as appropriate

Replace extracellular fluid deficit with IV saline, as appropriate

Irrigate NG tube with isotonic saline to avoid electrolyte washout, as appropriate

Monitor patient receiving digitalis for toxicity resulting from hypokalemia associated with metabolic alkalosis, as appropriate

Monitor for neurological and/or neuromuscular manifestations of metabolic alkalosis (e.g., seizures, confusion, stupor, coma, tetany, and hyperactive reflexes)

Assist with activities of daily living, as appropriate

Monitor for pulmonary manifestations of metabolic alkalosis (e.g., bronchospasm and hypoventilation)

Monitor for cardiac manifestations of metabolic alkalosis (e.g., arrhythmias, reduced contractility, and decreased cardiac output)

Monitor for GI manifestations of metabolic alkalosis (e.g., nausea, vomiting, and diarrhea)

Instruct the patient and/or family on actions instituted to treat the metabolic alkalosis

Continued

Background Readings:

Baer, C.L. (1993). Acid-base balance. In M.R. Kinney, D.R. Packa, & S.B. Dunbar (Eds.), AACN's clinical reference for critical-care nursing (pp. 209-216). St. Louis: Mosby.

Khanna, A., & Kurtzman, N.A. (2001). Metabloic alkalosis. Respiratory Care, 46(4), 354-365.

Shapiro, B., Peruzzi, W.T., Kozelowski-Templin, R. (1994). Clinical application of blood gases (5th ed.). St. Louis: Mosby.

Speakman, E. (2001). Fluid, electrolyte, and acid-base balances. In P.A. Potter & A. Perry (Eds.), Fundamentals of Nursing (5th ed.). St. Louis: Mosby.

Acid-Base Management: Respiratory Acidosis   1913

Definition: Promotion of acid-base balance and prevention of complications resulting from serum pCO_2 levels higher than desired

Activities:

Obtain ordered specimen for laboratory analysis of acid-base balance (e.g., ABG, urine, and serum levels), as appropriate

Monitor ABG levels for decreasing pH level, as appropriate

Monitor for indications of chronic respiratory acidosis (e.g., barrel chest, clubbing of nails, pursed-lips breathing, and use of accessory muscles), as appropriate

Monitor determinants of tissue oxygen delivery (e.g., PaO_2, SaO_2, and hemoglobin levels and cardiac output), if available

Monitor for symptoms of respiratory failure (e.g., low PaO_2 and elevated $PaCO_2$ levels and respiratory muscle fatigue)

Position patient for optimum ventilation-perfusion matching (e.g., good lung down, prone, semi-Fowlers), as appropriate

Maintain airway clearance (e.g., suction, insert or maintain artificial airway, chest physiotherapy, and cough-deep breath), as appropriate

Monitor respiratory pattern

Monitor work of breathing (e.g., respiratory rate, heart rate, use of accessory muscles, and diaphoresis)

Provide mechanical ventilatory support, if necessary

Provide low-carbohydrate, high-fat diet (e.g., Pulmocare feedings) to reduce CO_2 production, if indicated

Provide frequent oral hygiene

Monitor GI functioning and distention to prevent reduced diaphragmatic movement, as appropriate

Promote adequate rest periods (e.g., 90 minutes of undisturbed sleep, organize nursing care, limit visitors, and coordinate consults), as appropriate

Monitor neurological status (e.g., level of consciousness and confusion)

Instruct the patient and/or family on actions instituted to treat the respiratory acidosis

Contract with patient's visitors for limited visitation schedule to allow for adequate rest periods to reduce respiratory compromise, if indicated

Background Readings:

American Association of Critical Care Nurses. (1998). Core Curriculum for critical care nursing (5th ed.). Philadelphia: WB Saunders.

Baer, C.L. (1993). Acid-base balance. In C.L. Kinney, D.R. Packa, & S.B. Dunbar (Eds.), AACN's clinical reference for critical-care nursing (pp. 209-216). St. Louis: Mosby.

Shapiro, B., Peruzzi, W.T., Kozelowski-Templin, R. (1994). Clinical application of blood gases (5th ed.). St. Louis: Mosby.

A

Acid-Base Management: Respiratory Alkalosis   1914

Definition: Promotion of acid-base balance and prevention of complications resulting from serum pCO_2 levels lower than desired

Activities:

Obtain ordered specimen for laboratory analysis of acid-base balance (e.g., ABG, urine, and serum levels), as appropriate

Monitor ABG levels for increased pH level

Maintain patent IV access

Monitor intake and output

Maintain a patent airway

Monitor for hyperventilation resulting in respiratory alkalosis (e.g., hypoxemia, CNS injury, hypermetabolic states, GI distention, pain, and stress)

Monitor respiratory pattern

Monitor for indications of impending respiratory failure (e.g., low PaO_2 level, respiratory muscle fatigue, low SaO_2/SvO_2 level)

Monitor for hypophosphatemia associated with respiratory alkalosis, as appropriate

Monitor for neurological and/or neuromuscular manifestations of respiratory alkalosis (e.g., paresthesias, tetany, and seizures), as appropriate

Monitor for cardiopulmonary manifestations of respiratory alkalosis (e.g., arrhythmias, decreased cardiac output, and hyperventilation)

Provide oxygen therapy, if necessary

Provide mechanical ventilatory support, if necessary

Reduce oxygen consumption to minimize hyperventilation (e.g., promote comfort, control fever, and reduce anxiety), as appropriate

Promote adequate rest periods (e.g., 90 minutes of undisturbed sleep, organize nursing care, limit visitors, and coordinate consults), as appropriate

Administer sedatives, pain relief, neuromuscular-blocking agents (only if patient is mechanically ventilated), as appropriate

Promote stress reduction

Monitor mechanical ventilator settings for high-minute ventilation (i.e., rate, mode, and tidal volume), as appropriate

Provide frequent oral hygiene

Promote orientation

Instruct the patient and/or family on actions instituted to treat the respiratory alkalosis

Contract with patient's visitors for limited visitation schedule to allow for adequate rest periods to reduce respiratory compromise, if indicated

Background Readings:

Baer, C.L. (1993). Acid-base balance. In M.R. Kinney, D.R. Packa, & S.B. Dunbar (Eds.), AACN's clinical reference for critical-care nursing (pp. 209-216). St. Louis: Mosby.

Foster, G.T., Vaziri, N.D., Sassoon, C.S.H. (2001). Respiratory alkalosis. Respiratory Care, 46(4), 384-391.

Shapiro, B., Peruzzi, W.T., Kozelowski-Templin, R. (1994). Clinical application of blood gases (5th ed.). St. Louis: Mosby.

Acid-Base Monitoring   1920

Definition: Collection and analysis of patient data to regulate acid-base balance

Activities:

Obtain blood for determination of ABG levels, ensuring adequate circulation to the extremity before and after blood withdrawal

Place blood samples for ABG determination on ice, as appropriate, and send to the lab

Note patient's temperature and percent of oxygen administered at time blood was drawn

Note if arterial pH level is on the alkaline or acidotic side of the mean (7.4)

Note if $PaCO_2$ level shows respiratory acidosis, respiratory alkalosis, or normalcy

Note if the HCO_3 level shows metabolic acidosis, metabolic alkalosis, or normalcy

Examine the pH level in conjunction with the $PaCO_2$ and HCO_3 levels to determine whether the acidosis/alkalosis is compensated or uncompensated

Note the PaO_2, SaO_2, and hemoglobin levels to determine the adequacy of arterial oxygenation

Monitor end-tidal CO_2 level, as appropriate

Monitor for an increase in the anion gap (>14 mEq/L), signaling an increased production or decreased excretion of acid products

Monitor for signs and symptoms of HCO_3 deficit and metabolic acidosis: Kussmaul respirations, weakness, disorientation, headache, anorexia, coma, urinary pH level of <6, plasma HCO_3 level of <22 mEq/L, plasma pH level of <7.35, base excess of ≤2 mEq/L, associated hyperkalemia, and possible CO_2 deficit

Monitor for causes of possible HCO_3 deficit, such as diarrhea, renal failure, tissue hypoxia, lactic acidosis, diabetic ketoacidosis, malnutrition, and salicylate overdose

Administer oral or parenteral HCO_3 agents, if appropriate

Administer prescribed insulin and potassium for treatment of diabetic ketoacidosis, as appropriate

Monitor for signs and symptoms of HCO_3 excess and metabolic alkalosis: numbness and tingling of the extremities, muscular hypertonicity, shallow respirations with pause, bradycardia, tetany, urinary pH level of >7, plasma HCO_3 level of >26 mEq/L, plasma pH level of >7.45, BE of >2 mEq/L, associated hypokalemia, and possible CO_2 retention

Monitor for possible causes of HCO_3 excess, such as vomiting, gastric suction, hyperaldosteronism, diuretic therapy, hypochloremia, and excessive ingestion of medications containing HCO_3

Teach patient to avoid excessive use of medications containing HCO_3, as appropriate

Administer pharmacological agents to replace chloride, as appropriate

Monitor for signs and symptoms of carbonic acid deficit and respiratory alkalosis: frequent sighing and yawning, tetany, paresthesia, muscle twitching, palpitations, tingling and numbness, dizziness, blurred vision, diaphoresis, dry mouth, convulsions, pH level of >7.45, $PaCO_2$ <35 mm Hg, associated hyperchloremia, and possible HCO_3 deficit

Monitor for possible causes of carbonic acid deficits and associated hyperventilation, such as pain, CNS lesions, fever, and mechanical ventilation

Sedate patient to reduce hyperventilation, if appropriate

Administer pain medication, as appropriate

Treat fever, as appropriate

Administer parenteral chloride solutions to reduce HCO_3, while correcting the cause of respiratory alkalosis, as appropriate

Monitor for signs and symptoms of carbonic acid excess and respiratory acidosis: hand tremor with extensions of arms, confusion, drowsiness progressing to coma, headache, slowed verbal response,

Continued

A

Activities:—cont'd

nausea, vomiting, tachycardia, warm sweaty extremities, pH level of <7.35, $PaCO_2$ level of >45 mm Hg, associated hypochloremia, and possible HCO_3 excess

Monitor for possible causes of carbonic acid excess and respiratory acidosis, such as airway obstruction, depressed ventilation, CNS depression, neurological disease, chronic lung disease, musculoskeletal disease, chest trauma, infection, ARDS, cardiac failure, and use of respiratory depressant drugs

Support ventilation and airway patency in the presence of respiratory acidosis and rising $PaCO_2$ level, as appropriate

Administer oxygen therapy, as appropriate

Administer antimicrobial agents and bronchodilators, as appropriate

Administer low-flow oxygen and monitor for CO_2 narcosis in cases of chronic hypercapnia

---

Background Readings:

Coombs, M. (2001). Making sense of arterial blood gases. Nursing Times, 97(27), 6-38.

Paulson, W.D. (1999). Common causes of acid-base disorders. The Journal of Critical Illness, 14(2), 110-111.

Thelan, L.A., & Urden, L.D. (1993). Critical care nursing: Diagnosis and management (2nd ed.). St. Louis: Mosby.

Active Listening {4920}

Definition: Attending closely to and attaching significance to a patient's verbal and nonverbal messages

Activities:

Establish the purpose for the interaction

Display interest in the patient

Use questions or statements to encourage expression of thoughts, feelings, and concerns

Focus completely on the interaction by suppressing prejudice, bias, assumptions, preoccupying personal concerns, and other distractions

Display an awareness of and sensitivity to emotions

Use nonverbal behavior to facilitate communication (e.g., be aware of physical stance conveying nonverbal messages)

Listen for the unexpressed message and feeling, as well as content, of the conversation

Be aware of which words are avoided, as well as the nonverbal message that accompanies the expressed words

Be aware of the tone, tempo, volume, pitch, and inflection of the voice

Identify the predominant themes

Determine the meaning of the message by reflecting on attitudes, past experiences, and the current situation

Time a response so that it reflects understanding of the received message

Clarify the message through the use of questions and feedback

Verify understanding of messages through use of questions or feedback

Use a series of interactions to discover the meaning of behavior

Avoid barriers to active listening (e.g., minimizing feelings, offering easy solutions, interrupting, talking about self, and premature closure)

Use silence/listening to encourage the expression of feelings, thoughts, and concerns

Background Readings:

Audio Visual Campus. (1993). Active listening [Video]. San Diego: Levitz Sommer Productions.

Craven, R.F., & Hirnle, C.J. (2000) Fundamentals of nursing: Human health and function (3rd ed.) (pp. 336 338). Philadelphia. Lippincott

Helms, J. (1985). Active listening. In G.M. Bulechek & J.C. McCloskey (Eds.), Nursing interventions: Treatments for nursing diagnosis (pp. 328-337). Philadelphia: W.B. Saunders.

Johnson, B.S. (1993) Psychiatric–Mental Health Nursing (3rd ed.) (pp. 65-68). Philadelphia: Lippincott.

A

Activity Therapy   4310

> *Definition:* Prescription of and assistance with specific physical, cognitive, social, and spiritual activities to increase the range, frequency, or duration of an individual's (or group's) activity

Activities:

Collaborate with occupational, physical, and/or recreational therapists in planning and monitoring an activity program, as appropriate

Determine patient's commitment to increasing frequency and/or range of activity

Assist to explore the personal meaning of usual activity (e.g., work) and/or favorite leisure activities

Assist to choose activities consistent with physical, psychological, and social capabilities

Assist to focus on what patient can do, rather than on deficits

Assist to identify and obtain resources required for the desired activity

Assist to obtain transportation to activities, as appropriate

Assist patient to identify preferences for activities

Assist patient to identify meaningful activities

Assist patient to schedule specific periods for diversional activity into daily routine

Assist patient/family to identify deficits in activity level

Instruct patient/family regarding the role of physical, social, spiritual, and cognitive activity in maintaining function and health

Instruct patient/family how to perform desired or prescribed activity

Assist patient/family to adapt environment to accommodate desired activity

Provide activities to increase attention span in consultation with OT

Facilitate activity substitution when patient has limitations in time, energy, or movement

Refer to community centers or activity programs

Assist with regular physical activities (e.g., ambulation, transfers, turning, and personal care), as needed

Provide gross motor activities for hyperactive patient

Make environment safe for continuous large muscle movement, as indicated

Provide motor activity to relieve muscle tension

Provide noncompetitive, structured, and active group games

Promote engagement in recreational and diversional activities aimed at reducing anxiety: group singing; volleyball; table tennis; walking; swimming; simple, concrete tasks; simple games; routine tasks; housekeeping chores; grooming; puzzles and cards

Provide positive reinforcement for participation in activities

Assist patient to develop self-motivation and self-reinforcement

Monitor emotional, physical, social, and spiritual responses to activity

Assist patient/family to monitor patient's progress toward goal achievement

Background Readings:

Glick, O.J. (1992). Interventions related to activity and movement. In G.M. Bulechek & J.C. McCloskey (Eds.), *Symposium on Nursing Interventions. Nursing Clinics of North America,* 27(2), 541-568.

MacNeil, R., & Teague, M. (1987). *Aging and leisure: Vitality in later life.* Englewood Cliffs, NJ: Prentice-Hall.

McFarland, G.K., & McFarlane, E.A. (1997). *Nursing diagnosis and intervention.* (3rd ed.) St. Louis: Mosby.

Warnick, M.A. (1985). Acute care patients can stay active. *Journal of Gerontological Nursing,* 11(3), 31-35.

Acupressure 1320

Definition: Application of firm, sustained pressure to special points on the body to decrease pain, produce relaxation, and prevent or reduce nausea

Activities:

Screen for contraindications, such as contusions, scar tissue, infection, and serious cardiac conditions (also contraindicated for young children)

Decide on applicability of acupressure for treatment of a particular individual

Determine individual's degree of psychological comfort with touch

Determine desired outcomes

Refer to acupressure text to match the etiology, location, and symptomatology to appropriate acupoint after advanced training in the techniques of acupressure

Determine which acupoint(s) to stimulate, depending on desired outcome

Explain to individual that you will be searching for a tender area(s)

Encourage individual to relax during the stimulation

Probe deeply with finger, thumb, or knuckle for a very pressure-sensitive spot in the general location of the acupoint

Observe verbal or postural cues to identify desired point or location (such as wincing, "ouch")

Stimulate acupoint by pressing in with finger, thumb, or knuckle and using one's body weight to lean into the point to which pressure is applied

Use finger pressure or wristbands to apply pressure to selected acupoint for treating nausea

Apply steady pressure over hypertonic muscle tissue for pain until relaxation is felt or pain is reported to have decreased, usually 15 to 20 seconds

Repeat procedure over same point on opposite side of body

Treat the contralateral points first when there is extreme tenderness at any one point

Apply steady pressure until the nausea subsides or maintain wristbands indefinitely during actual or anticipated nausea

Observe for relaxation and verbalizations of decreases in discomfort or nausea

Use daily acupressure applications during the first week of treatment for pain

Recommend use of progressive relaxation techniques and/or stretching exercises between treatments

Teach family/significant other to provide acupressure treatments

Document action and individual response to acupressure

Background Readings:

Dibble, S.L., Chapman, J., Mack, K.A., & Shih, A. (2000). Acupressure for nausea: Results of a pilot study. Oncology Nursing Forum, 27(1), 41-47.

Lorenzi, E.A. (1999). Complementary/alternative therapies. So many choices. Geriatric Nursing, 20(3), 125-1336.

Mann E., (1999). Using acupuncture and acupressure to treat postoperative emesis. Professional Nurse, 14(10), 691-694.

Windle, P.E., Borromeo, A., Robles, H., & Ilacio-Uy, V. (2001). The effects of acupressure on the incidence of postoperative nausea and vomiting in postsurgical patients. Journal of Perianesthesia Nursing, 16(3), 158-162.

A

Admission Care   7310

Definition: Facilitating entry of a patient into a health care facility

Activities:

Introduce yourself and your role in providing care

Orient patient/family/significant others to expectations of care

Provide appropriate privacy for the patient/family/significant others

Orient patient/family/significant others to immediate environment

Orient patient/family/significant others to agency facilities

Obtain admission history including information on past medical illnesses, medications, and allergies

Perform admission physical assessment, as appropriate

Perform admission financial assessment, as appropriate

Perform admission psychosocial assessment, as appropriate

Perform admission religious assessment, as appropriate

Perform admission risk assessment (e.g., risk for falls, TB screening, skin assessment)

Provide patient with "Patient's Bill of Rights"

Obtain advance care directive information (i.e., Living Will and Durable Power of Attorney for Healthcare)

Document pertinent information

Maintain confidentiality of patient data

Identify patient at risk for readmission

Establish patient plan of care, nursing diagnoses, outcomes, and interventions

Begin discharge planning

Implement safety precautions, as appropriate

Label patient's chart, room door, and/or head of bed, as indicated

Notify physician of admission and patient status

Obtain physician's orders for patient care

Background Reading:

Perry, A., & Potter, P.A. (2002). Clinical nursing skill and techniques (5th ed.). St. Louis: Mosby.

Airway Insertion and Stabilization

3120

A

Definition: Insertion or assistance with insertion and stabilization of an artificial airway

Activities:

Select the correct size and type of oropharyngeal or nasopharyngeal airway

Insert oro/nasopharyngeal airway, ensuring that it reaches to the base of the tongue, supporting the tongue in a forward position

Tape the oro/nasopharyngeal airway in place

Monitor for dyspnea, snoring, or inspiratory crowing when oro/nasopharyngeal airway is in place

Change the oro/nasopharyngeal airway daily and inspect mucosa

Insert an esophageal obturator airway (EOA), as appropriate

Auscultate for breath sounds bilaterally before inflating the esophageal cuff of the EOA

Collaborate with the physician to select the correct size and type of endotracheal (ET) or tracheostomy tube

Select artificial airways with high-volume, low-pressure cuffs

Limit insertion of ET tubes and tracheostomies to qualified and credentialed personnel

Encourage physicians to place ET tubes via the oropharyngeal route, as appropriate

Assist with insertion of an endotracheal tube by gathering necessary intubation and emergency equipment, positioning patient, administering medications as ordered, and monitoring the patient for complications during insertion

Assist with emergent tracheostomy by setting up appropriate support equipment, administering medications, providing a sterile environment, and monitoring for changes in the patient's condition

Instruct patient and family about the intubation procedure

Auscultate the chest after intubation

Inflate endotracheal/tracheostomy cuff, using minimal occlusive volume technique or minimal leak technique

Stabilize endotracheal/tracheostomy tube with adhesive tape, twill tape, or commercially available stabilizing device

Mark endotracheal tube at the position of the lips or nares, using the centimeter markings on the ET tube, and document

Verify tube placement with a chest radiograph, ensuring cannulation of the trachea 2 to 4 cm above the carina

Minimize leverage and traction of the artificial airway by suspending ventilator tubing from overhead supports, using flexible catheter mounts and swivels, and supporting tubes during turning, suctioning, and ventilator disconnection/reconnection

Background Readings:

Heffner, J.E. (1990). Airway management in the critically ill patient. Critical Care Clinics, 6, 533-550.

Odom, J.L. (1993). Airway emergencies in the post anesthesia care unit. In K.L. Saleh & V. Binsko, (Eds.), Nursing Clinics of North America, 28(3), 483-493.

Thelan, L.A., & Urden, L.D. (1998). Critical care nursing: Diagnosis and management (3rd ed.). St. Louis: Mosby.

Titler, M.G., & Jones, G. (1992). Airway management. In G.M. Bulechek & J.C. McCloskey (Eds.), Nursing interventions: Essential nursing treatments (2nd ed.) (pp. 512-530). Philadelphia: W.B. Saunders.

Waugaman, W.R., Foster, S.D., & Rigor, B.M. (1992). Principles and practice of nurse anesthesia. Norwalk, CT: Appleton & Lange.

A

Airway Management

3140

Definition: Facilitation of patency of air passages

Activities:

Open the airway, using the chin lift or jaw thrust technique, as appropriate

Position patient to maximize ventilation potential

Identify patient requiring actual/potential airway insertion

Insert oral or nasopharyngeal airway, as appropriate

Perform chest physical therapy, as appropriate

Remove secretions by encouraging coughing or by suctioning

Encourage slow, deep breathing; turning; and coughing

Use fun techniques to encourage deep breathing for children (e.g., blow bubbles with bubble blower; blow on pinwheel, whistle, harmonica, balloons, party blowers; have blowing contest using ping-pong balls, feathers)

Instruct how to cough effectively

Assist with incentive spirometer, as appropriate

Auscultate breath sounds, noting areas of decreased or absent ventilation and presence of adventitious sounds

Perform endotracheal or nasotracheal suctioning, as appropriate

Administer bronchodilators, as appropriate

Teach patient how to use prescribed inhalers, as appropriate

Administer aerosol treatments, as appropriate

Administer ultrasonic nebulizer treatments, as appropriate

Administer humidified air or oxygen, as appropriate

Remove foreign bodies with McGill forceps, as appropriate

Regulate fluid intake to optimize fluid balance

Position to alleviate dyspnea

Monitor respiratory and oxygenation status, as appropriate

Background Readings:

American Association of Critical Care Nurses. (1998). Core curriculum for critical care nursing (5th ed.). Philadelphia: W.B. Saunders

Perry, A.G., & Potter, P.A. (2002). Clinical nursing skills and techniques (5th ed.). St. Louis: Mosby.

Racht, E.M. (2002). 10 pitfalls in airway management: how to avoid common airway management complications. JEMS: Journal of Emergency Medical Services, 27(3), 28-30, 32-4, 36-8.

Airway Suctioning   3160

Definition: Removal of airway secretions by inserting a suction catheter into the patient's oral airway and/or trachea

Activities:

Determine the need for oral and/or tracheal suctioning

Auscultate breath sounds before and after suctioning

Inform the patient and family about suctioning

Aspirate the nasopharynx with a bulb syringe or suction device, as appropriate

Provide sedation, as appropriate

Use universal precautions: gloves, goggles, and mask, as appropriate

Insert a nasal airway to facilitate nasotracheal suctioning, as appropriate

Instruct the patient to take several deep breaths before nasotracheal suctioning and use supplemental oxygen, as appropriate

Hyperoxygenate with 100% oxygen, using the ventilator or manual resuscitation bag

Hyperinflate at 1 to 1.5 times the preset tidal volume using the mechanical ventilator, as appropriate

Use sterile disposable equipment for each tracheal suction procedure

Select a suction catheter that is one half the internal diameter of the endotracheal tube, tracheostomy tube, or patient's airway

Instruct the patient to take slow, deep breaths during insertion of the suction catheter via the nasotracheal route

Leave the patient connected to the ventilator during suctioning, if a closed tracheal suction system or an oxygen insufflation device adaptor is being used

Use the lowest amount of wall suction necessary to remove secretions (e.g., 80 to 100 mm Hg for adults)

Monitor patient's oxygen status (SaO_2 and SvO_2 levels) and hemodynamic status (MAP level and cardiac rhythms) immediately before, during, and after suctioning

Base the duration of each tracheal suction pass on the necessity to remove secretions and the patient's response to suctioning

Hyperinflate and hyperoxygenate between each tracheal suction pass and after the final suction pass

Suction the oropharynx after completion of tracheal suctioning

Clean area around tracheal stoma after completion of tracheal suctioning, as appropriate

Stop tracheal suctioning and provide supplemental oxygen if patient experiences bradycardia, an increase in ventricular ectopy, and/or desaturation

Vary suctioning techniques, based on the clinical response of the patient

Note type and amount of secretions obtained

Send secretions for culture and sensitivity tests, as appropriate

Instruct the patient and/or family how to suction the airway, as appropriate

Continued

A

Background Readings:

Barnes, C., & Kirchhoff, K.T. (1986). Minimizing hypoxemia due to endotracheal suctioning: A review of the literature. Heart & Lung, 15, 164-176.

Craven, R. F., & Hirnle, C. J. (2000) Fundamentals of nursing: Human health and function (3rd ed.) (pp. 825-827). Philadelphia: Lippincott.

Nelson, D.M. (1992). Interventions related to respiratory care. In G.M. Bulechek & J.C. McCloskey (Eds.),

Symposium on Nursing Interventions. Nursing Clinics of North America, 27(2), 301-324.

Stone, K., & Turner, B. (1988). Endotracheal suctioning. Annual Review of Nursing Research, 7, 27-49.

Stone, K.S., Preusser, B.A., Groch, K.F., Karl, J.I., & Gronyon, D.S. (1991). The effect of lung hyperinflation and endotracheal suctioning on cardiopulmonary hemodynamics. Nursing Research, 40(2), 76-79.

Titler, M.G., & Jones, G. (1992). Airway management. In G.M. Bulechek & J.C. McCloskey (Eds.), Nursing interventions: Essential nursing treatments (2nd ed.) (pp. 512-530). Philadelphia: W.B. Saunders.

Allergy Management   6410

A

Definition: Identification, treatment, and prevention of allergic responses to food, medications, insect bites, contrast material, blood, and other substances

Activities:

Identify known allergies (e.g., medication, food, insect, environmental) and usual reaction

Notify caregivers and health care providers of known allergies

Document all allergies in clinical record, according to protocol

Place an allergy band on patient, as appropriate

Monitor patient for allergic reactions to new medications, formulas, foods, latex, and/or test dyes

Monitor the patient following exposures to agents known to cause allergic responses for signs of generalized flush, angioedema, urticaria, paroxysmal coughing, severe anxiety, dyspnea, wheezing, orthopnea, vomiting, cyanosis, or shock

Keep patient under observation for 30 minutes following administration of an agent known to be capable of inducing an allergic response

Instruct the patient with medication allergies to question all new prescriptions regarding potential for allergic reactions

Encourage patient to wear a medical alert tab, as appropriate

Identify immediately the level of threat an allergic reaction presents to patient's health status

Monitor for reoccurrence of anaphylaxis within 24 hours

Provide life-saving measures during anaphylactic shock or severe reactions

Provide medication to reduce or minimize an allergic response

Assist with allergy testing, as appropriate

Administer allergy injections, as needed

Watch for allergic responses during immunizations

Instruct patient/parent to avoid substances that cause allergic reactions, as appropriate

Instruct patient/parent in how to treat rashes, vomiting, diarrhea, or respiratory problems associated with exposure to allergy-producing substance

Instruct patient to avoid further use of substances causing allergic responses

Discuss methods to control environmental allergens (e.g., dust, mold, and pollen)

Instruct patient and caregiver(s) on how to avoid situations that put the patient at risk and how to respond if an anaphylactic reaction should occur

Instruct patient and caregiver on use of epinephrine pen

Background Readings:

Hendry, C., & Farley, A.H. (2001). Understanding allergies and their treatment. Nursing Standard, 15(35), 47-53.

Hoole, A., Pickard, C., Ouimette, R., Lohr, J., & Greenberg, R. (1995). Patient care guidelines for nurse practitioners (4th ed.). Philadelphia: J.B. Lippincott.

Lemone, P., & Burke, K. (1996). Medical surgical nursing: Critical thinking in client care. Menlo Park, CA: Addison-Wesley.

Trzcinski, K.M. (1993). Update on common allergic diseases. Pediatric Nursing, 19(4), 410-415.

A

Amnioinfusion   6700

Definition: Infusion of fluid into the uterus during labor to relieve umbilical cord compression or to dilute meconium-stained fluid

Activities:

Observe for signs of inadequate amniotic fluid volume (e.g., oligohydramnios, asymmetric intrauterine growth retardation, postdatism, known fetal urinary tract abnormalities, and prolonged rupture of membranes)

Recognize potential contraindications for amnioinfusion (e.g., amnionitis, polyhydramnios, multiple gestation, severe fetal distress, fetal scalp pH < 7.20, known fetal anomaly, known uterine anomaly)

Observe for variable or prolonged fetal heart rate decelerations during intrapartal electronic monitoring

Document presence of thick meconium fluid with rupture of membranes

Ensure informed consent

Prepare equipment needed for amnioinfusion

Flush intrauterine catheter with infusate

Use universal precautions

Place intrauterine catheter using sterile technique

Calibrate and flush catheter after placement using universal precautions

Infuse 500 to 1000 cc of isotonic IV solution rapidly into the uterine cavity per protocol or physician order

Place patient in Trendelenburg position, as appropriate

Maintain continuous infusion at prescribed rates

Monitor intrauterine pressure readings

Observe characteristics of return fluid

Change perineal pads, as appropriate

Document changes in intrapartal electronic monitor tracings

Observe for signs of adverse reaction (e.g., uterine overdistension, umbilical cord prolapse, and amniotic fluid embolism)

Determine cord blood gas levels at the time of delivery to evaluate effectiveness of intervention

Background Readings:

Longobucco, D., & Winkler, E. (1999). Amnioinfusion: Intrapartum indications and administration. Mother Baby Journal, 4(2), 13-18.

Snell, B.J. (1993). The use of amnioinfusion in nurse-midwifery practice. Journal of Nurse-Midwifery, 39(2), 62S-70S.

Weismiller, D.G. (1998). Transcervical amnioinfusion. American Family Physician, 1-9.

Amputation Care   3420

Definition: Promotion of physical and psychological healing before and after amputation of a body part

Activities:

Encourage the patient to participate in the decision to amputate, if possible, as patient participation is an important factor in postsurgical adjustment and rehabilitation

Ensure that the patient understands and accepts the need for amputation surgery prior to surgery, if possible

Provide information and support before and after surgery

Place a pressure-relieving mattress on the bed before surgery, as appropriate, to help prevent pressure sore development

Position stump in proper body alignment

Place a below-the-knee stump in an extended position

Avoid putting stump in a dependent position to decrease edema and vascular stasis

Avoid disturbing stump dressing immediately after surgery as long as there is no leakage or sign of infection

Wrap the stump, as required

Promote a smooth, conical-shaped stump through wrapping for a proper prosthesis fit

Monitor amount of edema present in stump

Monitor for phantom limb pain (burning, cramping, throbbing, crushing, or tingling pain where the limb was)

Explain that phantom limb pain may start several weeks after surgery and may be triggered by pressure on other areas

Administer various types of pain control (both pharmacological and nonpharmacological) as needed for comfort, both before and after surgery (e.g., TENS, phonophoresis, massage)

Monitor for psychological concerns related to change in body image, such as depression or anxiety

Teach patient to report signs and symptoms of impaired circulation (e.g., tingling, absent peripheral pulse, cool skin temperature)

Monitor wound healing at incision site

Place affected area in whirlpool bath, when appropriate

Inspect skin for signs of breakdown

Instruct patient on how to correctly perform range-of-motion exercises and why they are important after surgery

Assist patient with range-of-motion exercises, as needed

Instruct patient on endurance and strengthening exercises

Assist with endurance and strengthening exercises, as needed

Instruct patient to avoid sitting for long periods

Encourage use of a trapeze for movement in bed, as appropriate

Instruct in transfer techniques

Appraise a patient's adjustment to changes in body image

Accept initial need for concealment of stump

Provide gentle persuasion and support to view and handle altered body part

Continued

A

Activities:—cont'd

Assist patient with grieving process associated with the loss of the body part

Facilitate the identification of needed changes in lifestyle

Set mutual goals for progressive self-care

Encourage patient to practice self-care of stump

Provide appropriate education for self-care after discharge

Provide opportunities for interaction with persons with similar amputations, as appropriate

Provide appropriate information about prosthetic devices and mobilization techniques

Discuss need for long-range assistive devices (e.g., modifications to home and car), as appropriate

Discuss potential long-term goals for rehabilitation with patient, which may include walking without a support device (e.g., a cane or walker) or even jogging, as appropriate

Background Readings:

Bloomquist, T. (2001). Amputation and phantom limb pain: A pain-prevention model. AANA Journal, 69(3), 211-217.

Bryant, G. (2001). Stump care. AJN, 101(2), 67-71.

Esquenazi, A., & DiGiacomo, R. (2001). Rehabilitation after amputation. Journal of the American Podiatric Association, 91(1), 13-22.

Gibson, J (2001). Lower limb amputation. Nursing Standard, 15(28), 47-52.

Perry A.G., & Potter P.A. (2002). Clinical nursing skills and techniques (5th ed.) (pp. 1064-1067). St. Louis: Mosby.

Sjodahl, C., Jarnlo, G.-B., & Persson, B. (2001). Gait improvement in unilateral transfemoral amputees by a combined psychological and physiotherapeutic treatment. Journal of Rehabilitation Medicine, 33(3), 114-118.

Analgesic Administration   2210   A

Definition: Use of pharmacologic agents to reduce or eliminate pain

Activities:

Determine pain location, characteristics, quality, and severity before medicating patient

Check medical order for drug, dose, and frequency of analgesic prescribed

Check history for drug allergies

Evaluate the patient's ability to participate in selection of analgesic, route, and dose and involve the patient, as appropriate

Choose the appropriate analgesic or combination of analgesics when more than one is prescribed

Determine analgesic selections (narcotic, nonnarcotic, or NSAID), based on type and severity of pain

Determine the preferred analgesic, route of administration, and dosage to achieve optimal analgesia

Choose the IV route, rather than IM, for frequent pain medication injections, when possible

Sign out narcotics and other restricted drugs, according to agency protocol

Monitor vital signs before and after administering narcotic analgesics with first-time dose or if unusual signs are noted

Attend to comfort needs and other activities that assist in relaxation to facilitate response to analgesia

Administer analgesics around the clock to prevent peaks and troughs of analgesia, especially with severe pain

Set positive expectations regarding the effectiveness of analgesics to optimize patient response

Administer adjuvant analgesics and/or medications when needed to potentiate analgesia

Consider use of continuous infusion, either alone or in conjunction with bolus opioids, to maintain serum levels

Institute safety precautions for those receiving narcotic analgesics, as appropriate

Instruct patient to request PRN pain medication before the pain is severe

Inform the individual that with narcotic administration, drowsiness sometimes occurs during the first 2 to 3 days and then subsides

Correct misconceptions/myths patient or family members may hold regarding analgesics, particularly opioids (e.g., addiction and risks of overdose)

Evaluate the effectiveness of analgesic at regular frequent intervals after each administration, but especially after the initial doses, also observing for any signs and symptoms of untoward effects (e.g., respiratory depression, nausea and vomiting, dry mouth, and constipation)

Document response to analgesic and any untoward effects

Evaluate and document level of sedation for patients receiving opioids

Implement actions to decrease untoward effects of analgesics (e.g., constipation and gastric irritation)

Collaborate with the physician if drug, dose, route of administration, or interval changes are indicated, making specific recommendations based on equianalgesic principles

Teach about the use of analgesics, strategies to decrease side effects, and expectations for involvement in decisions about pain relief

Background Readings:

Clinton, P., & Eland, J.A. (1991). Pain. In M. Maas, K. Buckwalter, & M. Hardy (Eds.), Nursing diagnoses and interventions for the elderly (pp. 348-368). Redwood City, CA: Addison-Wesley.

Craven, R.F., & Hirnle, C.J. (2000). Fundamentals of nursing: Human health and function (3rd ed.) (pp. 1161-1168). Philadelphia: Lippincott

Herr, K.A., & Mobily, P.R. (1992). Interventions related to pain. In G.M. Bulechek & J.C. McCloskey (Eds.), Symposium on Nursing Interventions. Nursing Clinics of North America, 27(2), 347-370.

McCaffery, M., & Beebe, A. (1989). Pain. Clinical manual for nursing practice (pp. 42-123). St. Louis: Mosby.

Perry, A.G., & Potter, P.A. (1990). Clinical nursing skills and techniques (pp. 96-101). St. Louis: Mosby.

Analgesic Administration: Intraspinal 2214

Definition: Administration of pharmacologic agents into the epidural or intrathecal space to reduce or eliminate pain

Activities:

Check patency and function of catheter, port, and/or pump

Ensure that IV access is in place at all times during therapy

Label the catheter and secure it appropriately

Ensure that the proper formulation of the drug is used (e.g., correct concentration and preservative free)

Ensure narcotic antagonist availability for emergency administration and administer per physician order, as necessary

Start continuous infusion of analgesic agent after correct catheter placement has been verified, and monitor rate to ensure delivery of prescribed dosage of medication

Monitor temperature, blood pressure, respirations, pulse, and level of consciousness at appropriate intervals and record on flow sheet

Monitor level of sensory blockade at appropriate intervals and record on flow sheet

Monitor catheter site and dressings to check for a loose catheter or wet dressing, and notify appropriate personnel per agency protocol

Administer catheter site care according to agency protocol

Secure needle in place with tape and apply appropriate dressing according to agency protocol

Monitor for adverse reactions, including respiratory depression, urinary retention, undue somnolence, itching, seizures, nausea, and vomiting

Monitor orthostatic blood pressure and pulse before the first attempt at ambulation

Instruct patient to report side effects, alterations in pain relief, numbness of extremities, and need for assistance with ambulation if weak

Follow institutional policies for injection of intermittent analgesic agents into the injection port

Provide adjunct medications as appropriate (e.g., antidepressants, anticonvulsants, and nonsteroidal antiinflammatory agents)

Increase intraspinal dose, based on pain intensity score

Instruct and guide patient through nonpharmalogical measures (e.g., simple relaxation therapy, simple guided imagery, and biofeedback) to enhance pharmacological effectiveness

Instruct patient about proper home care for external or implanted delivery systems, as appropriate

Remove or assist with removal of catheter according to agency protocol

Background Readings:

Acute Pain Management Panel. (1992). Acute pain management: Operative or medical procedures and trauma. Clinical practice guideline. AHCPR Pub. No. 92-0032. Rockville, MD: Agency for Health Care Policy and Research, Public Health Service, U.S. Department of Health and Human Services.

American Nurses Association. (1992). ANA position statement: The role of the registered nurse in the management of analgesia by catheter techniques. SCI Nursing, 9(2), 54-55.

El-Baz, N., & Goldin, M. (1987). Continuous epidural infusion of morphine for pain relief after cardiac operations. Journal of Cardiovascular Surgery, 93, 878-883.

Keeney, S. (1993). Nursing care of the postoperative patient receiving epidural analgesia. MEDSURG Nursing, 2(3), 191-196.

Paice, J., & Magolan, J. (1991). Intraspinal drug therapy. Nursing Clinics of North America, 26(2), 477-498.

Wild, L., & Coyne, C. (1992). The basics and beyond: Epidural analgesia. American Journal of Nursing, 92(4), 26-34.

Anaphylaxis Management   6412

Definition: Promotion of adequate ventilation and tissue perfusion for an individual with a severe allergic (antigen-antibody) reaction

Activities:

Identify and remove source of allergen, if possible

Administer aqueous epinephrine 1:1000 subcutaneously with appropriate dosing for age

Place individual in a comfortable position

Apply tourniquet per protocol immediately proximal to the allergen point of entry (e.g., injection site, IV site, insect bite, etc.), when possible, as appropriate

Establish and maintain a patent airway

Administer oxygen at high flow rate (10-15 L/min)

Monitor vital signs

Start an IV infusion of normal saline, lactated Ringer's, or a plasma volume expander, as appropriate

Reassure the individual and the family members

Monitor for signs of shock, (e.g., respiratory difficulty, cardiac arrhythmias, seizures, and hypotension)

Monitor for self-reports of impending doom

Maintain flow sheet of activities, including vital signs and medication administration

Administer IV fluids rapidly (1000 ml/hr) to support blood pressure, per physician order or protocol

Administer spasmolytics, antihistamines, or corticosteroids as indicated if urticaria, angioedema, or bronchospasm present

Consult with other healthcare providers and refer, as needed

Monitor for recurrence of anaphylaxis within 24 hours

Instruct the individual and family on the use of an epinephrine injection pen

Instruct the individual and family on prevention of future episodes

Background Readings:

Hoole, A., Pickard, C., Ouimette, R., Lohr, J.H., & Greenberg, R. (1996). Individual care guidelines for nurse practitioners (4th ed.). Philadelphia: J.B. Lippincott.

Jevon, P. (2001), Anaphylaxis: Emergency treatments. Nursing Times 96(14), 39-40.

Lemone, P., & Burke, K. (1996). Medical surgical nursing: Critical care thinking in client care. Redwood City, CA: Addison-Wesley.

Project Team of the Resuscitation Council (UK). (1999). Emergency medical treatment of anaphylactic reaction. Journal of Accidental Emergency Medicine, 16, 243-247.

A

Anesthesia Administration   2840

Definition: Preparation for and administration of anesthetic agents and monitoring of patient responsiveness during administration

Activities:

Verify patient identification

Perform and document the patient's health history and physical assessment, evaluating preexisting conditions, allergies, and contraindications for specific anesthetic agents or techniques

Request appropriate consultations, as well as diagnostic and laboratory studies, based on the patient's health status and proposed surgery

Implement indicated preoperative activities to prepare patient physiologically for surgery and anesthesia

Develop and document an anesthetic plan appropriate for the patient and procedure

Collaborate with involved health care providers throughout all phases of anesthesia care

Inform the patient what to expect from anesthesia, answering any questions and concerns

Obtain informed consent

Perform a safety check on all anesthesia equipment before each anesthetic is administered

Ensure availability of essential emergency and resuscitation equipment

Start appropriate intravenous and invasive monitoring lines and initiate noninvasive monitoring modalities

Administer appropriate preanesthetic medications and fluids

Assist in the transfer of the patient from the stretcher to the operating room table

Position patient to prevent peripheral nerve damage and pressure injuries

Ensure proper placement of safety strap and continuous patient safety throughout all phases of anesthesia care

Deliver anesthetic consistent with each patient's physiological needs, patient's requests, clinical judgment, and Standards for Nurse Anesthesia Practice

Assess and maintain an adequate airway, ensuring adequate oxygenation during all phases of anesthesia care

Determine acceptable blood loss and administer blood, if needed

Calculate appropriate fluid needs and administer intravenous fluids, as indicated

Monitor vital signs, respiratory and circulatory adequacy, response to anesthesia, and other physiological parameters; measure and evaluate appropriate lab values

Administer adjunct drugs and fluids necessary to manage the anesthetic, maintain physiological homeostasis, and correct adverse or unfavorable responses to anesthesia and surgery

Provide eye protection

Assess and clinically manage emergence from anesthesia by administering indicated medications, fluids, and ventilatory support

Transfer patient to the postanesthesia or intensive care unit with appropriate monitoring and oxygen therapy

Provide comprehensive patient report to nursing staff on arrival in unit

Manage postoperative pain and anesthetic side effects

Ascertain patient recovery and stability in the immediate postoperative period before transfer of care

Provide postanesthesia follow-up evaluation and care related to anesthesia side effects and complications after discharge from postanesthesia care area

A

Background Readings:

American Association of Nurse Anesthetists. (1989). Professional practice manual for the certified registered nurse anesthetist. American Association of Nurse Anesthetists Monograph.

Barash, P.G., Cullen, B.F., & Stoeling, R.K. (1989). Handbook of clinical anesthesia. Philadelphia: J.B. Lippincott.

Waugaman, W.R., Foster, S.D., & Rigor, B.M. (1992). Principles and practice of nurse anesthesia. Norwalk, CT: Appleton & Lange.

A

Anger Control Assistance   4640

Definition: Facilitation of the expression of anger in an adaptive, nonviolent manner

Activities:

Establish basic trust and rapport with patient

Use a calm, reassuring approach

Determine appropriate behavioral expectations for expression of anger, given patient's level of cognitive and physical functioning

Limit access to frustrating situations until patient is able to express anger in an adaptive manner

Encourage patient to seek assistance from nursing staff or responsible others during periods of increasing tension

Monitor potential for inappropriate aggression and intervene before its expression

Prevent physical harm if anger is directed at self or others (e.g., restrain and remove potential weapons)

Provide physical outlets for expression of anger or tension (e.g., punching bag, sports, clay, and writing in a journal)

Provide reassurance to patient that nursing staff will intervene to prevent patient from losing control

Use external controls (e.g., physical or manual restraint, time outs, and seclusion) as needed, to calm patient who is expressing anger in a maladaptive manner

Provide feedback on behavior to help patient identify anger

Assist patient in identifying the source of anger

Identify the function that anger, frustration, and rage serve for the patient

Identify consequences of inappropriate expression of anger

Assist patient in planning strategies to prevent the inappropriate expression of anger

Identify with patient the benefits of expressing anger in an adaptive, nonviolent manner

Establish expectation that patient can control his/her behavior

Instruct on use of calming measures (e.g., time outs and deep breaths)

Assist in developing appropriate methods of expressing anger to others (e.g., assertiveness and use of feeling statements)

Provide role models who express anger appropriately

Support patient in implementing anger control strategies and in the appropriate expression of anger

Provide reinforcement for appropriate expression of anger

Background Readings:

Carpenito, L.J. (1993). Nursing diagnosis: Application to clinical practice (5th ed.). New York: J.B. Lippincott.

Haven, E., & Piscitello, V. (1989). The patient with violent behavior. In S. Lewis, R.D.K. Grainger, W.A. McDowell, et al. (Eds.), Manual of psychosocial nursing interventions: Promoting mental health in medical-surgical settings (pp. 187-204). Philadelphia: W.B. Saunders.

Kanak, M.F. (1992). Interventions related to safety. In G.M. Bulechek & J.C. McCloskey (Eds.), Symposium on nursing interventions. Nursing Clinics of North America, 27(2), 371-395.

Townsend, M.C. (1988). Nursing diagnoses in psychiatric nursing: A pocket guide for care plan construction. Philadelphia: F.A. Davis.

Animal-Assisted Therapy   4320

Definition: Purposeful use of animals to provide affection, attention, diversion, and relaxation

Activities:

Determine patient's acceptance of animals as therapeutic agents

Determine if patient has any allergies to animals

Teach patient/family purpose and rationale for having animals in a care environment

Enforce standards for screening, training, and grooming of animals in therapy program

Enforce standards for health maintenance of animals in therapy program

Fulfill health inspector's rules concerning animals in an institution

Develop/have protocol that outlines appropriate response to accident or injury as result of animal contact

Provide therapy animals for patient such as dogs, cats, horses, snakes, turtles, gerbils, guinea pigs, and birds

Avoid animal visits with unpredictable or violent patients

Monitor closely animal visits with patients with special conditions (e.g., open wounds, delicate skin, multiple IV lines, or other equipment)

Facilitate patient's holding and petting therapy animals

Encourage repeated stroking of the therapy animal

Facilitate patient's watching therapy animals

Encourage patient's expression of emotions to animals

Arrange for patient to exercise, as appropriate

Encourage patient to play with therapy animals

Encourage patient to feed/groom animals

Have patient and others who pet or contact an animal wash hands

Provide an opportunity to reminisce and share about previous experiences with pets/other animals

Background Readings:

Barba, B.E. (1995). The positive influence of animals: Animal assisted therapy in acute care. Clinical Nurse Specialist 9(4), 199-202.

Cole, K. M. (1999). Animal-assisted therapy. In G. M. Bulechek, J.C. McCloskey (Eds.), Nursing Interventions: Effective nursing treatments (3rd ed.) (pp. 508-519). Philadelphia: W.B. Saunders.

Giuliano, K., Bloniasz, E., Bell, J. (1999). Implementation of a pet visitation program in critical care. Critical Care Nurse, 19(3), 43-50.

Johnson, R.A. (Ed.). (2002) Special issue: Human-animal interaction research. Western Journal of Nursing Research, 24(6), 606-715

Jorgenson, J. (1997). Therapeutic use of companion animals in health care. Image 29(3), 249-254.

Owen, O.G. (2001). Paws for thought. Nursing Times, 97(9), 28-29.

A

Anticipatory Guidance 5210

Definition: Preparation of patient for an anticipated developmental and/or situational crisis

Activities:

Assist the patient to identify possible upcoming, developmental, and/or situational crisis and the effects the crisis may have on personal and family life

Instruct about normal development and behavior, as appropriate

Provide information on realistic expectations related to the patient's behavior

Determine the patient's usual methods of problem solving

Assist the patient to decide how the problem will be solved

Assist the patient to decide who will solve the problem

Use case examples to enhance the patient's problem-solving skills, as appropriate

Assist the patient to identify available resources and options for course of action, as appropriate

Rehearse techniques needed to cope with upcoming developmental milestone or situational crisis with the patient, as appropriate

Assist the patient to adapt to anticipated role changes

Provide a ready reference for the patient (e.g., educational materials/pamphlets), as appropriate

Suggest books/literature for the patient to read, as appropriate

Refer the patient to community agencies, as appropriate

Schedule visits at strategic developmental/situational points

Schedule extra visits for patient with concerns or difficulties

Schedule follow-up phone calls to evaluate success or reinforcement needs

Provide the patient with a phone number to call for assistance, if necessary

Include the family/significant others, as appropriate

Background Readings:

Craven, R. F., & Hirnle, C.J. (2000). Fundamentals of nursing: Human health and function (3rd ed.) (pp. 1269-1270). Philadelphia: Lippincott.

Denehy, J.A. (1990). Anticipatory guidance. In M.J. Craft & J.A. Denehy (Eds.), Nursing interventions for infants and children (pp. 53-68). Philadelphia: W.B. Saunders.

Rakel, B.A. (1992). Interventions related to patient teaching. In G.M. Bulechek & J.C. McCloskey (Eds.), Symposium on Nursing Interventions. Nursing Clinics of North America, 27(2), 397-424.

Schulman, J.L., & Hanley, K.K. (1987). Anticipatory guidance: An idea whose time has come. Baltimore: Williams & Wilkins.

Smith, C.E. (1987). Using the teaching process to determine what to teach and how to evaluate learning. In C.E. Smith (Ed.), Patient education: Nurses in partnership with other health professionals (pp. 61-95). Philadelphia: W.B. Saunders.

Anxiety Reduction 5820

Definition: Minimizing apprehension, dread, foreboding, or uneasiness related to an unidentified source of anticipated danger

Activities:

Use a calm, reassuring approach

Clearly state expectations for patient's behavior

Explain all procedures, including sensations likely to be experienced during the procedure

Seek to understand the patient's perspective of a stressful situation

Provide factual information concerning diagnosis, treatment, and prognosis

Stay with patient to promote safety and reduce fear

Encourage family to stay with patient, as appropriate

Provide objects that symbolize safeness

Administer back rub/neck rub, as appropriate

Encourage noncompetitive activities, as appropriate

Keep treatment equipment out of sight

Listen attentively

Reinforce behavior, as appropriate

Create an atmosphere to facilitate trust

Encourage verbalization of feelings, perceptions, and fears

Identify when level of anxiety changes

Provide diversional activities geared toward the reduction of tension

Help patient identify situations that precipitate anxiety

Control stimuli, as appropriate, for patient needs

Support the use of appropriate defense mechanisms

Assist patient to articulate a realistic description of an upcoming event

Determine patient's decision-making ability

Instruct patient in use of relaxation techniques

Administer medications to reduce anxiety, as appropriate

Observe for verbal and nonverbal signs of anxiety

Background Readings:

Badger, J.M. (1994). Calming the anxious patient. American Journal of Nursing, 94(5), 46-50.
Perry, A.G., & Potter, P.A. (2002). Clinical nursing skills and techniques (5th ed.). St. Louis: Mosby.

A

Area Restriction 6420

> *Definition:* Limitation of patient mobility to a specified area for purposes of safety or behavior management

Activities:

Obtain a physician's order, if required by institutional policy, to use a physically restrictive intervention

Restrict to designated area that is appropriate to needs

Identify for patient and significant others those behaviors that necessitated the intervention

Explain procedure, purpose, and time period of the intervention to patient and significant others in understandable and nonpunitive terms

Explain to patient and significant others the behaviors necessary for termination of the intervention

Use protective devices (e.g., restraints, side rails, locked doors, fences, and gates) to physically limit mobility or access to harmful situations

Provide appropriate level of supervision/surveillance to monitor patient and to allow for therapeutic actions, as needed

Give immediate feedback about inappropriate behavior that patient can control and that contributes to need for continued restrictive intervention

Identify appropriate behavior

Assist patient to modify inappropriate behavior, when possible

Provide verbal reminders, as necessary, to remain in designated area

Provide for patient's psychological comfort, as needed

Offer structured activities within designated area to facilitate patient cooperation with restriction

Administer PRN medications for anxiety or agitation

Monitor the patient's response to procedure

Provide positive reinforcement for patient cooperation with restriction

Evaluate, at regular intervals, patient's need for continued restrictive intervention

Involve patient, when appropriate, in making decisions to move to a more/less restrictive form of intervention

Process with the patient and staff on termination of the restrictive intervention, the circumstances that led to the use of the intervention, as well as any patient concerns about the intervention itself

Document the rationale for use of restrictive intervention, patient's response to the intervention, patient's physical condition, nursing care provided throughout the intervention, and rationale for terminating the intervention

Provide the next appropriate level of restrictive intervention (e.g., physical restraint or seclusion), as needed

Background Readings:

Craig, C., Ray, F., & Hix, C. (1989). Seclusion and restraint: Decreasing the discomfort. Journal of Psychosocial Nursing and Mental Health Services, 27(7), 16-19.

Kanak, M.F. (1992). Interventions related to safety. In G.M. Bulechek & J.C. McCloskey (Eds.), Symposium on Nursing Interventions. Nursing Clinics of North America, 27(2), 371-396.

Kozier, B., & Erb, G. (1991). Fundamentals of nursing: Concepts and procedures (4th ed.). Menlo Park, CA: Addison-Wesley.

Aromatherapy   1330

Definition: Administration of essential oils through massage, topical ointments or lotions, baths, inhalation, douches, or compresses (hot or cold) to calm and soothe, provide pain relief, enhance relaxation and comfort

Activities:

Obtain verbal consent for use of aromatherapy

Select appropriate essential oil or blend of essential oils to obtain desired outcome

Determine individual response to the selected aroma (e.g., like vs. dislike) prior to use

Use education and training in the background and philosophy in the use of essential oils, mode of action, and any contraindications

Monitor individual for discomfort and nausea before and after administration

Dilute essential oils with appropriate carrier oils prior to topical use

Monitor for contact dermatitis associated with possible allergy to essential oils

Monitor for exacerbation of asthma in conjunction with use of essential oils, as appropriate

Instruct individual on purposes and application of aromatherapy, as appropriate

Monitor baseline and follow-up vital signs, as appropriate

Monitor individual for preadministration and postadministration report of level of stress, mood, and anxiety, as appropriate

Administer essential oil using appropriate methods (e.g., massage, inhalation) and to appropriate areas of the body (e.g., feet, back)

Document physiological responses to aromatherapy, as appropriate

Evaluate and document response to aromatherapy

Background Readings:

Bryan-Brown, C. W., & Dracup, K. (1995). Alternative therapies. American Journal of Critical Care, 4(6), 416-418.

Buckle, J. (1998). Clinical aromatherapy and touch: Complementary therapies for nursing practice. Critical Care Nurse, 18(5), 54-61.

Buckle, J. (2001). The role of aromatherapy in nursing care. Nursing Clinics of North America, 36(1), 57-72.

Cooke, B., & Ernst, E. (2000). Aromatherapy: A systematic review. British Journal of General Practice, 50, 493-496.

Dunn, C., Sleep, J., & Collett, D. (1995). Sensing an improvement: An experimental study to evaluate the use of aromatherapy, massage and periods of rest in an intensive care unit. Journal of Advanced Nursing, 21, 34-40.

Petersen, D. (September/October 1997). Aromatherapy: Psychological effects of essential oils. Alternative Therapies in Clinical Practice, 4(5), 165-167.

Stevensen, C. J. (1994). The psychophysiological effects of aromatherapy massage following cardiac surgery. Complementary Therapies in Medicine, 2, 27-35.

Tate, S. (1997). Peppermint oil: A treatment for postoperative nausea. Journal of Advanced Nursing, 26, 543-549.

Wheeler Robins, J.L. (1999). The science and art of aromatherapy. Journal of Holistic Nursing, 17(1), 5-17.

A

Art Therapy

Definition: Facilitation of communication through drawings or other art forms

Activities:

Provide art supplies appropriate for developmental level and goals for therapy

Provide a quiet environment that is free from interruptions

Discuss description of drawing or artistic creation with patient

Provide a smooth, flat surface for drawing

Spend time with patient during the use of artistic medium

Observe patient's approach to artistic medium (e.g., hesitant, meticulous, or aggressive)

Record verbal comments made by patient during art therapy

Record observations made about approach to art therapy

Encourage patient to describe drawing or artistic creation

Record patient's interpretation of drawing or artistic creation

Discuss with patient what to draw, using direct or nondirect approach, as appropriate

Identify themes in artwork collected over a period of time

Copy patient's artwork for files, as needed and as appropriate

Use human figure drawings to determine patient's self-concept

Use Kinetic Family Drawings to determine family interaction patterns

Use drawings to determine the effects of stress events (e.g., hospitalization, divorce, or abuse) on patient

Compare artwork with patient's developmental level

Interpret meaning of significant aspects of the drawings, incorporating patient assessment data and literature on art therapy

Avoid reading meaning into drawings before having a complete history, baseline drawings, and a collection of drawings done over a period

Background Readings:

Denehy, J.A. (1990). Communicating with children through drawings. In M.J. Craft & J.A. Denehy (Eds.), Nursing Interventions for Infants and Children (pp. 111-126). Philadelphia: W.B. Saunders.

Kus, R.J., & Miller, M.A. (1992). Art therapy. In G.M. Bulechek & J.C. McCloskey (Eds.), Nursing Interventions: Essential Nursing Treatments (2nd ed.) (pp. 392-402). Philadelphia: W.B. Saunders.

Artificial Airway Management   3180

Definition: Maintenance of endotracheal and tracheostomy tubes and prevention of complications associated with their use

Activities:

Provide an oropharyngeal airway or bite block to prevent biting on the endotracheal tube, as appropriate

Provide 100% humidification of inspired gas/air

Provide adequate systemic hydration via oral or intravenous fluid administration

Inflate endotracheal/tracheostoma cuff using minimal occlusive volume technique or minimal leak technique

Maintain inflation of the endotracheal/tracheostoma cuff at 15 to 20 mm Hg during mechanical ventilation and during and after feeding

Suction the oropharynx and secretions from the top of the tube cuff before deflating cuff

Monitor cuff pressures every 4 to 8 hours during expiration using a three-way stopcock, calibrated syringe, and mercury manometer

Check cuff pressure immediately after delivery of any general anesthesia

Change endotracheal tapes/ties every 24 hours, inspect the skin and oral mucosa, and move ET tube to the other side of the mouth

Loosen commercial endotracheal tube holders at least once a day, and provide skin care

Auscultate for presence of lung sounds bilaterally after insertion and after changing endotracheal/tracheostomy ties

Note the centimeter reference marking on endotracheal tube to monitor for possible displacement

Assist with chest x-ray examination, as needed, to monitor position of tube

Minimize leverage and traction on the artificial airway by suspending ventilator tubing from overhead supports, using flexible catheter mounts and swivels, and supporting tubes during turning, suctioning, and ventilator disconnection and reconnection

Monitor for presence of crackles and rhonchi over large airways

Monitor for decrease in exhaled volume and increase in inspiratory pressure in patients receiving mechanical ventilation

Institute endotracheal suctioning, as appropriate

Institute measures to prevent spontaneous decannulation: secure artificial airway with tape/ties; administer sedation and muscle-paralyzing agent, as appropriate; and use arm restraints, as appropriate

Provide additional intubation equipment and ambu bag in a readily available location

Provide trachea care every 4 to 8 hours as appropriate: clean the inner cannula, clean and dry the area around the stoma, and change tracheostomy ties

Inspect skin around tracheal stoma for drainage, redness, and irritation

Maintain sterile technique when suctioning and providing tracheostomy care

Shield the tracheostomy from water

Provide mouth care and suction oropharynx, as appropriate

Tape the tracheostomy obturator to head of bed

Tape a second tracheostomy tube (same type and size) and forceps to head of bed

Institute chest physiotherapy, as appropriate

Ensure that endotracheal/tracheostomy cuff is inflated during feedings, as appropriate

Continued

A

Activities:—cont'd

Elevate head of the bed or assist patient to a sitting position in a chair during feedings, as appropriate

Add food coloring to enteral feedings, as appropriate

Background Readings:

Boggs, R.L., & Woolridge-Kim, M. (1993). AACN procedural manual for critical care (3rd ed). Philadelphia: W.B. Saunders.

Craven, R.F., & Hirnle, C. J. (2000) Fundamentals of Nursing: Human Health and Function (3rd ed.) (pp. 819-824). Philadelphia: Lippincott

Goodnough, S.K.C. (1988). Reducing tracheal injury and aspiration. Dimensions of Critical Care Nursing, 7, 324-331.

McHugh, J.M. (1985). Airway management. In S. Millar, L.K., Sampson, & M. Soukup (Eds.), AACN Procedural Manual for Critical Care (pp. 203-239). Philadelphia: W.B. Saunders.

Nelson, D.M. (1992). Interventions related to respiratory care. In G.M. Bulechek & J.C. McCloskey (Eds.), Symposium on Nursing Interventions. Nursing Clinics of North America, 27(2), 301-324.

Titler, M.G., & Jones, G. (1992). Airway management. In G.M. Bulechek & J.C. McCloskey (Eds.), Nursing Interventions: Essential Nursing Treatments (2nd ed.) (pp. 512-530). Philadelphia: W.B. Saunders.

Aspiration Precautions   3200

Definition: Prevention or minimization of risk factors in the patient at risk for aspiration

Activities:

Monitor level of consciousness, cough reflex, gag reflex, and swallowing ability

Monitor pulmonary status

Maintain an airway

Position upright 90 degrees or as far as possible

Keep tracheal cuff inflated

Keep suction setup available

Feed in small amounts

Check NG or gastrostomy tube placement before feeding

Check NG or gastrostomy tube residual before feeding

Avoid feeding, if residuals are high

Place "dye" in NG feeding tube

Avoid liquids or use thickening agent

Offer foods or liquids that can be formed into a bolus before swallowing

Cut food into small pieces

Request medication in elixir form

Break or crush pills before administration

Keep head of bed elevated 30 to 45 minutes after feeding

Suggest speech pathology consult, as appropriate

Suggest barium cookie swallow or video fluoroscopy, as appropriate

Background Readings:

Ackerman, L.L. (1992). Interventions related to neurological care. In G.M. Bulechek & J.C. McCloskey (Eds.), Symposium on Nursing Interventions. Nursing Clinics of North America, 27(2), 325-346.

American Nurses' Association Council in Medical-Surgical Nursing Practice & American Association of Neuroscience Nurses. (1985). Neuroscience nursing practice: Process and outcome for selected diagnoses. Kansas City, MO: American Nurses Association.

Maas, M.L., Buckwalter, K.C., Hardy, M.D., Reimer, T.T., Titler, M.G., & Specht, J.P. (2001) Nursing Care of Older Adults: Diagnoses, Outcomes, and Interventions (pp. 167-168). St. Louis: Mosby.

Sands, J.A. (1991). Incidence of pulmonary aspiration in intubated patients receiving enteral nutrition through wide- and narrow-bore nasogastric feeding tubes. Heart & Lung, 20(1), 75-80.

Schwartz-Cowley, R., & Gruen, A.K. (1988). Swallowing dysfunction in patients with altered mobility. In P.H. Mitchell, L.C. Hodges, M. Muwaswes, et al. (Eds.), AANN's Neuroscience Nursing (pp. 345-357). Norwalk, CT: Appleton & Lange.

Taylor, T. (1982). A comparison of two methods of nasogastric tube feedings. Journal of Neurosurgical Nursing, 14(1), 49-55.

A

Assertiveness Training 4340

Definition: Assistance with the effective expression of feelings, needs, and ideas while respecting the rights of others

Activities:

Determine barriers to assertiveness (e.g., developmental stage, chronic medical or psychiatric condition, and female socialization)

Help patient recognize and reduce cognitive distortions that block assertion

Differentiate between assertive, aggressive, and passive-aggressive behaviors

Help to identify personal rights, responsibilities, and conflicting norms

Help clarify problem areas in interpersonal relationships

Promote expression of thoughts and feelings, both positive and negative

Help identify self-defeating thoughts

Assist patient to distinguish between thought and reality

Instruct patient in the different ways to act assertively

Instruct patient about strategies for practicing assertive behavior (e.g., making requests, saying no to unreasonable requests, and initiating and concluding conversation)

Facilitate practice opportunities, using discussion, modeling, and role playing

Help practice conversational and social skills (e.g., use of "I" statements, nonverbal behaviors, openness, and accepting compliments)

Praise efforts to express feelings and ideas

Monitor anxiety level and discomfort related to behavioral change

Background Readings:

Barker, P. (1990). Breaking the shell. Nursing Times, 86(46), 36-38.

Craven, R.F., & Hirnle, C.J. (2000). Fundamentals of nursing: Human health and function (3rd ed.) (p. 1311). Philadelphia: Lippincott.

Pointer, P., & Lancaster, J. (1988). Assertiveness. In M. Stanhope & J. Lancaster (Eds.), Community health nursing (2nd ed.) (pp. 609-625). St. Louis: Mosby.

Sadler, A.G. (1985). Assertiveness training. In G.M. Bulechek & J.C. McCloskey (Eds.), Nursing interventions: Treatments for nursing diagnoses (pp. 234-254). Philadelphia: W.B. Saunders.

Smith, K.E., Schreiner, B., Jackson, C., & Travis, L.B. (1993). Teaching assertive communication skills to adolescents with diabetes: Evaluation of a camp curriculum. The Diabetes Educator, 19(2), 136-141.

Asthma Management 3210

Definition: Identification, treatment, and prevention of reactions to inflammation/constriction in the airway passages

Activities:

Determine baseline respiratory status to use as a comparison point

Document baseline measurements in clinical record

Compare current status with previous status to detect changes in respiratory status

Obtain spirometry measurements (FEV_1, FVC, FEV_1/FVC ratio) before and after the use of a short-acting bronchodilator

Monitor peak expiratory flow rate (PERF), as appropriate

Educate patient about the use of the PERF meter at home

Monitor for asthmatic reactions

Determine client/family understanding of disease and management

Instruct client/family on antiinflammatory and bronchodilator medications and their appropriate use

Teach proper techniques for using medication and equipment (e.g., inhaler, nebulizer, peak flow meter)

Determine compliance with prescribed treatments

Encourage verbalization of feelings about diagnosis, treatment, and impact on lifestyle

Identify known triggers and usual reaction

Teach client to identify and avoid triggers as possible

Establish a written plan with the client for managing exacerbations

Assist in the recognition of signs/symptoms of impending asthmatic reaction and implementation of appropriate response measures

Monitor rate, rhythm, depth, and effort of respiration

Note onset, characteristics, and duration of cough

Observe chest movement, including symmetry, use of accessory muscles, and supraclavicular and intercostal muscle retractions

Auscultate breath sounds, noting areas of decreased/absent ventilation and adventitious sounds

Administer medication as appropriate and/or per policy and procedural guidelines

Auscultate lung sounds after treatment to determine results

Offer warm fluids to drink, as appropriate

Coach in breathing/relaxation techniques

Use a calm, reassuring approach during asthma attack

Inform client/family about the policy and procedures for carrying and administration of asthma medications at school

Inform parent/guardian when child has needed/used PRN medication in school, as appropriate

Refer for medical assessment, as appropriate

Establish a regular schedule of follow-up care

Instruct and monitor pertinent school staff in emergency procedures

Prescribe and/or renew asthma medications, as appropriate

Continued

A

Background Readings:

American Academy of Allergy, Asthma and Immunology. (1999). Pediatric Asthma: Promoting Best Practice. Guide for Managing Asthma in Children. Milwaukee, WI: Author.

National Asthma Education and Prevention Program. Second Expert Panel. (1997). Guidelines for Diagnosis and Management of Asthma. NIH Publication No. 97-4051.

Silkworth, C.K. (1993). IHP: Asthma. In M.B. Haas, M.J.V. Gerber, W.R. Miller, K.M. Kalb, C.K. Silkworth, R.E. Leuhr, & S.I.S. Will. (Eds.), The School Nurse's Source Book of Individualized Healthcare Plans—Volume 1. (pp. 133-150). North Branch, MN: Sunrise River Press.

Szilagyi, P. & Kemper, K. (1999). Management of chronic childhood asthma in the primary care office. Pediatric Annals, 28(1), 43-52.

University of Michigan Health System. (2000). Asthma: Guidelines for clinical care. Available online: http://www.cme.med.umich.edu/ pdf/guideline/asthma.pdf

Yoos, H.L., & McMullen, A. (1999). Symptom monitoring in childhood asthma: How to use a peak flow meter. Pediatric Annals, 28(1), 31-39.

Attachment Promotion   6710

A

Definition: Facilitation of the development of the parent-infant relationship

Activities:

Discuss parent's reaction to pregnancy

Determine the image mother has of her unborn child

Ascertain before birth whether parent(s) has names picked out for both sexes

Provide parent(s) the opportunity to hear fetal heart tones as soon as possible

Discuss parental reaction to hearing fetal heart tones

Provide parent(s) the opportunity to see the ultrasound image of fetus

Identify body parts of infant on ultrasound image

Discuss parent's reaction to viewing ultrasound image of fetus

Encourage parent(s) to note fetal movement

Discuss parent's reaction to fetal movement

Encourage parent(s) to attend prenatal classes

Encourage father/significant other to participate in labor and delivery

Assist father/significant other during participation in labor and delivery

Place infant on mother's body immediately after birth

Encourage mother to hold, touch, and examine the infant while umbilical cord is being severed

Provide father opportunity to hold newborn in delivery area

Provide pain relief for mother

Provide opportunity for parent(s) to see, hold, and examine newborn immediately after birth

Encourage parent(s) to hold infant close to body

Share information gained from initial physical assessment of newborn with parent(s)

Inform parent(s) of care being given to newborn

Keep infant with parent(s) after birth, when possible

Provide family privacy during initial interaction with newborn

Encourage parent(s) to touch and speak to newborn

Assist parent(s) to participate in infant care

Encourage parent(s) to identify family characteristics observed in newborn

Encourage parents to massage infant

Reinforce eye contact with infant

Reinforce caregiver role behaviors

Provide assistance in self-care to maximize focus on infant

Provide rooming-in in hospitals

Encourage parent(s) to bring toys or clothing for newborn

Assist parent(s) in planning for early discharge

Phone parent to determine how family is coping with transition to home environment

Refer for further follow-up care, when appropriate

Continued

A

Activities:—cont'd

Explain equipment used to monitor infant in nursery

Encourage parent(s) to visit infant in the nursery

Demonstrate ways to touch infant confined to isolette

Place pictures of family in isolette so infant can "see" the family

Encourage parent(s) to bring personal items, such as toys or pictures, to be put in isolette or at bedside of infant

Provide parent(s) opportunity to hold and care for infant while in the nursery

Encourage parent(s) to see and touch newborn before transport

Take Polaroid picture of infant to leave with mother before transporting infant to another hospital

Encourage father and mother to accompany infant transferred to another hospital

Inform parent(s) of care being given to infant in another hospital

Inform parent(s) of behavioral characteristics infant exhibits while being cared for in another hospital

Give parent(s) footprint of infant to orientate to reality of size of newborn

Discuss infant behavioral characteristics with parent(s)

Point out infant state changes to parent(s)

Assist parent(s) in planning infant care during alert state

Point out infant cues that show responsiveness to parent(s)

Instruct parent(s) on signs of overstimulation

Reinforce normal aspects of infant with defect

Give parent lock of infant's hair when shaved for IV

Background Readings:

Denehy, J.A. (1992). Interventions related to parent-infant attachment. In G.M. Bulechek & J.C. McCloskey (Eds.), Symposium on Nursing Interventions. Nursing Clinics of North America, 27(2), 425-444.

Pressler, J.L. (1990). Promoting attachment. In M.J. Craft & J.A. Denehy (Eds.), Nursing Interventions for Infants and Children (pp. 4-17). Philadelphia: W.B. Saunders.

Wong, D.L., & Wilson, D. (1995). Whaley & Wong's Nursing Care of Infants and Children (5th ed.) (pp. 324-328). St. Louis: Mosby.

Autogenic Training   5840

Definition: Assisting with self-suggestions about feelings of heaviness and warmth for the purpose of inducing relaxation

Activities:

Choose a quiet, comfortable setting

Prepare a quiet environment

Take precautions to prevent interruptions

Instruct patient on purpose for the intervention

Seat patient in a reclining chair or place in recumbent position

Have patient wear comfortable, unrestricted clothing

Read a prepared script to patient, pausing for enough time for the statement to be internally repeated

Use statements in the script that elicit feelings of heaviness, lightness, or floating of specific body parts

Instruct patient to repeat statements to self and to elicit the feeling within the body part being directed

Rehearse with the script for about 15 to 20 minutes

Encourage patient to remain relaxed for another 15 to 20 minutes

Provide home instructions with a script or audiotape for patient to use

Proceed to elicit feelings of warmth after heaviness sensations have been mastered

Follow the procedure for eliciting heaviness using a prepared script or audiotape for eliciting warmth

Background Readings:

Scandrett, S., & Uecker, S. (1992). Relaxation training. In G.M. Bulechek & J.C. McCloskey (Eds.), Nursing interventions: Essential nursing treatments (2nd ed.) (pp. 434-461). Philadelphia: W.B. Saunders.

Tiernan, P.J. (1994). Independent nursing interventions: Relaxation and guided imagery in critical care. Critical Care Nurse, October, 47-51.

A

Autotransfusion

2860

Definition: Collecting and reinfusing blood that has been lost intraoperatively or postoperatively from clean wounds

Activities:

Screen for appropriateness of salvage (contraindications include sepsis or infection or tumor at the site, blood containing an irrigant that is not injectable, hemostatic agents, or microcrystalline collagen)

Determine the risk/benefit ratio

Obtain patient's informed consent

Instruct patient regarding procedure

Use appropriate blood retrieval system

Label collection device with the patient's name, hospital number, date, and time that collection was begun

Monitor patient and system frequently during retrieval

Maintain integrity of the system before, during, and after blood retrieval

Screen blood for appropriateness of reinfusion

Maintain integrity of blood between salvage and reinfusion

Prepare blood for reinfusion

Document time of initiation of collecting, condition of blood, type and amount of anticoagulants, and retrieval volume

Reinfuse transfusion within 6 hours of retrieval

Maintain universal precautions

Background Readings:

American Association of Blood Banks. (1990). Guidelines for blood salvage and reinfusion in surgery and trauma. Arlington, VA: The Association.

Arlington, R.G., Costigan, K.A., & Aievoli, C.P. (1992). Postoperative orthopaedic blood salvage and reinfusion. Orthopaedic Nursing, 11(3), 30-38.

Failla, S.D., & Radaslovich, N. (1993). Ask the OR. American Journal of Nursing, 93(6), 74.

LeMone, P., & Burke, K.M. (2000). Medical – Surgical Nursing: Critical Thinking in Client Care (2nd ed.) (p. 281). Upper Saddle River, NJ: Prentice Hall Health.

Peterson, K.J. (1992). Nursing management of autologous blood transfusion. Journal of Intravenous Nursing, 15(3), 128-134.

Bathing   1610

B

Definition: Cleaning of the body for the purposes of relaxation, cleanliness, and healing

Activities:

Assist with chair shower, tub bath, bedside bath, standing shower, or sitz bath, as appropriate or desired

Wash hair, as needed and desired

Bathe in water of a comfortable temperature

Use fun bathing techniques with children (e.g. wash dolls or toys; pretend a boat is a submarine; punch holes in bottom of plastic cup, fill with water, and let it "rain" on child)

Assist with perineal care, as needed

Assist with hygiene measures (e.g., use of deodorant or perfume)

Administer foot soaks, as needed

Shave patient, as indicated

Apply lubricating ointment and cream to dry skin areas

Offer hand washing after toileting and before meals

Apply drying powders to deep skin folds

Monitor skin condition while bathing

Monitor functional ability while bathing

Background Readings:

Perry, A.G., & Potter, P.A. (2002). Clinical nursing skills and techniques (5th ed.). St. Louis: Mosby.

Sloane, P.D., Rader, J., Barrick, A.L., Hoeffer, B., Dwyer, D., McKenzie, D., Lavelle, M., Buckwalter, K., Arrington, L., & Pruitt, T. (1995). Bathing persons with dementia. The Gerontologist, 35(5), 672-678.

Wong, D.L. (1995). Whaley and Wong's nursing care of infants and children (5th ed.). St. Louis: Mosby.

B

Bed Rest Care

0740

Definition: Promotion of comfort and safety and prevention of complications for a patient unable to get out of bed

Activities:

Explain reasons for requiring bed rest

Place on an appropriate therapeutic mattress/bed

Position in proper body alignment

Avoid using rough-textured bed linens

Keep bed linen clean, dry, and wrinkle free

Apply a footboard to the bed

Use devices on the bed (e.g., sheepskin) that protect the patient

Apply appliances to prevent footdrop

Raise siderails, as appropriate

Place bed-positioning switch within easy reach

Place the call light within reach

Place bedside table within patient's reach

Attach trapeze to the bed, as appropriate

Turn, as indicated by skin condition

Turn the immobilized patient at least every 2 hours, according to a specific schedule

Monitor skin condition

Teach bed exercises, as appropriate

Facilitate small shifts of body weight

Perform passive and/or active range-of-motion exercises

Assist with hygiene measures (e.g., use of deodorant or perfume)

Assist with activities of daily living

Apply antiembolism stockings

Monitor for constipation

Monitor for urinary function

Monitor pulmonary status

Background Readings:

Potter, P.A., & Perry, A. (1998). Fundamentals of nursing: Concepts, process and practice (4th ed.). St. Louis: Mosby.

Titler, M.G., Pettit, D., Bulechek, G.M., McCloskey, J.C., Craft, M.J., Cohen, M.Z., Crossley, J.D., Denehy, J.A., Glick, O.J., Kruckeberg, T.W., Maas, M.L., Prophet, C.M., & Tripp-Reimer, T. (1991). Classification of nursing interventions for care of the integument. Nursing Diagnosis, 2(2), 45-56.

Bedside Laboratory Testing 7610

Definition: Performance of laboratory tests at the bedside or point of care

Activities:

Obtain adequate training/orientation before performing testing

Participate in color blindness testing, as needed for particular test and as required by institution

Participate in proficiency testing programs, as required by institution

Follow institutional procedures for specimen collection and preservation, as appropriate

Label specimens immediately to minimize sample mix-ups, as appropriate

Obtain appropriate specimen for the bedside test being performed

Perform bedside testing on collected specimens in a timely manner

Use universal precautions when handling specimens for testing

Store reagents according to manufacturer's requirements or as stated in your institution's procedure manual

Check expiration date of any reagent preparation, including test strips and contents of commercial kits to avoid using expired reagents

Follow manufacturer's guidelines and institutional procedures for instrument calibration

Document instrument calibration, as required

Perform quality control checks according to manufacturer's recommendation or as stated in institutional procedure

Document quality control checks, as required

Perform test according to manufacturer's directions or as stated in institutional procedures

Ensure accurate timing with testing that requires prescribed times

Document results of tests, according to institutional procedure

Report abnormal or critical results to physician, as appropriate

Perform cleaning and maintenance of instruments according to manufacturer's guidelines or as stated in institutional procedure

Document cleaning and maintenance, as required

Report test results to patient, as appropriate

Background Readings:

College of American Pathologists, Commission on Laboratory Accreditation. (1993). Inspection checklist: Ancillary testing. Northfield, IL: College of Pathologists.

Corbett, J.V. (1992). Laboratory tests & diagnostic procedures with nursing diagnoses (3rd ed.). Norwalk, CT: Appleton & Lange.

Kee, J.L. (1991). Laboratory and diagnostic tests with nursing implications (3rd ed.). Norwalk, CT: Appleton & Lange.

Perry, A.C., & Potter, P.A. (1998). Clinical nursing skills & techniques (4th ed.). St. Louis: Mosby.

B

Behavior Management   **4350**

Definition: Helping a patient to manage negative behavior

Activities:

Hold the patient responsible for his/her behavior

Communicate expectation that patient will retain control

Consult with family to establish patient's cognitive baseline

Set limits with patient

Refrain from arguing or bargaining about the established limits with the patient

Establish routines

Establish shift-to-shift consistency in environment and care routine

Use consistent repetition of health routines as a means of establishing them

Avoid interruptions

Increase physical activity as appropriate

Limit number of caregivers

Use a soft, low speaking voice

Avoid cornering the patient

Redirect attention away from agitation source

Avoid projecting a threatening image

Avoid arguing with patient

Ignore inappropriate behavior

Discourage passive-aggressive behavior

Praise efforts at self-control

Medicate as needed

Apply wrist/leg/chest restraints as necessary

Background Readings:

Ackerman, L.L. (1992). Interventions related to neurological care. In G.M. Bulechek & J.C. McCloskey (Eds.), Symposium on nursing interventions. Nursing Clinics of North America, 27(2), 325-346.

American Nurses' Association Council in Medical-Surgical Nursing Practice & American Association of Neuroscience Nurses. (1985). Neuroscience nursing practice: Process and outcome for selected diagnoses. Kansas City, MO: American Nurses Association.

Coucouvanis, J.A. (1990). Behavior management. In M.J. Craft & J.A. Denehy (Eds.), Nursing interventions for infants and children (pp. 151-165). Philadelphia: W.B. Saunders.

Hinkle, J. (1988). Nursing care of patients with minor head injury. Journal of Neuroscience Nursing, 20(1), 8-14.

Phylar, P.A. (1989). Management of the agitated and aggressive head injury patient in an acute hospital setting. Journal of Neuroscience Nursing, 21(6), 353-356.

Woody, S. (1988). Episodic dyscontrol syndrome and head injury: A case presentation. Journal of Neuroscience Nursing, 20(3), 180-184.

Behavior Management: Overactivity/Inattention   4352

Definition: Provision of a therapeutic milieu that safely accommodates the patient's attention deficit and/or overactivity while promoting optimal function

Activities:

Provide a structured and physically safe environment, as necessary

Use a calm, matter-of-fact, reassuring approach

Determine appropriate behavioral expectations and consequences, given the patient's level of cognitive functioning and capacity for self-control

Develop a behavioral management plan that is carried out consistently by all care providers

Communicate rules, behavioral expectations, and consequences using simple language with visual cues, as necessary

Refrain from arguing or bargaining about established limits

Provide reassurance that staff will assist patient with managing his/her behavior, as necessary

Praise desired behaviors and efforts at self-control

Provide consistent consequences for both desired and undesired behavior(s)

Obtain patient's attention before initiating verbal interactions (e.g., call by name and make eye contact)

Give any instructions/explanations slowly, using simple and concrete language

Ask patient to repeat instructions before beginning tasks

Break multiple step instructions into simple steps

Allow patient to carry out one task before being given another

Provide assistance, as necessary, to complete task(s)

Provide positive feedback for completion of each step

Provide aids that will increase environmental structure, concentration, and attention to tasks (e.g., watches, calendars, signs, and step-by-step written instructions)

Decrease or withdraw verbal and physical cues, as they become unnecessary

Monitor and regulate level of activity and stimulation in environment

Maintain a routine schedule that includes a balance of structured time (e.g., physical and nonphysical activities) and quiet time

Limit choices, as necessary

Redirect or remove patient from source of overstimulation (e.g., a peer or a problem situation)

Use external controls, as necessary, to calm patient (e.g., time out, seclusion, and physical restraint)

Monitor physical status of overactive patient (e.g., body weight, hydration, and condition of feet in patient who paces)

Monitor fluid and nutritional intake

Provide high-protein, high-calorie finger foods and fluids that can be consumed "on the run"

Limit excessive intake of food and fluids

Limit intake of caffeinated food and fluids

Instruct in problem-solving skills

Encourage the expression of feelings in an appropriate manner

Teach/reinforce appropriate social skills

Continued

B

Activities:—cont'd

Set limits on intrusive, interruptive behavior(s)

Provide illness teaching to patient/significant others if the overactivity or inattention is illness-based (e.g., attention deficit disorder, hyperactivity, mania, and schizophrenia)

Administer medications (e.g., stimulants and antipsychotics) to promote desired behavior changes

Monitor patient for medication side effects and desired behavioral outcomes

Provide medication teaching to patient/significant others

Discuss reasonable behavioral expectations for patient with family/significant others

Teach behavioral management techniques to significant others

Assist patient and involved others (family, employers, and teachers) to adapt the home, work, or school environment(s) to accommodate limitations imposed by chronic inattention and overactivity

Facilitate family coping through support groups, respite care, and family counseling, as appropriate

Background Readings:
Cipkala-Gaffin, J.A., & Cipkala-Gaffin, G.L. (1989). Developmental disabilities and nursing interventions. In L.M. Birckhead (Ed.), Psychiatric mental health nursing. The therapeutic use of self (pp. 349-379). Philadelphia: J.B. Lippincott.
Fortinash, K.M., & Holoday-Worret, P.A. (1991). Psychiatric nursing care plans. St. Louis: Mosby.
Kendall, P.C., & Braswell, L. (1985). Cognitive-behavioral therapy for impulsive children. New York: The Guilford Press.
Stockard, S. (1987). Disorders of childhood. In J. Norris, M. Kunes-Connell, S. Stockard, P.M. Ehrhart, & G.R. Newton (Eds.), Mental health-psychiatric nursing. A Continuum of Care (pp. 657-691). New York: John Wiley & Sons.
Townsend, M.C. (1988). Nursing diagnoses in psychiatric nursing. A pocket guide for care plan construction. Philadelphia: F.A. Davis.

Behavior Management: Self-Harm   4354

Definition: Assisting the patient to decrease or eliminate self-mutilating or self-abusive behaviors

Activities:

Determine the motive/reason for the behavior(s)

Develop appropriate behavioral expectations and consequences, given the patient's level of cognitive functioning and capacity for self-control

Communicate behavioral expectations and consequences to patient

Remove dangerous items from the patient's environment

Apply, as appropriate, mitts, splints, helmets, or restraints to limit mobility and ability to initiate self-harm

Provide ongoing surveillance of patient and environment

Communicate risk to other care providers

Instruct patient in coping strategies (e.g., assertiveness training, impulse control training, and progressive muscle relaxation), as appropriate

Anticipate trigger situations that may prompt self-harm and intervene to prevent it

Assist patient to identify situations and/or feelings that may prompt self-harm

Contract with patient, as appropriate, for "no self-harm"

Encourage patient to seek out care providers to talk as urge to harm self occurs

Teach and reinforce patient for effective coping behaviors and appropriate expression of feelings

Administer medications, as appropriate, to decrease anxiety, stabilize mood, and decrease self-stimulation

Use a calm, nonpunitive approach when dealing with self-harmful behavior(s)

Avoid giving positive reinforcement to self-harmful behavior(s)

Provide the predetermined consequences if patient is engaging in self-harmful behaviors

Place patient in a more protective environment (e.g., area restriction and seclusion) if self-harmful impulses/behaviors escalate

Assist patient, as appropriate to level of cognitive functioning, to identify and assume responsibility for the consequences of behavior (e.g., dress own self-inflicted wound)

Assist patient to identify trigger situations and feelings that prompted self-harmful behavior

Assist patient to identify more appropriate coping strategies that could have been used and their consequences

Monitor patient for medication side effects and desired outcomes

Provide medication teaching to patient/significant others

Provide family/significant other with guidelines as to how self-harmful behavior can be managed outside the care environment

Provide illness teaching to patient/significant others if self-harmful behavior is illness based (e.g., borderline personality disorder or autism)

Monitor patient for self-harmful impulses that may progress to suicidal thoughts/gestures

Background Readings:

Fortinash, K.M., & Holoday-Worret, P.A. (1989). Psychiatric nursing care plans. St. Louis: Mosby.

Linehan, M., Armstrong, H., Suarez, A., Allmon, D., & Heard, H. (1991). Cognitive-behavioral treatment of chronically para-suicidal borderline patients. Archives of General Psychiatry, 48, 1060-1061.

Pawlicki, C.M., & Gaumer, C. (1993). Nursing care of the self-mutilating patient. Bulletin of the Menninger Clinic, 57(3), 380-389.

Continued

B

Background Readings:—cont'd

Spillers, G. (1991). Suicide potential. In G.K. McFarland & M.D. Thomas (Eds.), Psychiatric mental health nursing. Application of the nursing process (pp. 475-482). Philadelphia: J.B. Lippincott.

Stockard, S. (1987). Disorders of childhood. In J. Norris, M. Kunes-Connell, S. Stockard, P.M. Ehrhart, & G.R. Newton (Eds.), Mental health-psychiatric nursing. A continuum of care (pp. 657-691). New York: John Wiley & Sons.

Townsend, M.C. (1988). Nursing diagnoses in psychiatric nursing: A pocket guide for care plan construction. Philadelphia: F.A. Davis.

Valente, S.M. (1991). Deliberate self injury: Management in a psychiatric setting. Journal of Psychosocial Nursing and Mental Health Services, 29(12), 19-25.

Behavior Management: Sexual　　　　4356

Definition: Delineation and prevention of socially unacceptable sexual behaviors

Activities:

Identify sexual behaviors that are unacceptable, given the particular setting and patient population

Specify explicit expectations (based on level of cognitive functioning and capacity for self-control) related to sexual behavior or verbalizations that might be directed toward others or objects in the environment

Discuss with patient the consequences of socially unacceptable sexual behavior and verbalizations

Discuss the negative impact that socially unacceptable sexual behavior may have on others

Avoid assigning roommates with communication difficulties, history of inappropriate sexual activity, or heightened vulnerabilities (e.g., younger children)

Assign patient to a private room if assessed to be at high risk for socially unacceptable sexual behavior

Limit patient's physical mobility (e.g., area restriction), as needed, to decrease opportunity for socially unacceptable sexual behavior(s)

Communicate risk to other care providers

Provide appropriate level of supervision/surveillance to monitor patient

Use a calm, matter-of-fact approach when responding to socially unacceptable sexual remarks and behavior

Redirect from any socially unacceptable sexual behavior/verbalizations

Discuss with patient why the sexual behavior or verbalization is unacceptable

Provide the predetermined consequences for undesirable sexual behavior

Teach/reinforce appropriate social skills

Provide sex education, as appropriate to developmental level

Discuss with patient acceptable ways to fulfill individual sexual needs in privacy

Discourage initiation of sexual or intimate relationships while under severe stress

Encourage appropriate expression of feelings about past situational or traumatic crises

Provide counseling, as needed, for patient who has been sexually abused

Assist family with understanding of and management of unacceptable sexual behaviors

Provide opportunities for staff to process their feelings about patient sexual behavior that is socially unacceptable

Background Readings:

Cipkala-Gaffin, J.A., & Cipkala-Gaffin, G.L. (1989). Developmental disabilities and nursing interventions. In L.M. Birckhead (Ed.), Psychiatric mental health nursing. The therapeutic use of self (pp. 349-379). Philadelphia: J.B. Lippincott.

Hartley, R., & Robinson, C. (1987). Mental retardation. In J. Norris, M. Kunes-Connell, S. Stockard, P.M. Ehrhart, & G.R. Newton (Eds.), Mental health-psychiatric nursing. A continuum of care (pp. 495-525). New York: John Wiley & Sons.

Stockard, S., & Cullen, S. (1987). Personality disorders. In J. Norris, M. Kunes-Connell, S. Stockard, P.M. Ehrhart, & G.R. Newton (Eds.), Mental health-psychiatric nursing. A continuum of care (pp. 571-603). New York: John Wiley & Sons.

Thompson, J.M., McFarland, G.K., Hirsch, J.E., Tucker, S.M., & Bowers, A.C. (1989). Mosby's manual of clinical nursing (2nd ed.). St. Louis: Mosby.

Townsend, M.C. (1988). Nursing diagnoses in psychiatric nursing. A pocket guide for care plan construction. Philadelphia: F.A. Davis.

Behavior Modification   4360

Definition: Promotion of a behavior change

Activities:

Determine patient's motivation to change

Assist patient to identify strengths, and reinforce these

Encourage substitution of undesirable habits with desirable habits

Introduce patient to persons (or groups) who have successfully undergone the same experience

Maintain consistent staff behavior

Reinforce constructive decisions concerning health needs

Give feedback in terms of feelings when patient is noted to be free of symptoms and looks relaxed

Avoid showing rejection or belittlement as patient struggles with changing behavior

Offer positive reinforcement for patient's independently made decisions

Encourage patient to examine own behavior

Assist the patient in identifying even small successes

Identify the patient's problem in behavioral terms

Identify the behavior to be changed (target behavior) in specific, concrete terms

Break down behavior to be changed into smaller, measurable units of behavior (e.g., stopping smoking: number of cigarettes smoked)

Use specific time periods when measuring units of behavior (e.g., number of cigarettes smoked per day)

Determine whether the identified target behavior needs to be increased, decreased, or learned

Consider that it is easier to increase a behavior than to decrease a behavior

Establish behavioral objectives in written form

Develop a behavior change program

Establish a baseline occurrence of the behavior before initiating change

Develop a method (e.g., a graph or chart) for recording behavior and its changes

Encourage the patient to participate in recording behaviors

Discuss the behavior modification process with the patient/significant other

Facilitate the involvement of other health care providers in the modification process, as appropriate

Facilitate family involvement in the modification process, as appropriate

Administer positive reinforcers with behaviors that are to be increased

Withdraw positive reinforcers from behaviors that are to be decreased, and attach reinforcers to a more desirable replacement behavior

Encourage the patient to participate in the selection of reinforcers

Choose reinforcers that are meaningful to the patient

Choose reinforcers that can be controlled (e.g., used only when behavior to be changed occurs)

Consider nurse-given reinforcers (e.g., attention, time to talk, and reading to the patient)

Administer reinforcers promptly after a behavior occurs

Identify a schedule for delivery of reinforcers: may be continuous or intermittent

Coordinate a token or point system of reinforcement for complex or multiple behaviors

Develop a treatment contract with the patient to support implementation of the token/point system

Foster skills acquisition by systematically reinforcing simple components of the skill or task

Promote learning of desired behavior by using modeling techniques

Explore the possibility of using biofeedback to enhance patient's awareness of behavior changes

Evaluate changes in behavior by comparing baseline occurrences with postintervention occurrences of behavior

Document modification process, as necessary

Communicate intervention plan and modifications to treatment team on a regular basis

Follow up reinforcement over longer term (phone or personal contact)

Background Readings:

Haber, J., McMahon, A.L., Price-Hoskins, P., & Sideleau, B.F. (1992). Comprehensive psychiatric nursing (4th ed.). St. Louis: Mosby.

Kalish, H.I. (1981). From behavioral science to behavioral modification. St. Louis: McGraw-Hill.

LeBow, M.D. (1976). Applications of behavior modification in nursing practice. In M. Hersen, R.M. Eisler, & P.M. Miller (Eds.), Progress in behavior modification (Vol. 2). New York: Academic Press.

Simons, M.R. (1992). Interventions related to compliance. In G.M. Bulechek & J.C. McCloskey (Eds.), Symposium on Nursing Interventions. Nursing Clinics of North America, 27(2), 477-494.

Wilson, H.S., & Kneisl, C.R. (1992). Psychiatric nursing (4th ed.). Menlo Park, CA: Addison-Wesley.

Wong, D.L., & Wilson, D. (1995). Whaley & Wong's nursing care of infants and children (5th ed.) (p. 73). St. Louis: Mosby.

B

Behavior Modification: Social Skills   4362

Definition: Assisting the patient to develop or improve interpersonal social skills

Activities:

Assist patient to identify interpersonal problems resulting from social skill deficits

Encourage patient to verbalize feelings associated with interpersonal problems

Assist patient to identify desired outcomes for problematic interpersonal relationships or situations

Assist patient to identify possible courses of action and their social/interpersonal consequences

Identify a specific social skill(s) that will be the focus of training

Assist patient to identify the behavioral steps for the targeted social skill(s)

Provide models who demonstrate the behavioral steps in the context of situations that are meaningful to the patient

Assist patient to role play the behavioral steps

Provide feedback (e.g., praise or rewards) to patient about performance of targeted social skill(s)

Educate patient's significant others (e.g., family, peers, and employers), as appropriate, about the purpose and process of social skills training

Involve significant others in social skills training sessions (e.g., role playing) with patient, as appropriate

Provide feedback to patient and significant others about the appropriateness of their social responses in training situations

Encourage patient/significant others to self-evaluate outcomes of their social interactions, self-reward for positive outcomes, and problem solve less desirable outcomes

Background Readings:

Halford, W.K., & Hayes, R. (1991). Psychological rehabilitation of chronic schizophrenic patients: Recent findings on social skills training and family psychoeducation. Clinical Psychology Review, 11, 23-44.

Hartley, R., & Robinson, C. (1987). Mental retardation. In J. Norris, M. Kunes-Connell, S. Stockard, P.M. Ehrhart, & G.R. Newton (Eds.), Mental health–Psychiatric Nursing. A continuum of care (pp. 495-525). New York: John Wiley & Sons.

Hollinger, J.D. (1987). Social skills for behaviorally disordered children as preparation for mainstreaming: Theory, practice, and new directions. Remedial and Special Education, 8(4), 17-27.

Liberman, R.P., DeRisi, W.J., & Mueser, K.T. (1989). Social skills training with psychiatric patients. New York: Pergamon Press.

McGinnis, E., Goldstein, A.P., Sprafkin, R.P., & Gershaw, N.J. (1984). Skillstreaming the elementary school child. A structured learning approach to teaching prosocial skills. Champaign, IL: Research Press.

Westwell, J., & Martin, M.L. (1991). Social interaction, impaired. In G.K. McFarland, & M.D. Thomas (Eds.), Psychiatric mental health nursing. Application of the nursing process (pp. 437-443). Philadelphia: J.B. Lippincott.

Bibliotherapy   4680

Definition: Use of literature to enhance the expression of feelings and the gaining of insight

Activities:

Determine the particular needs of the situation

Set therapy goals

Select books that reflect the situation or feelings the patient is experiencing

Consult with a librarian who is skilled in book finding

Consult guides to recommended books from self-help groups

Make selections appropriate for reading level

Read aloud, as needed or feasible

Use pictures and illustrations

Encourage reading and rereading

Talk about the feelings expressed by the characters

Follow up reading sessions with play sessions or role modeling work, either individually or in therapy groups

Evaluate goal attainment

Background Readings:

Cohen, L.J. (1987). Bibliotherapy. Journal of Psychosocial Nursing and Mental Health Services, 25(10), 20-24.

Cohen, L.J. (1992). Bibliotherapy: The therapeutic use of books for women. Journal of Nurse-Midwifery, 37(2), 91-95.

Cohen, L.J. (1993). Discover the healing power of books. American Journal of Nursing, 93(10), 70-74.

Kus, R.J. (1989). Bibliotherapy and gay American men of Alcoholics Anonymous. Journal of Gay and Lesbian Psychotherapy, 1(2), 73-86.

B

Biofeedback

5860

Definition: Assisting the patient to modify a body function using feedback from instrumentation

Activities:

Analyze nature of the problem to be treated

Determine patient's acceptance of this type of treatment

Instruct patient about specific monitoring equipment used

Construct treatment plan to treat the problem

Connect patient to the instrumentation device, as needed

Assist patient to learn to modify bodily responses to equipment cues

Arrange therapy room so that patient cannot touch any conductive object

Instruct patient to check instrumentation before use to ensure proper functioning

Respond to fears and concerns related to the instrumentation

Discuss length of treatment session with patient/family

Establish an appropriate baseline against which to compare treatment effect

Identify appropriate criteria for reinforcement of patient's responses

Provide feedback on progress after each session

Set conditions with patient to evaluate therapeutic outcome

Background Readings:

Graves, P., & Lancaster, J. (1992). Stress management and crisis intervention. In M. Stanhope & J. Lancaster (Eds.), Community health nursing (3rd ed.) (pp. 612-631). St. Louis: Mosby.

Holmes, P. (1990). Mind over bladder. Nursing Times, 86(4), 16-17.

Good, M. (1998) Biofeedback. In M. Snyder & R. Lindquist. (Eds.), Complementary/alternative therapies in nursing (3rd ed.) (pp. 75-87). New York: Springer Publishing Company.

Kanfer, F.H., & Goldstein, A.P. (1985). Helping people change: A textbook of methods (3rd ed.). New York: Pergamon Press.

Snyder, M. (1988). Nursing management strategies: An overview. In P.H. Mitchell, L.C. Hodges, M. Muwasews, & C. Nalleck (Eds.), AANN's neuroscience nursing, phenomena and practice (pp. 41-54). Norwalk, CT: Appleton & Lange.

Bioterrorism Preparedness   8810

Definition: Preparing for an effective response to bioterrorism events or disaster

Activities:

Identify potential types of chemical agents that are likely terrorism agents (e.g., nerve agents, mustard agents, cyanide)

Identify potential types of biological agents that are likely terrorism agents (e.g., anthrax, smallpox, botulism, and plague)

Follow instructions regarding involvement in screening clients during a bioterrorism event

Integrate responses to biological and chemical terrorism into agency disaster preparedness planning and evaluation

Identify all community medical, emergency, and social agency resources available (e.g., World Health Organization [WHO], Federal Emergency Management Agency [FEMA], National Disaster Medical System [NDMS], Centers for Disease Control and Prevention [CDC], state and local public health agencies)

Consider current WHO and CDC recommended strategies to contain natural or deliberate disease and chemical exposures

Become familiar with signs and symptoms and common onset presentations of clients exposed to bioterrorism agents

Modify initial client assessment questions and history to be inclusive of exposure risk and physical symptoms of exposure

Monitor clients with vague flulike symptoms

Report symptoms suggestive of exposure to appropriate triage officers and health agencies

Consult appropriate epidemiology and infection control professionals, as necessary

Consider the reliability of information, especially in emergencies, potential disasters, or mass exposures

Maintain current knowledge of protective equipment, protective procedures, and isolation techniques

Ensure that protective equipment (e.g., hazmat suits, headgear, gloves, respirators) is available and in good working order

Be familiar with and follow all decontamination policies, procedures, and protocols

Participate in continuing education to maintain up to date knowledge

Background Readings:

Centers for Disease Control and Prevention (CDC). Bioterrorism preparedness and response—official statements. Retrieved April 15, 2002, from http://www.bt.cdc.gov/press/Hughes/05012001.asp

Federal Emergency Management Agency (FEMA). Planning health and medical needs in a terrorist incident. Retrieved April 15, 2002, from http://www.fema.gov/txt/onp/toolkit

Gebbie, K.M., & Qureshi, K. (2002). Emergency and disaster preparedness: Core competency for nurses. American Journal of Nursing, 102(1), 46-51.

Reilly, C.M., & Dleason, D. (2002). Smallpox. American Journal of Nursing, 102(2), 51-55.

U.S. Department of Health and Human Services, Office of Emergency Preparedness (OEP). Counter terrorism planning: Response planning. Retrieved April 15, 2002, from http://www.ndms.dhhs.gov/ct

Veenema, T.G. (2002). Chemical and biological terrorism: Current updates for nurse educators. Nursing Education Perspectives, 23(2), 62-71.

World Health Organization. (2001). Responding to the deliberate use of biological agents and chemicals as weapons. Retrieved April 15, 2002, from http://www.who.int/emc/deliberate_epi.html

World Health Organization (2001). Frequently asked questions regarding the deliberate use of biological agents and chemicals as weapons. Retrieved April 15, 2002, from http://www.who.int/emc/questions.html

B

Birthing   6720

Definition: Delivery of a baby

Activities:

Provide anticipatory guidance for delivery

Include support person(s) in birth experience, as appropriate

Perform vaginal exam to determine fetal position and station

Maintain patient modesty and privacy in a quiet environment during delivery

Adhere to patient's requests for management of delivery, when these requests are consistent with standards of perinatal care

Obtain permission of patient and partner when other health care personnel enter delivery area

Assist patient with position for delivery

Stretch perineal tissue, as appropriate, to minimize lacerations or episiotomy

Inform patient about the need for an episiotomy

Administer local anesthetic before delivery or episiotomy, as indicated

Perform episiotomy, as appropriate

Instruct patient on shallow breathing (e.g., "panting") with delivery of head

Deliver fetal head slowly, maintaining flexion until parietal bones are delivered

Support perineum during delivery

Check for the presence of a nuchal cord

Reduce nuchal cord, as appropriate (e.g., clamp and cut cord or slip over head)

Suction secretions from nares and mouth of infant with a bulb syringe after delivery of head

Suction for meconium-stained fluid, as appropriate

Cleanse and dry infant's head after delivery

Assist delivery of shoulders

Use maneuvers to release shoulder dystocia (e.g., suprapubic pressure or McRobert's maneuver), as appropriate

Deliver the body of infant slowly

Support infant body

Clamp and cut umbilical cord after pulsations have ceased, when not contraindicated

Obtain cord blood, if Rh negative or as needed for cord blood gas evaluation

Anticipate spontaneous expulsion of the placenta

Assign the 1-minute Apgar score

Apply controlled umbilical cord traction, while guarding the fundus of uterus

Inspect cervix for lacerations after delivery of placenta

Administer local anesthetic before surgical repair, when indicated

Suture episiotomy or lacerations, as appropriate

Perform rectal exam to ensure tissue integrity

Inspect placenta, membranes, and cord after delivery

Estimate blood loss after parturition

Cleanse perineum

Apply perineal pad

Praise maternal and support person efforts

Provide information about infant's appearance and condition

Encourage verbalization of questions or concerns about birth experience and newborn

Consult with attending physician about indicators of actual or potential complications

Document events of birth

Sign birth certificate, as appropriate

Background Readings:

Adams, C.J. (Ed.). (1983). Nurse-midwifery: Health care for women and newborns. New York: Grune & Stratton.

Mattson, S., & Smith, J.E. (Eds.). (1993). Core curriculum for maternal-newborn nursing. Philadelphia: W.B. Saunders.

Varney, H. (1987). Nurse-midwifery (2nd ed.). St. Louis: Mosby.

B

Bladder Irrigation

0550

Definition: Instillation of a solution into the bladder to provide cleansing or medication

Activities:

Determine whether the irrigation will be continuous or intermittent

Observe universal precautions

Explain the procedure to the client

Set up sterile irrigating supplies, maintaining sterile technique per agency protocol

Cleanse site of entry or end of Y-connector with alcohol wipe

Instill irrigating fluid, per agency protocol

Monitor and maintain correct flow rate, as necessary

Record amount of fluid used, characteristics of fluid, amount returned, and patient responsiveness, according to agency protocol

Background Readings:

Ellis, J.R., Nowlis, E.A., & Bentz, P.M. (1988). Modules for basic nursing skills (4th ed.). Boston: Houghton Mifflin.

Gilbert, V., & Gobbi, M. (1989). Making sense of bladder irrigation. Nursing Times, 85 (16), 40-42.

Potter, P., & Perry, A. (1998). Fundamentals of nursing: Concepts, process, and practice (4th ed.). St. Louis: Mosby.

Bleeding Precautions   4010

Definition: Reduction of stimuli that may induce bleeding or hemorrhage in at-risk patients

Activities:

Monitor the patient closely for hemorrhage

Note hemoglobin/hematocrit levels before and after blood loss, as indicated

Monitor for signs and symptoms of persistent bleeding (e.g., check all secretions for frank or occult blood)

Monitor coagulation studies, including prothrombin time (PT), partial thromboplastin time (PTT), fibrinogen, fibrin degradation/split products, and platelet counts, as appropriate

Monitor orthostatic vital signs, including blood pressure

Maintain bed rest during active bleeding

Administer blood products (e.g., platelets and fresh frozen plasma), as appropriate

Protect the patient from trauma, which may cause bleeding

Avoid injections (IV, IM, or SQ), as appropriate

Instruct the ambulating patient to wear shoes

Use soft toothbrush or toothettes for oral care

Use electric razor, instead of straight-edge, for shaving

Tell patient to avoid invasive procedures; if they are necessary, monitor closely for bleeding

Coordinate timing of invasive procedures with platelet or fresh frozen plasma transfusions, if appropriate

Refrain from inserting objects into a bleeding orifice

Avoid taking rectal temperatures

Tell patient to avoid lifting heavy objects

Administer medications (e.g., antacids), as appropriate

Instruct patient to avoid aspirin or other anticoagulants

Instruct patient to increase intake of foods rich in vitamin K

Use therapeutic mattress to minimize skin trauma

Avoid constipation (e.g., encourage fluid intake and stool softeners), as appropriate

Instruct the patient and/or family on signs of bleeding and appropriate actions (e.g., notify the nurse), should bleeding occur

Background Readings:

Cullen, L.M. (1992). Interventions related to circulatory care. In G.M. Bulechek & J.C. McCloskey (Eds.), Symposium on Nursing Interventions. Nursing Clinics of North America, 27(2), 445-476.

Jennings, B. (1991). The hematologic system. In J. Alspach (Ed.), AACN's core curriculum for critical care nursing (4th ed.) (pp. 675-747). Philadelphia: W.B. Saunders.

Johanson, B.C., Wells, S.J., Hoffmeister, D., & Dungca, C.U. (1988). Standards for critical care (3rd ed.). St. Louis: Mosby.

Thompson, J.M., McFarland, G.K., Hirsch, J.E., & Tucker, S.M. (1998). Mosby's clinical nursing (4th ed.). St. Louis: Mosby.

B

Bleeding Reduction   4020

Definition: Limitation of the loss of blood volume during an episode of bleeding

Activities:

Identify the cause of the bleeding

Monitor the patient closely for hemorrhage

Monitor the amount and nature of blood loss

Note hemoglobin/hematocrit levels before and after blood loss, as indicated

Monitor trends in blood pressure and hemodynamic parameters, if available (e.g., central venous pressure and pulmonary capillary/artery wedge pressure)

Monitor fluid status, including intake and output, as appropriate

Monitor coagulation studies, including prothrombin time (PT), partial thromboplastin time (PTT), fibrinogen, fibrin degradation/split products, and platelet counts, as appropriate

Monitor determinants of tissue oxygen delivery (e.g., PaO_2, SaO_2, and hemoglobin levels and cardiac output), if available

Instruct the patient and/or family on signs of bleeding and appropriate actions (e.g., notify the nurse), should further bleeding occur

Instruct the patient on activity restrictions, if appropriate

Instruct patient and family on severity of blood loss and appropriate actions being performed

Arrange availability of blood products for transfusion, if necessary

Maintain patent IV access

Administer blood products (e.g., platelets and fresh frozen plasma), as appropriate

Perform proper precautions in handling blood products or bloody secretions

Apply direct pressure or pressure dressing, if appropriate

Background Readings:

Cullen, L.M. (1992). Interventions related to circulatory care. In G.M. Bulechek & J.C. McCloskey (Eds.), Symposium on Nursing Interventions. Nursing Clinics of North America, 27(2), 445-476.

Jennings, B. (1991). The hematologic system. In J. Alspach (Ed.), AACN's core curriculum for critical care nursing (4th ed.) (pp. 675-747). Philadelphia: W.B. Saunders.

Johanson, B.C., Wells, S.J., Hoffmeister, D., & Dungca, C.U. (1988). Standards for critical care (3rd ed.). St. Louis: Mosby.

Thompson, J.M., McFarland, G.K., Hirsch, J.E., & Tucker, S.M. (1998). Mosby's clinical nursing (4th ed.). St. Louis: Mosby.

Bleeding Reduction: Antepartum Uterus   4021

Definition: Limitation of the amount of blood loss from the pregnant uterus during third trimester of pregnancy

Activities:

Obtain client history of blood loss (e.g., onset, amount, presence of pain, and presence of clots)

Review for risk factors related to late pregnancy bleeding (e.g., abruption, smoking, cocaine use, pregnancy-induced hypertension, and placenta previa)

Obtain an accurate estimate of fetal age by last menstrual period report, prior ultrasound dating reports, or obstetrical history, if available

Inspect perineum for amount and characteristic of bleeding

Monitor maternal vital signs, as needed, based on amount of blood loss

Monitor fetal heart rate electronically

Palpate for uterine contractions or increased uterine tone

Observe electronic fetal tracing for evidence of uteroplacental insufficiency (e.g., late decelerations, decreased long-term variability, and absent accelerations)

Initiate fetal resuscitation, as appropriate, for abnormal (nonreassuring) signs of uteroplacental insufficiency

Delay digital cervical exam until location of placenta has been verified (e.g., ultrasound report)

Perform ultrasound exam for placental location

Perform or assist with speculum exam to visualize blood loss and cervical status

Weigh Chux or pads to accurately estimate blood loss

Inspect clothing, sheets, and mattress pad in the event of hemorrhage

Initiate emergency procedures for antepartum hemorrhage, as appropriate (e.g., oxygen therapy, IV therapy, and type and cross)

Draw blood for diagnostic tests, as appropriate (e.g., Kleihauer-Betke, ABO, Rh, CBC, and clotting studies)

Administer Rho(D) immune globulin, as appropriate

Record intake and output

Elevate lower extremities to increase perfusion to vital organs and fetus

Administer blood products, as appropriate

Initiate safety measures (e.g., strict bed rest and lateral position)

Instruct patient to report increases in vaginal bleeding (e.g., gushes, clots, and trickles) during hospitalization

Teach patient to differentiate between old and fresh bleeding

Instruct client on lifestyle changes to reduce the chance of further bleeding, as appropriate (e.g., smoking cessation assistance, sexual abstinence, bed rest care, constipation management, nutrition management, and coping enhancement)

Provide discharge planning, including referral to home care nurses

Schedule follow-up antepartum fetal surveillance

Discuss reasons to return to the hospital

Discuss use of emergency medical system for transportation, as appropriate

Background Readings:

Littleton, L.Y., & Engebretson, J.C. (2002). Maternal, neonatal, and women's health nursing, (pp. 510-514). Albany, NY: Delmar.

Mattson, S., & Smith, J.E. (Eds.). (1993). Core curriculum for maternal-newborn nursing. Philadelphia: W.B. Saunders.

B

Bleeding Reduction: Gastrointestinal   4022

Definition: Limitation of the amount of blood loss from the upper and lower gastrointestinal tract and related complications

Activities:

Evaluate patient's psychological response to hemorrhage and perception of events

Monitor for signs and symptoms of persistent bleeding (e.g., check all secretions for frank or occult blood)

Hematest all excretions and observe for blood in emesis, sputum, feces, urine, NG tube drainage, and wound drainage, as appropriate

Monitor coagulation studies and complete blood count (CBC) with WBC differential

Monitor coagulation studies, including prothrombin time (PT), partial thromboplastin time (PTT), fibrinogen, fibrin degradation/split products, and platelet counts, as appropriate

Administer medications (e.g., lactulose or vasopressin), as appropriate

Insert nasogastric tube to suction and monitor secretions, if appropriate

Perform nasogastric lavage, as appropriate

Document color, amount, and character of stools

Maintain pressure in cuffed/balloon nasogastric tube

Avoid extremes in gastric pH level by administration of appropriate medication (e.g., antacids or histamine-blocking agent)

Establish a supportive relationship with the patient and family

Instruct the patient and family on activity restriction and progression

Promote stress reduction

Maintain a patent airway

Avoid administration of anticoagulants

Monitor the patient's nutritional status

Monitor determinants of tissue oxygen delivery (e.g., PaO_2, SaO_2, and hemoglobin levels and cardiac output), if available

Administer IV fluids, as appropriate

Instruct the patient and/or family on procedures (e.g., endoscopy, sclerosis, and surgery), if appropriate

Instruct the patient and/or family on the need for blood replacement, as appropriate

Instruct the patient and/or family to avoid the use of antiinflammatory medications (e.g., aspirin and ibuprofen)

Coordinate counseling for the patient and/or family (e.g., clergy, Alcoholics Anonymous), if appropriate

Background Readings:

Alspach, J.G. (Ed.) (1998). core curriculum for critical care nursing. American Association of Critical Care Nurses (p. 674). Philadelphia: W.B. Saunders Co.

Cullen, L.M. (1992). Interventions related to circulatory care. In G.M. Bulechek & J.C. McCloskey (Eds.), Symposium on Nursing Interventions. Nursing Clinics of North America, 27(2), 445-476.

Johanson, B.C., Wells, S.J., Hoffmeister, D., & Dungca, C.U. (1988). Standards for critical care (3rd ed.). St. Louis: Mosby.

Kaldor, P. (1988). Medical and surgical therapies for gastrointestinal problems. In M. R. Kinney, D.R. Packa, & S.B. Dunbar, (Eds.), AACN's clinical reference for critical-care nursing (pp. 1363-1366). New York: McGraw-Hill.

Bleeding Reduction: Nasal   4024

B

Definition: Limitation of the amount of blood loss from the nasal cavity

Activities:

Apply manual pressure over the bleeding or the potential bleeding area

Identify the cause of the bleeding

Monitor the amount and nature of blood loss

Monitor the amount of bleeding into the oropharynx

Apply ice pack to affected area

Place packing in nasal cavity, if appropriate

Administer blood products (e.g., platelets and fresh frozen plasma), as appropriate

Note hemoglobin/hematocrit levels before and after blood loss, as indicated

Instruct the patient on activity restrictions, if appropriate

Promote stress reduction

Provide pain relief/comfort measures

Maintain a patent airway

Instruct patient to avoid traumatizing nares (e.g., avoid scratching or touching nose)

Assist patient with oral care, as appropriate

Instruct the patient and/or family on signs of bleeding and appropriate actions (e.g., notify the nurse), should further bleeding occur

Background Readings:

Cullen, L.M. (1992). Interventions related to circulatory care. In G.M. Bulechek & J.C. McCloskey (Eds.), Symposium on Nursing Interventions. Nursing Clinics of North America, 27(2), 445-476.

Jennings, B. (1991). The hematologic system. In J. Alspach (Ed.), AACN's core curriculum for critical care nursing (4th ed.) (pp. 675-747). Philadelphia: W.B. Saunders.

Johanson, B.C., Wells, S.J., Hoffmeister, D., & Dungca, C.U. (1988). Standards for critical care (3rd ed.). St. Louis: Mosby.

Kitt, S., & Karser, J. (1990). Emergency nursing: A physiological and clinical perspective. Philadelphia: W.B. Saunders.

Thompson, J.M., McFarland, G.K., Hirsch, J.E., & Tucker, S.M. (1998). Mosby's clinical nursing (4th ed.). St. Louis: Mosby.

B

Bleeding Reduction: Postpartum Uterus   4026

Definition: Limitation of the amount of blood loss from the postpartum uterus

Activities:

Review obstetrical history and labor record for risk factors for postpartum hemorrhage (e.g., prior postpartum hemorrhage, long labor, induction, preeclampsia, prolonged second stage, assisted delivery, multiple birth, cesarean birth, or precipitous birth)

Apply ice to fundus

Increase frequency of fundal massage

Evaluate for bladder distention

Encourage voiding or catheterize distended bladder

Observe characteristics of lochia (e.g., color, clots, and volume)

Weigh amount of blood loss

Request additional nurses to help with emergency procedures and to assume care for newborn

Elevate legs

Initiate IV infusion

Start second IV line, as appropriate

Administer IV or IM oxytocics, per protocol or order

Notify primary practitioner of patient status

Monitor maternal vital signs every 15 minutes or more frequently, as appropriate

Cover with warm blankets

Monitor maternal color, level of consciousness, and pain

Initiate oxygen therapy at 6 to 8 L per face mask

Insert Foley catheter with urometer to monitor urine output

Order emergency laboratory tests or blood

Administer blood products, as appropriate

Assist primary practitioner with packing uterus, evacuating hematoma, or suturing lacerations, as appropriate

Keep patient and family informed of clinical condition and management

Provide perineal care, as needed

Prepare for emergency hysterectomy, as needed

Discuss events with nursing team for provision of adequate postpartum surveillance of maternal status

Background Readings:

Littleton, L.Y., & Engbertson, J.C. (2002). Maternal, neonatal, and women's health nursing, (pp. 908-911). Albany, NY: Delmar.

Mattson, S., & Smith, J.E. (Eds.). (1993). Core curriculum for maternal-newborn nursing. Philadelphia: W.B. Saunders.

Bleeding Reduction: Wound   4028

Definition: Limitation of the blood loss from a wound that may be a result of trauma, incisions, or placement of a tube or catheter

Activities:

Apply manual pressure over the bleeding or the potential bleeding area

Apply ice pack to affected area

Apply pressure dressing to site of bleeding

Use mechanical device (e.g., C-type clamp) for applying pressure for longer periods, if appropriate

Replace or reinforce pressure dressing, as appropriate

Place bleeding extremity in an elevated position

Monitor size and character of hematoma, if present

Monitor pulses distal to bleeding site

Instruct patient to apply pressure to site when sneezing, coughing, and so on

Instruct the patient on activity restrictions, if appropriate

Instruct the patient and/or family on signs of bleeding and appropriate actions (e.g., notify the nurse), should further bleeding occur

Background Readings:

Cullen, L.M. (1992). Interventions related to circulatory care. In G.M. Bulechek & J.C. McCloskey (Eds.), Symposium on Nursing Interventions. Nursing Clinics of North America, 27(2), 445-476.

Johanson, B.C., Wells, S.J., Hoffmeister, D., & Dungca, C.U. (1988). Standards for critical care (3rd ed.). St. Louis: Mosby.

Kitt, S., & Karser, J. (1990). Emergency nursing: A physiological and clinical perspective. Philadelphia: W.B. Saunders.

Thompson, J.M., McFarland, G.K., Hirsch, J.E., & Tucker, S.M. (1998). Mosby's clinical nursing (4th ed.). St. Louis: Mosby.

B

Blood Products Administration   4030

Definition: Administration of blood or blood products and monitoring of patient's response

Activities:

Verify physician's orders

Obtain patient's transfusion history

Obtain or verify patient's informed consent

Verify that blood product has been prepared, typed, and cross-matched (if applicable) for the recipient

Verify correct patient, blood type, Rh type, unit number, and expiration date; and record per agency protocol

Instruct patient about signs and symptoms of transfusion reactions (itching, dizziness, shortness of breath, and chest pain)

Assemble administration system with filter appropriate for blood product and recipient's immune status

Prime administration system with isotonic saline

Prepare an IV pump approved for blood product administration, if indicated

Perform venipuncture, using appropriate technique

Avoid transfusion of more than one unit of blood or blood product at a time, unless necessitated by recipient's condition

Monitor IV site for signs and symptoms of infiltration, phlebitis, and local infection

Monitor vital signs (e.g., baseline and throughout and after transfusion)

Monitor for transfusion reactions

Monitor for fluid overload

Monitor and regulate flow rate during transfusion

Refrain from administering IV medications or fluids, other than isotonic saline, into blood or blood product lines

Refrain from transfusing product removed from controlled refrigeration for more than 4 hours

Change filter and administration set at least every 4 hours

Administer saline when transfusion is complete

Document time frame of transfusion

Document volume infused

Stop transfusion if blood reaction occurs and keep veins open with saline

Obtain blood sample and first voided urine specimen after a transfusion reaction

Coordinate the return of the blood container to the lab after a blood reaction

Notify laboratory immediately, in the event of a blood reaction

Maintain universal precautions

Background Readings:

American Association of Blood Banks. (1994). Standards fro blood banks and transfusion services (126th ed.). Bethesda, MD: American Association of Blood Banks.

American Red Cross, Council of Community Blood Centers, and American Association of Blood Banks. (March, 1994). Circular of information for the use of human blood and blood components.

Perry, A.G., & Potter, P.A. (2002). Clinical nursing skills and techniques (5th ed.). St. Louis: Mosby.

Revised intravenous nursing standards of practice. (2000). Journal of Intravenous Nursing (Is-suppl), Nov-Dec.

Body Image Enhancement   5220

Definition: Improving a patient's conscious and unconscious perceptions and attitudes toward his/her body

Activities:

Determine patient's body image expectations based on developmental stage

Use anticipatory guidance to prepare patient for predictable changes in body image

Determine if perceived dislike for certain physical characteristics creates a dysfunctional social paralysis for teenagers and other high-risk groups

Assist patient to discuss changes caused by illness or surgery, as appropriate

Help patient determine the extent of actual changes in the body or its level of functioning

Determine if a recent physical change has been incorporated into patient's body image

Assist patient to separate physical appearance from feelings of personal worth, as appropriate

Assist patient to determine the influence of a peer group on the patient's perception of present body image

Assist patient to discuss changes caused by puberty as appropriate

Assist patient to discuss changes caused by a normal pregnancy, as appropriate

Assist patient to discuss changes caused by aging, as appropriate

Teach the patient the normal changes in the body associated with various stages of aging, as appropriate

Assist the patient to discuss stressors affecting body image due to congenital condition, injury, disease, or surgery

Identify the effects of the patient's culture, religion, race, sex, and age in terms of body image

Monitor frequency of statements of self-criticism

Monitor whether patient can look at the changed body part

Monitor for statements that identify body image perceptions concerned with body shape and body weight

Use self-picture drawing as a mechanism of evaluating a child's body image perceptions

Instruct children about the functions of the various body parts, as appropriate

Determine patient's and family's perceptions of the alteration in body image versus reality

Identify coping strategies used by parents in response to changes in child's appearance

Determine how child responds to parent's reactions, as appropriate

Teach parents the importance of their responses to the child's body changes and future adjustment, as appropriate

Assist parents to identify feelings prior to intervening with child, as appropriate

Determine if a change in body image has contributed to increased social isolation

Assist patient in identifying parts of his/her body that have positive perceptions associated with them

Identify means of reducing the impact of any disfigurement through clothing, wigs, or cosmetics, as appropriate

Assist patient to identify actions that will enhance appearance

Assist the hospitalized patient to apply cosmetics prior to seeing visitors, as appropriate

Facilitate contact with individuals with similar changes in body image

Identify support groups available to patient

Continued

B

Activities:—cont'd

Assist patient at risk for anorexia or bulimia to develop more realistic body image expectations

Use self-disclosure exercises with groups of teenagers or others distraught over normal physical attributes

Background Readings:

Blaesing, S., & Brockhaus, J. (1972). The development of body image in the child. Nursing Clinics of North America, 7(4), 597-607.

Haber, J., McMahon, A.L., Price-Hoskins, P., & Sideleau, B.F. (1997). Comprehensive psychiatric nursing (5th ed.). St. Louis: Mosby-Year Book.

Janelli, L.M. (1986). Body image in older adults: A review of the literature. Rehabilitation Nursing, 11(4), 6-8.

McBride, L.G. (1986). Teaching about body image: A technique for improving body satisfaction. Journal of School Health, 56(2), 76-77.

Nichols, P. (1996). Clear thinking: Clearing dark thoughts with new words and images. Iowa City, IA: River Lights Publishers.

Williams, M.L. (1987). The nursing diagnosis of body image disturbance in adolescents dissatisfied with their physical characteristics. Holistic Nursing Practice, 1(4), 52-59.

Wilson, H.S., & Kneisl, C.R. (1992). Psychiatric nursing (4th ed.). Menlo Park, CA: Addison-Wesley.

Vernon, A. (1989a). Thinking, feeling, behaving: An emotional education curriculum for adolescents (grades 1-6). Champaign, IL: Research Press.

Vernon, A. (1989b). Thinking, feeling, behaving: An emotional education curriculum for adolescents (grades 7-12). Champaign, IL: Research Press.

Body Mechanics Promotion   0140

Definition: Facilitating the use of posture and movement in daily activities to prevent fatigue and musculoskeletal strain or injury

Activities:

Determine patient's commitment to learning and using correct posture

Collaborate with physical therapy in developing a body mechanics promotion plan, as indicated

Determine patient's understanding of body mechanics and exercises (e.g., return demonstration of correct techniques while performing activities/exercises)

Instruct patient on structure and function of spine and optimal posture for moving and using the body

Instruct patient about need for correct posture to prevent fatigue, strain, or injury

Instruct patient how to use posture and body mechanics to prevent injury while performing any physical activities

Determine patient awareness of own musculoskeletal abnormalities and the potential effects of posture and muscle tissue

Instruct to use a firm mattress/chair or pillow, if appropriate

Instruct to avoid sleeping prone

Assist to demonstrate appropriate sleeping positions

Assist to avoid sitting in the same position for prolonged periods

Demonstrate how to shift weight from one foot to another while standing

Instruct patient to move feet first and then body when turning to walk from a standing position

Assist patient/family to identify appropriate posture exercises

Assist patient to select warm-up activities before beginning exercise or work not done routinely

Assist patient to perform flexion exercises to facilitate back mobility, as indicated

Instruct patient/family regarding frequency and number of repetitions for each exercise

Monitor improvement in patient's posture/body mechanics

Provide information about possible positional causes of muscle or joint pain

Background Readings:

Craven, R.F., & Hirnle, C.J. (2000) Fundamentals of nursing: Human health and function (3rd ed.) (pp. 738-739). Philadelphia: Lippincott.

Glick, O.J. (1992). Interventions related to activity and movement. In G.M. Bulechek & J.C. McCloskey (Eds.), Symposium on Nursing Interventions. Nursing Clinics of North America, 27(2), 541-568.

Lewis, C.B. (1989). Improving mobility in older persons. Rockville, MD: Aspen.

Sheahan, S. (1982). Assessment of low back pain. Nurse Practitioner, 7, 15-23.

Sweezey, S. (1988). Low back pain. Geriatrics, 43(2), 39-44.

B

Bottle Feeding 1052

Definition: Preparation and administration of fluids to an infant via a bottle

Activities:

Determine infant state prior to initiating feeding

Warm formula to room temperature before feeding

Hold infant during feeding

Position infant in a semi-Fowler's position for feeding

Burp the infant frequently during and after the feeding

Place nipple on top of tongue

Control fluid intake by regulating softness of nipple, size of the hole, and size of the bottle

Increase infant alertness by loosening infant's clothes, rubbing hands and feet, or talking to infant

Encourage sucking by stimulating the rooting reflex, if appropriate

Increase effectiveness of suck by compressing cheeks in unison with suck, if appropriate

Provide chin support to decrease leaking of formula and improve lip closure

Monitor fluid intake

Monitor/evaluate suck reflex during feeding

Monitor infant weight, as appropriate

Boil unpasteurized milk

Boil water used for preparing formula, if indicated

Instruct parent or caregiver on sterilization techniques for feeding equipment

Instruct parent or caregiver on proper dilution of concentrated formula

Instruct parent on proper storage of formula

Determine water source used to dilute concentrated or powdered formula

Determine fluoride content of water used to dilute concentrated or powdered formula and refer for flouride supplementation, if indicated

Caution parent or caregiver about using microwave oven to warm formula

Instruct and demonstrate to parent oral hygiene techniques appropriate to infant's dentition to be used after each feeding

Background Readings:

May, K.A., & Mahlmeister, L.R. (1994). Maternal and neonatal nursing: Family-centered care (3rd ed.). Philadelphia: Lippincott.

Olds, S.B., London, M.L., & Ladewig, P.A. (1992). Maternal-newborn nursing: A family centered approach (4th ed.). Menlo Park, CA: Addison-Wesley.

Bowel Incontinence Care   0410

Definition: Promotion of bowel continence and maintenance of perianal skin integrity

B

Activities:

Determine physical or psychological cause of fecal incontinence

Explain etiology of problem and rationale for actions

Determine goals of bowel management program with patient/family

Discuss procedures and expected outcomes with patient

Instruct patient/family to record fecal output, as appropriate

Wash perianal area with soap and water and dry it thoroughly after each stool

Use nonionic detergent preparation, such as Peri-Wash, for cleansing, as appropriate

Use powder and creams on perianal area with caution

Keep bed and clothing clean

Implement bowel training program, as appropriate

Monitor for adequate bowel evacuation

Monitor diet and fluid requirements

Monitor for side effects of medication administration

Use rectal pouch, as appropriate

Empty rectal pouch, as needed

Place on incontinent pads, as needed

Provide protective pants, as needed

Background Readings:

Bielefeldt, K., Enck, P., & Wienbeck, M. (1990). Diagnosis and treatment of fecal incontinence. Digestive Diseases, 8, 179-188.

Freedman, P. (1991). The rectal pouch: A safer alternative to rectal tubes. American Journal of Nursing, May, 105-106.

Lara, L.L., Troop, P.R., & Beadleson-Baird, M. (1990). The risk of urinary tract infection in bowel incontinent men. Journal of Gerontological Nursing, 16(5), 24-26.

Lincoln, R., & Roberts, R. (1989). Continence issues in acute care. Nursing Clinics of North America, 24(3), 741-754.

Maas, M.L., Buckwalter, K.C., Hardy, M.D., Reimer, T.T., Titler, M.G., & Specht, J.P. (2001) Nursing care of older adults: Diagnoses, outcomes, & interventions, (pp. 249-250). St. Louis: Mosby

McLane, A.M., & McShane, R.E. (1992). Bowel management. In G.M. Bulechek & J.C. McCloskey (Eds.), Nursing interventions: Essential nursing treatments (2nd ed.) (pp. 73-85). Philadelphia: W.B. Saunders.

B

Bowel Incontinence Care: Encopresis   0412

Definition: Promotion of bowel continence in children

Activities:

Gather information about toilet training history, duration of encopresis, and attempts made to eliminate the problem

Determine cause of soiling (e.g., constipation and fecal impaction), as appropriate

Order tests for physical causes (e.g., endoscopy, radiographic procedures, and stool analysis)

Prepare child and family for diagnostic tests

Perform rectal exam, as appropriate

Instruct family about physiology of normal defecation and toilet training

Recommend dietary changes or behavioral therapy, as appropriate

Conduct family psychosocial assessment, including responses of caregivers and self-esteem of child

Use play therapy to assist the child with working through feelings

Investigate family communication patterns, strengths, and coping abilities

Encourage parents to foster security by removing anxiety associated with toileting

Encourage parents to demonstrate love and acceptance at home to counteract peer ridicule

Discuss psychosocial dynamics of encopresis with parents (e.g., familial patterns, family disruption, self-esteem issues, and self-limiting characteristic)

Discuss ways to reward toileting behavior

Refer for family therapy, as appropriate

Background Readings:

Gleeson, R.M. (1990). Bowel continence for the child with a neurogenic bowel. Rehabilitation Nursing, 15(6), 319-321.

Mott, S.R., James, S.R., & Sperhac, A.M. (1990). Nursing care of children and families (2nd ed.). Redwood City, CA: Addison-Wesley.

Sprague-McRae, J.M., Lamb, W., & Homer, D. (1993). Encopresis: A study of treatment alternatives and historical behavioral characteristics. Nurse Practitioner, 18(10), 52-63.

Wong, D.L. (1997). Whaley & Wong's essentials of pediatric nursing (5th ed.). St. Louis: Mosby.

Bowel Irrigation

0420

Definition: Instillation of a substance into the lower gastrointestinal tract

Activities:

Determine reason for gastrointestinal cleansing

Avoid use if patient has a history of ulcerative colitis or regional enteritis

Check physician order for gastrointestinal cleansing

Choose appropriate type of enema

Explain procedure to patient

Provide for privacy

Inform patient that there may be abdominal cramping and urge to defecate

Assemble equipment

Position patient, as appropriate

Protect bed linens

Provide bedpan or commode, as appropriate

Ascertain appropriate temperature of irrigating substance

Lubricate tubing before insertion, as appropriate

Insert substance in rectum, as appropriate

Ascertain amount of substance return from body orifice

Monitor for side effects of irrigation solution or oral medication

Monitor for signs and symptoms of diarrhea, constipation, and impaction

Note if returns from enema or laxatives are not clear

Cleanse anal area

Background Readings:

Craven, R.F., & Hirnle, C.J. (2000) Fundamentals of nursing: Human health and function (3rd ed.) (pp. 1098-1101). Philadelphia: Lippincott.

Innes, B.S. (1986). Meeting bowel elimination needs. In K.C. Sorenson & J. Luckmann (Eds.), Basic nursing (pp. 827-851). Philadelphia: W.B. Saunders.

B

Bowel Management 0430

Definition: Establishment and maintenance of a regular pattern of bowel elimination

Activities:

Note date of last bowel movement

Monitor bowel movements including frequency, consistency, shape, volume, and color, as appropriate

Monitor bowel sounds

Report an increase in frequency of and/or high-pitched bowel sounds

Report diminished bowel sounds

Monitor for signs and symptoms of diarrhea, constipation, and impaction

Evaluate for fecal incontinence as necessary

Note preexistent bowel problems, bowel routine, and use of laxatives

Teach patient about specific foods that assist in promoting bowel regularity

Instruct patient/family members to record color, volume, frequency, and consistency of stools

Insert rectal suppository, as needed

Initiate a bowel training program, as appropriate

Encourage decreased gas-forming food intake, as appropriate

Instruct patient on foods high in fiber, as appropriate

Give warm liquids after meals, as appropriate

Evaluate medication profile for gastrointestinal side effects

Obtain a guaiac for stools, as appropriate

Refrain from doing rectal/vaginal examination if medical condition warrants

Background Readings:

Craft, M.J., & Denehy, J.A. (Eds.). (1990). Nursing interventions for infants and children. Philadelphia: W.B. Saunders.

Craven, R.F., & Hirnle, C.J. (2000) Fundamentals of nursing: Human health and function (3rd ed.) (pp. 1077-1114). Philadelphia: Lippincott.

Goetz, L.L., Hurvitz, E.A., Nelson, V.S., & Waring, W. (1998). Bowel management in children and adolescents with spinal cord injury. The Journal of Spinal Cord Medicine, 21(4), 335-341.

Hardy, M.A. (1991). Normal changes with aging. In M. Maas, K.C. Buckwalter, & M. Hardy (Eds.), Nursing diagnoses and interventions for the elderly (pp. 145-146). Redwood City, CA: Addison-Wesley.

McLane, A.M., & McShane, R.E. (1991). Constipation. In M. Maas, K. Buckwalter, & M. Hardy (Eds.), Nursing diagnoses and interventions for the elderly (pp. 147-158). Redwood City, CA: Addison-Wesley.

Mangan, P., & Thomas, L. (1988). Preserving dignity. Geriatric Nursing and Home Care, 8(9), 14.

Bowel Training   0440

B

Definition: Assisting the patient to train the bowel to evacuate at specific intervals

Activities:

Plan bowel program with patient and appropriate others

Consult with physician and patient regarding use of suppositories

Teach patient/family the principles of bowel training

Instruct patient about which foods are high in bulk

Provide foods high in bulk and/or that have been identified as assistive by the patient

Ensure adequate fluid intake

Ensure adequate exercise

Initiate an uninterrupted, consistent time for defecation

Ensure privacy

Administer suppository, as appropriate

Perform digital rectal dilatation, as necessary

Teach patient digital rectal dilatation, as appropriate

Evaluate bowel status regularly

Modify bowel program, as needed

Background Readings:

Innes, B.S. (1986). Meeting bowel elimination needs. In K.C. Sorenson & J. Luckmann (Eds.), Basic nursing (pp. 827-851). Philadelphia: W.B. Saunders.

Maas, M., & Specht, J. (1991). Bowel incontinence. In M. Maas, K.C. Buckwalter, & M. Hardy (Eds.), Nursing diagnoses and interventions for the elderly (pp. 169-180). Redwood City, CA: Addison-Wesley.

Maas, M.L., Buckwalter, K.C., Hardy, M.D., Reimer, T.T., Titler, M.G., & Specht, J.P. (2001). Nursing care of older adults: Diagnoses, outcomes, & interventions, (pp. 248-249). St. Louis: Mosby.

McLane, A.M., & McShane, R.E. (1992). Bowel management. In G.M. Bulecheck & J.C. McCloskey (Eds.), Nursing interventions: Essential nursing treatments (2nd ed.) (pp. 73-85). Philadelphia: W.B. Saunders.

B

Breast Examination   6522

Definition: Inspection and palpation of the breasts and related areas

Activities:

Determine possible risk factors for the development of breast cancer, including age, age at first pregnancy, age at menarche, age at menopause, family history, history of breast disease, parity status, and history of breastfeeding

Ascertain whether patient has noticed any pain, lump, thickening, or tenderness of the breast or discharge, distortion, retraction, or scaling of the nipple

Assist patient to positions of comfort as exam proceeds, always allowing privacy and sensitivity as needed

Explain specific steps of exam as you proceed

Conduct exam while patient is in upright then supine position

Instruct patient to remove gown

Inspect the breasts for size, shape, changes in skin texture or color, including any redness, dimpling, puckering, scaling, or retraction of the skin

Note symmetry and contour of the breasts and the position of the nipples bilaterally for any deviation or abnormality

Instruct patient to assume four different positions for visual inspection—arms at sides, hands at waist and pushing inward toward hips, hands behind the head, and arms across waist with chest falling forward

Assess for nipple discharge by gently squeezing each nipple

Inspect and palpate lymph node chains, including the supraclavicular, infraclavicular, lateral, central, subscapular, and anterior nodes for any abnormalities

Note the number, size, location, consistency, and mobility of nodes

Place a small pillow or towel under the shoulder blade of the breast to be examined, abduct the arm on the same side of that breast, and place the patient's hand behind her head

Using a systematic approach, palpate breast tissue with the palmar surface of the first three fingers of your dominant hand

Move in a rotary fashion and compress the breast tissue against the chest wall

Examine all four quadrants of the breast, including the axillary tail

Note any masses, including location, shape, size (in cm), tenderness, mobility, and consistency

Observe mastectomy scar site for presence of a rash, edema, thickening, and erythema, as appropriate

Repeat same process with other breast

Document all findings

Report abnormalities to physician or nurse in charge, as appropriate

Encourage patient to demonstrate self-palpation during and after clinical breast examination

Instruct the patient about the importance of regular, breast self-examination

Advise regular mammograms as appropriate for age, condition, and risk

Background Readings:

American Cancer Society. (1993). Guidelines for the cancer-related checkup: An update. Atlanta: American Cancer Society.

American Nurses Foundation. (1994). Clinician's handbook of preventive services. Waldorf, MD: American Nurses Publishing.

Champion, V.L. (1995). Results of a nurse-delivered intervention on proficiency and nodule detection with breast self-examination. Oncology Nursing Forum, 22(5), 819-824.

Edge, V., & Miller, M. (1994). Women's health care. St. Louis: Mosby-Year Book.

Perry, A.G., & Potter, P.A. (1998). Clinical nursing skills and techniques. (4th ed.). St. Louis: Mosby–Year Book.

Shaw, S.L. (1994). The role of the nurse in a comprehensive breast center. Journal of Oncology Management, 3(6), 49-51.

Breastfeeding Assistance   1054

Definition: Preparing a new mother to breastfeed her infant

Activities:

Discuss with parents an estimate of effort and length of time they would like to put toward breastfeeding

Provide early mother/infant contact opportunity to breastfeed within two hours after birth

Assist parents in identifying infant arousal cues as opportunities to practice breastfeeding

Monitor infant's ability to suck

Encourage mother to ask for assistance with early attempt to nurse, accomplishing 8-10 feedings in 24 hours

Observe infant at breast to determine correct positioning, audible swallowing and suck/swallow pattern

Monitor infant's ability to grasp the nipple correctly (e.g., "latch-on" skills)

Instruct mother to monitor infant's suck

Encourage comfort and privacy in early attempts to breastfeed

Encourage nonnutritive sucking at breast

Encourage mother to offer both breasts at each feeding

Encourage mother to allow infant to breastfeed as long as interested

Instruct mother on proper positioning

Instruct proper technique to break suction of nursing infant

Monitor skin integrity of nipples

Instruct on nipple care including how to prevent nipple soreness

Discuss the use of a breast pump if newborn is unable to breastfeed initially

Monitor increased filling of breasts in response to nursing and/or pumping

Inform mother of pump options available if needed to maintain lactation

Instruct on how to control breast congestion with timely emptying by nursing or pumping

Instruct on storage and warming of breast milk

Provide formula supplementation only when necessary

Instruct mother on how to burp newborn

Instruct mother on normal characteristics of infant voiding and stooling

Monitor letdown reflex

Instruct mother on well-balanced diet during lactation

Encourage mother to drink fluids to satisfy thirst

Instruct mother about infant growth spurts

Encourage use of comfortable, cotton, supportive nursing bra

Instruct to avoid using plastic lined nursing pads

Encourage mother to contact healthcare practitioner before taking any medication while breastfeeding

Encourage mother to avoid use of birth control pills while breastfeeding

Discuss alternative methods of contraception

Encourage mother to avoid cigarettes while breastfeeding

Identify maternal support system for maintaining lactation

Continued

Activities:—cont'd

Encourage frequent rest periods

Encourage continued lactation upon return to work or school

Provide written material to reinforce instruction at home

Refer parents to appropriate classes or support groups for breastfeeding

Refer mother to a lactation consultant as appropriate

Background Readings:

Hill, P., & Aldag, J. (1996). Smoking and breastfeeding status. Research in Nursing & Health, 19, 125-126.

Olds, S.B., London, M.L., & Ladewig, P.A. (1992). Maternal-newborn nursing: A family centered approach (4th ed.). Menlo Park, CA: Addison-Wesley.

Riordan, J., & Auerbach, K. (1993). Breastfeeding and human lactation. Boston: Jones & Bartlett Publishers.

Calming Technique   5880

Definition: Reducing anxiety in patient experiencing acute distress

Activities:

Hold and comfort an infant or child

Rock an infant, as appropriate

Speak softly or sing to an infant or child

Offer pacifier to infant, as appropriate

Maintain eye contact with patient

Provide "time out" in room, as appropriate

Maintain calm, deliberate manner

Sit and talk with patient

Encourage slow, purposeful deep breathing

Facilitate the patient's expression of anger in a constructive manner

Rub forehead, as appropriate

Reduce or eliminate stimuli creating fear or anxiety

Identify significant others whose presence can assist patient

Reassure patient of personal safety or security

Stay with patient

Use distraction, as appropriate

Offer warm fluids or milk

Offer back rub, as appropriate

Offer warm bath or shower

Provide antianxiety medications, as needed

Instruct patient on methods to decrease anxiety, as appropriate

Instruct patient on techniques to use to calm a crying infant (e.g., speaking to infant, placing hand on belly, restraining arms, picking up, and holding and rocking)

Background Readings:

Beck, C.K., Rawlins, R.P., & Williams, S.R. (1988). Mental health–psychiatric nursing. St. Louis: Mosby.

Brazelton, T.B. (1984). Neonatal behavioral assessments scale (2nd ed.). Philadelphia: J.B. Lippincott.

Luckmann, J., & Sorensen, K.C. (1987). Medical-surgical nursing (3rd ed.). Philadelphia: W.B. Saunders.

C

Capillary Blood Sample 4035

Definition: Obtaining an arteriovenous sample from a peripheral body site, such as the heel, finger, or other transcutaneous site

Activities:

Verify correct patient identification

Minimize anxiety for the patient using age-appropriate procedures

Maintain standard precautions

Select puncture site (e.g., outer lower aspect of heel, sides of distal fingers or toes, alternative sites such as the forearm)

Puncture outer aspect of heel no deeper than 2.4 mm on infants

Warm the site for approximately 5 minutes if specimen is to be an arterialized sample, according to agency protocol

Use aseptic technique during skin puncture

Puncture skin manually with a lancet or an approved penetration device according to manufacturer's specifications

Wipe off first drop of blood with dry gauze, per manufacturer's specifications or agency protocol

Collect blood in manner appropriate to test being performed (e.g., allow a drop of blood to fall onto manufacturer's specified area of filter paper or test strips, draw blood into tubes by capillary action as droplets form)

Apply intermittent pressure as far away from the puncture site as possible to promote blood flow

Avoid hemolysis caused by excessive squeezing or "milking" of puncture site

Follow manufacturer's guidelines regarding timing of tests and preservation of blood sample (e.g., sealing blood tubes), as necessary

Label specimen as necessary, according to agency protocol

Send specimen to laboratory, as necessary

Bandage site, as necessary

Teach and monitor self-sampling capillary blood, as appropriate

Dispose of equipment properly

Document completion of capillary blood sampling

Background Readings:

Escalante-Kanashiro, R., & Tatalean-Da-Fieno, J. (2000). Capillary blood gases in a pediatric intensive care unit. Critical Care Medicine, 28(1), 224-226.

Fletcher, M., & MacDonald, M.G. (1993). Atlas of procedures in neonatology (2nd ed.). Philadelphia, PA: J.B. Lippincott.

Meehan, R.M. (1998). Heelsticks in neonates for capillary blood sampling [corrected]. Neonatal Network—Journal of Neonatal Nursing, 17(1), 12-27.

Perry, A.G., & Potter, P.A. (2002). Clinical nursing skills and techniques (5th ed.). St. Louis: Mosby.

Pettersen, M.D., Driscoll, D.J., Moyer, T.P., Dearani, J.A., & McGregor, C.G. (1999). Measurement of blood serum cyclosporine levels using capillary "fingerstick" sampling: A validation study. Transplant International, 12(6), 429-432.

Wong, D.L., Perry, S.E., & Hockenberry, M.J. (2002). Maternal child nursing care. St. Louis: Mosby.

Yum, S.I., & Roe, J. (1999). Capillary blood sampling for self-monitoring of blood glucose. Diabetes Technology and Therapeutics, 1(1), 29-37.

Cardiac Care   4040

Definition: Limitation of complications resulting from an imbalance between myocardial oxygen supply and demand for a patient with symptoms of impaired cardiac function

Activities:

Evaluate chest pain (e.g., intensity, location, radiation, duration, and precipitating and alleviating factors)

Perform a comprehensive appraisal of peripheral circulation (e.g., check peripheral pulses, edema, capillary refill, color, and temperature of extremity)

Document cardiac dysrhythmias

Note signs and symptoms of decreased cardiac output

Monitor vital signs frequently

Monitor cardiovascular status

Monitor for cardiac dysrhythmias, including disturbances of both rhythm and conduction

Monitor respiratory status for symptoms of heart failure

Monitor abdomen for indications of decreased perfusion

Monitor fluid balance (e.g., intake/output and daily weight)

Monitor appropriate laboratory values (e.g., cardiac enzymes, electrolyte levels)

Monitor pacemaker functioning, if appropriate

Recognize presence of blood pressure alterations

Recognize psychological effects of underlying condition

Evaluate the patient's response to ectopy or dysrhythmias

Provide antiarrhythmic therapy according to unit policy (e.g., antiarrhythmic medication, cardioversion, or defibrillation), as appropriate

Monitor patient's response to antiarrhythmic medications

Instruct the patient and family on activity restriction and progression

Arrange exercise and rest periods to avoid fatigue

Monitor the patient's activity tolerance

Monitor for dyspnea, fatigue, tachypnea, and orthopnea

Promote stress reduction

Establish a supportive relationship with the patient and family

Instruct the patient on the importance of immediately reporting any chest discomfort

Offer spiritual support to the patient and/or family (e.g., contact clergy), as appropriate

Background Readings:

American Association of Critical-Care Nurses. (1990). Outcome standards for nursing care of the critically ill. Laguna Niguel, CA: AACN.

Cullen, L.M. (1992). Interventions related to circulatory care. In G.M. Bulechek & J.C. McCloskey (Eds.), Symposium on Nursing Interventions. Nursing Clinics of North America, 27(2), 445-476.

DeAngelis, R. (1991). The cardiovascular system. In J. Alspach (Ed.), AACN core curriculum for critical care nursing (4th ed.) (pp. 132-314). Philadelphia: W.B. Saunders.

Johanson, B.C., Wells, S.J., Hoffmeister, D., & Dungca, C.U. (1988). Standards for critical care (3rd ed.). St. Louis: Mosby.

LeMone, P., & Burke, K.M. (2000). Medical-surgical nursing: critical thinking in client care (2nd ed.) (pp. 1083-1098). Upper Saddle River, NJ: Prentice Hall Health.

Riegel, B. (1988). Acute myocardial infarction: Nursing interventions to optimize oxygen supply and demand. In L. Kern (Ed.), Cardiac critical care nursing (pp. 59-90). Rockville, MD: Aspen.

U.S. Department of Health and Human Services. (1994). Unstable angina: Diagnosis and management. Rockville, MD: Agency for Health Care Policy and Research.

C

Cardiac Care: Acute   4044

Definition: Limitation of complications for a patient recently experiencing an episode of an imbalance between myocardial oxygen supply and demand resulting in impaired cardiac function

Activities:

Evaluate chest pain (e.g., intensity, location, radiation, duration, and precipitating and alleviating factors)

Provide immediate and continuous means to summon nurse, and let the patient and family know calls will be answered immediately

Monitor cardiac rhythm and rate

Auscultate heart sounds

Recognize the frustration and fright caused by inability to communicate and exposure to strange machinery and environment

Auscultate lungs for crackles or other adventitious sounds

Monitor neurological status

Monitor intake/output, urine output, and daily weight, if appropriate

Select best EKG lead for continuous monitoring, if appropriate

Obtain 12-lead EKG, if appropriate

Determine serum CK, LDH, and AST levels, as appropriate

Monitor renal function (e.g., BUN and Cr levels), if appropriate

Monitor liver function, if appropriate

Monitor lab values for electrolytes, which may increase the risk of dysrhythmias (e.g., serum potassium and magnesium), as appropriate

Obtain chest x-ray, if appropriate

Monitor trends in blood pressure and hemodynamic parameters, if available (e.g., central venous pressure and pulmonary capillary/artery wedge pressure)

Provide small, frequent meals

Limit intake of caffeine, sodium, cholesterol, food high in fat, and so on

Monitor the effectiveness of oxygen therapy, if appropriate

Monitor determinants of oxygen delivery (e.g., PaO_2 and hemoglobin levels and cardiac output), if appropriate

Maintain an environment conducive to rest and healing

Instruct the patient to avoid activities that result in the Valsalva maneuver (e.g., straining during bowel movement)

Administer medications that will prevent episodes of the Valsalva maneuver (e.g., stool softeners, antiemetics), as appropriate

Refrain from taking rectal temperatures

Prevent peripheral thrombus formation (e.g., turn every 2 hours and administer low-dose anticoagulants)

Administer medications to relieve/prevent pain and ischemia, as needed

Monitor effectiveness of medication

Background Readings:

American Association of Critical-Care Nurses. (1990). Outcome standards for nursing care of the critically ill. Laguna Niguel, CA: AACN.

Bines, A.S., & Landron, S.L. (1993). Cardiovascular emergencies in the post anesthesia care unit. In K.L. Saleh & V. Brinsko (Eds.), Nursing Clinics of North America, 28(3), 493-506.

Cullen, L.M. (1992). Interventions related to circulatory care. In G.M. Bulechek & J.C. McCloskey (Eds.), Symposium on Nursing Interventions. Nursing Clinics of North America, 27(2), 445-476.

DeAngelis, R. (1991). The cardiovascular system. In J. Alspach (Ed.), AACN core curriculum for critical care nursing (4th ed.) (pp. 132-314). Philadelphia: W.B. Saunders.

Johanson, B.C., Wells, S.J., Hoffmeister, D., & Dungca, C.U. (1988). Standards for critical care (3rd ed.). St. Louis: Mosby.

LeMone, P., & Burke, K.M. (2000). Medical-surgical nursing: Critical thinking in client care, (2nd ed.) (pp. 1083-1098). Upper Saddle River, NJ: Prentice Hall Health.

Lewis, S.M., & Collier, I.C. (1996). Medical-surgical nursing: Assessment and management of clinical problems (4th ed.). St. Louis: Mosby.

U.S. Department of Health and Human Services. (1994). Unstable angina: Diagnosis and management. Rockville, MD: Agency for Health Care Policy and Research.

Woo, M.A. (1992). Clinical management of the patient with an acute infarction. Nursing Clinics of North America, 27(1), 189-204.

C

C

Cardiac Care: Rehabilitative 4046

Definition: Promotion of maximum functional activity level for a patient who has experienced an episode of impaired cardiac function that resulted from an imbalance between myocardial oxygen supply and demand

Activities:

Monitor the patient's activity tolerance

Maintain ambulation schedule, as tolerated

Encourage realistic expectations for the patient and family

Instruct the patient and family on appropriate prescribed and over-the-counter medications

Instruct the patient and family on cardiac risk factor modification (e.g., smoking cessation, diet, and exercise), as appropriate

Instruct the patient on self-care for chest pain (e.g., take sublingual nitroglycerine every 5 minutes three times; if chest pain is unrelieved, seek emergency medical care)

Instruct the patient and family on the exercise regimen, including warm-up, endurance, and cool-down, as appropriate

Instruct the patient and family on any lifting/pushing weight limitations, if appropriate

Instruct the patient and family on any special considerations regarding activities of daily living (e.g., isolate activities and allow rest periods), if appropriate

Instruct the patient and family on wound care and precautions (e.g., sternal incision or catheterization site), if appropriate

Instruct the patient and family on follow-up care

Coordinate patient referrals (e.g., dietary, social services, and physical therapy)

Instruct the patient and family on access to emergency services available in their community, as appropriate

Background Readings:

Allen, J., Becker, D., & Swank, R. (1990). Factors related to functional status after coronary artery bypass surgery. Heart & Lung, 19(4), 337-343.

Craven, R.F., & Hirnle, C.J. (2000). Fundamentals of nursing: Human health and function (3rd ed.) (pp. 873-874). Philadelphia: Lippincott.

Cullen, L.M. (1992). Interventions related to circulatory care. In G.M. Bulechek & J.C. McCloskey (Eds.), Symposium on Nursing Interventions. Nursing Clinics of North America, 27(2), 445-476.

Lamb, J., & Carlson, V. (1986). Handbook for cardiovascular nursing. Philadelphia: J.B. Lippincott.

Miller, P., Wikoff, R., McMahon, M., et al. (1989). Personal adjustments and regimen compliance one year after myocardial infarction. Heart & Lung, 18(4), 339-346.

Miller, P., Wikoff, R., McMahon, M., et al. (1988). Influence of a nursing interaction on regimen adherence and societal adjustment post myocardial infarction. Nursing Research, 37(5), 297-301.

Murdaugh, C. (1988). The nurse's role in education of the cardiac patient. In L. Kern (Ed.), Cardiac critical care nursing (pp. 251-280). Rockville, MD: Aspen.

Murdaugh, C., & Verran, J. (1987). Theoretical modeling to predict physiological indicants of cardiac preventive behaviors. Nursing Research, 36(5), 284-291.

U.S. Department of Health and Human Services. (1995). Cardiac rehabilitation. Rockville, MD: Agency for Health Care Policy and Research.

Weeks, L. (1986). Advanced cardiovascular nursing. Boston: Blackwell Scientific Publications.

Cardiac Precautions   4050

Definition: Prevention of an acute episode of impaired cardiac function by minimizing myocardial oxygen consumption or increasing myocardial oxygen supply

Activities:

Avoid causing intense emotional situations

Avoid overheating or chilling the patient

Discourage decision making when the patient is under severe stress

Refrain from giving oral stimulants

Refrain from inserting a rectal tube

Refrain from taking rectal temperatures

Refrain from doing a rectal/vaginal examination

Limit environmental stimuli

Delay bathing, if appropriate

Restrict smoking

Refrain from arguing

Provide small, frequent meals

Substitute artificial salt and limit sodium intake, if appropriate

Identify the patient's readiness to learn lifestyle modification

Discuss modifications in sexual activity with patient and significant other, if appropriate

Encourage noncompetitive activities

Instruct the patient on progressive exercise

Instruct patient/family on symptoms of cardiac compromise indicating need for rest

Identify the patient's methods of handling stress

Promote effective techniques for reducing stress

Perform relaxation therapy, if appropriate

Background Readings:

American Association of Critical-Care Nurses. (1990). Outcome standards for nursing care of the critically ill. Laguna Niguel, CA: AACN.

Cullen, L.M. (1992). Interventions related to circulatory care. In G.M. Bulechek & J.C. McCloskey (Eds.), Symposium on Nursing Interventions. Nursing Clinics of North America, 27(2), 445-476.

DeAngelis, R. (1991). The cardiovascular system. In J. Alspach (Ed.), AACN core curriculum for critical care nursing (4th ed.) (pp. 132-314). Philadelphia: W.B. Saunders.

Futrell, A., Forst, S., Harell, J., et al. (1991). Effects of occupied and unoccupied bed making on myocardial work in healthy subjects. Heart & Lung, 20(2), 161-167.

Kirchhoff, K.T. (1981). An examination of the physiologic basis for coronary precautions. Heart & Lung, 10(5), 874-879.

Kirchhoff, K.T. (1990). Electrocardiographic response to ice water ingestion. Heart & Lung, 19(1), 41-48.

Weeks, L. (1986). Advanced cardiovascular nursing. Boston: Blackwell Scientific Publications.

Caregiver Support 7040

> *Definition:* Provision of the necessary information, advocacy, and support to facilitate primary patient care by someone other than a health care professional

Activities:

Determine caregiver's level of knowledge

Determine caregiver's acceptance of role

Accept expressions of negative emotion

Acknowledge difficulties of caregiving role

Explore with the caregiver strengths and weaknesses

Acknowledge dependency of patient on caregiver, as appropriate

Make positive statements about caregiver's efforts

Encourage caregiver to assume responsibility, as appropriate

Provide support for decisions made by caregiver

Encourage the acceptance of interdependency among family members

Monitor family interaction problems related to care of patient

Provide information about patient's condition in accordance with patient preferences

Teach caregiver the patient's therapy in accordance with patient preferences

Teach caregiver techniques to improve security of patient

Provide for follow-up health caregiver assistance through phone calls and/or community nurse care

Monitor for indicators of stress

Explore with caregiver how she/he is coping

Teach caregiver stress management techniques

Educate caregiver about the grieving process

Support caregiver through grieving process

Encourage caregiver participation in support groups

Teach caregiver health care maintenance strategies to sustain own physical and mental health

Foster caregiver social networking

Identify sources of respite care

Inform caregiver of health care and community resources

Teach caregiver strategies to access and maximize health care and community resources

Act for caregiver if overburdening becomes apparent

Notify emergency services agency/personnel about the patient's stay at home, health status, and technologies in use with consent of patient and family

Discuss caregiver limits with patient

Provide encouragement to caregiver during times of setback for patient

Support caregiver in setting limits and taking care of self

Background Readings:

Craft, M.J., & Denehy, J.A. (1990). Nursing interventions for infants and children. Philadelphia: W.B. Saunders.

Craft, M.J., & Willadsen, J.A. (1992). Interventions related to family. In G.M. Bulechek & J.C. McCloskey (Eds.), Symposium on Nursing Interventions. Nursing Clinics of North America, 27(2), 517-540.

Maas, M.L., Buckwalter, K.C., Hardy, M.D., Reimer, T.T., Titler, M.G., & Specht, J.P. (2001). Nursing care of older adults: Diagnoses, outcomes, & interventions (pp. 686-693). St. Louis: Mosby.

Moore, L.W., Marocco, G., Schmidt, S.M., Guo, L., & Estes, J. (2002). Perspectives of caregivers of stroke survivors: Implications for nursing, MEDSURG Nursing, 11(6), 289-295.

C

C

Case Management

7320

Definition: Coordinating care and advocating for specified individuals and patient populations across settings to reduce cost, reduce resource use, improve quality of health care, and achieve desired outcomes

Activities:

Identify individuals or patient populations who would benefit from case management (e.g., high cost, high volume, and/or high risk)

Identify payment source for case management service

Explain the role of the case manager to patient and family

Explain the cost of service to patient and/or family before rendering care

Obtain patient or family's permission to be enrolled in a case management program, as appropriate

Develop relationships with patient, family, and other health care providers, as needed

Use effective communication skills with patient, family, and other health care providers

Treat patient and family with dignity and respect

Maintain patient and family confidentiality and privacy

Assess patient's physical health status, mental status, functional capability, formal and informal support systems, financial resources, and environmental conditions, as needed

Determine treatment plan with input from patient and/or family

Explain critical paths to patient and family

Individualize critical path for patient

Determine outcomes to be obtained with input from patient and/or family

Discuss plan of care and intended outcomes with patient's physician

Negotiate work schedule with the nurse manager (head nurse) to attend weekly group practice meetings, as needed

Integrate care management information and revised interventions (processes) into intershift report and group practice meetings, as needed

Evaluate progress toward established goals on a continual basis

Revise interventions and goals as necessary to meet patient's needs

Identify resources and/or services needed

Coordinate provision of needed resources or services

Coordinate care with other pertinent health care providers (e.g., other nurses, physician(s), social worker, third-party payer(s), physical therapist)

Provide direct care as necessary

Educate patient and/or family on importance of self-care

Encourage appropriate patient and/or family decision-making activities

Document all case management activities

Monitor plan for quality, quantity, timeliness, and effectiveness of services

Facilitate access to necessary health and social services

Assist patient and/or family with access to the health care delivery system

Guide patient and/or family through the health care delivery system

Assist patient and/or family in making informed decisions regarding health care

Advocate for patient as necessary

Recognize need to merge patient, clinical, and financial concerns

Notify patient and/or family of change in service, termination of service, and discharge from case management program

Promote efficient use of resources

Monitor cost-effectiveness of care

Modify care to increase cost-effectiveness, as needed

Establish quality improvement program to evaluate case management activities

Document cost-effectiveness of case management

Report outcomes to insurers and other third-party payers

Market services to individuals, families, insurers, and employers

Background Readings:

Bower, K. (1988). Case management by nurses. Washington, DC: American Nurses Publishing.

Crummer, M.B., & Carter, V. (1993). Critical pathways–the pivotal tool. Journal of Cardiovascular Nursing, 7(4), 30-37.

Davis, V. (1996). Staff development for nurse case management. In E.L. Cohen (Ed.), Nurse case management in the 21st century (pp. 189-196). St. Louis: Mosby.

Flarey, D.L., & Blancett, S.S. (1996). Handbook of nursing case management: Health care delivery in a world of managed care. Gaithersburg, MD: Aspen Publishers, Inc.

Newell, M. (1996). Using case management to improve health outcomes. Gaithersburg, MD: Aspen Publishers, Inc.

Zander, K. (1993). The impact of managing care on the role of a nurse. Series on Nursing Administration, 5, 65-82.

C

Cast Care: Maintenance 0762

Definition: Care of a cast after the drying period

Activities:

Apply sodium bicarbonate (baking soda) to an odiferous cast

Inspect cast for signs of drainage from wounds under the cast

Mark the circumference of any drainage as a gauge for future assessments

Apply plastic to cast if close to groin

Instruct patient not to scratch skin under the cast with any objects

Avoid getting a plaster cast wet

Position cast on pillows to lessen strain on other body parts

Check for cracking or breaks in the cast

Apply an arm sling for support, if appropriate

Pad rough cast edges and traction connections, as appropriate

Background Readings:

Beck, C.K., Rawlins, R.P., & Williams, S.R. (1988). Mental health-psychiatric nursing. St. Louis: Mosby.

Farrell, J. (1986). Illustrated guide to orthopedic nursing (3rd ed.). Philadelphia: J.B. Lippincott.

Feller, N.G., Stroup, K., & Christian, L. (1989). Helping staff nurses become mini-specialists: Cast care. American Journal of Nursing, 89(7), 991-992.

Kozier, B., & Erb, G. (1989). Techniques in clinical nursing (3rd ed.). Menlo Park, CA: Addison-Wesley.

Perry, A.G., & Potter, P.A. (1998). Clinical nursing skills and techniques. (4th ed.) St. Louis: Mosby.

Smith, S., & Duell, D. (1992). Clinical nursing skills (3rd ed.). Los Altos, CA: National Nursing Review.

Cast Care: Wet 0764

Definition: Care of a new cast during the drying period

Activities:

Expose the drying cast to air

Monitor circulation and color of fingers/toes on injured extremity

Support the cast with pillows during the drying period

Inform the patient that the cast will feel warm as the cast dries

Monitor capillary refill by applying pressure to a fingernail or toenail

Apply plastic to cast if close to groin

Maintain the angles of the cast during the drying period

Inspect cast for signs of drainage from wounds under the cast

Mark the circumference of any drainage as a gauge for future assessments

Explain the need for limited activity while cast dries

Identify any change in sensation or increased pain at the fracture site

Background Readings:

Perry, A.G., & Potter, P.A. (1998). Clinical nursing skills and techniques. (4th ed.). St. Louis: Mosby.
Smith, S., & Duell, D. (1992). Clinical nursing skills (3rd ed.). Los Altos, CA: National Nursing Review.

C

C

Cerebral Edema Management 2540

Definition: Limitation of secondary cerebral injury resulting from swelling of brain tissue

Activities:

Monitor for confusion, changes in mentation, complaints of dizziness, syncope

Monitor neurologic status closely and compare with baseline

Monitor vital signs

Monitor CSF drainage characteristics: color, clarity, consistency

Record CSF drainage

Monitor CVP, PAWP, and PAP, as appropriate

Monitor ICP and CPP

Analyze ICP waveform

Monitor respiratory status: rate, rhythm, depth of respirations; PaO_2, pCO_2, pH, bicarbonate

Allow ICP to return to baseline between nursing activities

Monitor patient's ICP and neurological responses to care activities

Decrease stimuli in patient's environment

Plan nursing care to provide rest periods

Give sedation, as needed

Note patient's change in response to stimuli

Screen conversation within patient's hearing

Administer anticonvulsants, as appropriate

Avoid neck flexion or extreme hip/knee flexion

Avoid Valsalva maneuvers

Administer stool softeners

Position with head of bed up 30° or greater

Avoid use of PEEP

Administer paralyzing agent, as appropriate

Encourage family/significant other to talk to patient

Restrict fluids

Avoid use of hypotonic IV fluids

Adjust ventilator settings to keep $PaCO_2$ at prescribed level

Limit suction passes to less than 15 seconds

Monitor lab values: serum and urine osmolality, sodium, potassium

Monitor volume pressure indices

Perform passive range-of-motion excercises

Monitor intake and output

Maintain normothermia

Administer loop-active or osmotic diuretics

Implement seizure precautions

Titrate barbiturate to achieve suppression or burst-suppression of EEG as ordered

Establish means of communication: ask yes or no questions; provide magic slate, paper and pencil, picture board, flashcards, VOCAID device

Background Readings:

American Association of Critical-Care Nurses (1998). Core curriculum for critical care nursing (5th ed.). Philadelphia: W.B. Saunders.

American Academy of Pediatrics. (1999). The management of minor closed head injury in children. Pediatrics, 104(6), 1407-15.

Orfanelli, L. (2001). Neurologic examination of the toddler. American Journal of Nursing, 101(12), 24CC-24FF.

Yanko, J.R., & Mitcho, K. (2001). Acute care management of severe traumatic brain injuries. Critical Care Nursing Quarterly, 23(4), 1-23.

C

Cerebral Perfusion Promotion 2550

Definition: Promotion of adequate perfusion and limitation of complications for a patient experiencing or at risk for inadequate cerebral perfusion

Activities:

Consult with physician to determine hemodynamic parameters, and maintain hemodynamic parameters within this range

Induce hypertension with volume expansion or inotropic or vasoconstrictive agents, as ordered, to maintain hemodynamic parameters and maintain/optimize cerebral perfusion pressure (CPP)

Administer and titrate vasoactive drugs, as ordered, to maintain hemodynamic parameters

Administer agents to expand intravascular volume, as appropriate (e.g., colloid, blood products, and crystalloid)

Administer volume expanders to maintain hemodynamic parameters, as ordered

Monitor prothrombin time (PT) and partial thromboplastin time (PTT), if using hetastarch as a volume expander

Administer rheologic agents (e.g., low-dose mannitol or low-molecular-weight dextrans [LMDs]), as ordered

Keep hematocrit level around 33% for hypervolemic hemodilution therapy

Phlebotomize patient, as appropriate, to maintain hematocrit level in desired range

Maintain serum glucose level within normal range

Consult with physician to determine optimal head of bed (HOB) placement (e.g., 0, 15, or 30 degrees) and monitor patient's responses to head positioning

Avoid neck flexion or extreme hip/knee flexion

Keep pCO_2 level at 25 mm Hg or greater

Administer calcium channel blockers, as ordered

Administer vasopressin, as ordered

Administer and monitor effects of osmotic and loop-active diuretics and corticosteroids

Administer pain medication, as appropriate

Administer anticoagulant medication, as ordered

Administer antiplatelet medications, as ordered

Administer thrombolytic medications, as ordered

Monitor patient's prothrombin time (PT) and partial thromboplastin time (PTT) to keep 1 to 2 times normal, as appropriate

Monitor for anticoagulant therapy side effects

Monitor for signs of bleeding (e.g., test stool and NG tube drainage for blood)

Monitor neurological status

Calculate and monitor cerebral perfusion pressure (CPP)

Monitor patient's ICP and neurological responses to care activities

Monitor mean arterial pressure (MAP)

Monitor CVP

Monitor PAWP and PAP

Monitor respiratory status (e.g., rate, rhythm, and depth of respirations; pO_2, pCO_2, pH, and bicarbonate levels)

Auscultate lung sounds for crackles or other adventitious sounds

Monitor for signs of fluid overload (e.g., rhonchi, jugular venous distention [JVD], edema, and increase in pulmonary secretions)

Monitor determinants of tissue oxygen delivery (e.g., $PaCO_2$, SaO_2, and hemoglobin levels and cardiac output), if available

Monitor lab values for changes in oxygenation or acid-base balance, as appropriate

Monitor intake and output

Background Readings:

Bronstein, K.S., Popovich, J.M., & Stewart-Amidei, C. (1991). Promoting stroke recovery: A research-based approach for nurses. St. Louis: Mosby.

Hickey, J.V. (1992). The clinical practice of neurological and neurosurgical nursing. Philadelphia: J.B. Lippincott.

Hummel, S.K. (1989). Cerebral vasospasm: Current concepts of pathogenesis and treatment. Journal of Neuroscience Nursing, 21(4), 216-224.

Mitchell, S.K., & Yates, R.R. (1986). Cerebral vasospasm: Theoretical causes, medical management and nursing implications. Journal of Neuroscience Nursing, 18(6), 315-323.

Stewart-Amidei, C. (1989). Hypervolemic hemodilution: A new approach to subarachnoid hemorrhage. Heart & Lung, 18(6), 590-598.

C

C

Cesarean Section Care

6750

Definition: Preparation and support of patient delivering a baby by cesarean section

Activities:

Determine patient's perception of and preparation for cesarean section, as appropriate

Explain reasons for unplanned cesarean section, as appropriate

Encourage patient to express feelings about unplanned cesarean section

Give information about procedure and sensations that will be experienced

Set up for cesarean delivery

Prepare abdomen for cesarean delivery

Encourage father to observe delivery, as appropriate

Provide emotional support to patient during cesarean section

Give information about how procedure is proceeding

Give information about infant

Provide opportunity to see or hold infant after birth, as appropriate

Take patient to recovery room, if indicated

Inspect condition of surgical incision, as appropriate

Assist in performing leg exercises until effects of anesthetic wear off

Encourage patient to continue leg exercises until ambulatory

Give pain medication to facilitate rest, relaxation, lactation, and child care, as appropriate

Give TENS therapy to breastfeeding mother to minimize the use of medications, as appropriate

Discuss patient's and significant other's feelings about cesarean delivery

Background Readings:

Littleton, L.Y., & Engbretson, J.C. (2002). Maternal, neonatal, and women's health nursing (pp. 694-695). Albany, NY: Delmar.

Olds, S.B., London, M.L., & Ladewig, P.A. (1992). Maternal-newborn nursing: A family centered approach (4th ed.). Menlo Park, CA: Addison-Wesley.

Chemical Restraint   6430

Definition: Administration, monitoring, and discontinuation of psychotropic agents used to control an individual's extreme behavior

Activities:

Implement alternative interventions to attempt to eliminate the need for restraint

Provide diversionary activities prior to the use of restraints (e.g., television, visitors)

Identify for the patient and significant others those behaviors that necessitated the intervention (e.g., agitation, violence)

Explain the procedure, purpose, and duration of the intervention to patient and significant others in understandable terms

Follow the 5 rights of medication administration

Note patient's medical history and history of allergies

Monitor the patient's response to the medication

Monitor level of consciousness

Monitor vital signs

Provide appropriate level of supervision/surveillance to monitor patient and to allow for therapeutic actions, as needed

Provide for patient's psychological comfort, as needed

Monitor skin color, temperature, sensation, and condition

Provide for movement and exercise, according to patient's level of self-control, condition, and abilities

Position patient to facilitate comfort and prevent aspiration and skin breakdown

Assist with periodic changes in body position

Assist with needs related to nutrition, elimination, hydration, and personal hygiene

Evaluate, at regular intervals, patient's need for continued restrictive intervention

Involve patient, when appropriate, in making decisions to move to a more/less restrictive form of intervention

Background Readings:

Kow, J.V., & Hogan, D.B. (2000). Use of physical and chemical restraints in medical teaching units. Canadian Medical Association Journal, 162(3), 339-340.

Middleton, H., Keene, R.G., Johnson, C., Elkins, A.D., & Keem A.E. (1999). Physical and pharmacologic restraints in long-term care facilities. Journal of Gerontological Nursing, 25(7), 26-33.

Chemical Restraint Guidelines Draft. (12/00). Retrieved March 8, 2002, from http://www.ascp.com/public/pr/hcfadraftchem.shtml

Chemotherapy Management   2240

Definition: Assisting the patient and family to understand the action and minimize side effects of antineoplastic agents

Activities:

Monitor for side effects and toxic effects of chemotherapeutic agents

Provide information to patient and family on how antineoplastic drugs work on cancer cells

Teach patient and family about the effects of chemotherapy on bone marrow functioning

Instruct patient and family on ways to prevent infection, such as avoiding crowds and using good hygiene and hand-washing techniques

Instruct patient to promptly report fevers, chills, nosebleeds, excessive bruising, and tarry stools

Instruct patient and family to avoid the use of aspirin products

Institute neutropenic and bleeding precautions

Determine the patient's previous experience with chemotherapy-related nausea and vomiting

Administer antiemetic drugs for nausea and vomiting

Minimize stimuli from noises, light, and odors (especially food odors)

Teach the patient relaxation and imagery techniques to use before, during, and after treatments, as appropriate

Offer the patient a bland and easily digested diet

Administer chemotherapeutic drugs in the late evening, so the patient may sleep at the time emetic effects are greatest

Ensure adequate fluid intake to prevent dehydration and electrolyte imbalance

Monitor the effectiveness of measures to control nausea and vomiting

Teach patient and family to monitor for signs and symptoms of stomatitis

Instruct patient on proper oral hygiene techniques

Teach patient to use oral nystatin suspension to control fungal infection, as appropriate

Teach patient to avoid temperature extremes and chemical treatments of the hair while receiving chemotherapy

Teach patient to comb hair gently and to sleep on a silk pillowcase to minimize hair loss

Inform patient that hair loss is expected, as determined by type of chemotherapeutic agent used

Assist patient in obtaining a wig or other head-covering device, as appropriate

Offer six small feedings daily, as tolerated

Instruct patient to avoid hot, spicy foods

Provide nutritious, appetizing foods of patient's choice

Monitor nutritional status and weight

Teach patient and family to monitor for organ toxicity, as determined by type of chemotherapeutic agent used

Discuss with patient the possibility of sterility and other reproductive system impairments, as appropriate

Instruct long-term survivors and their families of the possibility of second malignancies and the importance of reporting increased susceptibility to infection, fatigue, or bleeding

Follow recommended guidelines for safe handling of parenteral antineoplastic drugs during drug preparation and administration

C

Background Readings:

Doane, L.S. (1993). Administering intraperitoneal chemotherapy using a peritoneal port. Nursing Clinics of North America, 28(4), 885-898.

LeMone, P., & Burke, K.M. (2000). Medical-surgical nursing: Critical thinking in client care (2nd ed.) (pp. 338-344). Upper Saddle River, NJ: Prentice Hall Health.

Miaskowski, C. (1991). Chemotherapy update. Nursing Clinics of North America, 26(2), 331-340.

Patrick, M.L., Woods, S.L., Craven, R.F., Rokosky, J.S., & Bruno, P.M. (1991). Medical-surgical nursing pathophysiological concepts (2nd ed.). Philadelphia: J.B. Lippincott.

Wegeneka, M.H. (1999) Chemotherapy management. In G. Bulechek & J. McCloskey (Eds). Nursing interventions: Effective nursing treatments (3rd ed.) (pp. 285-296). Philadelphia: W.B. Saunders Company.

Wheeler, V. (1991). Cancer therapy and principles of nursing management. In M.L. Patrick, S.L. Woods, R.F. Craven, J.S. Rokosky, & P.M. Bruno (Eds.), Medical-surgical nursing: Pathophysiological concepts (2nd ed.) (pp. 333-347). Philadelphia: J.B. Lippincott.

Chest Physiotherapy 3230

Definition: Assisting the patient to move airway secretions from peripheral airways to more central airways for expectoration and/or suctioning

Activities:

Determine presence of contraindications for use of chest physical therapy

Determine which lung segment(s) needs to be drained

Position patient with the lung segment to be drained in uppermost position

Use pillows to support patient in designated position

Use percussion with postural drainage by cupping hands and clapping the chest wall in rapid succession to produce a series of hollow sounds

Use chest vibration in combination with postural drainage, as appropriate

Use an ultrasonic nebulizer, as appropriate

Use aerosol therapy, as appropriate

Administer bronchodilators, as appropriate

Administer mucokinetic agents, as appropriate

Monitor amount and type of sputum expectoration

Encourage coughing during and after postural drainage

Monitor patient tolerance by means of SaO_2, respiratory rhythm and rate, cardiac rhythm and rate, and comfort levels

Background Readings:

Brooks-Brunn, J. (1986). Respiration. In L. Abels (Ed.), Critical care nursing: A physiologic approach (pp. 168-253). St. Louis: Mosby.

Craven, R.F., & Hirnle, C.J. (2000) Fundamentals of nursing: Human health and function. (3rd ed.) (pp. 810-813). Philadelphia: Lippincott.

Kiriloff, L.H., Owens, G.R., Rogers, R.M., & Mazzocco, M.C. (1985). Does chest physical therapy work? Chest, 88, 436-444.

Nelson, D.M. (1992). Interventions related to respiratory care. In G.M. Bulechek & J.C. McCloskey (Eds.), Symposium on Nursing Interventions. Nursing Clinics of North America, 27(2), 301-324.

Sutton, P., Parker, R., Webber, B., Newman, S., Garland, N., Lopez-Vidriera, M., Pavia, D., & Clark, S.W. (1983). Assessment of forced expiration technique, postural drainage, and directed coughing in chest physiotherapy. European Journal of Respiratory Disease, 64, 62-68.

Childbirth Preparation

6760

Definition: Providing information and support to facilitate childbirth and to enhance the ability of an individual to develop and perform the role of parent

Activities:

Prepare patient and partner for labor and delivery

Explore options for prenatal care and labor and delivery with patient

Inform patient about option for delivery over an intact perineum and circumstances dictating the need for an episiotomy

Instruct patient on steps to be taken if desire is to avoid episiotomy, such as perineal massage, Kegel exercises, optimal nutrition, and prompt treatment of vaginitis

Educate patient about delivery options if complications arise

Teach patient and partner breathing and relaxation techniques to be used during labor and delivery

Teach partner measures to comfort patient during labor (e.g., back rub, back pressure, and positioning)

Prepare partner to coach mother during labor and delivery

Discuss arrangement for sibling care during hospitalization

Discuss advantages and disadvantages of breastfeeding and bottle feeding

Instruct patient to prepare nipples for breastfeeding, as indicated

Determine patient's knowledge and attitudes about parenting

Promote patient's self-esteem in taking on parental role

Provide anticipatory guidance for parenthood

Determine how parent(s) prepared sibling(s) for coming of new baby, as appropriate

Assist patient in planning strategies to prepare siblings for newborn

Refer parent(s) to sibling preparation class

Assist parent to select a physician or clinic to perform child health supervision for newborn

Encourage patient to get infant car seat to take newborn home from hospital

Background Readings:

Department of Health and Human Services. (1989). Caring for our future: The content of prenatal care: A report of the Public Health Service Panel on the Content of Prenatal Care. No. 90-3182. Washington, DC: U.S. Government Printing Office.

Fawcett, J., Pollio, N., Tully, A., Baron, M., Henklein, J.C., & Jones, R.C. (1993). Effects of information on adaptation to cesarean birth. Nursing Research, 42(1), 49-53.

Littleton, L.Y., & Engebertson, J.C. (2002). Maternal, neonatal, and women's health nursing (pp. 477-489). Albany, NY: Delmar.

Olds, S.B., London, M.L., & Ladewig, P.A. (1992). Maternal-newborn nursing: A family centered approach (4th ed.). Menlo Park, CA: Addison-Wesley.

Circulatory Care: Arterial Insufficiency 4062

Definition: Promotion of arterial circulation

Activities:

Perform a comprehensive appraisal of peripheral circulation (e.g., check peripheral pulses, edema, capillary refill, color, and temperature)

Determine the ankle-brachial index (ABI), as appropriate

Evaluate peripheral edema and pulses

Inspect skin for arterial ulcers or tissue breakdown

Monitor degree of discomfort or pain with exercise, at night, or while resting

Place extremity in a dependent position, as appropriate

Administer antiplatelet or anticoagulant medications, as appropriate

Change the patient's position at least every 2 hours, as appropriate

Encourage the patient to exercise as tolerated

Protect the extremity from injury (e.g., sheepskin under feet and lower legs, footboard/bed cradle at foot of bed; well-fitted shoes)

Provide warmth (e.g., additional bed clothes, increasing the room temperature), as appropriate

Instruct the patient on factors that interfere with circulation (e.g., smoking, restrictive clothing, exposure to cold temperatures, and crossing of legs and feet)

Instruct the patient on proper foot care

Avoid applying direct heat to the extremity

Maintain adequate hydration to decrease blood viscosity

Monitor fluid status, including intake and output

Implement wound care, as appropriate

Background Readings:

Anonymous. (2001). Clinical management extra: Vascular ulcers. Arterial vs. venous ulcers: Diagnosis and treatment. Advances in Skin & Wound Care, 14(3), 146-149.

Hayward, L. (2002). Wound care. Patient-centered leg ulcer care. Nursing Times, 98(2), 59, 61.

Hiatt, W.R., & Regensteiner, J.G. (1993). Nonsurgical management of peripheral arterial disease. Hospital Practice, 28(2), 59-70.

Circulatory Care: Mechanical Assist Device   4064

Definition: Temporary support of the circulation through the use of mechanical devices or pumps

Activities:

Perform a comprehensive appraisal of peripheral circulation (e.g., check peripheral pulses, edema, capillary refill, color, and temperature of extremity)

Monitor sensorium and cognitive abilities

Monitor degree of chest discomfort or pain

Evaluate pulmonary artery pressures, systemic pressures, cardiac output, and systemic vascular resistance, as indicated

Assist with insertion or implantation of the device

Observe for hemolysis as indicated by blood in the urine, hemolyzed blood specimens, increase in daily serum hemoglobin, frank bleeding, and hyperkalemia

Observe cannulas for kinks or disconnections

Determine activated clotting times every hour, as appropriate

Administer anticoagulants or antithrombolytics, as ordered

Monitor the device regularly to ensure proper functioning

Have back-up equipment available at all times

Administer positive inotropic agents, as appropriate

Monitor coagulation profiles every 6 hours, as appropriate

Administer blood products, as appropriate

Monitor urine output every hour

Monitor electrolytes, BUN, and creatinine daily

Monitor weight daily

Monitor intake and output

Obtain chest x-ray daily

Use strict aseptic technique in changing dressings

Administer prophylactic antibiotics

Monitor for fever and leukocytosis

Collect blood, urine, sputum, and wound cultures for temperatures greater than 38° C, as appropriate

Administer antifungal oral solutions

Administer total parenteral nutrition, as appropriate

Administer pain medications, as needed

Teach patient and family about the device

Provide emotional support for the patient and family

Background Readings:

LeMone, P., & Burke, K.M. (2000) Medical-surgical nursing: Critical thinking in client care (2nd ed.) (pp. 1110-1112). Upper Saddle River, NJ: Prentice Hall Health.

Ruzevich, S. (1993). Cardiac assist devices. In J.M. Clochesy, C. Breu, S. Cardin, E.B. Rudy, & A.A. Whittaker (Eds.), Critical care nursing (pp. 183-192). Philadelphia: W.B. Saunders.

C

Circulatory Care: Venous Insufficiency   4066

Definition: Promotion of venous circulation

Activities:

Perform a comprehensive appraisal of peripheral circulation (e.g., check peripheral pulses, edema, capillary refill, color, and temperature)

Evaluate peripheral edema and pulses

Inspect skin for stasis ulcers and tissue breakdown

Implement wound care (debridement, antimicrobial therapy), as needed

Apply dressing appropriate for wound size and type, as appropriate

Monitor degree of discomfort or pain

Instruct the patient on the importance of compression therapy

Apply compression therapy modalities (short-stretch or long-stretch bandages), as appropriate

Elevate affected limb 20 degrees or greater above the level of the heart, as appropriate

Change the patient's position at least every 2 hours, as appropriate

Encourage passive or active range-of-motion exercises especially of the lower extremities, during bed rest

Administer antiplatelet or anticoagulant medications, as appropriate

Protect the extremity from injury (e.g., sheepskin under feet and lower legs, footboard/bed cradle at foot of bed; well-fitted shoes)

Instruct the patient on proper foot care

Maintain adequate hydration to decrease blood viscosity

Monitor fluid status, including intake and output

Background Readings:

Anonymous. (2001). Clinical management extra: Vascular ulcers. Arterial vs. venous ulcers: Diagnosis and treatment. Advances in Skin & Wound Care, 14(3), 146-149.

Hayward, L. (2002). Wound care. Patient-centered leg ulcer care. Nursing Times, 98(2), 59, 61.

Hess, C. T. (2001). Clinical management extra: Management of a venous ulcer: A case study approach. Advances in Skin & Wound Care, 14(3), 148-149.

Kunimoto, B. T. (2001). Management and prevention of venous leg ulcers: A literature-guided approach. Ostomy/Wound Management, 47(6), 36-49.

Circulatory Precautions   4070

Definition: Protection of a localized area with limited perfusion

Activities:

Perform a comprehensive appraisal of peripheral circulation (e.g., check peripheral pulses, edema, capillary refill, color, and temperature of extremity)

Do not start an IV or draw blood in the affected extremity

Refrain from taking blood pressure in affected extremity

Refrain from applying pressure or tourniquet to affected extremity

Maintain adequate hydration to prevent increased blood viscosity

Avoid injury to affected area

Prevent infection in wounds

Instruct the patient to test bath water before entering to avoid burning skin

Instruct patient on foot and nail care

Instruct patient and family on protection from injury of affected area

Monitor extremities for areas of heat, redness, pain, or swelling

Background Readings:

American Association of Critical-Care Nurses. (1990). Outcome standards for nursing care of the critically ill. Laguna Niguel, CA: AACN.

Cullen, L.M. (1992). Interventions related to circulatory care. In G.M. Bulechek & J.C. McCloskey (Eds.), Symposium on Nursing Interventions. Nursing Clinics of North America, 27(2), 445-476.

DeAngelis, R. (1991). The cardiovascular system. In J. Alspach (Ed.), AACN core curriculum for critical care nursing (4th ed.) (pp. 132-314). Philadelphia: W.B. Saunders.

Doyle, J., Johantgen, M., & Vitello-Cicciu, J. (1993). Vascular disease. In M.R. Kinney, D.R. Packa, & S.B. Dunbar (Eds.), AACN's clinical reference for critical-care nursing (pp. 607-634). St. Louis: Mosby.

LeMone, P., & Burke, K.M. (2000). Medical-surgical nursing: Critical thinking in client care (2nd ed.) (pp. 1253-1257). Upper Saddle River, NJ: Prentice Hall Health.

Circumcision Care

3000

Definition: Preprocedural and postprocedural support to males undergoing circumcision

Activities:

Verify that the surgical consent form is properly signed

Verify correct patient identification

Administer preprocedure pain control approximately 1 hour prior to the procedure (e.g., acetaminophen)

Position the patient in a comfortable position during the procedure

Use a padded circumcision seat for infants

Use a radiant warmer to maintain body temperature during the procedure

Shield infant's eyes from direct light

Use a pacifier dipped in sucrose during the procedure and until the next feeding, with permission from parent/guardian

Swaddle the infant's upper body during the circumcision

Play soft, appropriate music during the procedure

Monitor vital signs

Administer a topical local analgesic agent (e.g., EMLA), as ordered

Assist the physician with the dorsal penile nerve block, as appropriate

Apply white petroleum jelly and/or dressing, as appropriate

Monitor for bleeding every 30 minutes for a least 2 hours after the procedure

Provide postprocedure pain control every 4 to 6 hours for 24 hours (e.g., acetaminophen)

Instruct the patient/parent of signs and symptoms to report to the physician (e.g., increased temperature, bleeding, swelling, inability to urinate)

Arrange for cultural accommodations

Background Readings:

Alkalay, A.L., & Sola, A. (2000). Analgesia and local anesthesia for non-ritual circumcision in stable healthy newborns. Neonatal Intensive Care, 13(2), 19-22.

Joyce, B.A., Keck, J. F., & Gerkensmeyer, J. (2001). Evaluation of pain management interventions for neonatal circumcision pain. Journal of Pediatric Health Care, 15, 105-114.

Williamson, M.L. (1997). Circumcision anesthesia: A study of nursing implications for dorsal penile nerve block. Pediatric Nursing 12(1), 59-63.

University of Iowa Hospital and Clinics. (2000). Children's and Women's Services. Department of Nursing. Circumcision standard of practice. Iowa City, IA: University of Iowa Hospital and Clinics.

Code Management   6140

Definition: Coordination of emergency measures to sustain life

Activities:

Ensure that the airway is open, artificial respirations are administered, and cardiac compressions are being delivered

Call a code according to agency standard

Bring the code cart to the bedside

Attach the cardiac monitor and determine the rhythm

Deliver cardioversion or defibrillation, as indicated

Ensure that someone is oxygenating the patient and assisting with intubation, as indicated

Initiate an IV line and administer IV fluids, as indicated

Ensure that someone is (1) setting up medications; (2) delivering medications; (3) interpreting EKG and delivering cardioversion/defibrillation, as needed; and (4) documenting care

Remind personnel of current Advanced Cardiac Life Support, as appropriate

Ensure that someone is attending to needs of the family, if present

Ensure that someone is coordinating care of other patients in the unit

Review actions after code to identify areas of strength and those that need to be improved

Background Readings:

Biggers, V. (1992). Codes for a code. American Journal of Nursing, May, 57-61.
Thelan, L.A., & Urden, L.D. (1998). Critical care nursing: Diagnosis and management (3rd ed.). St. Louis: Mosby.

C

Cognitive Restructuring   4700

Definition: Challenging a patient to alter distorted thought patterns and view self and the world more realistically

Activities:

Help the patient accept the fact that self-statements mediate emotional arousal

Help patient understand that inability to attain desirable behaviors frequently results from irrational self-statements

Assist patient in changing irrational self-statements to rational self-statements

Point out styles of dysfunctional thinking (e.g., polarized thinking, overgeneralization, magnification, personalization)

Assist patient in labeling the painful emotion (e.g., anger, anxiety, hopelessness) that he/she is feeling

Assist patient in identifying the perceived stressors (e.g., situations, events, interactions with other people) that contributed to his/her stress

Assist patient to identify own faulty interpretations about the perceived stressors

Assist patient in recognizing the irrationality of certain beliefs compared with actual reality

Assist patient to replace faulty interpretations with more reality-based interpretations of stressful situations, events, interactions

Make statement/ask question that challenges patient's perception/behavior, as appropriate

Make statement that describes alternative way of looking at situation

Assist patient to identify belief system that affects health status

Make use of patient's usual belief system to see situation in different way

Background Readings:

McKay, M., Davis, M., & Fanning, P. (1981). Thoughts and feelings: The art of cognitive stress intervention. Richmond, CA: New Harbenger Publications.

Pender, N. (1996). Health promotion in nursing practice (3rd ed.) Stamford, CT: Appleton & Lange.

Scandrett-Hibdon, S. (1992). Cognitive reappraisal. In G.M. Bulechek & J.C. McCloskey (Eds.), Nursing interventions: Essential nursing treatments (2nd ed.) (pp. 462-471). Philadelphia: W.B. Saunders.

Cognitive Stimulation   4720

Definition: Promotion of awareness and comprehension of surroundings by utilization of planned stimuli

Activities:

Consult with family to establish patient's preinjury cognitive baseline

Inform patient of recent nonthreatening news events

Offer environmental stimulation through contact with varied personnel

Present change gradually

Provide a calendar

Stimulate memory by repeating patient's last expressed thought

Orient to time, place, and person

Talk to patient

Provide planned sensory stimulation

Use TV, radio, or music as part of planned stimuli program

Allow for rest periods

Place familiar objects and photographs in patient's environment

Use repetition to present new material

Vary methods of presentation of material

Use memory aids: checklists, schedules, and reminder notices

Reinforce or repeat information

Present information in small, concrete portions

Ask patient to repeat information

Use touch therapeutically

Provide verbal and written instructions

Background Readings:

Ackerman, L.L. (1992). Interventions related to neurological care. In G.M. Bulechek & J.C. McCloskey (Eds.), Symposium on Nursing Interventions. Nursing Clinics of North America, 27(2), 325-346.

American Nurses Association Council in Medical-Surgical Nursing Practice & American Association of Neuroscience Nursing. (1985). Neuroscience nursing practice: Process and outcome for selected diagnoses. Kansas City, MO: ANA.

Craven, R.F., & Hirnle, C.J. (2000) Fundamentals of nursing: Human health and function (3rd ed.) (pp. 1215-1220). Philadelphia: Lippincott.

Guentz, S.J. (1987). Cognitive rehabilitation of the head-injured patient. Critical Care Nursing Quarterly, 10(3), 51-57.

Kater, K.M. (1989). Response of head-injured patients to sensory stimulation. Western Journal of Nursing Research, 11(1), 20-33.

Phylar, P.A. (1989). Management of the agitated and aggressive head injury patient in an acute hospital setting. Journal of Neuroscience Nursing, 21(6), 353-356.

Rosenthal, M., & Griffith, E.R. (1990). Rehabilitation of the adult and child with traumatic brain injury. Philadelphia: F.A. Davis.

Communicable Disease Management   8820

Definition: Working with a community to decrease and manage the incidence and prevalence of contagious diseases in a specific population

Activities:

Monitor at-risk populations for compliance with prevention and treatment regimen

Monitor adequate continuation of immunization in targeted populations

Provide vaccine to targeted populations as available

Monitor incidence of exposure to communicable diseases during known outbreak

Monitor sanitation

Monitor environmental factors that influence the transmission of communicable diseases

Provide information about adequate preparation and storage of food, as needed

Provide information about adequate control of vectors and animal reservoir hosts, as needed

Inform the public regarding disease and activities associated with management, as needed

Promote access to adequate health education related to prevention and treatment of communicable diseases and prevention of recurrence

Improve surveillance systems for communicable diseases, as needed

Promote legislation that ensures appropriate monitoring of and treatment for communicable diseases

Report activities to appropriate agencies, as required

Background Readings:

Benenson, A. (Ed.). (1995). Control of communicable diseases manual (16th ed.). Washington, DC: American Public Health Association.

McEwen, M. (1998). Community based nursing. Philadelphia: W.B. Saunders.

Stanhope, M., & Lancaster, J. (1996). Community health nursing: Promoting health of aggregates, families and individuals. (4th ed.). St. Louis: Mosby.

Communication Enhancement: Hearing Deficit   4974

Definition: Assistance in accepting and learning alternate methods for living with diminished hearing

Activities:

Facilitate appointment for hearing examination, as appropriate

Facilitate use of hearing aids, as appropriate

Teach patient that sounds will be experienced differently with the use of a hearing aid

Keep hearing aid clean

Check hearing aid batteries routinely

Give one simple direction at a time

Listen attentively

Refrain from shouting at patient with communication disorders

Move close to less affected ear

Face the client directly, speak slowly, clearly, and concisely

Use simple words and short sentences, as appropriate

Increase voice volume as appropriate

Do not cover your mouth, smoke, talk with a full mouth, or chew gum when speaking

Obtain patient's attention through touch

Validate understanding of messages by asking the patient to repeat what was said

Use paper, pencil, or computer communication when necessary

Facilitate location of resources for hearing aids

Facilitate location of telephone adapted for the hearing impaired, as appropriate

Background Readings:

Lindblade, D., & McDonald, M. (1995). Removing communication barriers for the hearing-impaired elderly. MEDSURG Nursing, 4 (5), 377-385

Maas, M.L., Buckwalter, K.C., Hardy, M.D., Reimer, T.T., Titler, M.G., & Specht, J.P. (Eds.). (2001). Nursing care of older adults: Diagnoses, outcomes, & interventions (p. 485). St. Louis: Mosby

Styker, R. (1977). Rehabilitative aspects of acute and chronic nursing care. Philadelphia: W.B. Saunders.

C

Communication Enhancement: Speech Deficit   4976

Definition: Assistance in accepting and learning alternate methods for living with impaired speech

Activities:

Solicit family's assistance in understanding patient's speech, as appropriate

Allow patient to hear spoken language frequently, as appropriate

Provide verbal prompts/reminders

Give one simple direction at a time, as appropriate

Listen attentively

Use simple words and short sentences, as appropriate

Refrain from shouting at patient with communication disorders

Refrain from dropping your voice at the end of a sentence

Stand in front of patient when speaking

Use picture board, if appropriate

Use hand gestures, as appropriate

Perform prescriptive speech-language therapies during informal interactions with patient

Teach esophageal speech, as appropriate

Instruct patient and family on use of speech aids (e.g., tracheal-esophageal prosthesis and artificial larynx)

Encourage patient to repeat words

Provide positive reinforcement and praise, as appropriate

Carry on one-way conversations, as appropriate

Reinforce need for follow-up with speech pathologist after discharge

Use interpreter, as necessary

Background Readings:

Buckwalter, K.C., Cusack, D., Kruckeberg, T., & Shoemaker, A. (1991). Family involvement with communication impaired residents in long term care settings. Applied Nursing Research, 4(2), 77-84.

Buckwalter, K.C., Cusack, D., Sidles, E., Wadle, K., & Beaver, M. (1989). Increasing communication ability in aphasic/dysarthric patients. Western Journal of Nursing Research, 11(6), 736-747.

Carlisle, D. (1990). An understanding profession . . . speech therapist. Nursing Times, 86(10), 52-53.

Emuk-Herring, B. Impaired communication. (2001). In Maas, M.L., Buckwalter, K.C., Hardy, M.D., Reimer, T.T., Titler, M.G., & Specht, J.P. (Eds.). Nursing care of older adults: Diagnoses, outcomes, & interventions (pp. 664-678). St. Louis: Mosby.

Labreche, J., Loughrey, L., & Roberts, P. (1993). Rehabilitation nurses and speech therapy: The effects of two teaching techniques on recognition and use of function words by aphasic stroke patients. Rehabilitation Nursing, 18(1), 54-55.

Phipps, W.J. (1993). The patient with nose and throat problems. In B.C. Long, W.J. Phipps, & V.L. Cassmeyer (Eds.), Medical-surgical nursing: A nursing process approach (3rd ed.) (pp. 498-507). St. Louis: Mosby.

Communication Enhancement: Visual Deficit   4978

Definition: Assistance in accepting and learning alternate methods for living with diminished vision

Activities:

Identify yourself when you enter the patient's space

Note patient's reaction to diminished vision (e.g., depression, withdrawal, or denial)

Accept patient's reaction to diminished vision

Assist patient in setting new goals to learn how to "see" with other senses

Build on patient's remaining vision, as appropriate

Walk one or two steps ahead of the patient, with patient's hand on your elbow

Describe environment to patient

Do not move items in patient's room without informing patient

Read mail, newspaper, and other pertinent information to patient

Identify items on food tray in relation to numbers on a clock

Fold paper money in different ways for easy identification

Inform patient where to locate radio or talking books

Provide a magnifying glass or prism eyeglasses, as appropriate, for reading

Provide Braille reading material, as appropriate

Initiate occupational therapy referral, as appropriate

Refer patient with visual problems to appropriate agency

Background Readings:

Craven, R.F., & Hirnle, C.J. (2000). Fundamentals of nursing: Human health and function (3rd ed.) (p. 1186). Philadelphia: Lippincott.

Maas, M.L., Buckwalter, K.C., Hardy, M.D., Reimer, T.T., Titler, M.G., & Specht, J.P. (Eds.), (2001). Nursing care of older adults: Diagnoses, outcomes, & interventions (pp. 483-485). St. Louis: Mosby.

Styker, R. (1977). Rehabilitative aspects of acute and chronic nursing care. Philadelphia: W.B. Saunders.

C

Community Disaster Preparedness   8840

Definition: Preparing for an effective response to a large-scale disaster

Activities:

Identify potential types of disasters for area (e.g., weather-related, industrial, environmental)

Work with other agencies in planning for a disaster (e.g., law enforcement, fire department, Red Cross, Salvation Army, ambulance services, social service agencies)

Develop plans for specific types of disasters (e.g., multiple-casualty incident, bomb, tornado, hurricane, flood, chemical spill), as appropriate

Identify all community medical and social service agency resources available to respond to a disaster

Develop a disaster notification network to alert personnel

Develop triage procedures

Establish prearranged roles during a disaster

Identify rendezvous site for assisting disaster victims

Identify alternate rendezvous sites for health care personnel

Know where disaster equipment and supplies are stored

Conduct periodic checks of equipment

Check and restock supplies routinely

Educate health care personnel on disaster plan(s) on a routine basis

Encourage community preparation for disaster events

Educate community members on safety, self-help, and first aid measures

Encourage community members to have a personal preparedness plan (e.g., emergency telephone numbers, battery-operated radio, working flashlight, first aid kit, medical information, physician information, list of persons to be notified in an emergency)

Assist in preparation of shelters and emergency aid stations

Conduct mock disaster drills annually or as appropriate

Evaluate performance of disaster personnel after a disaster or mock disaster drill

Identify mechanism for debriefing for health care personnel after a disaster

Sensitize health care personnel to the potential psychological effects (e.g., depression, sadness, fear, anger, phobias, guilt, irritability, anxiety) of a disaster

Identify postdisaster referral resources (e.g., rehabilitation, convalescence, counseling)

Identify postdisaster needs (e.g., ongoing disaster-related health care needs, collection of epidemiological data, assessment of cause of disaster, steps for prevention of reoccurrence)

Update disaster plans, as needed

Background Readings:

Grant, H.D., Murray, R.H., & Bergeron, J.D. (1994). Emergency care (6th ed.). Englewood Cliffs, NJ: Prentice-Hall, Inc.

Ossler, C.C. (1992). The community health nurse in occupational health. In M. Stanhope & J. Lancaster (Eds.), Community health nursing: Process and practice for promoting health (pp. 731-746). St. Louis: Mosby.

Santamaria, B. (1995). Nursing in a disaster. In C.M. Smith & F.A. Maurer (Eds.), Community health nursing: Theory and practice (pp. 382-400). Philadelphia: W.B. Saunders.

Community Health Development   8500

Definition: Assisting members of a community to identify a community's health concerns, mobilize resources, and implement solutions

Activities:

Identify health concerns, strengths, and priorities with community partners

Provide opportunities for participation by all segments of the community

Assist community members in raising awareness of health problems and concerns

Engage in dialogue to define community health concerns and develop action plans

Facilitate implementation and revision of community plans

Assist community members with resource development and procurement

Enhance community support networks

Identify and mentor potential community leaders

Maintain open communication with community members and agencies

Strengthen contacts between individuals and groups to discuss common and competing interests

Provide an organizational framework through which people can enhance communication and negotiation skills

Provide an environment in which individuals and groups feel safe expressing their views

Develop strategies for managing conflict

Unify community members behind a common mission

Ensure that community members maintain control of decision making

Build commitment to the community by demonstrating how participation will influence individual lives and improve outcomes

Develop mechanisms for member involvement in local, state, and national activities related to community health concerns

Background Readings:

Denhan, A., Quinn, S., & Gamble, D. (1998). Community organizing for health promotion in the rural South: An exploration of community competence. Family and Community Health, 2(1), 1-21.

Eng, E., & Parker, E. (1994). Measuring community competence in the Mississippi Delta: The interface between program evaluation and empowerment. Health Education Quarterly, 21(2), 119-120.

May, K., Mendelson, C., & Ferketich, S. (1995). Community empowerment in rural health care. Public Health Nursing, 12(1), 25-30.

Spradley, B., & Allender, J. (1996). Community health nursing: Concepts and practice. (4th ed.). Philadelphia: Lippincott.

Stanhope, M., & Lancaster, J. (1996). Community health nursing: Promoting health of aggregates, families, and individuals. (4th ed.). St. Louis: Mosby.

Complex Relationship Building   5000

Definition: Establishing a therapeutic relationship with a patient who has difficulty interacting with others

Activities:

Identify own attitude toward the patient and the situation

Set limits on what you will do for patient

Set aside personal feelings evoked by the patient that may have a negative impact on therapeutic interactions

Create climate of warmth and acceptance

Provide for physical comfort before interactions

Discuss confidentiality of information shared, as appropriate

Monitor patient's nonverbal messages

Seek clarification of nonverbal messages, as appropriate

Respond to patient's nonverbal messages, as appropriate

Adjust physical distance between you and patient, as appropriate

Maintain open body posture

Use periods of silence to communicate interest, as appropriate

Develop special ways of communicating (images, other words)

Return conversation to main subject as required

Reassure patient of your interest in him/her as a person, as appropriate

Use self-disclosure, as appropriate

Establish a mutually acceptable agreement on time and length of meetings, as appropriate

Assist patient to identify feelings such as anger, anxiety, hostility, or sadness that impede ability to interact with others

Encourage patient to take the time needed to express himself/herself

Set limits of acceptable behavior during therapeutic sessions, as appropriate

Reflect the main ideas back to the patient in your own words

Identify topics of mutual interest

Introduce yourself to patient's significant others, as appropriate

Establish time of next interaction before leaving each time

Summarize conversation at the end of the discussion

Use summary as a starting point for future conversations

Return at the established time to demonstrate your interest in patient

Discuss responsibilities of patient in the one-to-one, nurse-patient relationship

Prepare for termination of relationship, as appropriate

Convey recognition of accomplishments during relationship

Facilitate patient's attempts to review therapeutic relationship experiences

Support patient's efforts to interact with others in a positive manner

Background Readings:

Craven, R.F., & Hirnle, C.J. (2000) Fundamentals of nursing: Human health and function (3rd ed.) (pp. 335-336). Philadelphia: Lippincott.

Egan, G.G. (1986). The skilled helper: A systematic approach to effective helping. Monterey, CA: Brooks/Cole Publishing.

McFarland, G.K., Wasli, E.L., & Kelchner, E. (1992). Nursing diagnoses and process in psychiatric mental health nursing. New York: J.B. Lippincott.

Conflict Mediation   5020

Definition: Facilitation of constructive dialogue between opposing parties with a goal of resolving disputes in a mutually acceptable manner

Activities:

Provide a private, neutral setting for conversation

Allow parties to voice personal concerns

Offer guidance through the process

Maintain own neutrality throughout the process

Employ a variety of communication techniques (e.g., active listening, questioning, paraphrasing, reflecting)

Facilitate defining the issues

Assist parties to identify possible solutions to the issues

Facilitate search for outcomes acceptable to both parties

Support the efforts of the participants to foster resolution

Monitor flow of mediation process

Background Readings:

Arnold, E., & Boggs, K.U. (1995). Interpersonal relationships: Professional communication skills for nurses. (2nd ed.) Philadelphia: Saunders.

Schwebel, A.I., & Clement, J.A. (1996) Mediation as a mental health service: Consumer's and family members' perceptions. Psychiatric Rehabilitation Journal, 20(1), 55-58.

Severson, M.M. (1995). Social work and the pursuit of justice through mediation. Social Work, 40(5), 683-691.

Sullivan, E.J., & Decker, P.J. (1992). Effective management in nursing. Redwood City, CA: Addison-Wesley Nursing.

C

Constipation/Impaction Management   0450

Definition: Prevention and alleviation of constipation/impaction

Activities:

Monitor for signs and symptoms of constipation

Monitor for signs and symptoms of impaction

Monitor bowel movements, including frequency, consistency, shape, volume, and color, as appropriate

Monitor bowel sounds

Consult with physician about a decrease/increase in frequency of bowel sounds

Monitor for signs and symptoms of bowel rupture and/or peritonitis

Explain etiology of problem and rationale for actions to patient

Identify factors (e.g., medications, bed rest, and diet) that may cause or contribute to constipation

Institute a toileting schedule, as appropriate

Encourage increased fluid intake, unless contraindicated

Evaluate medication profile for gastrointestinal side effects

Instruct patient/family to record color, volume, frequency, and consistency of stools

Teach patient/family how to keep a food diary

Instruct patient/family on high-fiber diet, as appropriate

Instruct patient/family on appropriate use of laxatives

Instruct patient/family on the relationship of diet, exercise, and fluid intake to constipation/impaction

Evaluate recorded intake for nutritional content

Advise patient to consult physician if constipation or impaction persists

Suggest use of laxative/stool softener, as appropriate

Inform patient of procedure for manual removal of stool, if necessary

Remove the fecal impaction manually, if necessary

Administer enema or irrigation, as appropriate

Weigh patient regularly

Teach patient or family about normal digestive processes

Teach patient/family about time frame for resolution of constipation

Background Readings:

Battle, E., & Hanna, C. (1980). Evaluation of a dietary regimen for chronic constipation: Report of a pilot study. Journal of Gerontological Nursing, 6(9) 527-532.

Craven, R.F., & Hirnle, C.J. (2000) Fundamentals of nursing: Human health and function (3rd ed.) (pp. 1084-1085). Philadelphia: Lippincott.

McLane, A.M., & McShane, R.E. (2001). Constipation. In Maas, M.L., Buckwalter, K.C., Hardy, M.D., Reimer, T.T., Titler, M.G., & Specht, J.P. (Eds.), Nursing diagnoses and interventions for the elderly (pp. 220-237). Redwood City, CA: Addison-Wesley.

Taylor, C.M. (1987). Nursing diagnosis cards. Springhouse, PA: Springhouse Corporation.

Yakabowich, M. (1990). Prescribe with care: The role of laxatives in treatment of constipation. Journal of Gerontological Nursing, 16(7), 4-11.

Consultation 7910

Definition: Using expert knowledge to work with those who seek help in problem solving to enable individuals, families, groups, or agencies to achieve identified goals

Activities:

Identify the purpose for consultation

Collect data and identify problem that is focus of consultation

Identify and clarify expectations of all parties involved

Provide expert knowledge for those seeking help

Involve those who are seeking help throughout the consulting process

Identify accountability structure

Determine the appropriate model of consultation to be used (e.g., purchase of expertise model, process consultation model)

Identify fee expectations, as appropriate

Develop a written contract to define agreement and avoid misunderstandings

Promote ability of those seeking help to progress with more self-direction and responsibility

Prepare a final report of recommendations

Respond professionally to acceptance or rejection of ideas

Background Readings:

Clemen-Stone, S., McGuire, S., & Eigisti, D. (1997). Comprehensive community health nursing: Family, aggregate, and community practice. St. Louis: Mosby.

Hau, M.L. (1997). Ten common mistakes to avoid as an independent consultant. American Association of Occupational Health Nurses Journal, 45(1), 17-24.

Hoffman, S. (1998). Professional practice consultation—opportunity or opportunism. Journal of Professional Nursing, 14(2), 67.

Iglesias, G.H. (1998). Role evolution of the mental health clinical nurse specialist in home care. Clinical Nurse Specialist, 12(1), 38-44.

Mastroianni, I., & Machles, D. (1997). What are consulting services worth? Applying cost analysis techniques to evaluate effectiveness. American Association of Occupational Health Nurses Journal, 45(1), 35-45.

Stackhouse, J. (1998). Into the community: Nursing in ambulatory and home care. Philadelphia: Lippincott.

Stanhope, M., & Lancaster, J. (1996). Community health nursing: Promoting health of aggregates, families, and individuals. (4th ed.). St. Louis: Mosby.

Contact Lens Care

1620

Definition: Prevention of eye injury and lens damage by proper use of contact lenses

Activities:

Wash hands thoroughly before touching the lenses

Clean lenses with the recommended sterile solution

Use recommended solutions to wet lenses

Store in a clean storage kit

Remove lenses at bedtime or at appropriate intervals for patient who cannot do this for self

Instruct patient how to examine lenses for damage

Instruct the patient to avoid irritating eye makeup

Avoid use of chemicals (e.g., soaps, lotions, creams, and sprays) near lenses because they may damage the lenses

Make referral to eye specialist, as appropriate

Background Reading:

Perry, A.G., & Potter, P.A. (2002). Clinical nursing skills and techniques (5th ed.). St. Louis: Mosby.

Controlled Substance Checking

7620

Definition: Promoting appropriate use and maintaining security of controlled substances

C

Activities:

Account for controlled substance cabinet keys at all times

Follow agency protocol for dispensing and administering controlled substances

Count all controlled substances with an RN on opposite shift

Inspect packaging of controlled substances for signs of tampering

Report discrepancy(ies) immediately, per agency policy

Follow agency protocol for resolving discrepancy(ies)

Lock controlled substances cabinet after count is finished

Document accuracy of count on appropriate form

Count controlled substances received from pharmacy

Return controlled substances not in routine use to pharmacy

Document wasting of controlled substances

Monitor for evidence of misadministration or diversion of controlled substances

Report suspected misadministration or diversion of controlled substances, according to agency policy

Background Readings:

Carlson, G.M., Castile, J.A., & Janousek, J.P. (1988). Guidelines for the prevention and detection of controlled substance diversion. Hospital Pharmacy, 23(12), 1057-1059.

Craven, R.F., & Hirnle, C.J. (2000). Fundamentals of nursing: Human health and function (3rd ed.) (pp. 503-505). Philadelphia: Lippincott.

Coping Enhancement 5230

Definition: Assisting a patient to adapt to perceived stressors, changes, or threats that interfere with meeting life demands and roles

Activities:

Appraise a patient's adjustment to changes in body image, as indicated

Appraise the impact of the patient's life situation on roles and relationships

Encourage patient to identify a realistic description of change in role

Appraise the patient's understanding of the disease process

Appraise and discuss alternative responses to situation

Use a calm, reassuring approach

Provide an atmosphere of acceptance

Assist the patient in developing an objective appraisal of the event

Help patient to identify the information he/she is most interested in obtaining

Provide factual information concerning diagnosis, treatment, and prognosis

Provide the patient with realistic choices about certain aspects of care

Encourage an attitude of realistic hope as a way of dealing with feelings of helplessness

Evaluate the patient's decision-making ability

Seek to understand the patient's perception of a stressful situation

Discourage decision making when the patient is under severe stress

Encourage gradual mastery of the situation

Encourage patience in developing relationships

Encourage relationships with persons who have common interests and goals

Encourage social and community activities

Encourage the acceptance of limitations of others

Acknowledge the patient's spiritual/cultural background

Encourage the use of spiritual resources, if desired

Explore patient's previous achievements

Explore patient's reasons for self-criticism

Confront patient's ambivalent (angry or depressed) feelings

Foster constructive outlets for anger and hostility

Arrange situations that encourage patient's autonomy

Assist patient in identifying positive responses from others

Encourage the identification of specific life values

Explore with the patient previous methods of dealing with life problems

Introduce patient to persons (or groups) who have successfully undergone the same experience

Support the use of appropriate defense mechanisms

Encourage verbalization of feelings, perceptions, and fears

Discuss consequences of not dealing with guilt and shame

Encourage the patient to identify own strengths and abilities

Assist the patient in identifying appropriate short- and long-term goals

Assist the patient in breaking down complex goals into small, manageable steps

Assist the patient in examining available resources to meet the goals

Reduce stimuli in the environment that could be misinterpreted as threatening

Appraise patient's needs/desires for social support

Assist the patient to identify available support systems

Determine the risk of the patient inflicting self-harm

Encourage family involvement, as appropriate

Encourage the family to verbalize feelings about ill family member

Provide appropriate social skills training

Assist the patient to identify positive strategies to deal with limitations and manage needed lifestyle or role changes

Assist the patient to solve problems in a constructive manner

Instruct the patient on the use of relaxation techniques, as needed

Assist the patient to grieve and work through the losses of chronic illness and/or disability, if appropriate

Assist the patient to clarify misconceptions

Encourage the patient to evaluate own behavior

Background Readings:
Clark, S. (1987). Nursing diagnosis: Ineffective coping: A theoretical framework. Heart & Lung, 16(6), 670-675.
Clark, S. (1987). Nursing diagnosis: Ineffective coping: Planning care. Heart & Lung, 16(6), 677-683.
Musil, C.M., & Abraham, I.L. (1986). Coping, thinking, and mental health nursing: Cognitions and their application to psychosocial intervention. Issues in Mental Health Nursing, 8(3), 191-201.
Panzarine, S. (1985). Coping: Conceptual and methodological issues. Advances in Nursing Science, 7(4), 49-57.
Robinson, L. (1990). Stress and anxiety. Nursing Clinics of North America, 25(4), 935-944.
Simons, M.R. (1992). Interventions related to compliance. In G.M. Bulechek & J.C. McCloskey (Eds.), Symposium on Nursing Interventions. Nursing Clinics of North America, 27(2), 477-494.
Wilberding, J.Z. (1991). Ineffective individual coping. In M. Maas, K. Buckwalter, & M. Hardy (Eds.), Nursing diagnoses and interventions for the elderly (pp. 587-594). Redwood City, CA: Addison-Wesley.

Cost Containment 7630

Definition: Management and facilitation of efficient and effective use of resources

Activities:

Use supplies, and equipment efficiently and effectively

Document current or previously utilized resources

Determine the appropriate health care setting (e.g., home care, urgent care, emergency department, clinic, acute care, long-term care) needed to provide services

Assign personnel within budget according to patient acuity

Communicate and coordinate patient care needs with other departments, so care is delivered in a timely manner

Evaluate necessity of health care (e.g., procedures, laboratory tests, specialty care)

Consult and negotiate with other disciplines to prevent unnecessary/duplicative tests and procedures

Discharge patients as soon as appropriate

Investigate competitive prices for supplies and equipment

Determine if supplies should be disposable or reusable

Determine if supplies should be purchased or leased

Secure supplies and equipment at competitive prices

Use standardized documentation (i.e., critical paths) to contain costs and maintain quality, as appropriate

Collaborate with interdisciplinary teams to contain costs and maintain quality, as appropriate

Use/refer to quality improvement programs to monitor delivery of quality patient care in a cost-effective manner

Evaluate services and programs for cost-effectiveness on an ongoing basis

Identify mechanisms to reduce costs

Inform patient of the cost and alternatives of when and where to obtain health care services

Inform patient of the cost, time, and alternatives involved in a specific test or procedure

Encourage patient/family to ask questions about services and charges

Discuss patient's financial situation

Explore with patient creative options to secure needed resources

Background Readings:

DeBour, L.M. (1990). Organizations as financial systems. In J. Dienemann (Ed.), Nursing administration: Strategic perspectives and application (pp. 263-297). Norwalk, CT: Appleton & Lange.

Gillies, D.A. (1994). Nursing management: A systems approach (3rd ed.). Philadelphia: W.B. Saunders.

Lound, J.L. (1994). Managing fiscal resources. In L.M. Simms, S.A. Price, & N.E. Ervin (Eds.), The professional practice of nursing administration (pp. 173-184). Albany, NY: Delmar.

Marquis, B.L., & Huston, C.J. (1992). Leadership roles and management functions in nursing: Theory and application. Philadelphia: J.B. Lippincott.

Swansburg, R.C. (1993). Introductory management and leadership for clinical nurses: A text-workbook. Boston: Jones and Bartlett Publishers.

Tappen, R.M. (1995). Nursing leadership and management: Concepts and practice (3rd ed.). Philadelphia: F.A. Davis.

Cough Enhancement   3250

Definition: Promotion of deep inhalation by the patient with subsequent generation of high intrathoracic pressures and compression of underlying lung parenchyma for the forceful expulsion of air

Activities:

Monitor results of pulmonary function tests, particularly vital capacity, maximal inspiratory force, forced expiratory volume in 1 second (FEV_1), and FEV_1/FVC, as appropriate

Assist patient to a sitting position with head slightly flexed, shoulders relaxed, and knees flexed

Encourage patient to take several deep breaths

Encourage patient to take a deep breath, hold it for 2 seconds, and cough two or three times in succession

Instruct patient to inhale deeply, bend forward slightly, and perform three or four huffs (against an open glottis)

Instruct patient to inhale deeply several times, to exhale slowly, and to cough at the end of exhalation

Initiate lateral chest wall rib spring techniques during the expiration phase of the cough maneuver, as appropriate

Compress abdomen below the xiphoid with the flat hand, while assisting the patient to flex forward as the patient coughs

Instruct patient to follow coughing with several maximal inhalation breaths

Encourage use of incentive spirometry, as appropriate

Promote systemic fluid hydration, as appropriate

Assist patient to use a pillow or rolled blanket as a splint against incision when coughing

Background Readings:

Perry, A.G., & Potter, P.A. (2002). Clinical nursing skills and techniques (5th ed.). St. Louis: Mosby.

Thelan, L.A., & Urden, L.D. (1993). Critical care nursing: Diagnosis and management (2nd ed.). St. Louis: Mosby.

Counseling   5240

Definition: Use of an interactive helping process focusing on the needs, problems, or feelings of the patient and significant others to enhance or support coping, problem solving, and interpersonal relationships

Activities:

Establish a therapeutic relationship based on trust and respect

Demonstrate empathy, warmth, and genuineness

Establish the length of the counseling relationship

Establish goals

Provide privacy and ensure confidentiality

Provide factual information as necessary and appropriate

Encourage expression of feelings

Assist patient to identify the problem or situation that is causing the distress

Use techniques of reflection and clarification to facilitate expression of concerns

Ask patient/significant others to identify what they can/cannot do about what is happening

Assist patient to list and prioritize all possible alternatives to a problem

Identify any differences between patient's view of the situation and the view of the health care team

Determine how family behavior affects patient

Verbalize the discrepancy between the patient's feelings and behaviors

Use assessment tools (e.g., paper and pencil measures, audiotape, videotape, interactional exercises with other people) to help increase patient's self-awareness and counselor's knowledge of situation, as appropriate

Reveal selected aspects of your own experiences or personality to foster genuineness and trust as appropriate

Assist patient to identify strengths, and reinforce these

Encourage new skill development as appropriate

Encourage substitution of undesirable habits with desirable habits

Reinforce new skills

Discourage decision making when the patient is under severe stress, when possible

Background Readings:

Banks, L.J. (1992). Counseling. In G.M. Bulechek & J.C. McCloskey (Eds.), Nursing interventions: Essential nursing treatments (pp. 279-291). Philadelphia: W.B. Saunders.

Corey, G. (1991). Theory and practice of counseling and psychotherapy. (4th ed.). Pacific Grove, CA: Brooks/Cole Publishing Company.

Crisis Intervention   6160

Definition: Use of short-term counseling to help the patient cope with a crisis and resume a state of functioning comparable to or better than the pre-crisis state

Activities:

Provide atmosphere of support

Determine whether patient presents safety risk to self or others

Initiate necessary precautions to safeguard the patient or others at risk for physical harm

Encourage expression of feelings in a nondestructive manner

Assist in identification of the precipitants and dynamics of the crisis

Assist in identification of past/present coping skills and their effectiveness

Assist in identification of personal strengths and abilities that can be used in resolving the crisis

Assist in development of new coping and problem-solving skills, as needed

Assist in identification of available support systems

Provide guidance about how to develop and maintain support system(s)

Introduce patient to persons (or groups) who have successfully undergone the same experience

Assist in identification of alternative courses of action to resolve the crisis

Assist in evaluation of the possible consequences of the various courses of action

Assist patient to decide on a particular course of action

Assist in formulating a time frame for implementation of chosen course of action

Evaluate with patient whether crisis has been resolved by chosen course of action

Plan with patient how adaptive coping skills can be used to deal with crises in the future

Background Readings:

Aguilera, D.C. (1974). Crisis intervention: Theory and methodology. St. Louis: Mosby.

Johnson, B.C., Wells, S.J., Hoffmeister, D., & Dungca, C.U. (1988). Standards for critical care (3rd ed.). St. Louis: Mosby.

Kanak, M.F. (1992). Interventions related to patient safety. In G.M. Bulechek & J.C. McCloskey (Eds.), Symposium on Nursing Interventions. Nursing Clinics of North America, 27(2), 371-396.

Kus, R.J. (1992). Crisis intervention. In G.M. Bulechek & J.C. McCloskey (Eds.), Nursing interventions: Essential Nursing treatments (2nd ed.) (pp. 179-190). Philadelphia: W.B. Saunders.

Morley, W.E., Messick, J.M., & Aguilera, D.C. (1967). Crisis: Paradigms of intervention. Journal of Psychiatric Nursing, 5(6), 531-544.

Critical Path Development   7640

Definition: Constructing and using a timed sequence of patient care activities to enhance desired patient outcomes in a cost-efficient manner

Activities:

Conduct chart audit to determine current patterns of care for patient population

Review current standards of practice related to patient population

Collaborate with other health professionals to develop the critical path

Identify appropriate intermediate and final outcomes with time frames

Identify appropriate interventions with time frames

Share critical path with patient and family, as appropriate

Evaluate patient progress toward identified outcomes at defined intervals

Calculate variances and report them through appropriate channels

Document patient progress toward identified outcomes, per agency policy

Document reason for variances from planned interventions and expected outcomes

Implement corrective action(s) for variance(s), as appropriate

Revise critical path, as appropriate

Background Readings:

Huber, D. (1996). Leadership & nursing core management (pp. 321-322). Philadelphia: W.B. Saunders Company.

Mosher, C., Cronk, P., Kidd, A., McCormick, P., Stockton, S., & Sulla, C. (1992). Upgrading practice with critical pathways. American Journal of Nursing, 92(1), 41-44.

Spath, P.L. (1994). Clinical paths: Tools for outcomes management. Chicago: American Hospital Association.

Thompson, K.S., Caddick, K., Mathie, J., & Abraham, T. (1991). Building a critical path for ventilator dependent patients. American Journal of Nursing, 91(7), 28-31.

Culture Brokerage   7330

Definition: The deliberate use of culturally competent strategies to bridge or mediate between the patient's culture and the biomedical health care system

Activities:

Determine the nature of the conceptual differences that the patient and nurse have of the health problem or treatment plan

Promote open discussion of cultural differences and similarities

Identify, with the patient, cultural practices that may negatively impact health so the patient can make informed choices

Discuss discrepancies openly and clarify conflicts

Negotiate, when conflicts cannot be resolved, an acceptable compromise regarding treatment based on biomedical knowledge, knowledge of the patient's belief systems, and ethical standards

Allow more than the usual time to process the information and work through a decision

Appear relaxed and unhurried in interactions with the patient

Use nontechnical language

Arrange for cultural accommodation (e.g., late kitchen during Ramadan)

Include the family, when appropriate, in the plan for adherence with the prescribed regimen

Accommodate involvement of family to give support or direct care

Translate the patient's symptom terminology into health care language that other professionals can more easily understand

Facilitate intercultural communication (e.g., use of a translator, bilingual written materials/media, accurate nonverbal communication; avoid stereotyping)

Provide information to the patient about the health care system

Provide information to other health care providers about the patient's culture

Assist other health care providers to understand and accept patient's reasons for nonadherence

Alter the therapeutic environment by incorporating appropriate cultural elements

Modify typical interventions (e.g., patient teaching) in culturally competent ways

Background Readings:

Caudle, P. (1993). Providing culturally sensitive health care to Hispanic clients. Nurse Practitioner, 18(12), 40-51.

Gorman, D. (1995). Multiculturalism and transcultural nursing in Australia. Journal of Transcultural Nursing, 6(2), 27-33.

Jackson, L.E. (1993). Understanding, eliciting, and negotiating clients' multicultural health beliefs. Nurse Practitioner, 18(4), 36-42.

Leininger, M. (1994). Culturally competent care: Visible and invisible. Journal of Transcultural Nursing, 6(1), 23-25.

Rairdan B., & Higgs, Z.R. (1992). When your patient is a Hmong refugee. American Journal of Nursing, 92(3), 52-55.

Sloat, A.R., & Matsuura, W. (1990). Intercultural communication. In M.J. Craft & J.A. Denehy (Eds.), Nursing interventions for infants and children (pp. 166-180). Philadelphia: W.B. Saunders.

Tripp-Reimer, T., Brink, P.J., & Pinkam, C. (1999). Culture brokerage. In G.M. Bulechek & J.C. McCloskey (Eds.), Nursing interventions: Effective nursing treatments. (3rd ed.). Philadelphia: W.B. Saunders.

C

Cutaneous Stimulation   1340

Definition: Stimulation of the skin and underlying tissues for the purpose of decreasing undesirable signs and symptoms such as pain, muscle spasm, or inflammation

Activities:

Discuss various methods of skin stimulation, their effects on sensation, and expectations of patient during activity

Select a specific cutaneous stimulation strategy, based on the individual's willingness to participate, ability to participate, preference, support of significant others, and contraindications

Select the most appropriate type of cutaneous stimulation for the patient and the condition (e.g., massage, cold, ice, heat, menthol, vibration, or TENS)

Instruct on indications for, frequency of, and procedure for application

Apply stimulation directly on or around the affected site, as appropriate

Select stimulation site, considering alternate sites when direct application is not possible (e.g., adjacent to, distal to, between affected areas and the brain)

Consider acupressure points as sites of stimulation, as appropriate

Determine the duration and frequency of stimulation, based on method chosen

Encourage the use of an intermittent method of stimulation, as appropriate

Allow the family to participate, as much as possible

Select alternate method or site of stimulation, if altered sensation is not achieved

Discontinue stimulation, if increased pain or skin irritation occurs

Evaluate and document response to stimulation

Background Readings:

Herr, K.A., & Mobily, P.R. (1992). Interventions related to pain. In G.M. Bulechek & J.C. McCloskey (Eds.), Symposium on Nursing Interventions. Nursing Clinics of North America, 27(2), 347-370.

McCaffery, M., & Beebe, A. (1989). Pain. Clinical manual for nursing practice (pp. 130-171). St. Louis: Mosby.

Decision-Making Support   5250

Definition: Providing information and support for a patient who is making a decision regarding health care

Activities:

Determine whether there are differences between the patient's view of own condition and the view of health care providers

Inform patient of alternative views or solutions

Help patient identify the advantages and disadvantages of each alternative

Establish communication with patient early in admission

Facilitate patient's articulation of goals for care

Obtain informed consent, when appropriate

Facilitate collaborative decision making

Be familiar with institution's policies and procedures

Respect patient's right to receive or not to receive information

Provide information requested by patient

Help patient explain decision to others, as needed

Serve as a liaison between patient and family

Serve as a liaison between patient and other health care providers

Refer to legal aid, as appropriate

Refer to support groups, as appropriate

Background Readings:

Donahue, M.P. (1985). Advocacy. In G.M. Bulechek & J.C. McCloskey (Eds.), Nursing interventions: Treatments for nursing diagnosis (pp. 338-351). Philadelphia: W.B. Saunders.

Kohnke, M.F. (1982). Advocacy: Risk and reality. St. Louis: Mosby.

O'Heath, K. (1991). Powerlessness. In M. Maas, K. Buckwalter, & M. Hardy (Eds.), Nursing Diagnoses and interventions for the elderly (pp. 449-459). Redwood City, CA: Addison-Wesley.

Sime, M. (1992). Decisional control. In M. Snyder (Ed.), Independent nursing interventions (2nd ed.) (pp. 110-114). Albany, NY: Delmar Publishers.

D

Delegation   7650

Definition: Transfer of responsibility for the performance of patient care while retaining accountability for the outcome

Activities:

Determine the patient care that needs to be completed

Identify the potential for harm

Evaluate the complexity of the care to be delegated

Determine the problem-solving and innovative skills required

Consider the predictability of the outcome

Evaluate the competency and training of the health care worker

Explain task to the health care worker

Determine the level of supervision needed for the specific delegated intervention or activity (e.g., physically present or immediately available)

Institute controls, so that the nurse can review the interventions or activities of the health care worker and intervene as necessary

Follow up with health care workers on a regular basis to evaluate their progress in completing the specific tasks

Evaluate the outcome of the delegated intervention or activity and the performance of the health care worker

Monitor patient's and family's satisfaction with care

Background Readings:

American Association of Critical-Care Nurses. (1991). Consider this: Delegation. Journal of Nursing Administration, 21(7/8), 11, 13.

Blegen, M., Gardner, D., & McCloskey, J.C. (1992). Who helps you with your work? American Journal of Nursing, 92(1), 26-31.

Brown, S.T. (1985). Don't hesitate to delegate! Nursing Success Today, 2(12), 27-29.

Cronenwett, L., & Sanders, E.M. (1992). Progress report on unlicensed assistive personnel. Informational Report No. CNP-CNE-B. Washington, D.C.: American Nurses Association.

Hansten, R., & Washburn, M. (1992). Working with people: What do you say when you delegate work to others? American Journal of Nursing, 92(7), 48, 50.

Jung, F. (1991). Teaching registered nurses how to supervise nursing assistants. Journal of Nursing Administration, 21(4), 32-36.

Delirium Management

6440

Definition: Provision of a safe and therapeutic environment for the patient who is experiencing an acute confusional state

Activities:

Identify etiological factors causing delirium

Initiate therapies to reduce or eliminate factors causing the delirium

Monitor neurological status on an ongoing basis

Provide unconditional positive regard

Verbally acknowledge the patient's fears and feelings

Provide optimistic but realistic reassurance

Allow the patient to maintain rituals that limit anxiety

Provide patient with information about what is happening and what can be expected to occur in the future

Avoid demands for abstract thinking, if patient can think only in concrete terms

Limit need for decision making, if frustrating/confusing to patient

Administer PRN medications for anxiety or agitation

Encourage visitation by significant others, as appropriate

Recognize and accept the patient's perceptions or interpretation of reality (hallucinations or delusions)

State your perception in a calm, reassuring, and nonargumentative manner

Respond to the theme/feeling tone, rather than the content, of the hallucination or delusion

Remove stimuli, when possible, that create misperception in a particular patient (e.g., pictures on the wall or television)

Maintain a well-lit environment that reduces sharp contrasts and shadows

Assist with needs related to nutrition, elimination, hydration, and personal hygiene

Maintain a hazard-free environment

Place identification bracelet on patient

Provide appropriate level of supervision/surveillance to monitor patient and to allow for therapeutic actions, as needed

Use physical restraints, as needed

Avoid frustrating patient by quizzing with orientation questions that cannot be answered

Inform patient of person, place, and time, as needed

Provide a consistent physical environment and daily routine

Provide caregivers who are familiar to the patient

Use environmental cues (e.g., signs, pictures, clocks, calendars, and color coding of environment) to stimulate memory, reorient, and promote appropriate behavior

Provide a low-stimulation environment for patient in whom disorientation is increased by overstimulation

Encourage use of aids that increase sensory input (e.g., eyeglasses, hearing aids, and dentures)

Approach patient slowly and from the front

Address the patient by name when initiating interaction

Reorient the patient to the health care provider with each contact

Communicate with simple, direct, descriptive statements

Continued

Activities:—cont'd

Prepare patient for upcoming changes in usual routine and environment before their occurrence

Provide new information slowly and in small doses, with frequent rest periods

Focus interpersonal interactions on what is familiar and meaningful to the patient

Background Readings:

Batt, L.J. (1989). Managing delirium. Implications for geropsychiatric nurses. Journal of Psychosocial Nursing, 27(5), 22-25.

Boss, B.J. (1984). The nervous system. In J. Howe, E.J. Dickason, D.A. Jones, & M.J. Snider (Eds.), The handbook of nursing (pp. 669-788). New York: John Wiley & Sons.

Coyne, P.J., Lyne, M.E., & Watson, A.C. (2002). Symptom management in people with AIDS. American Journal of Nursing, 102(9), 48-56

Curl, A. (1989). Agitation and the older adult. Journal of Psychosocial Nursing, 27(12), 12-14.

Ludwig, L.M. (1989). Acute brain failure in the critically ill patient. Critical Care Nursing, 9(10), 62-75.

Sullivan, N., & Fogel, B.S. (1986). Could this be delirium? American Journal of Nursing, 86(12), 1359-1363.

Wakefield, B., Mentes, J., Mobily, P., Tripp-Reimer, T., Culp, K.R., Rapp, C.G., Gasper, P., Kundrat, M., Wadle, K.R., & Akins, J. Acute confusion. In M.L. Maas, K.C. Buckwalter, M.D. Hardy, T.T. Reiner, M.G. Titler, & J.P. Specht (Eds.), Nursing care of older adults: Diagnoses, outcomes, & interventions (pp. 442-454). St. Louis: Mosby.

Delusion Management   6450

Definition: Promoting the comfort, safety, and reality orientation of a patient experiencing false, fixed beliefs that have little or no basis in reality

Activities:

Establish a trusting, interpersonal relationship with patient

Provide patient with opportunities to discuss delusions with caregivers

Avoid arguing about false beliefs; state doubt matter-of-factly

Avoid reinforcing delusional ideas

Focus discussion on the underlying feelings, rather than the content of the delusion ("It appears as if you may be feeling frightened.")

Provide comfort and reassurance

Encourage patient to validate delusional beliefs with trusted others (e.g., reality testing)

Encourage patient to verbalize delusions to caregivers before acting on them

Assist patient to identify situations in which it is socially unacceptable to discuss delusions

Provide recreational, diversionary activities that require attention or skill

Monitor self-care ability

Assist with self-care, as needed

Monitor physical status of patient

Provide for adequate rest and nutrition

Monitor delusions for presence of content that is self-harmful or violent

Protect the patient and others from delusionally based behaviors that might be harmful

Maintain a safe environment

Provide appropriate level of surveillance/supervision to monitor patient

Reassure the patient of safety

Provide for the safety and comfort of patient and others when patient is unable to control behavior (e.g., limit setting, area restriction, physical restraint, or seclusion)

Decrease excessive environmental stimuli, as needed

Assist patient to avoid or eliminate stressors that precipitate delusions

Maintain a consistent daily routine

Assign consistent caregivers on a daily basis

Administer antipsychotic and antianxiety medications on a routine and as-needed basis

Provide medication teaching to patient/significant others

Monitor patient for medication side effects and desired therapeutic effects

Educate family and significant others about ways to deal with patient who is experiencing delusions

Provide illness teaching to patient/significant others, if delusions are illness-based (e.g., delirium, schizophrenia, or depression)

Continued

D

Background Readings:

Aromando, L. (1989). Mental health and psychiatric nursing. Springhouse, PA: Springhouse.

Beck, C.K., Rawlins, R.P., & Williams, S.R. (1988). Mental health psychiatric nursing (2nd ed.). St. Louis: Mosby.

Birckhead, L.M. (1989). Thought disorder and nursing interventions. In L.M. Birckhead (Ed.), Psychiatric-mental health nursing: The therapeutic use of self (pp. 311-347). Philadelphia: J.B. Lippincott.

Eklund, E.S. (1991). Perception/cognition, altered. In G.K. McFarland & M.D. Thomas (Eds.), Psychiatric mental health nursing: Application to the Nursing Process (pp. 332-357). Philadelphia: J.B. Lippincott.

Norris, J. (1987). Schizophrenia and schizophreniform disorders. In J. Norris, M. Kunes-Connell, S. Stockard, P.M. Ehrhart, & G.R. Newton (Eds.), Mental health–psychiatric nursing: A continuum of care (pp. 785-811). New York: John Wiley & Sons.

Varcarolis, E.M. (2000) Psychiatric nursing clinical guide (pp. 234-235). Philadelphia: W.B. Saunders Company.

D

Dementia Management   6460

Definition: Provision of a modified environment for the patient who is experiencing a chronic confusional state

Activities:

Include family members in planning, providing, and evaluating care, to the extent desired

Identify usual patterns of behavior for such activities as sleep, medication use, elimination, food intake, and self-care

Determine physical, social, and psychological history of patient, usual habits, and routines

Determine type and extent of cognitive deficit(s), using standardized assessment tool

Monitor cognitive functioning, using a standardized assessment tool

Determine behavioral expectations appropriate for patient's cognitive status

Provide a low-stimulation environment (e.g., quiet, soothing music; nonvivid and simple, familiar patterns in decor; performance expectations that do not exceed cognitive processing ability; and dining in small groups)

Provide adequate but nonglare lighting

Identify and remove potential dangers in environment for patient

Place identification bracelet on patient

Provide a consistent physical environment and daily routine

Prepare for interaction with eye contact and touch, as appropriate

Introduce self when initiating contact

Address the patient distinctly by name when initiating interaction, and speak slowly

Give one simple direction at a time

Speak in a clear, low, warm, respectful tone of voice

Use distraction, rather than confrontation, to manage behavior

Provide unconditional positive regard

Avoid touch and proximity, if this causes stress or anxiety

Provide caregivers that are familiar to the patient (e.g., avoid frequent rotations of staff assignments)

Avoid unfamiliar situations, when possible (e.g., room changes and appointments without familiar people present)

Provide rest periods to prevent fatigue and reduce stress

Monitor nutrition and weight

Provide space for safe pacing and wandering

Avoid frustrating patient by quizzing with orientation questions that cannot be answered

Provide cues—such as current events, seasons, location, and names—to assist orientation

Seat patient at small table in groups of three to five for meals, as appropriate

Allow patient to eat alone, if appropriate

Provide finger foods to maintain nutrition for patient who will not sit and eat

Provide patient a general orientation to the season of the year by using appropriate cues (e.g., holiday decorations, seasonal decorations and activities, and access to contained, out-of-doors area)

Decrease noise levels by avoiding paging systems and call lights that ring or buzz

Select television or radio programs based on cognitive processing abilities and interests

Continued

D

Activities:—cont'd

Select one-to-one and group activities geared to the patient's cognitive abilities and interests

Label familiar photos with names of the individuals in photos

Select artwork for patient rooms featuring landscapes, scenery, or other familiar images

Ask family members and friends to see the patient one or two at a time, if needed, to reduce stimulation

Discuss with family members and friends how best to interact with the patient

Assist family to understand that it may be impossible for patient to learn new material

Limit number of choices patient has to make, so not to cause anxiety

Provide boundaries, such as red or yellow tape on the floor, when low-stimulus units are not available

Place patient's name in large block letters in room and on clothing, as needed

Use symbols, other than written signs, to assist patient to locate room, bathroom, or other area

Monitor carefully for physiological causes of increased confusion that may be acute and reversible

Remove or cover mirrors, if patient is frightened or agitated by them

Discuss home safety issues and interventions

Background Readings:

Aronson, M.K. (Ed.). (1994). Reshaping dementia care. Thousand Oaks, CA: Sage Publications.

Burgener, S.C., Twigg, P. (2002). Interventions for persons with irreversible dementia. Annual Review of Nursing Research, 20, 89-124.

Perry, A.G., & Potter, P.A. (2002). Clinical nursing skills and techniques (5th ed.). St. Louis: Mosby.

Stolley, J.M., Gerdner, L.A., & Buckwalter, K.C. (1999). Dementia management. In G.M. Bulechek & J.C. McCloskey (Eds.), Nursing interventions: Effective nursing treatments (3rd ed.) (pp. 533-548). Philadelphia: W.B. Saunders.

Dementia Management: Bathing   6462

D

Definition: Reduction of aggressive behavior during cleaning of the body

Activities:

Personalize bath according to patient's usual bathing preferences and/or cultural traditions

Use a flexible approach by providing choices and control over time of day and type of bath (shower, tub, or sponge bath)

Avoid terms "bath" and "shower," if possible, to reduce anxiety

Ensure privacy and safety while undressing and bathing

Simulate homelike environment as much as possible (e.g., wall treatment, soft music, aromatherapy, soft lighting)

Provide comfortable environment (e.g., temperature, soft lighting, reduced noise)

Give a reason for the bath (e.g., "Let's get your bath done before your daughter comes.")

Avoid rapid transportation to the bathroom

Introduce to bath slowly by first letting water trickle on hand

Allow time to perform care in an unrushed fashion

Undress patient gradually in the bathroom while discussing something of interest other than the bath

Use familiar bath products to promote relaxation

Ensure water is appropriate temperature

Reduce feelings of being cold by providing warm towels, washing face and hair last, wash feet first or have beautician shampoo hair

Place warm towel over patient's head and shoulders while washing lower extremities

Massage a soothing lotion into skin following bath

View the patient as a whole person by focusing on the person rather than the task

Assign a trusted caregiver with a friendly attitude

Respond appropriately to patient's perceptions (e.g. temperature, pain, and fear of drowning)

Use gentle persuasion, not coercion

Use soft, reassuring tone of voice

Discuss topics of interest to patient with a pleasant, calm approach

Use gentle touch

Give short, simple directions

Encourage patient to assist with bath as able

Use distraction rather than confrontation to manage behavior

Maintain a quiet, peaceful environment

Assign caregiver of same sex, if available

Identify antecedents or "triggers" if aggressive behavior occurs

Monitor for verbal and nonverbal warning signs of increasing agitation

Give pain medication prior to bath if movement is painful

Offer sponge bath if other methods produce agitation

Remove dentures or offer patient something to eat to prevent biting during the bath

Continued

D

Activities:—cont'd
Provide a washcloth or something to hold for grabbing during the bath

Use comfortable bathing equipment

Background Readings:
Anderson, M.A., Wendler, M.C., & Congdon, J. (1998). Entering the world of dementia: CNA interventions for nursing home residents. Journal of Gerontological Nursing, 24(11), 31-37.
Hoeffer, B., Rader, J., McKenzie, D., Lavelle, M., & Stewart, B. (1997). Reducing aggressive behavior during bathing cognitively impaired nursing home residents. Journal of Gerontological Nursing, 23(5), 16-23, 53-59
Miller, M. F. (1997). Physically aggressive resident behavior during hygienic care. Journal of Gerontological Nursing, 23(5), 24-39, 53-59.
Sloane, P.D., Rader, J., Barrick, A.L., Hoeffer, B., Dwyer, D., McKenzie, D., Lavelle, M., Buckwalter, K., Arrington, L., & Pruitt, T. (1995). Bathing persons with dementia. The Gerontologist, 35(5), 672-678.

Deposition/Testimony   7930

Definition: Provision of recorded sworn testimony for legal proceedings based upon knowledge of the case

Activities:

Contact your employer and malpractice carrier, as appropriate, when notice of deposition or subpoena for testimony is received

Retain an attorney to represent you individually, as necessary

Discuss the case only with the attorney(s) representing you at the deposition

Avoid discussing the case with co-workers, physicians, and others involved without your attorney present

Request that your attorney explain the deposition process

Prepare by reviewing the clinical chart and reading or rereading any documents to be presented during the deposition

Avoid taking any notes, documents, or reports into the deposition unless instructed to do so by your attorney

Prepare to admit mistakes that occurred

Listen carefully to the entire question and understand it before you attempt to answer

Listen to the questions asked and answer the questions directly and truthfully

Ask for clarification if a question is unclear

Avoid second guessing a question or looking for traps

Answer a question only if the person asking is finished; do not interject words while a question is being asked

Answer questions based only on personal and professional knowledge; do not guess or speculate

Answer "I do not remember" or "I don't recall," if you do not remember a fact

Answer only the questions asked and do not volunteer any unsolicited information

Respond to questions with a "yes" or "no" answer if possible

Provide an explanation only if your attorney asks you for it

Testify only about documents you have read

Avoid answering a question to which your attorney objects

Correct the opposing lawyer, particularly if facts are misstated

Be respectful, courteous, and polite and do not argue with the other attorney

Speak calmly, clearly, and with confidence, but do not be pompous or self-satisfied

Spell unusual words after clearly enunciating them, if requested

Ask to talk with your attorney privately if necessary

Avoid offering to produce documents; let your attorney take the lead

Communicate with the opposing counsel or the opposing party only with your attorney present

Speak up and talk clearly so that all can be heard

If tired, ask to get up to take a break

Avoid taking any documents marked as exhibits

Continued

D

D

Background Readings:

Buppert, C. (1999). Nurse practitioner's business practice & legal guide. Gaithersburg, MD: Aspen Publishers.

Cady, R. (1999). Preparing to give a deposition. American Journal of Maternal-Child Nursing, 24(2), 108.

Cady, R. (2000). Testifying at a trial: What you need to know. American Journal of Maternal-Child Nursing, 25(4), 219.

Cohn, S. (1993). Glossary of legal terms. The complete lawyer, Seattle, WA: Law Seminars International, 41-43.

Dempski, K. (2000). If you have to give a deposition. RN, 63(1), 59-60.

Johnson, L.G. (1992). The deposition guide: A practical handbook for witnesses. Seattle, WA: Law Seminars International. 17-21.

Maggiore, W.A. (1999). 9 tips for surviving a deposition. Journal of Emergency Medical Services, 24(12), 84-85.

Riffle, S.H. (1993). Going to court. The complete lawyer. Seattle, WA: Law Seminars International, 22-26.

Scott, R.W. (1999). Health care malpractice: A primer on legal issues for professionals. New York: McGraw-Hill Publishers.

Sullivan, G.H. (1995). Giving a deposition. RN, 58(9), 57-61.

Developmental Care   8250

Definition: Structuring the environment and providing care in response to the behavioral cues and states of the preterm infant

Activities:

Create a therapeutic and supportive relationship with parents

Provide space for parents in unit and at infant's bedside

Provide parents with accurate, factual information regarding the infant's condition, treatment, and needs

Inform parents about developmental concerns and issues for preterm infants

Assist parents in becoming acquainted with their infant in a comfortable, nonhurried environment

Teach parents to recognize infant cues and states

Demonstrate infant capabilities to parents when administering Assessment of Preterm Infant Behavior (APIB) scale or other neurobehavior observation tools

Demonstrate how to elicit infant's visual or auditory attention

Assist parents in planning care responsive to infant cues and states

Point out infant's self-regulatory activities (e.g., hand to mouth, sucking, use of visual or auditory stimulus)

Provide "time out" when infant exhibits signs of stress (e.g., finger splaying, poor color, fluctuation of heart and respiratory rates)

Teach parent how to console infant using behavioral quieting techniques (e.g., placing hand on infant, positioning, swaddling, etc.)

Create individualized development plan for each infant and update regularly

Avoid overstimulation by stimulating one sense at a time (e.g., avoid talking while handling, looking at infant while feeding)

Assist parents to have realistic expectations for infant's behavior and development

Provide boundaries that maintain flexion of extremities while still allowing room for extension (e.g., nesting, swaddling, bunting, hammock, hat, clothing)

Provide supports to maintain positioning and prevent deformities (e.g., back rolls, nesting, bunting, head donuts)

Reposition infant frequently

Provide midline orientation of arms to facilitate hand-to-mouth activities

Provide water mattress and sheepskin, as appropriate

Use smallest diaper to prevent hip abduction

Monitor stimuli (e.g., light, noise, handling, procedures) in infant's environment and reduce as appropriate

Decrease environmental ambient light

Shield eyes of infant when using lights with high foot-candles wattage

Alter environmental lighting to provide diurnal rhythmicity

Decrease environmental noise (e.g., turn down and respond quickly to monitor alarms and telephones, move conversation away from bedside)

Position incubator away from source of noise (e.g., sinks, doors, telephone, areas of high activity, radio, traffic pattern)

Time infant care and feeding around sleep/wake cycle

Gather and prepare equipment needed away from bedside

Cluster care to promote longest possible sleep interval and energy conservation

Continued

D

Activities:—cont'd

Provide comfortable chair in quiet area for feeding

Use slow, gentle movements when handling, feeding, or caring for infant

Feed infant without looking at or talking to infant if this overstimulates infant

Position and support infant infant throughout feeding, maintaining flexion and midline position (e.g., shoulder and truncal support, foot bracing, hand holding, use of bunting, or swaddling)

Feed in upright position to promote tongue extension and swallowing

Promote parent participation in feeding

Support breastfeeding if mother desires

Use a pacifier for nonnutritive sucking if feeding via gavage and between feedings, as appropriate

Provide quiet environment after feeding to avoid gagging, hiccoughs, spitting, aspiration

Facilitate state transition and calming during painful, stressful but necessary procedures

Establish consistent and predictable routines to promote regular sleep/wake cycles

Provide stimulation using recorded instrumental music, mobiles, massage, rocking and touch, as appropriate

Background Readings:

Als, H., Lawhorn, G., Brown, E., Gibes, R, Duffy, F.H., McAnulty, G., & Blickman, J.G., (1986). Individualized behavioral and environmental care for the very low birth weight preterm infant at high risk for brochopulmonary dysplasia: Neonatal intensive care unit and developmental outcome. Pediatrics, 78(6), 1123-1132.

Becker, P.T., Grunwald, P.C., Moorman, J., & Stuhr, S. (1991). Outcomes of developmentally supportive nursing care for very low birth weight infants. Nursing Research, 40(3), 150-155.

Blackburn, S.T., & VandenBerg, K.A. (1993). Assessment and management of neonatal neurobehavioral development. In C. Kenner, A. Brueggemeyer, & L.P. Gunderson (Eds.), Comprehensive neonatal care: A physiologic perspective (pp. 1094-1123) Philadelphia: W.B. Saunders, Co.

Cole, J.G., Begish-Duddy, A., Judas, M.L., Jorgensen., K.M. (1990). Changing the NICU environment: The Boston City Hospital model. Neonatal Network, 9(2), 15-23.

Jorgensen, K.M. (1993). Developmental care of the preterm infant. South Weymouth, MA: Children's Medical Ventures.

Lawhorn, G., & Melzer, A. (1988). Developmental care of the very low birth weight infant. Journal of Perinatal & Neonatal Nursing, 2(1), 56-65.

Shogan, M.G., & Schumann, L.L. (1993). The effect of environmental lighting on the oxygen saturation of preterm infants in the NICU. Neonatal Network, 12(5), 7-13.

Zahr, L.K., Parker, S., & Cole, J. (1992). Comparing the effects of neonatal intensive care unit intervention on premature infants at different weights. Developmental and Behavioral Pediatrics, 13(3), 165-172.

Developmental Enhancement: Adolescent   8272

Definition: Facilitating optimal physical, cognitive, social, and emotional growth of individuals during the transition from childhood to adulthood

Activities:

Build a trusting relationship with adolescent and adolescent caregiver(s)

Encourage adolescent to be actively involved in decisions regarding his/her own health care

Discuss normal developmental milestones and associated behaviors with adolescent and caregiver(s)

Screen for health problems relevant to the adolescent and/or suggested by patient history (e.g., anemia; hypertension; hearing and vision disorders; hyperlipidemia; oral health problems; abnormal sexual maturation; abnormal physical growth; body image disturbances; eating disorders; poor nutrition; alcohol, tobacco or drug use; unhealthy sexual behavior; infectious disease; poor self-concept; low self-esteem; depression; difficult relationships; abuse; learning problems; or work problems)

Provide appropriate immunizations (e.g., measles, mumps, rubella, diphtheria, tetanus, hepatitis B)

Provide health counseling and guidance to adolescent and adolescent caregiver(s)

Promote personal hygiene and grooming

Encourage participation in safe exercise on a regular basis

Promote a healthy diet

Facilitate development of sexual identity

Encourage responsible sexual behavior

Provide contraceptives with instruction for use, if needed

Promote avoidance of alcohol, tobacco, and drugs

Promote vehicle safety

Facilitate decision-making ability

Enhance communication skills

Enhance assertiveness skills

Facilitate a sense of responsibility for self and others

Encourage nonviolent responses to conflict resolution

Encourage adolescents to set goals

Encourage development and maintenance of social relationships

Encourage participation in school, extracurricular, and community activities

Enhance parental effectiveness of adolescents

Refer for counseling as needed

Background Readings:

Archer, S. (Ed.). (1994). Interventions for adolescent identity development. Thousand Oaks, CA: Sage Publications.

American Nurses Association (1994). Clinician's handbook of preventive services. Waldorf, MD: American Nurses Publishing.

Papalia, D., & Olds, S. (1995). Human development. (6th ed.). New York: McGraw-Hill, Inc.

Rice, F. (1997). Child and adolescent development. Upper Saddle River, NJ: Prentice Hall.

D

Developmental Enhancement: Child 8274

Definition: Facilitating or teaching parents/caregivers to facilitate the optimal gross motor, fine motor, language, cognitive, social and emotional growth of preschool and school-aged children

Activities:

Build a trusting relationship with child

Establish one-on-one interaction with child

Assist each child to become aware he/she is important as an individual

Identify special needs of child and adaptations required, as appropriate

Build a trusting relationship with caregivers

Teach caregivers about normal developmental milestones and associated behaviors

Demonstrate activities that promote development to caregivers

Facilitate caregivers' contact with community resources; as appropriate

Refer caregivers to support group; as appropriate

Facilitate integration of child with peers

Make sure body language agrees with verbal communication

Encourage child to interact with others by role modeling interaction skills

Provide activities that encourage interaction among children

Assist child with sharing and taking turns

Encourage child to express self through positive rewards or feedback for attempts

Hold or rock and comfort child, especially when upset

Foster cooperation, not competition, among children

Create a safe, well-defined space for child to explore and learn

Teach child how to seek help from others, when needed

Encourage dreaming or fantasy, when appropriate

Offer age-appropriate toys or materials

Help child learn self-help skills (e.g., feeding, toileting, brushing teeth, washing hands, dressing)

Listen to and discuss music

Sing and talk to child

Encourage child to sing and dance

Teach child to follow directions

Facilitate role playing of daily activities of adults in child's world (e.g., playing store, etc.)

Be consistent and structured with behavior management/modification strategies

Redirect attention, when needed

Have child who is misbehaving "take breaks" or "time outs"

Provide opportunity and materials for building, drawing, clay modeling, painting, and coloring

Assist with cutting out and gluing various shapes

Provide opportunity for doing puzzles and mazes

Teach child to recognize and manipulate shapes

Activities:—cont'd

Teach child to write name/recognize first letter/recognize name, as appropriate

Name objects in environment

Tell or read stories to child

Work on ordering and sequencing of letters, numbers, and objects

Assist with spatial organization

Teach planning by encouraging child to guess what will happen next and have child list other possible choices, and so on

Provide opportunities for and encourage exercise, large motor activities

Teach child to jump over objects

Teach child to perform somersaults

Provide opportunity to play on playground

Go on walks with child

Monitor prescribed medication regimen, as appropriate

Ensure that medical tests and/or treatments are done in a timely manner, as appropriate

Background Readings:

American Public Health Association and the American Academy of Pediatrics. (1992). Caring for our children—National health and safety performance standards: Guidelines for out-of-home child care programs. Washington, DC: American Public Health Association and the American Academy of Pediatrics.

Kane, M. (1984). Cognitive styles of thinking and learning. Part 1. Academic Therapy, 19(5), 527-536.

Peck, J. (1989). Using storytelling to promote language and literacy development. The Reading Teacher, 43(2), 138-141.

Phillips, S., & Hartley, J.T. (1988). Developmental differences and interventions for blind children. Pediatric Nursing, 14(3), 201-204.

Dialysis Access Maintenance   4240

Definition: Preservation of vascular (arterial-venous) access sites

Activities:

Monitor catheter exit site for migration

Monitor access site for redness, edema, heat, drainage, bleeding, hematoma, and decreased sensation

Apply sterile gauze, ointment, and dressing to central venous dialysis catheter site with each treatment

Monitor for AV fistula patency at frequent intervals (e.g., palpate for thrill and auscultate for bruit)

Heparinize newly inserted central venous dialysis catheters

Reheparinize central venous dialysis catheters after dialysis or every 72 hours

Avoid mechanical compression of peripheral access sites

Avoid mechanical compression of patient's limbs near central dialysis catheter

Teach patient to avoid mechanical compression of peripheral access site

Teach patient how to care for dialysis access site

Avoid venipuncture and blood pressure measurement in peripheral access extremity

Background Readings:

Eisenbud, M.D. (1996). The handbook of dialysis access. Columbus, OH: Anadem Publishing.

Gutch, C.F., Stoner, M.H., Carea, A.L. (1993). Review of hemodialysis for nurses and dialysis personnel (5th ed.). St. Louis: Mosby–Year Book.

Lancaster, L.E. (Ed.) (1995). ANNA's core curriculum for nephrology nurses. (3rd ed.) (Section X). Pitman, NJ: Janetti, Inc.

Levine, D.Z. (1997). Caring for the real patient. (3rd ed.). Philadelphia: W.B. Saunders.

Diarrhea Management   0460

Definition: Management and alleviation of diarrhea

Activities:

Determine history of diarrhea

Obtain stool for culture and sensitivity if diarrhea continues

Evaluate medication profile for gastrointestinal side effects

Teach patient appropriate use of antidiarrheal medications

Instruct patient/family members to record color, volume, frequency, and consistency of stools

Evaluate recorded intake for nutritional content

Encourage frequent, small feedings, adding bulk gradually

Teach patient to eliminate gas-forming and spicy foods from diet

Suggest trial elimination of foods containing lactose

Identify factors (e.g., medications, bacteria, tube feedings) that may cause or contribute to diarrhea

Monitor for signs and symptoms of diarrhea

Instruct patient to notify staff of each episode of diarrhea

Observe skin turgor regularly

Monitor skin in perianal area for irritation and ulceration

Measure diarrhea/bowel output

Weigh patient regularly

Notify physician of an increase in frequency or pitch of bowel sounds

Consult physician if signs and symptoms of diarrhea persist

Instruct in low-fiber, high-protein, high-calorie diet, as appropriate

Instruct in avoidance of laxatives

Teach patient/family how to keep a food diary

Teach patient stress-reduction techniques, as appropriate

Assist patient in performing stress-reduction techniques

Monitor safe food preparation

Perform actions to rest the bowel (e.g., NPO, liquid diet)

Background Readings:

Hogan, C.M. (1998) The nurse's role in diarrhea management, Oncology Nurse Forum, 25(5), 879-886.

Taylor, C.M. (1987). Nursing diagnosis cards. Springhouse, PA: Springhouse Corporation.

Wadle, K. (2001) Diarrhea. In Maas, M.L., Buckwalter, K.C., Hardy, M.D., Reimer, T.T., Titler, M.G., & Specht, J.P. (Eds.). (2001) Nursing care of older adults: Diagnoses, outcomes, & interventions (pp. 227-237). St. Louis: Mosby.

Williams, M.S., Harper, R., Magnuson, B., Loan, T., Kearney, P. (1998). Diarrhea management in enterally fed patients. Nutrition in Clinical Problems, 13, 225-229.

Diet Staging 1020

Definition: Instituting required diet restrictions with subsequent progression of diet as tolerated

Activities:

Determine presence of bowel sounds

Institute NPO, as needed

Clamp NG tube and monitor tolerance, as appropriate

Monitor for alertness and presence of gag reflex, as appropriate

Monitor tolerance to ingestion of ice chips and water

Determine if patient is passing flatus

Collaborate with other health care team members to progress diet as rapidly as possible without complications

Progress diet from clear liquid, full liquid, soft, to regular or special diet, as tolerated, for adults and children

Progress from glucose water or oral electrolyte solution, half-strength formula, to full-strength formula for babies

Monitor tolerance to diet progression

Offer six small feedings, rather than three meals, as appropriate

Post the diet restrictions at bedside, on chart, and in care plan

Background Readings:

Burtis, G., Davis, J., & Martin, S. (1988). Applied nutrition and diet therapy. Philadelphia: W.B. Saunders.

Craven, R.F., & Hirnle, C.J. (2000) Fundamentals of nursing: Human health and function (3rd ed.) (pp. 941-944). Philadelphia: Lippincott.

Dietary Department, The University of Iowa Hospitals and Clinics. (1989). Recent advances in therapeutic diets (4th ed.). Ames, IA: Iowa State University Press.

Nolan, E.M. (1985). Nausea, vomiting, and dehydration. In M.M. Jacobs & W. Geels (Eds.), Signs and symptoms in nursing (pp. 373-403). Philadelphia: J.B. Lippincott.

Discharge Planning   7370

> *Definition:* Preparation for moving a patient from one level of care to another within or outside the current health care agency

Activities:

Assist patient/family/significant others to prepare for discharge

Collaborate with the physician, patient/family/significant others, and other health team members in planning for continuity of health care

Coordinate efforts of different health care providers to ensure a timely discharge

Identify patient's and primary caregiver's understanding of knowledge or skills required after discharge

Identify patient teaching needed for postdischarge care

Monitor readiness for discharge

Communicate patient's discharge plans, as appropriate

Document patient's discharge plans on chart

Formulate a maintenance plan for postdischarge follow-up

Assist patient/family/significant others in planning for the supportive environment necessary to provide the patient's posthospital care

Develop a plan that considers the health care, social, and financial needs of patient

Arrange for postdischarge evaluation, as appropriate

Encourage self-care, as appropriate

Arrange discharge to next level of care

Arrange for caregiver support, as appropriate

Discuss financial resources, if arrangements for health care are needed after discharge

Coordinate referrals relevant to linkages among health care providers

Background Readings:

Lowenstein, A.J., & Hoff, P.S. (1994). Discharge planning. A study of nursing staff involvement. Journal of Nursing Administration, 24(4), 45-50.

Luckmann, J., & Sorensen, K.C. (1987). Medical-surgical nursing (3rd ed.). Philadelphia: W.B. Saunders.

McClelland, E., Kelly, K., & Buckwalter, K.C. (1985). Continuity of care: Advancing the concept of discharge planning. New York: Harcourt Brace Jovanovich.

McKeehan, K.M. (1981). Continuing care. St. Louis: Mosby

Remer, D., Buckwalter, K.C., & Maas, M.L. (1991). Translocation syndrome. In M.L. Maas, K.C. Buckwalter, & M.A. Hardy (Eds.), Nursing diagnoses and interventions for the elderly (pp. 493-504). Redwood City, CA: Addison-Wesley.

D

Distraction 5900

Definition: Purposeful focusing of attention away from undesirable sensations

Activities:

Encourage the individual to choose the distraction technique(s) desired, such as music, engaging in conversation or telling a detailed account of event or story, guided imagery, or humor

Instruct the patient on the benefits of stimulating a variety of senses (e.g., through music, counting, television, and reading)

Consider distraction techniques as play, activity therapy, reading stories, singing songs, or rhythm activities for children that are novel, appeal to more than one sense, and do not require literacy or thinking ability

Suggest techniques consistent with energy level, ability, age appropriateness, developmental level, and effective use in the past

Individualize the content of the distraction technique, based on those used successfully in the past and age or developmental level

Advise patient to practice the distraction technique before the time needed, if possible

Instruct patient how to engage in the distraction (use of equipment or materials) prior to the time needed, if possible

Encourage participation of family and significant others and provide teaching, as necessary

Use distraction alone or in conjunction with other measures or distractions (multiple sensory distraction), as appropriate

Evaluate and document response to distraction

Background Readings:

Cason, C.L., & Grissom, N.L. (1997). Ameliorating adults' acute pain during phlebotomy with a distraction intervention. Applied Nursing Research, 10(4), 168-173.

Fanurik, D., Koh, J.L., & Schmitz, M.L. (2000). Distraction techniques combined with EMLA: Effects on IV insertion pain and distress in children. Children's Health Care, 29(2), 87-101.

Herr, K.A., & Mobily, P.R. (1992). Interventions related to pain. In G.M. Bulechek & J.C. McCloskey (Eds.), Symposium on Nursing Interventions. Nursing Clinics of North America, 27(2), 347-370.

Kleiber, C., Craft-Rosenberg, M., & Harper, D.C. (2001). Parents as distraction coaches during IV insertion: A randomized study. Journal of Pain and Symptom Management, 22(4), 851-861.

Kleiber, C., & Harper, D.C. (1999). Effects of distraction on children's pain and distress during medical procedures: A meta-analysis. Nursing Research, 48(1), 44-49.

Schneider, S.M., & Workman, M.L. (2000). Virtual reality as a distraction intervention for older children receiving chemotherapy. Pediatric Nursing, 26(6), 593-597.

Documentation   7920

Definition: Recording of pertinent patient data in a clinical record

Activities:

Record complete assessment findings in initial record

Document nursing assessments, nursing diagnoses, nursing interventions, and outcomes of care provided

Use guidelines as provided by the standards of practice for documentation in the setting

Use standardized, systematic, and prescribed format needed/required by setting

Use standardized forms as indicated for federal and state regulations and reimbursement.

Chart baseline assessments and care activities using agency-specific forms/flow sheets

Record all entries as promptly as possible

Avoid duplication of information in record

Record precise date and time of procedures or consultations by other health care providers

Describe patient behaviors objectively and accurately

Document evidence of client's specific claims (e.g., Medicare, workers' compensation, insurance, or litigation-related claims)

Document and report situations, as mandated by law, for adult or child abuse

Document use of major equipment or supplies, as appropriate

Record ongoing assessments, as appropriate

Record patient's response to nursing interventions

Document that physician was notified of change in patient status

Chart deviations from expected outcomes, as appropriate

Record use of safety measures such as side rails, as appropriate

Record specific patient behavior using patient's exact words

Record involvement of significant others, as appropriate

Record observations of family interactions and home environment, as appropriate

Record resolution/status of identified problems

Ensure that record is complete at time of discharge, as appropriate

Summarize patient status at the conclusion of nursing services

Sign record, using legal signature and title

Maintain confidentiality of record

Use documentation data in quality assurance and accreditation

Background Readings:

Brent, N.J. (1998). Legalities in home care. Home care fraud & abuse: Dishonest documentation. Home Healthcare Nurse, 16(3), 196-198.

Cline, A. (1989). Streamlined documentation through exceptional charting. Nursing Management, 20(2), 62-64.

Coles, M.C., & Fullenwider, S.D. (1988). Documentation: Managing the dilemma. Nursing Management, 19(12), 65-66, 70, 72.

Edelstein, J. (1990). A study of nursing documentation. Nursing Management, 21(11), 40-43, 46.

Mandell, M.S. (1987). Charting: How it can keep you out of court. Nursing Life, 7(5), 46-48.

Miller, P., & Pastoring, C. (1990). Daily nursing documentation can be quick and thorough. Nursing Management, 21(11), 47-49.

Southard, P., & Frankel, P. (1989). Trauma care documentation: A comprehensive guide. Journal of Emergency Nursing, 15(5), 393-398.

Dressing   1630

Definition: Choosing, putting on, and removing clothes for a person who cannot do this for self

Activities:

Identify areas in which patient needs assistance in dressing

Monitor patient's ability to dress self

Dress patient after personal hygiene is completed

Encourage participation in selection of clothing

Encourage use of self-care devices, as appropriate

Dress affected extremity first, as appropriate

Dress in nonrestrictive clothing, as appropriate

Dress in personal clothing, as appropriate

Change patient's clothing at bedtime

Select shoes/slippers conducive to walking and safe ambulation

Offer to launder clothing, as necessary

Give assistance until the patient is fully able to assume responsibility for dressing self

Background Readings:

Engleman, K.K., Mathews, R.M., & Altus, D.E. (2002). Restoring dressing independence in persons with Alzheimer's disease: A pilot study. American Journal of Alzheimer's Disease & Other Dementias, 17(1), 37-43.

Sorensen, K., & Luckmann, J. (1986). Basic nursing: A psychophysiologic approach (2nd ed.). Philadelphia: W.B. Saunders.

Stryker, R. (1977). Rehabilitative aspects of acute and chronic nursing care. Philadelphia: W.B. Saunders.

Dying Care   5260

Definition: Promotion of physical comfort and psychological peace in the final phase of life

Activities:

Reduce demand for cognitive functioning when patient is ill or fatigued

Monitor patient for anxiety

Monitor mood changes

Communicate willingness to discuss death

Encourage patient and family to share feelings about death

Support patient and family through stages of grief

Monitor pain

Minimize discomfort, when possible

Medicate by alternate route when swallowing problems develop

Postpone feeding when patient is fatigued

Offer fluids and soft foods frequently

Offer culturally appropriate foods

Monitor deterioration of physical and/or mental capabilities

Provide frequent rest periods

Assist with basic care, as needed

Stay physically close to frightened patient

Respect the need for privacy

Modify the environment, based on patient's needs and desires

Identify the patient's care priorities

Facilitate obtaining spiritual support for patient and family

Respect the patient's and family's specific care requests

Support the family's efforts to remain at the bedside

Include the family in care decisions and activities, as desired

Facilitate discussion of funeral arrangements

Background Readings:
Jones, K. (2001). Last touch. Nursing 2001, 31(10), 44-45.
Perry, A.G., & Potter, P.A. (2002). Clinical nursing skills and techniques (5th ed.). (pp. 559-616). St. Louis: Mosby.

Dysreflexia Management 2560

Definition: Prevention and elimination of stimuli that cause hyperactive reflexes and inappropriate autonomic responses in a patient with a cervical or high thoracic cord lesion

Activities:

Identify and minimize stimuli that may precipitate dysreflexia: bladder distention, renal calculi, infection, fecal impaction, rectal examination, suppository insertion, skin breakdown, and constrictive clothing or bed linen

Monitor for signs and symptoms of autonomic dysreflexia: paroxysmal hypertension, bradycardia, tachycardia, diaphoresis above the level of injury, facial flushing, pallor below the level of injury, headache, nasal congestion, engorgement of temporal and neck vessels, conjunctival congestion, chills without fever, pilomotor erection, and chest pain

Investigate and treat or remove offending cause (e.g., distended bladder, fecal impaction, skin lesions, and constricting bed clothes)

Place head of bed in upright position, as appropriate, if hyperreflexia occurs

Stay with patient and monitor status every 3 to 5 minutes if hyperreflexia occurs

Administer antihypertensive agents intravenously, as ordered

Instruct patient and family about causes, symptoms, treatment, and prevention of dysreflexia

Background Readings:

Hickey, J.V. (1992). The clinical practice of neurological and neurosurgical nursing (3rd ed.). Philadelphia: J.B. Lippincott.
Thelan, L.A., & Urden, L.D. (1993). Critical care nursing: Diagnosis and management (2nd ed.). St. Louis: Mosby.

Dysrhythmia Management 4090

Definition: Preventing, recognizing, and facilitating treatment of abnormal cardiac rhythms

Activities:

Ascertain patient and family history of heart disease and dysrhythmias

Monitor for and correct oxygen deficits, acid-base imbalances, and electrolyte imbalances, which may precipitate dysrhythmias

Apply EKG electrodes and connect to a cardiac monitor

Set alarm parameters on the EKG monitor

Ensure ongoing monitoring of bedside EKG by qualified individuals

Monitor EKG changes that increase risk of dysrhythmia development: prolonged QT interval, frequent premature ventricular contractions, and ectopy close to the T wave

Facilitate acquisition of a 12-lead EKG, as appropriate

Note activities associated with the onset of dysrhythmias

Note frequency and duration of dysrhythmia

Monitor hemodynamic response to the dysrhythmia

Determine whether patient has chest pain or syncope associated with the dysrhythmia

Ensure ready access to emergency dysrhythmia medications

Initiate and maintain IV access, as appropriate

Administer Advanced Cardiac Life Support, as indicated

Administer prescribed IV fluids and vasoconstrictor agents, as indicated, to facilitate tissue perfusion

Assist with insertion of temporary transvenous or external pacemaker, as appropriate

Teach patient and family the risks associated with the dysrhythmia(s)

Prepare patient and family for diagnostic studies (e.g., cardiac catheterization or electrical physiological studies)

Assist patient and family in understanding treatment options

Teach patient and family about actions and side effects of prescribed medications

Teach patient and family self-care behaviors associated with use of permanent pacemakers and AICD devices, as indicated

Teach patient and family measures to decrease the risk of recurrence of the dysrhythmia(s)

Teach patient and family how to access the emergency medical system

Teach a family member CPR, as appropriate

Background Readings:

Kenner, C.V., Guzetta, C.E., & Dossey, B.M. (1985). Critical care nursing: Body, mind and spirit (2nd ed.). Boston: Little, Brown & Co.

Thelan, L.A., & Urden, L.D. (1993). Critical care nursing: Diagnosis and management (2nd ed.). St. Louis: Mosby.

Ear Care   1640

Definition: Prevention or minimization of threats to ear or hearing

Activities:

Position infant so ears remain flat to head

Monitor for drainage from ears, as appropriate

Irrigate the ear, as appropriate

Avoid placing sharp objects in the ear

Administer eardrops, as appropriate

Instruct parents how to cleanse infant's ears

Instruct parents to monitor child with nasal congestion for ear infections

Explain the relationship between balance and the inner ear, as appropriate

Monitor for episodes of dizziness associated with ear problems, as appropriate

Instruct parents how to observe for ear infections in infant

Instruct parents about importance of completing antibiotic regimen

Instruct parents to hold baby upright when bottle feeding to avoid reflux into eustachian tubes

Determine if cerumen in the ear canal is causing pain or hearing loss

Instill mineral oil in the ear to soften impacted cerumen before irrigation

Irrigate the ear canal with a Water-Pik (or similar device) on a low setting using warm water ($80°$ to $90°$ F), as appropriate

Demonstrate proper technique for ear irrigation to parents/caregiver, as appropriate

Monitor frequency of ear infections

Instruct parents about tubes as a medical treatment, as appropriate

Instruct parents to avoid immersing child's ears in water with tubes present

Instruct parents how to administer eardrops, as appropriate

Instruct parents about the importance of routine hearing testing

Instruct children not to put foreign objects in ears

Instruct how to monitor and regulate high-volume noise exposure

Instruct patient to wear hearing protection for exposure to high-intensity noise

Instruct teenager concerning the potential danger of exposure to high-volume music, especially with headphones

Instruct patient with pierced ears how to avoid infection at the insertion site

Encourage use of ear plugs for swimming, if patient is susceptible to ear infections

Background Readings:

Perry, A.G., & Potter, P.A. (1998). Clinical nursing skills and techniques. (4th ed.). St. Louis: Mosby.

Smith, S., & Duell, D. (1992). Clinical nursing skills (3rd ed.). Los Altos, CA: National Nursing Review.

Watkins, S., Moore, T.H., & Phillips, J. (1984). Clearing impacted ears. American Journal of Nursing, 84(9), 1107.

Eating Disorders Management   1030

Definition: Prevention and treatment of severe diet restriction and overexercising or binging and purging of food and fluids

Activities:

Collaborate with other members of health care team to develop a treatment plan; involve patient and/or significant others as appropriate

Confer with team and patient to set a target weight if patient is not within a recommended weight range for age and body frame

Establish the amount of daily weight gain that is desired

Confer with dietician to determine daily caloric intake necessary to attain and/or maintain target weight

Teach and reinforce concepts of good nutrition with patient (and significant others as appropriate)

Encourage patient to discuss food preferences with dietician

Develop a supportive relationship with patient

Monitor physiological parameters (vital signs, electrolytes), as needed

Weigh patient on a routine basis (e.g., at same time of day and after voiding)

Monitor intake and output of fluids, as appropriate

Monitor daily caloric food intake

Encourage patient self-monitoring of daily food intake and weight gain/maintenance, as appropriate

Establish expectations for appropriate eating behaviors, intake of food/fluid, and amount of physical activity

Use behavioral contracting with patient to elicit desired weight gain or maintenance behaviors

Restrict food availability to scheduled, pre-served meals and snacks

Observe patient during and after meals/snacks to ensure that adequate intake is achieved and maintained

Accompany patient to bathroom during designated observation times following meals/snacks

Limit time spent in bathroom during periods when not under observation

Monitor patient for behaviors related to eating, weight loss, and weight gain

Use behavior modification techniques to promote behaviors that contribute to weight gain and to limit weight loss behaviors, as appropriate

Provide reinforcement for weight gain and behaviors that promote weight gain

Provide remedial consequences in response to weight loss, weight loss behaviors, or lack of weight gain

Provide support (e.g., relaxation therapy, desensitization exercises, opportunities to talk about feelings) as patient integrates new eating behaviors, changing body image, and lifestyle changes

Encourage patient to use daily logs to record feelings, as well as circumstances surrounding urge to purge, vomit, overexercise

Limit physical activity as needed to promote weight gain

Provide a supervised exercise program when appropriate

Allow opportunity to make limited choices about eating and exercise as weight gain progresses in desirable manner

Assist patient (and significant others, as appropriate) to examine and resolve personal issues that may contribute to the eating disorder

Assist patient to develop self-esteem that is compatible with a healthy body weight

Confer with health care team on routine basis about patient's progress

Continued

Activities:—cont'd

Initiate maintenance phase of treatment when patient has achieved target weight and has consistently shown desired eating behaviors for designated period of time

Monitor patient's weight on routine basis

Determine acceptable range of weight variation in relation to target range

Place responsibility for choices about eating and physical activity with patient, as appropriate

Provide support and guidance, as needed

Assist patient to evaluate the appropriateness/consequences of choices about eating and physical activity

Reinstitute weight gain protocol if patient is unable to remain in target weight range

Institute a treatment program and follow-up care (medical, counseling) for home management

Background Readings:

Anderson, A.A., Morse, C., & Santmeyer, K. (1985). Inpatient treatment for anorexia nervosa. In D.M. Garner & P.E. Garfinkel (Eds.), Handbook of psychotherapy for anorexia nervosa and bulimia (pp. 311-343). New York: Guilford Press.

Crisp, A.H. (1990). Anorexia nervosa. Philadelphia: W.B. Saunders.

Garner, D.M., Rockert, W., Olmstead, M.P., Johnson, C., & Cosina, D.V. (1985). Psychoeducational principles in the treatment of bulimia and anorexia nervosa. In D.M. Garner & P.E. Garfinkel (Eds.), Handbook of psychotherapy for anorexia nervosa and bulimia (pp. 147-158). New York: Guilford Press.

Halmi, K. (1985). Behavioral management for anorexia nervosa. In D.M. Garner & P.E. Garfinkel (Eds.), Handbook of psychotherapy for anorexia nervosa and bulimia (pp. 147-159). New York: Guilford Press.

Love, C.C., & Seaton, H. (1991). Eating disorders. Highlights of nursing assessment and therapeutics. Nursing Clinics of North America, 26(3), 677-698.

Palmer, T.A. (1990). Anorexia nervosa, bulimia nervosa: Causal theories and treatment. Nurse Practitioner, 15(4), 13-21.

Plehn, K.W. (1990). Anorexia nervosa and bulimia: Incidence and diagnosis. Nurse Practitioner, 15(4), 22-31.

Wooley, S.C., & Wooley, W.O. (1985). Intensive outpatient and residential treatment for bulimia. In D.M. Garner & P.E. Garfinkel (Eds.), Handbook of psychotherapy for anorexia nervosa and bulimia (pp. 391-430). New York: Guilford Press.

Electroconvulsive Therapy (ECT) Management   2570

Definition: Assisting with the safe and efficient provision of electroconvulsive therapy in the treatment of psychiatric illness

Activities:

Encourage patient (and significant others, as appropriate) to express feelings regarding the prospect of ECT

Instruct patient and/or significant others about the treatment

Provide emotional support to patient and/or significant others, as needed

Ensure that the patient (or the legal designee if the patient is unable to give informed consent) has adequate understanding of ECT when the physician seeks informed consent to administer ECT

Confirm that there is a written order and signed consent form for ECT

Record patient's height and weight in the medical record

Discontinue or taper medications contraindicated for ECT per physician order

Review medication instructions with the outpatient who will be receiving ECT

Inform the physician of any laboratory abnormalities for the patient

Ensure that the patient receiving ECT has complied with the NPO requirement and medication instructions as ordered by the physician

Assist patient to dress in loose fitting clothing (i.e., preferably hospital pajamas) that can be opened in front to allow placement of monitoring equipment

Perform routine preoperative preparation (e.g., removal of dentures, jewelry, glasses, contact lenses; obtain vital signs; have patient void)

Ensure that patient's hair is clean, dry, and devoid of hair ornaments in preparation for electrode placement

Obtain a fasting blood glucose reading before and after procedure for those patients who have insulin-dependent diabetes

Ensure that patient is wearing an identification band

Administer medications prior to and throughout the treatment as ordered by the physician

Document the specifics of pretreatment preparation

Verbally communicate unusual vital signs, physical complaints/symptoms, or unusual occurrences to the ECT nurse or ECT psychiatrist prior to the treatment

Assist the treatment team in placing leads for various monitors (e.g., EEG, ECG) and monitoring equipment (e.g., pulse oximeter, blood pressure cuff, peripheral nerve stimulator) on the patient

Place a bite block in patient's mouth, and support chin allowing for airway patency during delivery of the electrical stimulus

Document the time elapsed, as well as the type and amount of movement, during the seizure

Document treatment-related data (e.g., medications given, patient response)

Position the unconscious patient on his/her side on the stretcher with side rails raised

Perform routine postoperative assessments (e.g., monitor vital signs, mental status, pulse oximeter, ECG)

Administer oxygen, as ordered

Suction oropharyngeal secretions, as needed

Administer intravenous fluids, as ordered

Provide supportive care and behavior management for postictal disorientation and agitation

Continued

Activities:—cont'd

Notify the anesthesia provider or ECT psychiatrist if patient's condition is destabilizing or if patient is failing to recover as expected

Document care provided and patient's response

Observe patient in recovery area until fully awake, oriented to time/place, and able to independently perform self-care activities

Assist patient, when adequately alert, oriented, physically stable, to return to the inpatient nursing unit or another recovery area

Provide the nursing staff who receive the post-ECT patient with a report on the treatment and patient's response to the treatment

Determine level of observation needed by patient upon return to the unit or recovery area

Provide that level of observation in the inpatient nursing unit or recovery area

Institute fall precautions, as needed

Observe the patient the first time that he/she attempts to ambulate independently to ensure that full muscle control has returned since receiving a muscle relaxant during ECT

Ensure that the patient's gag reflex has returned prior to offering oral medications, food, or fluids

Monitor patient for potential side effects of ECT (e.g., muscle soreness, headache, nausea, confusion, disorientation)

Administer medications (e.g., analgesics, antiemetics), as ordered for the treatment of side effects

Treat disorientation by restricting environmental stimulation and frequently reorienting patient

Encourage patient to verbalize feelings about the experience of ECT

Remind the amnesic patient that he/she had ECT

Provide emotional support to the patient, as needed

Reinforce teaching on ECT with patient and significant others, as appropriate

Update significant others on patient's status, as appropriate

Discharge the outpatient recipient of ECT to a responsible adult when patient has adequately recovered from the treatment per agency protocol

Collaborate with treatment team to evaluate the effectiveness of the ECT (e.g., mood, cognitive status) and modify patient's treatment plan, as needed

Background Readings:

American Psychiatric Association. Committee on Electroconvulsive Therapy (2001). The practice of electroconvulsive therapy. Recommendations for treatment, training, and privileging: A task force report of the American Psychiatric Association (2nd ed.). Washington, DC: American Psychiatric Association.

Scott, C.M. (2000). Mood disorders. In V.B. Carson (Ed.), Mental health nursing. The nurse-patient journey (pp. 679-720). Philadelphia: W.B. Saunders Company.

Sherr, J. (2000). Psychopharmacology and other biologic therapies. In K.M. Fortinash & P.A. Holoday-Worret (Eds.), Psychiatric mental health nursing. (pp. 536-571). St. Louis: Mosby.

Frisch, N.C. (2001). Complementary and somatic therapies. In N.C. Frisch & L.E. Frisch (Eds.), Psychiatric mental health nursing (2nd ed.) (pp. 743-757). Clifton Park, NY: Delmar Learning.

Stuart, G. (1998). Somatic therapies. In G.W. Stuart & M.T. Laraia (Eds.), Principles and practice of psychiatric nursing (6th ed.). (pp. 604-617). St. Louis: Mosby.

Townsend, M.C. (2000). Psychiatric mental health nursing. Concepts of care (3rd ed.) (pp. 283-290). Philadelphia: F.A. Davis Company.

University of Iowa Hospital & Clinics. Department of Nursing. (2001). Electroconvulsive therapy—Pre-treatment. Behavioral Health Service (BHS)–Psychiatric. Section II (7-10, 12).

Electrolyte Management   2000

Definition: Promotion of electrolyte balance and prevention of complications resulting from abnormal or undesired serum electrolyte levels

Activities:

Monitor for abnormal serum electrolyte levels, as available

Monitor for manifestations of electrolyte imbalance

Maintain patent IV access

Give fluids, as appropriate

Maintain accurate intake and output record

Maintain intravenous solution containing electrolyte(s) at constant flow rate, as appropriate

Administer supplemental electrolytes (e.g., oral, NG, and IV) as prescribed, if appropriate

Consult physician about administration of electrolyte-sparing medications (e.g., spiranolactone), as appropriate

Administer electrolyte-binding or -excreting resins (e.g., Kayexalate) as prescribed, if appropriate

Obtain ordered specimens for laboratory analysis of electrolyte levels (e.g., ABG, urine, and serum levels), as appropriate

Monitor for loss of electrolyte-rich fluids (e.g., nasogastric suction, ileostomy drainage, diarrhea, wound drainage, and diaphoresis)

Institute measures to control excessive electrolyte loss (e.g., by resting the gut, changing type of diuretic, or administering antipyretics), as appropriate

Irrigate nasogastric tubes with normal saline

Minimize the amount of ice chips consumed or oral intake by patients with gastric tubes connected to suction

Provide diet appropriate for patient's electrolyte imbalance (e.g., potassium-rich, low-sodium, and low-carbohydrate foods)

Instruct the patient and/or family on specific dietary modifications, as appropriate

Provide a safe environment for the patient with neurological and/or neuromuscular manifestations of electrolyte imbalance

Promote orientation

Teach patient and family about the types, causes and treatments of electrolyte imbalance, as appropriate

Consult physician if signs and symptoms of fluid and/or electrolyte imbalance persist or worsen

Monitor patient's response to prescribed electrolyte therapy

Monitor for side effects of prescribed supplemental electrolytes (e.g., GI irritation)

Monitor closely the serum potassium levels of patients taking digitalis and diuretics

Attach cardiac monitor, as appropriate

Treat cardiac arrhythmias, according to policy

Prepare patient for dialysis (e.g., assist with catheter placement for dialysis), as appropriate

Continued

Background Readings:

Askanazi, J., Starker, P., & Wissman, C. (1986). Fluid and electrolyte management in critical care. Boston: Butterworths.

Baer, C.L. (1993). Fluid & electrolyte balance. M.R. Kinney, D.R. Packa, & S.B. Dunbar (Eds.), AACN's clinical reference for critical-care nursing (pp. 173-208). St. Louis: Mosby.

Chan, J., & Gill, J. (1990). Kidney electrolyte disorders. New York: Churchill Livingston.

Cullen, L.M. (1992). Interventions related to fluid and electrolyte balance. In G.M. Bulechek & J.C. McCloskey (Eds.), Symposium on Nursing Interventions. Nursing Clinics of North America, 27(2), 569-598.

Horne, M., & Swearingen, P. (1997). Pocket guide to fluids and electrolytes (3rd ed.). St. Louis: Mosby.

Kokko, J., & Tannen, R. (1990). Fluids and electrolytes (2nd ed.). Philadelphia: W.B. Saunders.

Melillo, K.D. (1993). Interpretation of laboratory values in older adults. Nurse Practitioner, 18(7), 59-67.

E

Electrolyte Management: Hypercalcemia   2001

Definition: Promotion of calcium balance and prevention of complications resulting from serum calcium levels higher than desired

Activities:

Monitor intake and output

Monitor renal function (e.g., BUN and Cr levels), if appropriate

Monitor for digitalis toxicity (e.g., report serum levels above therapeutic range, monitor heart rate and rhythm before administering dose, and monitor for side effects), as appropriate

Monitor trends in serum levels of calcium (e.g., ionized calcium), as available

Monitor for electrolyte imbalances associated with hypercalcemia (e.g., hypo- or hyperphosphatemia, hyperchloremic acidosis, and hypokalemia from diuresis), as appropriate

Administer prescribed medications to reduce serum ionized calcium levels (e.g., phosphate, sodium bicarbonate, and glucocorticoids), as appropriate

Administer prescribed medications to promote renal excretion of calcium (e.g., IV fluid hydration with normal saline or half-normal saline and diuretics), as appropriate

Monitor for fluid overload resulting from hydration therapy (e.g., daily weight, urine output, jugular vein distention, lung sounds, and right atrial pressure), as appropriate

Avoid administration of vitamin D (e.g., calcifediol or ergocalciferol), which facilitates GI absorption of calcium, as appropriate

Discourage intake of calcium (e.g., dairy products, seafood, nuts, broccoli, spinach, and supplements), as appropriate

Avoid medications that prevent renal calcium excretion (e.g., lithium carbonate and thiazide diuretics), as appropriate

Monitor for indications of kidney stone formation (e.g., intermittent pain, nausea, vomiting, and hematuria) resulting from calcium accumulation, as appropriate

Encourage diet rich in fruits (e.g., cranberries, prunes, or plums) to increase urine acidity and reduce the risk of calcium stone formation, as appropriate

Monitor for CNS manifestations of hypercalcemia (e.g., lethargy, depression, loss of memory, headache, confusion, coma, and personality changes)

Monitor for neuromuscular manifestations of hypercalcemia (e.g., weakness, malaise, paresthesias, myalgia, hypotonia, decreased deep tendon reflexes, and poor coordination)

Monitor for GI manifestations of hypercalcemia (e.g., anorexia, nausea, vomiting, abdominal pain, and constipation)

Monitor for cardiovascular manifestations of hypercalcemia (e.g., shortened ST segment and QT interval, prolonged PR interval, cone-shaped T wave, sinus bradycardia, heart blocks, hypertension, and cardiac arrest)

Monitor for causes of increasing calcium levels (e.g., indications of severe dehydration and renal failure), as appropriate

Monitor patient at risk for increasing calcium levels due to bone resorption (e.g., spinal cord injury, solid tumor, and renal transplant), as appropriate

Administer indomethacin (Indocin), calcitonin, or plicamycin (Mithracin), as appropriate

Encourage mobilization to prevent bone resorption

Instruct patient and/or family in medications to avoid in hypercalcemia (e.g., certain antacids)

Instruct patient and/or family on measures instituted to treat hypercalcemia

Continued

E

Activities:—cont'd

Monitor for rebound hypocalcemia resulting from aggressive treatment of hypercalcemia

Monitor for recurring hypercalcemia 1 to 3 days after cessation of therapeutic measures

Obtain specimens for laboratory analysis of calcium and associated electrolyte levels (e.g., ABG, urine, and serum levels), as appropriate

Background Readings:

Askanazi, J., Starker, P., & Wissman, C. (1986). Fluid and electrolyte management in critical care. Boston: Butterworths.

Baer, C.L. (1993). Fluid and electrolyte balance. In M.R. Kinney, D.R. Packa, & S.B. Dunbar (Eds.), AACN's clinical reference for critical-care nursing (pp. 173-208). St. Louis: Mosby.

Chan, J., & Gill, J. (1990). Kidney electrolyte disorders. New York: Churchill Livingston.

Cullen, L.M. (1992). Interventions related to fluid and electrolyte balance. In G.M. Bulechek & J.C. McCloskey (Eds.), Symposium on Nursing Interventions. Nursing Clinics of North America, 27(2), 569-597.

Horne, M., & Swearingen, P. (1997). Pocket guide to fluids and electrolytes (3rd ed.). St. Louis: Mosby.

Kokko, J., & Tannen, R. (1990). Fluids and electrolytes (2nd ed.). Philadelphia: W.B. Saunders.

Rice, V. (1983). Magnesium, calcium and phosphate imbalances: Their clinical significance. Critical Care Nurse, May/June, 90-112.

Stark, J. (1991). The renal system. In J. Alspach (Ed.), American Association of Critical-Care Nurses core curriculum for critical-care nursing (4th ed.) (pp. 472-608). Philadelphia: W.B. Saunders.

Electrolyte Management: Hyperkalemia   2002

Definition: Promotion of potassium balance and prevention of complications resulting from serum potassium levels higher than desired

Activities:

Obtain specimens for laboratory analysis of potassium levels and associated electrolyte imbalances (e.g., ABG, urine, and serum levels), as appropriate

Monitor cause(s) of increasing serum potassium levels (e.g., renal failure, excessive intake, and acidosis), as appropriate

Administer electrolyte-binding and -excreting resins (e.g., Kayexalate) as prescribed, if appropriate

Monitor lab values for changes in oxygenation or acid-base balance, as appropriate

Administer prescribed medications to shift potassium into the cell (e.g., 50% dextrose and insulin, sodium bicarbonate, calcium chloride, and calcium gluconate), as appropriate

Insert rectal catheter for administration of cation-exchanging or -binding resins (e.g., Kayexalate per rectum), as appropriate

Avoid potassium-sparing medications (e.g., spironolactone [Aldactone] and triamterene [Dyrenium], as appropriate

Maintain potassium restrictions

Monitor for symptoms of inadequate tissue oxygenation (e.g., pallor, cyanosis, and sluggish capillary refill)

Maintain patent IV access

Monitor renal function (e.g., BUN and Cr levels), if appropriate

Administer prescribed diuretics, as appropriate

Monitor fluid status, including intake and output, as appropriate

Insert urinary catheter, if appropriate

Monitor for fluid overload resulting from associated renal failure, as appropriate

Provide food low in potassium (e.g., fruits, beef, gelatin, and olives)

Instruct patient on appropriate use of salt substitutes, as necessary

Monitor for digitalis toxicity (e.g., report serum levels above therapeutic range, monitor heart rate and rhythm before administering dose, and monitor for side effects), as appropriate

Monitor for unintentional potassium intake (e.g., penicillin G potassium or dietary potassium), as appropriate

Monitor for therapeutic effect of diuretic (e.g., increased urine output, decreased CVP/PCWP, and decreased adventitious breath sounds)

Monitor potassium levels after diuresis

Prepare patient for dialysis (e.g., assist with catheter placement for dialysis), as appropriate

Monitor patient's hemodynamic response to dialysis, as appropriate

Monitor infused and returned volume of peritoneal dialysate, as appropriate

Monitor neurological manifestations of hyperkalemia (e.g., muscle weakness, reduced sensation, hyporeflexia, and paresthesias)

Monitor cardiac manifestations of hyperkalemia (e.g., decreased cardiac output, heart blocks, peaked T waves, fibrillation, or asystole)

Instruct the patient and/or family on measures instituted to treat the hyperkalemia

Monitor for rebound hypokalemia (e.g., excessive diuresis, excessive use of cation-exchanging resins)

Continued

Activities:—cont'd

Monitor for hyperkalemia associated with a blood reaction, if appropriate

Request the freshest blood for transfusion, if the patient is to receive multiple blood transfusions

Respond to cardiac arrest

Anticipate use of pacemaker (e.g., check pacemaker settings and connections or make an insertion tray available), if indicated

Teach patient the rationale for use of diuretic therapy

Background Readings:

Askanazi, J., Starker, P., & Wissman, C. (1986). Fluid and electrolyte management in critical care. Boston: Butterworths.

Baer, C.L. (1993). Fluid and electrolyte balance. In M.R. Kinney, D.R. Packa, & S.B. Dunbar (Eds.), AACN's clinical reference for critical-care nursing (pp. 173-208). St. Louis: Mosby.

Chan, J., & Gill, J. (1990). Kidney electrolyte disorders. New York: Churchill Livingston.

Cullen, L.M. (1992). Interventions related to fluid and electrolyte balance. In G.M. Bulechek & J.C. McCloskey (Eds.), Symposium on Nursing Interventions. Nursing Clinics of North America, 27(2), 569-598.

Horne, M., & Swearingen, P. (1997). Pocket guide to fluids and electrolytes (3rd ed.). St. Louis: Mosby.

Kokko, J., & Tannen, R. (1990). Fluids and electrolytes (2nd ed.). Philadelphia: W.B. Saunders.

Olin, B.R. (Ed.). (1993). Facts and comparisons. St. Louis: Wolters Kluwer.

Rice, V. (1982). The role of potassium in health and disease. Critical Care Nurse, May/June, 54-74.

Stark, J. (1991). The renal system. In J. Alspach (Ed.), American Association of Critical-Care Nurses core curriculum for critical-care nursing (4th ed.) (pp. 472-608). Philadelphia: W.B. Saunders.

Electrolyte Management: Hypermagnesemia   2003

Definition: Promotion of magnesium balance and prevention of complications resulting from serum magnesium levels higher than desired

Activities:

Obtain specimens for laboratory analysis of magnesium level, as appropriate

Monitor trends in magnesium levels, as available

Monitor for electrolyte imbalances associated with hypermagnesemia (e.g., elevated BUN and Cr levels), as appropriate

Monitor for causes of increasing magnesium levels (e.g., renal failure, hyperalimentation, and frequent magnesium sulfate enemas)

Monitor for cardiopulmonary manifestations of hypermagnesemia (e.g., hypotension, flushing, bradycardia, respiratory depression, apnea, and heart blocks)

Position patient to facilitate ventilation

Administer prescribed calcium chloride (10% solution) IV to antagonize neuromuscular effects of hypermagnesemia, as appropriate

Monitor for CNS manifestations of hypermagnesemia (e.g., drowsiness, lethargy, and coma)

Monitor for neuromuscular manifestations of hypermagnesemia (e.g., weak to absent deep tendon reflexes, muscle paralysis, and flaccid muscles)

Administer prescribed anticholinergic medications (e.g., neostigmine or pentylenetetrazol) to potentiate neuromuscular transmission, as appropriate

Maintain bed rest and limit activities

Alternate high- and low-magnesium antacids (e.g., Maalox and AlternaGEL), as appropriate

Prepare patient for dialysis (e.g., assist with catheter placement for dialysis), as appropriate

Instruct patient and/or family on measures instituted to treat the hypermagnesemia

Provide comfort measures for the GI effects of hypermagnesemia

Background Readings:

Askanazi, J., Starker, P., & Wissman, C. (1986). Fluid and electrolyte management in critical care. Boston: Butterworths.

Baer, C.L. (1993). Fluid and electrolyte balance. In M.R. Kinney, D.R. Packa, & S.B. Dunbar (Eds.), AACN's clinical reference for critical-care nursing (pp. 173-208). St. Louis: Mosby.

Chan, J., & Gill, J. (1990). Kidney electrolyte disorders. New York: Churchill Livingstone.

Cullen, L.M. (1992). Interventions related to fluid and electrolyte balance. In G.M. Bulechek & J.C. McCloskey (Eds.), Symposium on Nursing Interventions. Nursing Clinics of North America, 27(2), 569-598.

Kokko, J., & Tannen, R. (1990). Fluids and electrolytes (2nd ed.). Philadelphia: W.B. Saunders.

Rice, V. (1983). Magnesium, calcium and phosphate imbalances: Their clinical significance. Critical Care Nurse, May/June, 90-112.

Stark, J. (1991). The renal system. In J. Alspach (Ed.), American Association of Critical-Care Nurses core curriculum for critical-care nursing (4th ed.) (pp. 472-608). Philadelphia: W.B. Saunders.

E

Electrolyte Management: Hypernatremia   2004

Definition: Promotion of sodium balance and prevention of complications resulting from serum sodium levels higher than desired

Activities:

Obtain specimens for lab analysis of altered sodium levels (e.g., serum and urine sodium, serum and urine chloride, urine osmolality, and urine specific gravity), as appropriate

Monitor for indications of dehydration (e.g., decreased sweating, decreased urine, decreased skin turgor, and dry mucous membranes)

Monitor for insensible fluid loss (e.g., diaphoresis and respiratory tract infection)

Monitor vital signs, as appropriate

Weigh patient daily and monitor trends

Provide comfort measures to decrease thirst

Monitor for side effects resulting from rapid corrections or overcorrections of hypernatremia (e.g., cerebral edema and seizures)

Maintain patent IV access

Monitor renal function (e.g., BUN and Cr levels), if appropriate

Monitor intake and output

Administer prescribed diuretics in conjunction with hypertonic fluids for hypernatremia associated with hypervolemia, as appropriate

Monitor hemodynamic status, including CVP, MAP, PAP, and PCWP, if available

Provide frequent oral hygiene

Promote skin integrity (e.g., monitor areas at risk for breakdown, promote frequent weight shifts, prevent shearing, and promote adequate nutrition), as appropriate

Administer normal saline and plasma expanders in the presence of hypernatremia associated with hypovolemia

Administer isotonic (.9%) saline, hypotonic (.45%) saline, hypotonic (5%) dextrose, or diuretics, as appropriate, based on fluid status and urine osmolality

Administer prescribed antidiuretic agents (e.g., desmopressin or vasopressin [Pitressin] in the presence of diabetes insipidus, as appropriate

Avoid administration/intake of high-sodium medications (e.g., Kayexalate, sodium bicarbonate, and hypertonic saline)

Maintain sodium restrictions

Instruct patient on appropriate use of salt substitutes, as necessary

Instruct the patient/family about foods and over-the-counter medications that are high in sodium (e.g., canned foods and selected antacids)

Monitor lab values associated with hypernatremia (e.g., hyperchloremia and hyperglycemia), as appropriate

Monitor for neurological and/or neuromuscular manifestations of hypernatremia (e.g., lethargy, irritability, seizures, coma, muscle rigidity, tremors, and hyperreflexia)

Institute seizure precautions

Monitor for cardiac manifestations of hypernatremia (e.g., tachycardia, orthostatic hypotension, and flat neck veins)

Instruct the patient and/or family on measures instituted to treat the hypernatremia

Instruct the family or significant other on signs and symptoms of hypovolemia (if hypernatremia is related to abnormal fluid loss)

Background Readings:

Askanazi, J., Starker, P., & Wissman, C. (1986). Fluid and electrolyte management in critical care. Boston: Butterworths.

Baer, C.L. (1993). Fluid and electrolyte balance. In M.R. Kinney, D.R. Packa, & S.B. Dunbar (Eds.), AACN's clinical reference for critical-care nursing (pp. 173-208). St. Louis: Mosby.

Chan, J., & Gill, J. (1990). Kidney electrolyte disorders. New York: Churchill Livingstone.

Cullen, L.M. (1992). Interventions related to fluid and electrolyte balance. In G.M. Bulechek & J.C. McCloskey (Eds.), Symposium on Nursing Interventions. Nursing Clinics of North America, 27(2), 569-598.

Horne, M., & Swearingen, P. (1997). Pocket guide to fluids and electrolytes (3rd ed.). St. Louis: Mosby.

Kokko, J., & Tannen, R. (1990). Fluids and electrolytes (2nd ed.). Philadelphia: W.B. Saunders.

Stark, J. (1991). The renal system. In J. Alspach (Ed.), American Association of Critical-Care Nurses core curriculum for critical-care nursing (4th ed.) (pp. 472-608). Philadelphia: W.B. Saunders.

Verbalis, J., & Robinson, A. (1984). Hypernatremia and hyponatremia. Topics of Emergency Medicine, January, 79-89.

E

Electrolyte Management: Hyperphosphatemia   2005

Definition: Promotion of phosphate balance and prevention of complications resulting from serum phosphate levels higher than desired

Activities:

Obtain specimens for laboratory analysis of phosphate and associated electrolyte levels (e.g., ABG, urine, and serum levels), as appropriate

Monitor for electrolyte imbalances associated with hyperphosphatemia (e.g., hypomagnesemia, hypocalcemia, respiratory acidosis, serum and urine phosphate levels, serum and urine calcium and magnesium levels), as appropriate

Monitor renal failure resulting in increasing serum phosphate levels

Administer prescribed phosphate-binding and diuretic medications (e.g., Amphojel, Phos-Lo cookie, and Basajel) with food to decrease absorption of dietary phosphate, as appropriate

Prevent constipation resulting from phosphate-binding medications

Provide comfort measures for the GI effects of hyperphosphatemia

Administer prescribed calcium and vitamin D supplements to reduce phosphate levels, as appropriate

Avoid phosphate-rich foods (e.g., dairy products, whole-grain cereal, nuts, dried fruits or vegetables, and organ meats), as appropriate

Prepare patient for dialysis (e.g., assist with catheter placement for dialysis), as appropriate

Institute seizure precautions

Instruct the patient and/or family on measures instituted to treat the hyperphosphatemia

Background Readings:

Askanazi, J., Starker, P., & Wissman, C. (1986). Fluid and electrolyte management in critical care. Boston: Butterworths.

Baer, C.L. (1993). Fluid and electrolyte balance. In M.R. Kinney, D.R. Packa, & S.B. Dunbar (Eds.), AACN's clinical reference for critical-care nursing (pp. 173-208). St. Louis: Mosby.

Chan, J., & Gill, J. (1990). Kidney electrolyte disorders. New York: Churchill Livingstone.

Cullen, L.M. (1992). Interventions related to fluid and electrolyte balance. In G.M. Bulechek & J.C. McCloskey (Eds.), Symposium on Nursing Interventions. Nursing Clinics of North America, 27(2), 569-598.

Kokko, J., & Tannen, R. (1990). Fluids and electrolytes (2nd ed.). Philadelphia: W.B. Saunders.

Rice, V. (1983). Magnesium, calcium, and phosphate imbalances: Their clinical significance. Critical Care Nurse, May/June, 90-112.

Stark, J. (1991). The renal system. In J. Alspach (Ed.), American Association of Critical-Care Nurses core curriculum for critical-care nursing (4th ed.) (pp. 472-608). Philadelphia: W.B. Saunders.

Electrolyte Management: Hypocalcemia   2006

Definition: Promotion of calcium balance and prevention of complications resulting from serum calcium levels lower than desired

Activities:

Monitor trends in serum levels of calcium (e.g., ionized calcium), as available

Monitor calcium levels closely in the patient receiving large numbers of blood transfusions

Monitor for electrolyte imbalances associated with hypocalcemia (e.g., hyperphosphatemia, hypomagnesemia, and alkalosis), as appropriate

Monitor for decreasing levels of serum ionized calcium (e.g., hemodilution, chronic diarrhea, pancreatitis, cardiopulmonary bypass, and small bowel disease)

Monitor for continued calcium loss (e.g., loop-diuretics, renal tubular dysfunction, and loss of exudates through burns or infection), as appropriate

Monitor fluid status, including intake and output, as appropriate

Monitor renal function (e.g., BUN and Cr levels), if appropriate

Maintain patent IV access

Administer appropriate prescribed calcium salt (e.g., calcium carbonate, calcium chloride, and calcium gluconate), as indicated

Monitor for side effects of IV administration of ionized calcium (e.g., calcium chloride), such as thrombophlebitis, soft tissue damage with extravasation, clotting, and thrombus formation, as appropriate

Avoid administration of medications decreasing serum ionized calcium (e.g., bicarbonate and citrated blood), as appropriate

Avoid administration of calcium salts with bicarbonate to prevent precipitation

Encourage intake of calcium (e.g., dairy products, seafood, nuts, broccoli, spinach, and supplements), as appropriate

Provide adequate intake of vitamin D (e.g., vitamin supplement and organ meats) to facilitate GI absorption of calcium, as appropriate

Monitor for neuromuscular manifestations of hypocalcemia (e.g., tetany, muscle twitching, cramping, grimacing, seizure, altered deep tendon reflexes, and spasm)

Monitor for acute laryngeal spasm and tetany requiring emergency airway management

Monitor for exacerbation of tetany resulting from hyperventilation or pressure on efferent nerves (e.g., from crossing legs), as appropriate

Monitor for CNS manifestations of hypocalcemia (e.g., personality disturbances, anxiety, irritability, depression, and psychosis)

Monitor for cardiovascular manifestations of hypocalcemia (e.g., decreased contractility, decreased cardiac output, hypotension, lengthened ST segment, and prolonged QT interval)

Monitor for GI manifestations of hypocalcemia (e.g., nausea, vomiting, constipation, and abdominal pain from muscle spasm)

Monitor for integument manifestations of hypocalcemia (e.g., scaling, eczema, alopecia, and hyperpigmentation)

Provide pain relief/comfort measures

Monitor for overcorrection and hypercalcemia

Instruct the patient and/or family on measures instituted to treat the hypocalcemia

Continued

Background Readings:

Askanazi, J., Starker, P., & Wissman, C. (1986). Fluid and electrolyte management in critical care. Boston: Butterworths.

Baer, C.L. (1993). Fluid and electrolyte balance. In M.R. Kinney, D.R. Packa, & S.B. Dunbar (Eds.), AACN's clinical reference for critical-care nursing (pp. 173-208). St. Louis: Mosby.

Chan, J., & Gill, J. (1990). Kidney electrolyte disorders. New York: Churchill Livingstone.

Cullen, L.M. (1992). Interventions related to fluid and electrolyte balance. In G.M. Bulechek & J.C. McCloskey (Eds.), Symposium on Nursing Interventions. Nursing Clinics of North America, 27(2), 569-598.

Horne, M., & Swearingen, P. (1997). Pocket guide to fluids and electrolytes (3rd ed.). St. Louis: Mosby.

Kokko, J., & Tannen, R. (1990). Fluids and electrolytes (2nd ed.). Philadelphia: W.B. Saunders.

Rice, V. (1983). Magnesium, calcium, and phosphate imbalances: Their clinical significance. Critical Care Nurse, May/June, 90-112.

Stark, J. (1991). The renal system. In J. Alspach (Ed.), American Association of Critical-Care Nurses core curriculum for critical-care nursing (4th ed.) (pp. 472-608). Philadelphia: W.B. Saunders.

E

Electrolyte Management: Hypokalemia   2007

Definition: Promotion of potassium balance and prevention of complications resulting from serum potassium levels lower than desired

Activities:

Obtain specimens for laboratory analysis of potassium levels and associated electrolyte imbalances (e.g., ABG, urine, and serum levels), as appropriate

Monitor lab values associated with hypokalemia (e.g., elevated glucose, metabolic alkalosis, reduced urine osmolality, urine potassium, hypochloremia, and hypocalcemia)

Monitor intracellular shifts causing decreasing serum potassium levels (e.g., metabolic alkalosis; dietary, especially carbohydrate, intake; and administration of insulin), as appropriate

Monitor renal cause(s) of decreasing serum potassium levels (e.g., diuretics, diuresis, metabolic alkalosis, and potassium-losing nephritis), as appropriate

Monitor GI cause(s) of decreasing serum potassium levels (e.g., diarrhea, fistulas, vomiting, and continuous NG suction), as appropriate

Monitor dilutional cause(s) of decreasing serum potassium levels (e.g., administration of hypotonic solutions and increased water retention, secondary to inappropriate ADH), as appropriate

Administer prescribed supplemental potassium (PO, NG, or IV), per policy

Consider appropriate potassium preparations when supplementing potassium (e.g., chloride-associated hypochloremia; gluconate; acetate; citrate; bicarbonate, decreased chloride levels and decreased serum potassium; sugar-free, for extracellular increases; or non–sugar-free, for intracellular increases), as appropriate

Monitor renal functions, EKG, and serum potassium levels during replacement, as appropriate

Prevent/reduce irritation from potassium supplement (e.g., administer PO or NG potassium supplements during or after meals to minimize GI irritation, dilute IV potassium adequately, administer IV supplement slowly, and apply topical anesthetic to IV site), as appropriate

Administer potassium-sparing diuretics (e.g., spironolactone [Aldactone] or triamterene [Dyrenium]), as appropriate

Monitor for digitalis toxicity (e.g., report serum levels above therapeutic range, monitor heart rate and rhythm before administering dose, and monitor for side effects), as appropriate

Avoid administration of alkaline substances (e.g., IV sodium bicarbonate and PO or NG antacids), as appropriate

Monitor neurological manifestations of hypokalemia (e.g., muscle weakness, altered level of consciousness, drowsiness, apathy, lethargy, confusion, and depression)

Monitor cardiac manifestations of hypokalemia (e.g., hypotension, broad T wave, U wave, ectopy, tachycardia, and weak pulse)

Monitor renal manifestations of hypokalemia (e.g., acidic urine, reduced urine osmolality, nocturia, polyuria, and polydipsia)

Monitor GI manifestations of hypokalemia (e.g., anorexia, nausea, cramps, constipation, distention, and paralytic ileus)

Monitor pulmonary manifestations of hypokalemia (e.g., hypoventilation and respiratory muscle weakness)

Position patient to facilitate ventilation

Monitor for symptoms of respiratory failure (e.g., low PaO_2 and elevated $PaCO_2$ levels and respiratory muscle fatigue)

Monitor for rebound hyperkalemia

Monitor for excessive diuresis

Continued

Activities:—cont'd

Instruct patient and/or family on measures instituted to treat the hypokalemia

Maintain patent IV access

Monitor fluid status, including intake and output, as appropriate

Provide foods rich in potassium (e.g., salt substitutes, dried fruits, bananas, green vegetables, tomatoes, yellow vegetables, chocolate, and dairy products), as appropriate

Background Readings:

Anonymous. (2000). Incredibly easy! Understanding hypokalemia. Nursing, 30(11), 74-76.

Baer, C.L. (1993). Fluid and electrolyte balance. In M.R. Kinney, D.R. Packa, & S.B. Dunbar (Eds.), AACN's clinical reference for critical-care nursing (pp. 173-208). St. Louis: Mosby.

Cullen, L.M. (1992). Interventions related to fluid and electrolyte balance. In G.M. Bulechek & J.C. McCloskey (Eds.), Symposium on Nursing Interventions. Nursing Clinics of North America, 27(2), 569-598.

Metheny, N.M. (Ed.). (2000). Fluid and electrolyte balance: Nursing considerations (4th ed.). Philadelphia: Lippincott, Williams, & Wilkins.

Pestana, C. (2000). Fluids and electrolytes in the surgical patient. Philadelphia: Lippincott, Williams, & Wilkins.

Springhouse Corporation. (2002). Fluids & electrolytes made incredibly easy (2nd ed.). Springhouse, PA: Springhouse.

Electrolyte Management: Hypomagnesemia   2008

Definition: Promotion of magnesium balance and prevention of complications resulting from serum magnesium levels lower than desired

Activities:

Obtain specimens for laboratory analysis of magnesium level, as appropriate

Monitor trends in magnesium levels, as available

Monitor for electrolyte imbalances associated with hypomagnesemia (e.g., hypokalemia, hypocalcemia, and hypochloremic alkalosis), as appropriate

Monitor for reduced intake through malnutrition or prolonged hyperalimentation without supplementation, as appropriate

Monitor for decreasing levels of magnesium resulting from decreased absorption of magnesium (e.g., surgical resection of bowel, pancreatic insufficiency, and increased dietary intake of calcium), as appropriate

Monitor for increasing excretion of magnesium (e.g., diuretics, renal disorders, renal excretion after transplant, hypercalcemia, diarrhea, fistulas, prolonged NG suction, burns, hyperglycemia, hyperthyroidism, and prolonged cardiopulmonary bypass), as appropriate

Administer magnesium supplement 250 mg (12.5 mEq) to 500 mg (25 mEq) orally four times daily, or 4 to 10 g IV in a 24-hour period, or per policy, as appropriate

Monitor for side effects of IV magnesium replacement (e.g., flushing, sweating, sensation of heat, and hypocalcemia), as appropriate

Administer magnesium-containing antacids (e.g., Mylanta, Maalox, Di Gel, or Milk of Magnesia) in combination with antidiarrheal medications (to prevent further loss of magnesium), as appropriate

Keep calcium gluconate available during rapid magnesium replacement in case of associated hypocalcemic tetany or apnea, as appropriate

Monitor deep tendon reflexes during rapid magnesium replacement, as precursor to cardiopulmonary side effects

Avoid administration of magnesium-depleting medications (e.g., furosemide [Lasix], ethacrynic acid [Edecrin], mannitol, gentamycin, tobramycin, carbenicillin, amphotericin B, digoxin, and cisplatin), as appropriate

Offer foods rich in magnesium (e.g., cocoa powder, nuts, cereals, seafood, meats, and legumes), as appropriate

Monitor for CNS manifestations of hypomagnesemia (e.g., altered mental status, insomnia, auditory and visual hallucinations, agitation, and personality change)

Monitor for neuromuscular manifestations of hypomagnesemia (e.g., muscle twitching, paresthesias, hyperactive reflexes, positive Babinski reflex, dysphagia, nystagmus, seizures, and tetany)

Monitor for GI manifestations of hypomagnesemia (e.g., nausea, vomiting, anorexia, diarrhea, and abdominal distention)

Monitor for cardiac manifestations of hypomagnesemia (e.g., ectopy; tachycardia; ventricular tachycardia; broad, flat, or inverted T wave; depressed ST segment; prolonged QT interval; digitalis intoxication; decreased cardiac output; hypotension)

Monitor for rebound hypermagnesemia, as appropriate

Instruct patient and/or family on measures instituted to treat the hypomagnesemia

Continued

Background Readings:

Askanazi, J., Starker, P., & Wissman, C. (1986). Fluid and electrolyte management in critical care. Boston: Butterworths.

Baer, C.L. (1993). Fluid and electrolyte balance. In M.R. Kinney, D.R. Packa, & S.B. Dunbar (Eds.), AACN's clinical reference for critical-care nursing (pp. 173-208). St. Louis: Mosby.

Chan, J., & Gill, J. (1990). Kidney electrolyte disorders. New York: Churchill Livingstone.

Cullen, L.M. (1992). Interventions related to fluid and electrolyte balance. In G.M. Bulechek & J.C. McCloskey (Eds.), Symposium on Nursing Interventions. Nursing Clinics of North America, 27(2), 569-598.

Keller, P., & Aronson, R. (1990). The role of magnesium in cardiac arrhythmias. Progress in Cardiovascular Disease, 32(6), 433-448.

Kokko, J., & Tannen, R. (1990). Fluids and electrolytes (2nd ed.). Philadelphia: W.B. Saunders.

Rice, V. (1983). Magnesium, calcium, and phosphate imbalances: Their clinical significance. Critical Care Nurse, May/June, 90-112.

Stark, J. (1991). The renal system. In J. Alspach (Ed.), American Association of Critical-Care Nurses core curriculum for critical-care nursing (4th ed.) (pp. 472-608). Philadelphia: W.B. Saunders.

E

Electrolyte Management: Hyponatremia   2009

Definition: Promotion of sodium balance and prevention of complications resulting from serum sodium levels lower than desired

Activities:

Obtain lab specimens for analysis of altered sodium levels (e.g., serum and urine sodium, serum and urine chloride, urine osmolality, and urine specific gravity), as appropriate

Monitor for electrolyte imbalances associated with hyponatremia (e.g., hypokalemia, metabolic acidosis, and hypoglycemia), as appropriate

Monitor for renal loss of sodium (oliguria)

Monitor renal function (e.g., BUN and Cr levels), if appropriate

Monitor intake and output

Weigh patient daily and monitor trends

Monitor for indications of fluid overload/retention (e.g., crackles, elevated CVP or PCWP, edema, neck vein distention, and ascites), as appropriate

Monitor hemodynamic status, including CVP, MAP, PAP, and PCWP, if available

Administer normal saline and plasma expanders in the presence of hypovolemia, as appropriate

Administer hypertonic (3% to 5%) saline at 3 ml/kg/hr or per policy for rapid correction of hyponatremia, as appropriate

Avoid excessive administration of hypotonic IV fluids, especially in the presence of SIADH, as appropriate

Administer diuretics only as indicated (e.g., thiazides, loop diuretics similar to furosemide, or ethacrynic acid), as appropriate

Teach patient the rationale for use of diuretic therapy

Prevent rapid correction or overcorrection of hyponatremia (e.g., serum sodium level of greater than 125 mEq/L and hypokalemia)

Limit patient activities to conserve energy, as appropriate

Maintain fluid restriction, as appropriate

Monitor for neurological and/or neuromuscular manifestations of hyponatremia (e.g., lethargy, increased ICP, confusion, headache, seizures, coma, fatigue, tremors, apprehension, muscle weakness, and hyperreflexia)

Institute seizure precautions

Monitor for cardiovascular manifestations of hyponatremia (e.g., elevated blood pressure, cold and clammy skin, and hypo- or hypervolemia)

Monitor for GI manifestations of hyponatremia (e.g., anorexia, nausea, vomiting, abdominal cramps, and diarrhea)

Encourage foods/fluids high in sodium, if appropriate

Instruct the patient and/or family on measures instituted to treat the hyponatremia

Background Readings:

Askanazi, J., Starker, P., & Wissman, C. (1986). Fluid and electrolyte management in critical care. Boston: Butterworths.

Baer, C.L. (1993). Fluid and electrolyte balance. In M.R. Kinney, D.R. Packa, & S.B. Dunbar (Eds.), AACN's clinical reference for critical-care nursing (pp. 173-208). St. Louis: Mosby.

Chan, J., & Gill, J. (1990). Kidney electrolyte disorders. New York: Churchill Livingstone.

Cullen, L.M. (1992). Interventions related to fluid and electrolyte balance. In G.M. Bulechek & J.C. McCloskey (Eds.), Symposium on Nursing Interventions. Nursing Clinics of North America, 27(2), 569-598.

Horne, M., & Swearingen, P. (1997). Pocket guide to fluids and electrolytes (3rd ed.). St. Louis: Mosby.

Kokko, J., & Tannen, R. (1990). Fluids and electrolytes (2nd ed.). Philadelphia: W.B. Saunders.

Stark, J. (1991). The renal system. In J. Alspach (Ed.), American Association of Critical-Care Nurses core curriculum for critical-care nursing (4th ed.) (pp. 472-608). Philadelphia: W.B. Saunders.

Verbalis, J., & Robinson, A. (1984). Hypernatremia and hyponatremia. Topics of Emergency Medicine, January, 79-89.

Electrolyte Management: Hypophosphatemia 2010

Definition: Promotion of phosphate balance and prevention of complications resulting from serum phosphate levels lower than desired

Activities:

Obtain specimens for laboratory analysis of phosphate and associated electrolyte levels (e.g., ABG, urine, and serum levels), as appropriate

Monitor for electrolyte imbalances associated with hypophosphatemia (e.g., hypokalemia; hypomagnesemia; respiratory alkalosis; metabolic acidosis; and serum and urine phosphate, calcium, and magnesium levels), as appropriate

Monitor for decreasing levels of phosphate resulting from reduced intake and absorption (e.g., starvation, hyperalimentation without phosphate, vomiting, small bowel or pancreatic disease, diarrhea, and ingestion of aluminum or magnesium hydroxide antacids)

Monitor for decreasing phosphate levels resulting from renal loss (e.g., hypokalemia, hypomagnesemia, heavy metal poisoning, alcohol, hemodialysis with phosphate-poor dialysate, thiazide diuretics, and vitamin D deficiency)

Monitor for decreasing phosphate levels resulting from extracellular to intracellular shifts (e.g., glucose administration, insulin administration, alkalosis, and hyperalimentation)

Administer prescribed phosphate supplements IV or PO, as appropriate

Monitor for rapid correction or overcorrection of hypophosphatemia (e.g., hyperphosphatemia, hypocalcemia, hypotension, hyperkalemia, hypernatremia, and tetany)

Monitor renal function during parenteral phosphate supplementation, as appropriate

Avoid phosphate-binding and diuretic medications (e.g., Amphojel, Phos-Lo cookie, and Basaljel)

Encourage increased oral intake of phosphate (e.g., dairy products, whole-grain cereal, nuts, dried fruits or vegetables, and organ meats), as appropriate

Monitor for neuromuscular manifestations of hypophosphatemia (e.g., weakness, lassitude, malaise, tremors, paresthesias, ataxia, increased creatinine phosphokinase, abnormal EMG, and rhabdomyolysis)

Conserve muscle strength (e.g., assist with passive or active range-of-motion exercises)

Monitor for CNS manifestations of hypophosphatemia (e.g., memory loss, reduced attention span, confusion, convulsions, coma, abnormal EEG, decreased reflexes, impaired sensory function, and cranial nerve palsies)

Monitor for skeletal manifestations of hypophosphatemia (e.g., aching bone pain, fractures, and joint stiffness)

Monitor for cardiovascular manifestations of hypophosphatemia (e.g., decreased contractility, decreased cardiac output, heart failure, and ectopy)

Monitor for pulmonary manifestations of hypophosphatemia (e.g., rapid, shallow respirations; decreased tidal volume; and decreased minute ventilation)

Monitor for GI manifestations of hypophosphatemia (e.g., nausea, vomiting, anorexia, impaired liver function, and portal hypertension)

Monitor for hematological manifestations of hypophosphatemia (e.g., anemia, increased hemoglobin affinity with oxygen leading to increased SaO_2, increased risk of infection resulting from impaired WBC functioning, and thrombocytopenia and hemorrhage resulting from platelet dysfunction)

Instruct the patient and/or family on measures instituted to treat the hypophosphatemia

Background Readings:

Askanazi, J., Starker, P., & Wissman, C. (1986). Fluid and electrolyte management in critical care. Boston: Butterworths.

Baer, C.L. (1993). Fluid and electrolyte balance. In M.R. Kinney, D.R. Packa, & S.B. Dunbar (Eds.), AACN's clinical reference for critical-care nursing (pp. 173-208). St. Louis: Mosby.

Chan, J., & Gill, J. (1990). Kidney electrolyte disorders. New York: Churchill Livingstone.

Cullen, L.M. (1992). Interventions related to fluid and electrolyte balance. In G.M. Bulechek & J.C. McCloskey (Eds.), Symposium on Nursing Interventions. Nursing Clinics of North America, 27(2), 569-598.

Kokko, J., & Tannen, R. (1990). Fluids and electrolytes (2nd ed.). Philadelphia: W.B. Saunders.

Rice, V. (1983). Magnesium, calcium, and phosphate imbalances: Their clinical significance. Critical Care Nurse, May/June, 90-112.

E

Electrolyte Monitoring 2020

Definition: Collection and analysis of patient data to regulate electrolyte balance

Activities:

Monitor the serum level of electrolytes

Monitor serum albumin and total protein levels, as indicated

Monitor for associated acid-base imbalances

Identify possible causes of electrolyte imbalances

Recognize and report presence of electrolyte imbalances

Monitor for fluid loss and associated loss of electrolytes, as appropriate

Monitor for Chvostek and/or Trousseau sign

Monitor for neurological manifestation of electrolyte imbalance (e.g., altered sensorium and weakness)

Monitor adequacy of ventilation

Monitor serum and urine osmolality levels

Monitor EKG tracings for changes related to abnormal potassium, calcium, and magnesium levels

Note changes in peripheral sensation, such as numbness and tremors

Note muscle strength

Monitor for nausea, vomiting, and diarrhea

Identify treatments that can alter electrolyte status, such as GI suctioning, diuretics, antihypertensives, and calcium channel blockers

Monitor for underlying medical disease that can lead to electrolyte imbalance

Monitor for signs and symptoms of hypokalemia: muscular weakness, cardiac irregularities (PVC), prolonged QT interval, flattened or depressed T wave, depressed ST segment, presence of U wave, paresthesia, decreased reflexes, anorexia, decreased GI motility, dizziness, confusion, increased sensitivity to digitalis, and depressed respirations

Monitor for signs/symptoms of hyperkalemia: irritability, restlessness, anxiety, nausea, vomiting, abdominal cramps, weakness, flaccid paralysis, circumoral numbness and tingling, tachycardia progressing to bradycardia, ventricular tachycardia/fibrillation, tall peaked T waves, flattened P wave, broad slurred QRS complex, and heart block progressing to asystole

Monitor for signs/symptoms of hyponatremia: disorientation, muscle twitching, nausea and vomiting, abdominal cramps, headaches, seizures, lethargy and withdrawal, and coma

Monitor for signs and symptoms of hypernatremia: extreme thirst; fever; dry, sticky mucous membranes; altered mentation; and seizures

Monitor for signs and symptoms of hypocalcemia: irritability, muscle tetany, muscle cramps, decreased cardiac output, prolonged ST segment and QT interval, bleeding, and fractures

Monitor for signs and symptoms of hypercalcemia: deep bone pain, excessive thirst, anorexia, lethargy, weakened muscles, shortened QT segment, wide T wave, widened QRS complex, and prolonged P-R interval

Monitor for signs and symptoms of hypomagnesemia: respiratory muscle depression, mental apathy, confusion, facial tics, spasticity, and cardiac dysrhythmias

Monitor for signs and symptoms of hypermagnesemia: muscle weakness, inability to swallow, hyporeflexia, hypotension, bradycardia, CNS depression, respiratory depression, lethargy, coma, and depression

Monitor for signs and symptoms of hypophosphatemia: bleeding tendencies, muscle weakness, paresthesia, hemolytic anemia, depressed white cell function, nausea, vomiting, anorexia, and bone demineralization

Activities:—cont'd

Monitor for signs and symptoms of hyperphosphatemia: tachycardia, nausea, diarrhea, abdominal cramps, muscle weakness, flaccid paralysis, and increased reflexes

Monitor for signs and symptoms of hypochloremia: hyperirritability, tetany, muscular excitability, slow respirations, and hypotension

Monitor for signs and symptoms of hyperchloremia: weakness; lethargy; deep, rapid breathing; and coma

Administer prescribed supplemental electrolytes, as appropriate

Provide diet appropriate for patient's electrolyte imbalance (e.g., potassium-rich foods or low-sodium diet)

Teach patient ways to prevent or minimize electrolyte imbalance

Instruct patient and/or family on specific dietary modifications, as appropriate

Consult physician, if signs and symptoms of fluid and/or electrolyte imbalance persist or worsen

E

Background Readings:

Melillo, K.D. (1993). Interpretation of laboratory values in older adults. Nurse Practitioner, 18(7), 59-60.

Thelan, L.A., & Urden, L.D. (1998). Critical care nursing: Diagnosis and management (3rd ed.). St. Louis: Mosby.

Thompson, J.M., McFarland, G.K., Hirsch, J.E., & Tucker, S.M. (1998). Mosby's clinical nursing (4th ed.). St. Louis: Mosby.

Titler, M.G. (1992). Interventions related to surveillance. In G.M. Bulechek & J.C. McCloskey (Eds.), Symposium on Nursing Interventions. Nursing Clinics of North America, 27(2), 495-516.

E

Electronic Fetal Monitoring: Antepartum 6771

Definition: Electronic evaluation of fetal heart rate response to movement, external stimuli, or uterine contractions during antepartal testing

Activities:

Review obstetrical history, if available, to determine obstetrical or medical risk factors requiring antepartum testing of fetal status

Determine patient's knowledge of reasons for antepartum testing

Provide written patient education material for antepartum tests (e.g., nonstress, oxytocin challenge, and biophysical profile tests), as well as electronic fetal monitor

Take maternal vital signs

Inquire about oral intake, including diet, cigarette smoking, and medication use

Label monitor strip per protocol

Review prior antepartum tests

Verify maternal and fetal heart rates before initiation of electronic fetal monitoring

Instruct patient about the reason for electronic monitoring, as well as the types of information obtainable

Perform Leopold maneuver to determine fetal position(s), as appropriate

Apply tocotransducer snugly to observe contraction frequency and duration

Apply ultrasound transducer(s) to area of uterus where fetal heart sounds are audible and trace clearly

Differentiate among multiple fetuses by documenting on the tracing when simultaneous tracings are conducted, using one electronic fetal monitor

Distinguish among multiple fetuses by comparing data when simultaneous tracings are conducted, using two different fetal monitors

Discuss appearance of rhythm strip with mother and support person

Reassure about normal fetal heart rate signs, including such typical features as artifact, loss of signal with fetal movement, high rate, and irregular appearance

Adjust monitors to achieve and maintain clarity of the tracing(s)

Obtain baseline tracing of fetal heart rate(s) per protocol for specific testing procedure

Interpret electronic monitor strip for baseline heart rate(s); long-term variability; and presence of spontaneous accelerations, decelerations, or contractions

Provide vibroacoustic stimulation, per protocol or physician or midwife order

Initiate IV infusion per protocol to begin oxytocin challenge test, as appropriate, per physician or midwife order

Increase oxytocin infusion, per protocol, until the appropriate number of contractions is achieved (e.g., usually three contractions in 10 minutes)

Observe monitor strip for the presence or absence of late decelerations

Interpret tracing based on protocol for nonstress or oxytocin challenge test criteria

Perform ultrasound exam for biophysical profile testing, per protocol or physician or midwife order

Score ultrasound exam based on protocol for biophysical profile criteria

Communicate test results to primary practitioner or midwife

Provide anticipatory guidance for abnormal test results (e.g., nonreassuring nonstress test, positive oxytocin challenge test, or low biophysical profile score)

Reschedule antepartum testing, per protocol or physician or midwife order

Activities:—cont'd

Provide written discharge instructions to remind patient of future testing times and other reasons to return for care (e.g., labor onset, spontaneous leaking of the bag of waters, bleeding, and decreased fetal movement)

Clean equipment, including abdominal belts

Background Readings:

Chez, B.F., Skurnick, J.H., Chez, R.A., et al. (1990). Interpretations of nonstress tests by obstetric nurses. Journal of Obstetric, Gynecologic and Neonatal Nursing, 19(3), 227-232.

Eganhouse, D.J. (1992). Fetal monitoring of twins. Journal of Obstetric, Gynecologic and Neonatal Nursing, 21(1), 16-22.

Fresquez, M.L., & Collins, D.E. (1992). Advancement of the nursing role in antepartum fetal evaluation. Journal of Perinatal and Neonatal Nursing, 5(4), 16-22.

Gregor, C.L., Paine, L.L., & Johnson, T.R.B. (1991). Antepartum fetal assessment. A nurse-midwifery perspective. Journal of Nurse-Midwifery, 36(3), 153-167.

Nurses Association of the American College of Obstetricians and Gynecologists. (1991). Nursing practice competencies and educational guidelines: Antepartum fetal surveillance and intrapartum fetal heart monitoring (2nd ed.). Washington: NAACOG.

Sabey, P.L., & Clark, S.L. (1992). Establishing an antepartum testing unit: The nurse's role. Journal of Perinatal and Neonatal Nursing, 5(4), 23-32.

E

Electronic Fetal Monitoring: Intrapartum 6772

Definition: Electronic evaluation of fetal heart rate response to uterine contractions during intrapartal care

Activities:

Verify maternal and fetal heart rates before initiation of electronic fetal monitoring

Instruct woman and support person(s) about the reason for electronic monitoring, as well as information to be obtained

Perform Leopold maneuver to determine fetal position(s)

Apply tocotransducer snugly to observe contraction frequency and duration

Palpate to determine contraction intensity with tocotransducer use

Apply ultrasound transducer(s) to area of uterus where fetal heart sounds are audible and trace clearly

Differentiate among multiple fetuses by documenting on the tracing when simultaneous tracings are conducted, using one electronic fetal monitor (e.g., baby A, baby B)

Distinguish among multiple fetuses by comparing data when simultaneous tracings are conducted, using two separate fetal monitors

Discuss appearance of rhythm strip with mother and support person

Reassure about normal fetal heart rate signs, including such typical features as artifact, loss of signal with fetal movement, high rate, and irregular appearance

Adjust monitors to achieve and maintain clarity of the tracing

Interpret strip when at least a 10-minute tracing of the fetal heart and uterine activity signals has been obtained

Document elements of the external tracing, including baseline heart rate(s), oscillatory patterns, long-term variability, accelerations, decelerations, and contraction frequency and duration

Document relevant intrapartal care (e.g., vaginal exams, medication administration, and maternal vital signs) directly on the monitor strip, as appropriate

Remove electronic monitors, as needed for ambulation, after verifying that the tracing is normal (e.g., reassuring)

Use intermittent or telemetry fetal monitoring, if available, to facilitate maternal ambulation and comfort

Initiate fetal resuscitation interventions to treat abnormal (e.g., nonreassuring) fetal heart patterns, as appropriate

Document changes in fetal heart patterns after resuscitation

Calibrate equipment, as appropriate, for internal monitoring with a spiral electrode and/or intrauterine pressure catheter

Use universal precautions

Apply internal fetal electrode after rupture of membranes, when necessary for reducing artifact or for evaluation of short-term variability

Apply internal uterine pressure catheter after rupture of membranes, when necessary for obtaining pressure data for uterine contractions and resting tone

Document maternal response to application of internal monitors, including degree of discomfort or pain, appearance of amniotic fluid, and presence of bleeding

Document fetal response to internal monitor placement, including short-term variability, accelerations, or decelerations of the fetal heart rate

Keep physician informed of pertinent changes in the fetal heart rate, interventions for nonreassuring patterns, subsequent fetal response, labor progress, and maternal response to labor

Activities:—cont'd

Continue electronic monitoring through second-stage labor or up to the time of cesarean delivery

Remove internal monitors before cesarean delivery to prevent maternal infection

Document monitor interpretation, according to institutional policy

Provide safekeeping of intrapartal strip as part of the permanent patient record

Background Readings:

Association of Women's Health, Obstetric, and Neonatal Nurses. (1993). Fetal heart monitoring principles & practices. Washington, DC: AWHONN.

Carlton, L.L. (1990). Module 6: Basic intrapartum fetal monitoring. In E.J. Martin (Ed.) Intrapartum management modules (pp. 151-234). Baltimore: Williams & Wilkins.

Eganhouse, D.J. (1991). Electronic fetal monitoring: Education and quality assurance. Journal of Obstetric, Gynecologic, and Neonatal Nursing, 20(1), 16-22.

Eganhouse, D.J. (1992). Fetal monitoring of twins. Journal of Obstetric, Gynecologic, and Neonatal Nursing, 21(1), 16-22.

Gilbert, E.S., & Harmon, J.S. (1998). Manual of high-risk pregnancy & delivery. (2nd ed.). St. Louis: Mosby.

Murray, M. (1988). Essentials of electronic fetal monitoring: Antepartal and intrapartal fetal monitoring. Washington, DC: NAACOG.

Tucker, S.M. (1992). Pocket guide to fetal monitoring (3rd ed.). St. Louis: Mosby.

E

E

Elopement Precautions 6470

Definition: Minimizing the risk of a patient leaving a treatment setting without authorization when departure presents a threat to the safety of patient or others

Activities:

Monitor patient for indicators of elopement potential (e.g., verbal indicators, loitering near exits, multiple layers of clothing, disorientation, separation anxiety, and homesickness)

Clarify the legal status of patient (e.g., minor or adult and voluntary or court-ordered treatment)

Communicate risk to other care providers

Familiarize patient with environment and routine to decrease anxiety

Limit patient to a physically secure environment (e.g., locked or alarmed doors at exits and locked windows), as needed

Provide adaptive devices to limit mobility, as needed (e.g., cribs, gates, Dutch doors, and physical restraint)

Provide appropriate level of supervision/surveillance to monitor patient

Increase supervision/surveillance when patient is outside secure environment (e.g., hold hands and increase staff-to-patient ratio)

Provide adaptive devices that monitor patient's physical location (e.g., electronic sensors placed on patient that trigger alarms or locks)

Record physical description (e.g., height, weight, eye/hair/skin color, and any distinguishing characteristics) for reference, should patient elope

Provide patient with identification band

Assign consistent caregivers on a daily basis

Encourage patient to seek out care providers for assistance when experiencing feelings (e.g., anxiety, anger, and fear) that may lead to elopement

Provide reassurance and comfort

Discuss with patient why he/she desires to leave the treatment setting

Identify with patient, when appropriate, the positive and negative consequences of leaving treatment setting

Identify with patient, when possible, any variables that may be altered to make the patient feel more comfortable with remaining in the treatment setting

Encourage patient, when appropriate, to make a commitment to continue treatment (e.g., contracting)

Background Readings:

Cipkala-Gaffin, J.A., & Cipkala-Gaffin, G.L. (1989). Developmental disabilities and nursing interventions. In L.M. Birckhead (Ed.), Psychiatric mental health nursing. The therapeutic use of self (pp. 349-379). Philadelphia: J.B. Lippincott.

Holnsteiner, M.G. (1991). Elopement, potential for. In G.K. McFarland, & M.D. Thomas (Eds.), Psychiatric mental health nursing. Application of the nursing process (pp. 222-227). Philadelphia: J.B. Lippincott.

McIndoe, K.I. (1986). Elope. Why psychiatric patients go AWOL. Journal of Psychosocial Nursing, 26(1), 16-20.

Embolus Care: Peripheral   4104

Definition: Limitation of complications for a patient experiencing, or at risk for, occlusion of peripheral circulation

Activities:

Perform a comprehensive appraisal of peripheral circulation (e.g., check peripheral pulses, edema, capillary refill, color, and temperature of extremity)

Monitor for pain in affected area

Appraise for presence of Homans' sign (pain when foot is forcefully dorsiflexed)

Monitor for signs of decreased venous circulation, including increased extremity circumference, painful swelling and tenderness, pain worsening in dependent position, palpable hard vein, severe cramping, redness and warmth, numbness and tingling, and fever

Administer anticoagulant medication, as appropriate

Monitor patient's prothrombin time (PT) and partial thromboplastin time (PTT) to keep 1 to 2 times normal, as appropriate

Keep protamine sulfate and/or vitamin K available in case of emergency

Monitor for signs of bleeding; for example, test stool and NG tube drainage for blood

Administer antacids and analgesics, as appropriate

Maintain patient on bedrest and change position every 2 hours

Elevate bed sheets by using bed cradle over the affected extremity, if appropriate

Monitor neurological status

Perform passive or active range-of-motion to unaffected extremities

Provide pain relief/comfort measures

Instruct the patient not to massage the affected area

Monitor for side effects from anticoagulant medications, if appropriate

Background Readings:

American Association of Critical-Care Nurses. (1990). Outcome standards for nursing care of the critically ill. Laguna Niguel, CA: AACN.

Cullen, L.M. (1992). Interventions related to circulatory care. In G.M. Bulechek & J.C. McCloskey (Eds.), Symposium on Nursing Interventions. Nursing Clinics of North America, 27(2), 445-476.

Doyle, J., Johantgen, M., & Vitello-Cicciu, J. (1993). Vascular disease. In M.R. Kinney, D.R. Packa, & S.B. Dunbar (Eds.). AACN's clinical reference for critical-care nursing (pp. 607-634). St. Louis: Mosby.

Johanson, B.C., Wells, S.J., Hoffmeister, D., & Dungca, C.U. (1988). Standards for critical care (3rd ed.). St. Louis: Mosby.

Neagley, S. (1991). The pulmonary system. In J. Alspach (Ed.), AACN core curriculum for critical care nursing (4th ed.) (pp. 98-101). Philadelphia: W.B. Saunders.

Embolus Care: Pulmonary 4106

Definition: Limitation of complications for a patient experiencing, or at risk for, occlusion of pulmonary circulation

Activities:

Evaluate chest pain (e.g., intensity, location, radiation, duration, and precipitating and alleviating factors)

Auscultate lung sounds for crackles or other adventitious sounds

Monitor respiratory pattern for symptoms of respiratory difficulty (e.g., dyspnea, tachypnea, and shortness of breath)

Monitor determinants of tissue oxygen delivery (e.g., PaO_2, SaO_2, and hemoglobin levels and cardiac output), if available

Monitor for symptoms of inadequate tissue oxygenation (e.g., pallor, cyanosis, and sluggish capillary refill)

Monitor for symptoms of respiratory failure (e.g., low PaO_2 and elevated $PaCO_2$ levels and respiratory muscle fatigue)

Encourage good ventilation (e.g., incentive spirometry and cough and deep breath every 2 hours)

Monitor lab values for changes in oxygenation or acid-base balance, as appropriate

Instruct the patient and/or family regarding diagnostic procedures (e.g., V/Q scan), as appropriate

Encourage the patient to relax

Determine arterial blood gas levels, if appropriate

Administer anticoagulants, as appropriate

Monitor side effects of anticoagulant medications, if appropriate

Avoid overwedging of pulmonary artery catheter to prevent pulmonary artery rupture, if appropriate

Monitor pulmonary artery tracing for spontaneous wedge of catheter, if appropriate

Reposition spontaneously wedged pulmonary artery catheter, if appropriate

Background Readings:

Cullen, L.M. (1992). Interventions related to circulatory care. In G.M. Bulechek & J.C. McCloskey (Eds.), Symposium on Nursing Interventions. Nursing Clinics of North America, 27(2), 445-476.

Doyle, J., Johantgen, M., & Vitello-Cicciu, J. (1993). Vascular disease. In M.R. Kinney, D.R. Packa, & S.B. Dunbar (Eds.), AACN's clinical reference for critical-care nursing (pp. 607-634). St. Louis: Mosby.

Johanson, B.C., Wells, S.J., Hoffmeister, D., & Dungca, C.U. (1988). Standards for critical care (3rd ed.). St. Louis: Mosby.

Neagley, S. (1991). The pulmonary system. In J. Alspach (Ed.), AACN's core curriculum for critical care nursing (4th ed.) (pp. 98-101). Philadelphia: W.B. Saunders.

Embolus Precautions   4110

Definition: Reduction of the risk of an embolus in a patient with thrombi or at risk for thrombus formation

Activities:

Perform a comprehensive appraisal of peripheral circulation (e.g., check peripheral pulses, edema, capillary refill, color, and temperature of extremity)

Elevate affected limb 20 degrees or greater, above the level of the heart, to improve venous return, as appropriate

Apply antiembolism stockings (e.g., elastic or pneumatic stockings), if appropriate

Remove antiembolism stockings for 15 to 20 minutes every 8 hours

Assist patient with passive or active range of motion, as appropriate

Change patient position every 2 hr, or ambulate as tolerated

Prevent injury to vessel lumen by preventing local pressure, trauma, infection, or sepsis

Refrain from massaging or compressing leg muscles

Instruct patient not to cross legs

Administer prophylactic low-dose anticoagulant and/or antiplatelet medication (e.g., heparin, aspirin, dipyridamole [Persantine], and dextran)

Instruct the patient to avoid activities that result in the Valsalva maneuver (e.g., straining during bowel movement)

Administer medications that will prevent episodes of the Valsalva maneuver (e.g., stool softeners and antiemetics), as appropriate

Instruct the patient and/or family on appropriate precautions

Encourage smoking cessation

Background Readings:

American Association of Critical-Care Nurses. (1990). Outcome standards for nursing care of the critically ill. Laguna Niguel, CA: AACN.

Cullen, L.M. (1992). Interventions related to circulatory care. In G.M. Bulechek & J.C. McCloskey (Eds.), Symposium on Nursing Interventions. Nursing Clinics of North America, 27(2), 445-476.

Doyle, J., Johantgen, M., & Vitello-Cicciu, J. (1993). Vascular disease. In M.R. Kinney, D.R. Packa, & S.B. Dunbar (Eds.), AACN's Clinical Reference for critical-care nursing (pp. 607-634). St. Louis: Mosby.

Johanson, B.C., Wells, S.J., Hoffmeister, D., & Dungca, C.U. (1988). Standards for critical care (3rd ed.). St. Louis: Mosby.

Neagley, S. (1991). The pulmonary system. In J. Alspach (Ed.), AACN core curriculum for critical care nursing (4th ed.) (pp. 98-101). Philadelphia: W.B. Saunders.

E

Emergency Care   6200

Definition: Providing life-saving measures in life-threatening situations

Activities:

Act quickly and methodically, giving care to the most urgent conditions

Activate the emergency medical system

Instruct others to call for help, if needed

Maintain an open airway

Perform cardiopulmonary resuscitation, as appropriate

Perform the Heimlich maneuver, as appropriate

Move patient to a safe location, as appropriate

Check for medical alert tags

Apply manual pressure over bleeding site, as appropriate

Apply a pressure dressing, as needed

Monitor the amount and nature of blood loss

Check for signs and symptoms of pneumothorax or flailing chest

Elevate injured part, as appropriate

Apply MAST trousers, as appropriate

Monitor vital signs

Determine the history of the accident from the patient or others in the area

Determine whether an overdose of a drug or other substance is involved

Determine whether toxic or poisonous substances are involved

Send drugs believed to be affecting patient to treatment facility, as appropriate

Monitor level of consciousness

Immobilize fractures, large wounds, and any injured part

Monitor neurological status for possible head or spinal injuries

Apply a cervical collar, as appropriate

Maintain body alignment in suspected spinal injuries

Provide reassurance and emotional support to patient

Initiate medical transport, as appropriate

Transport using a back board, as appropriate

Background Readings:

Beaver, B.M. (1990). Care of the multiple trauma victim: The first hour. Nursing Clinics of North America, 25(1), 11-22.

Laskowski-Jones, L. (2000) Responding to summer emergencies-education STATPack, Dimensions of Critical Care Nursing, 19(4), 11-12, July-August.

Smith, S., & Duell, D. (1992). Clinical nursing skills (3rd ed.). Los Altos, CA: National Nursing Review.

Sorensen, K., & Luckmann, J. (1986). Basic nursing: A psychophysiologic approach (2nd ed.). Philadelphia: W.B. Saunders.

Emergency Cart Checking   7660

Definition: Systematic review of the contents of an emergency cart at established time intervals

Activities:

Compare equipment on cart with list of designated equipment

Locate all designated equipment and supplies on cart

Ensure that equipment is operational

Clean equipment, as needed

Verify current expiration date on all supplies and medications

Replace missing or outdated supplies and equipment

Document cart check, per agency policy

Replace equipment, supplies, and medications as technology and guidelines are updated

Instruct new nursing staff on proper emergency cart checking procedures

Background Readings:

Copeland, W.M. (1990). Be prepared. Hospitals should develop methods to ensure emergency equipment is workable and available. Health Progress, 71(6), 80-81.

Shanaberger, C.J. (1988). Equipment failure is often human failure. Journal of Emergency Medical Services, 13(1), 124-125.

Emotional Support 5270

Definition: Provision of reassurance, acceptance, and encouragement during times of stress

Activities:

Discuss with the patient the emotional experience(s)

Explore with patient what has triggered emotions

Make supportive or empathetic statements

Embrace or touch patient supportively

Support the use of appropriate defense mechanisms

Assist patient in recognizing feelings such as anxiety, anger, or sadness

Encourage the patient to express feelings of anxiety, anger, or sadness

Discuss consequences of not dealing with guilt and shame

Listen to/encourage expressions of feelings and beliefs

Facilitate patient's identification of usual response pattern in coping with fears

Provide support during denial, anger, bargaining, and acceptance phases of grieving

Identify the functions that anger, frustration, and rage serve for the patient

Encourage talking or crying as means to decrease the emotional response

Stay with the patient and provide assurance of safety and security during periods of anxiety

Provide assistance in decision making

Reduce demand for cognitive functioning when patient is ill or fatigued

Refer for counseling, as appropriate

Background Readings:

Ahrens, J. (2002). Giving care & comfort in the aftermath of tragedy. Caring Magazine, 21(1), 10-11.

Arnold, E., & Boggs, K. (1989). Interpersonal relationships: Professional communication skills for nurses. Philadelphia: W.B. Saunders.

Boyle, K., Moddeman, G., & Mann, B. (1989). The importance of selected nursing activities to patients and their nurses. Applied Nursing Research, 2(4), 173-177.

Moore, J.C., & Hartman, C.R. (1988). Developing a therapeutic relationship. In C.K. Beck, R.P. Rawlins, & W.R. Williams (Eds.), Mental health-psychiatric nursing: A holistic life-cycle approach (2nd ed.) (pp. 92-117). St. Louis: Mosby.

Endotracheal Extubation   3270

Definition: Purposeful removal of the endotracheal tube from the nasopharyngeal or oropharyngeal airway

Activities:

Position the patient for best use of ventilatory muscles, usually with the head of the bed elevated 75 degrees

Instruct patient about the procedure

Hyperoxygenate the patient and suction the endotracheal airway

Suction the oral airway

Deflate the endotracheal cuff and remove the endotracheal tube

Encourage the patient to cough and expectorate sputum

Administer oxygen as ordered

Encourage coughing and deep breathing

Suction the airway, as needed

Monitor for respiratory distress

Observe for signs of airway occlusion

Monitor vital signs

Encourage voice rest for 4 to 8 hours, as appropriate

Monitor ability to swallow and talk

Background Readings:

Boggs, R.L. (1993). Airway management. In R.L. Boggs & M. Woodridge-King (Eds.), AACN procedure manual for critical care (3rd ed.) (pp. 1-65). Philadelphia: W.B. Saunders.

Elmquist, L. (1992). Decision-making for extubation of the post-anesthetic patient. Critical Care Nursing Quarterly, 15(1), 82-86.

E

Energy Management   0180

Definition: Regulating energy use to treat or prevent fatigue and optimize function

Activities:

Determine patient's physical limitations

Determine patient's/significant other's perception of causes of fatigue

Encourage verbalization of feelings about limitations

Determine causes of fatigue (e.g., treatments, pain, and medications)

Determine what and how much activity is required to build endurance

Monitor nutritional intake to ensure adequate energy resources

Consult with dietitian about ways to increase intake of high-energy foods

Monitor patient for evidence of excess physical and emotional fatigue

Monitor cardiorespiratory response to activity (e.g., tachycardia, other dysrhythmias, dyspnea, diaphoresis, pallor, hemodynamic pressures, and respiratory rate)

Monitor/record patient's sleep pattern and number of sleep hours

Monitor location and nature of discomfort or pain during movement/activity

Reduce physical discomforts that could interfere with cognitive function and self-monitoring/regulation of activity

Set limits with hyperactivity when it interferes with others or with the patient

Limit environmental stimuli (e.g., light and noise) to facilitate relaxation

Limit number of visitors and interruptions by visitors, as appropriate

Promote bed rest/activity limitation (e.g., increase number of rest periods)

Encourage alternate rest and activity periods

Arrange physical activities to reduce competition for oxygen supply to vital body functions (e.g., avoid activity immediately after meals)

Use passive and/or active range-of-motion exercises to relieve muscle tension

Provide calming diversionary activities to promote relaxation

Encourage an afternoon nap, if appropriate

Assist patient to schedule rest periods

Avoid care activities during scheduled rest periods

Plan activities for periods when the patient has the most energy

Assist patient to sit on side of bed ("dangle"), if unable to transfer or walk

Assist with regular physical activities (e.g., ambulation, transfers, turning, and personal care), as needed

Monitor administration and effect of stimulants and depressants

Encourage physical activity (e.g., ambulation or performance of activities of daily living, consistent with patient's energy resources)

Monitor patient's oxygen response (e.g., pulse rate, cardiac rhythm, and respiratory rate) to self-care or nursing activities

Teach patient and significant other techniques of self-care that will minimize oxygen consumption (e.g., self-monitoring and pacing techniques for performance of activities of daily living)

Instruct patient/significant other to recognize signs and symptoms of fatigue that require reduction in activity

Activities:—cont'd

Instruct patient/significant other to notify health care provider if signs and symptoms of fatigue persist

Assist the patient to understand energy conservation principles (e.g., the requirement for restricted activity or bed rest)

Assist the patient to identify tasks that family and friends can perform in the home to prevent/relieve fatigue

Teach activity organization and time management techniques to prevent fatigue

Assist the patient in assigning priority to activities to accommodate energy levels

Assist the patient/significant other to establish realistic activity goals

Assist patient to identify preferences for activity

Encourage patient to choose activities that gradually build endurance

Assist patient to limit daytime sleep by providing activity that promotes wakefulness, as appropriate

Evaluate programmed increases in levels of activities

Assist patient to self-monitor by developing and using a written record of calorie intake and energy expenditure, as appropriate

Background Readings:

Deiriggi, P.M. (1990). Effects of waterbed flotation on indicators of energy expenditure in preterm infants. Nursing Research, 39(3), 140-146.

Donohue, K., Miller, C., & Craig, B. (1988). Chronic alterations in mobility. In P.H. Mitchell, L.C. Hodges, M. Muwaswes, et al. (Eds.), AANN's neuroscience nursing: Phenomena and practice (pp. 319-343). Norwalk, CT: Appleton & Lange.

Glick, O.J. (1992). Interventions related to activity and movement. In G.M. Bulechek & J.C. McCloskey (Eds.), Symposium on Nursing Interventions. Nursing Clinics of North America, 27(2), 541-569.

Lubkin, I. (1990). Chronic illness: Impact and intervention (2nd ed.). Boston: Jones & Bartlett.

McFarland, G.K., & McFarlane, E.A. (1989). Nursing diagnosis and intervention. St. Louis: Mosby.

Potempa, K.M. (1992). Chronic fatigue. In J.J. Fritzpatrick, R.L. Taunton, & A.K. Jacox (Eds.), Annual review of nursing research, 10 (pp. 57-76). New York: Springer.

Enteral Tube Feeding   1056

Definition: Delivering nutrients and water through a gastrointestinal tube

Activities:

Explain the procedure to the patient

Insert a nasogastric, nasoduodenal, or nasojejunal tube according to agency protocol

Apply anchoring substance to skin and secure feeding tube with tape

Monitor for proper placement of the tube by inspecting oral cavity, checking for gastric residual, or listening while air is injected and withdrawn according to agency protocol

Mark the tubing at the point of exit to maintain proper placement

Confirm tube placement by x-ray examination prior to administering feedings or medications via the tube per agency protocol

Monitor for presence of bowel sounds every 4 to 8 hours, as appropriate

Monitor fluid and electrolyte status

Consult with other health care team members in selecting the type and strength of enteral feeding

Elevate head of the bed 30 to 45 degrees during feedings

Offer pacifier to infant during feeding, as appropriate

Hold and talk to infant during feeding to simulate usual feeding activities

Discontinue feedings 30 to 60 minutes before putting patient in a head-down position

Turn off the tube feeding 1 hour prior to a procedure or if the patient needs to be in a position with the head less than 30 degrees

Irrigate the tube every 4 to 6 hours as appropriate during continuous feedings and after every intermittent feeding

Use clean technique in administering tube feedings

Check gravity drip rate or pump rate every hour

Slow tube feeding rate and/or decrease strength to control diarrhea

Monitor for sensation of fullness, nausea, and vomiting

Check residual every 4 to 6 hours for the first 24 hours, then every 8 hours during continuous feedings

Check residual before each intermittent feeding

Hold tube feedings if residual is greater than 150 cc or more than 110% to 120% of the hourly rate in adults

Keep cuff of endotracheal or tracheostomy tube inflated during feeding, as appropriate

Keep open containers of enteral feeding refrigerated

Change insertion site and infusion tubing according to agency protocol

Wash skin around skin level device daily with mild soap and dry thoroughly

Check water level in skin level device balloon according to equipment protocol

Discard enteral feeding containers and administration sets every 24 hours

Refill feeding bag every 4 hours, as appropriate

Monitor for presence of bowel sounds every 4 to 8 hours, as appropriate

Monitor fluid and electrolyte status

Monitor for growth (height/weight) changes monthly, as appropriate

Monitor weight 3 times weekly initially, decreasing to once a month

Monitor for signs of edema or dehydration

Monitor fluid intake and output

Monitor calorie, fat, carbohydrate, vitamin, and mineral intake for adequacy (or refer to dietitian) 2 times weekly initially, decreasing to once a month

Monitor for mood changes

Prepare individual and family for home tube feedings, as appropriate

Monitor weight at least three times a week, as appropriate for age

E

Background Readings:

Fellows, L.S., Miller, E.H., Frederickson, M, Bly, B., & Felt, P. (2000). Evidence-based practice for enteral feedings and aspiration prevention: Strategies, bedside detection and practice change. MEDSUR6 Nursing, 9(1), 27-31.

Mahan, K.L., & Escott-Stump, S. (2000) In Krause's food, nutrition & diet therapy (9th ed.). Philadelphia: W.B. Saunders.

Methany, N.A. & Titler, M.G. (2001). Assessing placement of feeding tubes. American Journal of Nursing, 101(5), 6-45.

Perry, A.G., & Potter, P.A. (2002). Clinical nursing skills and techniques (5th ed.) (pp. 559-616). St. Louis: Mosby.

Environmental Management   6480

Definition: Manipulation of the patient's surroundings for therapeutic benefit, sensory appeal, and psychological well-being

Activities:

Create a safe environment for the patient

Identify the safety needs of patient, based on level of physical and cognitive function and history of behavior

Remove environmental hazards (e.g., loose rugs and small, movable furniture)

Remove harmful objects from the environment

Safeguard with side rails/side-rail padding, as appropriate

Escort patient during off-ward activities, as appropriate

Provide low-height bed, as appropriate

Provide adaptive devices (e.g., step stools or handrails), as appropriate

Place furniture in room in an appropriate arrangement that best accommodates patient or family disabilities

rovide sufficiently long tubing to allow freedom of movement, as appropriate

Place frequently used objects within reach

Provide single room, as indicated

Consider the aesthetics of the environment when selecting furnishings

Provide a clean, comfortable bed and environment

Provide a firm mattress

Provide linens and gown in good repair, free of residual stains

Place bed-positioning switch within easy reach

Neatly arrange supplies and linens that must remain in the patient's view

Block the patient's view of the bathroom, commode, or other equipment used for elimination

Remove materials used during dressing changes and elimination, as well as any residual odors prior to visitation and meals

Reduce environmental stimuli, as appropriate

Avoid unnecessary exposure, drafts, overheating, or chilling

Adjust environmental temperature to meet patient's needs, if body temperature is altered

Control or prevent undesirable or excessive noise, when possible

Provide music of choice

Provide headphones for private listening when music may disturb others

Manipulate lighting for therapeutic benefit

Provide attractively arranged meals and snacks

Clean areas used for eating and drinking utensils prior to patient use

Limit visitors

Individualize visiting restrictions to meet patient's and/or family's/significant other's needs

Individualize daily routine to meet patient's needs

Bring familiar objects from home

Facilitate use of personal items such as pajamas, robes, and toiletries

Activities:—cont'd

Maintain consistency of staff assignment over time

Provide immediate and continuous means to summon nurse, and let the patient and family know they will be answered immediately

Allow family/significant other to stay with patient

Educate patient and visitors about the changes/precautions, so they will not inadvertently disrupt the planned environment

Provide family/significant other with information about making home environment safe for patient

Promote fire safety, as appropriate

Control environmental pests, as appropriate

Provide room deodorizers, as needed

Provide care for flowers/plants

Assist patient or patient's family to arrange cards, flowers, and gifts to enhance the patient's visual appreciation

Background Readings:

Ackerman, L.L. (1992). Interventions related to neurological care. In G.M. Bulechek & J.C. McCloskey (Eds.), Symposium on Nursing Interventions. Nursing Clinics of North America, 27(2), 325-346.

Drury, J., & Akins, J. (1991). Sensory/perceptual alterations. In M. Maas, K. Buckwalter, & M. Hardy (Eds.), Nursing diagnoses and interventions for the elderly (pp. 369-389). Redwood City, CA: Addison-Wesley.

Gerdner, L., & Buckwalter, K. (1999). Music therapy. In G. Bulechek & J. McCloskey (Eds.), Nursing interventions: Effective nursing treatments (3rd ed.) (pp. 451-468). Philadelphia: W.B. Saunders.

Phylar, P.A. (1989). Management of the agitated and aggressive head injury patient in an acute hospital setting. Journal of Neuroscience Nursing, 21(6), 353-356.

Schuster, E., & Keegan, L. (2000). Envirionment. In B. Dossey, L. Keegan, & C. Guzzetta. Holistic nursing: A handbook for practice (3rd ed.) (pp. 249-282). Gaithersburg, MD: Aspen Publishers.

Stoner, N. (1999). Feeding. In G. Bulechek & J. McCloskey (Eds.) Nursing interventions: Effective nursing treatments (3rd ed.) (pp. 31-46). Philadelphia: W.B. Saunders.

E

E

Environmental Management: Attachment Process   6481

Definition: Manipulation of the patient's surroundings to facilitate the development of the parent-infant relationship

Activities:

Create a homelike environment

Provide a clean, comfortable bed

Create environment that fosters privacy

Place in private room, if possible

Provide primary nurse

Limit number of people in delivery room

Maintain consistency of staff assignment over time

Individualize daily routine to meet patient's needs

Provide accessible nutrition or snack center

Place infant bassinet at head of mother's bed

Maintain warm body temperature of newborn

Provide sufficiently long tubing to allow freedom of movement, as appropriate

Provide rocking chair

Provide comfortable chair for father/significant other

Maintain low level of stimuli in patient and family environment

Decrease number of people in the environment

Protect family from interruptions by visitors

Explain options and then let family choose hospital environment and visitation plan that best meets their needs

Allow for family visitation, as desired

Permit father/significant other to sleep in room with mother

Limit visiting hours to promote rest for mother

Reduce interruptions by phone calls

Reduce interruptions by hospital personnel

Develop policies that permit presence of significant others as much as desired

Background Readings:

Denehy, J.A. (1992). Interventions related to parent-infant attachment. In G.M. Bulechek & J.C. McCloskey (Eds.), Symposium on Nursing Interventions. Nursing Clinics of North America, 27(2), 425-444.

Pressler, J.L. (1990). Promoting attachment. In M.J. Craft & J.A. Denehy (Eds.), Nursing interventions for infants and children (pp. 4-17). Philadelphia: W.B. Saunders.

Environmental Management: Comfort   6482

Definition: Manipulation of the patient's surroundings for promotion of optimal comfort

Activities:

Select roommate with similar environmental concerns, when possible and as appropriate

Limit visitors

Prevent unnecessary interruptions and allow for rest periods

Determine sources of discomfort, such as damp or constrictive dressings, positioning of tubing, wrinkled bed linens, and environmental irritants

Provide a clean, comfortable bed

Adjust room temperature to that most comfortable for the individual, if possible

Provide or remove blankets to promote temperature comfort, as indicated

Avoid unnecessary exposure, drafts, overheating, or chilling

Adjust lighting to meet needs of individual activities, avoiding direct light in eyes

Control or prevent undesirable or excessive noise, when possible

Facilitate hygiene measures to keep the individual comfortable (e.g., wiping brow; applying skin creams; or cleaning body, hair, and oral cavity)

Position patient to facilitate comfort (e.g., using principles of body alignment, support with pillows, support joints during movement, splint over incisions, and immobilize painful body part)

Monitor skin, especially over body prominences, for signs of pressure or irritation

Avoid exposing skin or mucous membranes to irritants (e.g., diarrheal stool and wound drainage)

Background Readings:

Herr, K.A., & Mobily, P.R. (1992). Interventions related to pain. In G.M. Bulechek & J.C. McCloskey (Eds.), Symposium on Nursing Interventions. Nursing Clinics of North America, 27(2), 347-370.

Sorensen, K., & Luckmann, J. (1986). Basic nursing: A psychophysiologic approach (2nd ed.) (pp. 449-451). Philadelphia: W.B. Saunders.

E

Environmental Management: Community 6484

Definition: Monitoring and influencing of the physical, social, cultural, economic, and political conditions that affect the health of groups and communities

Activities:

Initiate screening for health risks from the environment

Participate in multidisciplinary teams to identify threats to safety in the community

Monitor status of known health risks

Participate in community programs to deal with known risks

Collaborate in the development of community action programs

Promote governmental policy to reduce specified risks

Encourage neighborhoods to become active participants in community safety

Coordinate services to at-risk groups and communities

Conduct educational programs for targeted risk groups

Work with environmental groups to secure appropriate governmental regulations

Background Readings:

Bracht, N. (1990). Health promotion at the community level. Newbury Park, CA: Sage Publications.

Dever, G. (1991). Community health analysis. Gaithersburg, MD: Aspen Publications.

Salazar, M.K., & Primomo, J. (1994). Taking the lead in environmental health. American Association of Occupational Health Nurses (AAOHN), 42(7), 317-324.

Stevens, P., & Hall, J. (1993). Environmental health in community health nursing. In J.F. Swanson & M. Albrecht (Eds.), Community health nursing: Promoting the health of aggregates (pp. 567-596). Philadelphia: W.B. Saunders.

Environmental Management: Home Preparation   6485

Definition: Preparing the home for safe and effective delivery of care

Activities:

Consult with patient and caregivers concerning preparation for care delivery at home

Check layout of home and eliminate obstacles

Order and validate operation of any equipment needed

Order and confirm delivery of any medication and supplies needed

Prepare teaching plans for use in the home to coincide with any earlier teaching already accomplished

Arrange scheduling of support personnel

Confirm that emergency plans are in place

Confirm date and time of transfer to home

Confirm arrangements for transportation to home with accompanying escort, as needed

Follow up to ensure that plans were feasible and carried out

Provide written materials regarding medications, supplies, and assistive devices as guides for caregivers, as needed

Provide documentation to meet agency guidelines

Background Readings:

Humphrey, C J., & Milone-Nuzzo, P. (1996). Orientation to home care nursing. Gaithersburg, MD: Aspen Publishers.

Kelly, K., & McClelland, E. (1989). Discharge planning: Home care considerations. In I. Martinson & A. Widmer (Eds.), Home care nursing. Philadelphia: W.B. Saunders.

McClelland, E., & Tarbox, M. (1998). Discharge planning: Home care considerations. In I. Martinson, A. Widmer, & C. Portillo (Eds.), Home care nursing (2nd ed.). Philadelphia: W.B. Saunders.

E

E

Environmental Management: Safety   6486

Definition: Monitoring and manipulation of the physical environment to promote safety

Activities:

Identify the safety needs of patient, based on level of physical and cognitive function and history of behavior

Identify safety hazards in the environment (i.e., physical, biological, and chemical)

Remove hazards from the environment, when possible

Modify the environment to minimize hazards and risk

Provide adaptive devices (e.g., step stools and handrails) to increase the safety of the environment

Use protective devices (e.g., restraints, side rails, locked doors, fences, and gates) to physically limit mobility or access to harmful situations

Notify agencies authorized to protect the environment (e.g., health department, environmental services, EPA, and police)

Provide patient with emergency phone numbers (e.g., police, local health department, and poison control center)

Monitor the environment for changes in safety status

Assist patient in relocating to safer environment (e.g., referral for housing assistance)

Initiate and/or conduct screening programs for environmental hazards (e.g., lead and radon)

Educate high-risk individuals and groups about environmental hazards

Collaborate with other agencies (e.g., health department, police, and EPA) to improve environmental safety

Background Readings:

Clark, M.J. (1992). Environmental influences on community health. In M.J. Clark (Ed.), Nursing in the community (pp. 342-365). Norwalk, CT: Appleton & Lange.

Kanak, M.F. (1992). Interventions related to safety. In G.M. Bulechek & J.C. McCloskey (Eds.), Symposium on Nursing Interventions. Nursing Clinics of North America, 27(2), 371-396.

Kozier, B., & Erb, G. (1991). Fundamentals of nursing: Concepts and procedures (4th ed.). Menlo Park, CA: Addison-Wesley.

Lancaster, J. (1992). Environmental health and safety. In M. Stanhope & J. Lancaster (Eds.), Community health nursing (3rd ed.) (pp. 293-309). St. Louis: Mosby.

U.S. Department of Health and Human Services. (1991). Healthy People 2000: National health promotion and disease prevention objectives. Washington, DC: US Government Printing Office.

Environmental Management: Violence Prevention   6487

Definition: Monitoring and manipulation of the physical environment to decrease the potential for violent behavior directed toward self, others, or environment

Activities:

Remove potential weapons from environment (e.g., sharps and ropelike objects)

Search environment routinely to maintain it as hazard free

Search patient and belongings for weapons/potential weapons during inpatient admission procedure, as appropriate

Monitor the safety of items being brought to the environment by visitors

Instruct visitors and other caregivers about relevant patient safety issues

Limit patient's use of potential weapons (e.g., sharps and ropelike objects)

Monitor patient during use of potential weapons (e.g., razor)

Place patient with potential for self-harm with a roommate to decrease isolation and opportunity to act on self-harm thoughts, as appropriate

Assign single room to patient with potential for violence toward others

Place patient in bedroom located near nursing station

Limit access to windows, unless locked and shatterproof, as appropriate

Lock utility and storage rooms

Provide paper dishes and plastic utensils at meals

Place patient in least restrictive environment that allows for necessary level of observation

Provide ongoing surveillance of all patient access areas to maintain patient safety and therapeutically intervene, as needed

Remove other individuals from the vicinity of a violent or potentially violent patient

Maintain a designated safe area (e.g., seclusion room) for patient to be placed when violent

Apply mitts, splints, helmets, or restraints to limit mobility and ability to initiate self-harm, as appropriate

Provide plastic, rather than metal, clothes hangers, as appropriate

Background Readings:

Carpenito, L.J. (1989). Nursing diagnosis: Application to clinical practice (3rd ed.) New York: J.B. Lippincott.

Goldstein, A.P. (1983). Prevention and control of aggression. New York: Pergammon Press.

Haven, E., & Piscitello, V. (1989). The patient with violent behavior. In S. Lewis, R.D.K. Grainger, W.A. McDowell, et al. (Eds.), Manual of psychosocial nursing interventions: Promoting mental health in medical-surgical settings (pp. 187-204). Philadelphia: W.B. Saunders.

Howells, K., & Hollin, C.R. (1992). Clinical approaches to violence. New York: John Wiley & Sons.

Kanak, M.F. (1992). Interventions related to safety. In G.M. Bulechek & J.C. McCloskey (Eds.), Symposium on Nursing Interventions. Nursing Clinics of North America, 27(2), 371-396.

Lewis, S., McDowell, W.A., & Gregory, R.J. (1989). The patient with suicidal ideation. In S. Lewis, R.D.K. Grainger, W.A. McDowell, et al. (Eds.), Manual of psychosocial nursing interventions: Promoting mental health in medical-surgical settings (pp. 173-175). Philadelphia: W.B. Saunders.

Munns, D., & Nolan, L. (1991). Potential for violence: Self-directed or directed at others. In M. Maas, K. Buckwalter, & M. Hardy (Eds.), Nursing diagnoses and interventions for the elderly (pp. 551-560). Redwood City, CA: Addison-Wesley.

Townsend, M.C. (1988). Nursing diagnoses in psychiatric nursing: A pocket guide for care plan construction. Philadelphia: F.A. Davis.

Environmental Management: Worker Safety 6489

Definition: Monitoring and manipulation of the worksite environment to promote safety and health of workers

Activities:

Maintain confidential health records on employees

Determine employee's fitness for work

Identify worksite environmental hazards and stressors (i.e., physical, biological, chemical, and ergonomic)

Identify applicable OSHA standards and worksite compliance with standards

Inform workers of their rights and responsibilities under OSHA (i.e., OSHA poster, copies of Act, and copies of standards)

Inform workers of hazardous substances to which they may be exposed

Use labels or signs to warn workers of potential worksite hazards

Maintain records of occupational injuries and illnesses on forms acceptable to OSHA, and participate in OSHA inspections

Keep log of occupational injuries and illnesses for workers

Identify risk factors for occupational injuries and illnesses through reviewing records for patterns of injuries and illnesses

Initiate modification of the environment to eliminate or minimize hazards (e.g., training programs to prevent back injuries)

Initiate worksite screening programs for early detection of work-related and nonoccupational illnesses and injuries (e.g., blood pressure, hearing and vision, and pulmonary function tests)

Initiate worksite health promotion programs based on health risk assessments (e.g., smoking cessation, stress management, and immunizations)

Identify and treat acute conditions at worksite

Develop emergency protocols and train selected employees on emergency care

Coordinate follow-up care for work-related injuries and illnesses

Background Readings:

American Association of Occupational Health Nurses. (1988). Standards for occupational health nursing practice. Atlanta: AAOHN.

Centers for Disease Control. (1986). Leading work-related diseases and injuries–United States. Morbidity and Mortality Weekly Report, 35, 113-116.

Clemen-Stone, S., Eigsti, D.G., & McGuire, S.L. (1991). Occupational health nursing. In S. Clemen-Stone, D.G. Eigsti, & S.L. McGuire (Eds.), Comprehensive family and community health nursing (3rd ed.) (pp. 616-657). St. Louis: Mosby.

Department of Health and Human Services. (1991). Healthy People 2000: National health promotion and disease prevention objectives (DHHS Publication No. PHS 91-50213). Washington, DC: U.S. Government Printing Office.

Department of Labor, Occupational Safety and Health Administration. (1994). All about OSHA. Washington, DC: U.S. Government Printing Office.

Environmental Risk Protection

8880

Definition: Preventing and detecting disease and injury in populations at risk from environmental hazards

E

Activities:

Assess environment for potential and actual risk

Analyze the level of risk associated with the environment (e.g. living habits, work, atmosphere, water, housing, food, waste, radiation, and violence)

Inform populations at risk about the environmental hazards

Monitor incidents of illness and injury related to environmental hazards

Maintain knowledge associated with specific environmental standards (e.g., Environmental Protection Agency (EPA) and Occupation Safety and Health Administration (OSHA) Regulations)

Notify agencies authorized to protect the environment about known hazards

Collaborate with other agencies to improve environmental safety

Advocate for safer environmental designs, protection systems, and use of protective devices

Support programs to disclose environmental hazards

Screen populations at risk for evidence of exposure to environmental hazards

Participate in data collection related to incidence and prevalence of exposure to environmental hazards

Background Readings:

Humphrey, C.J., & Milone Nuzzo, P. (1996). Orientation to home care nursing. Gaithersburg, MD: Aspen Publishers.

Klainberg, M., Holzemer, S., Leonard, M., & Arnold, J. (1998). Community health nursing: An alliance for health. New York: McGraw-Hill.

Kuss, T., Proulx-Girouard, L., Lovitt, S., Katz, C.B., & Kennelly, P. (1997). A public health nursing model. Public Health Nursing, 14(2), 81-91.

Nestel, R.M. (1996). Occupational safety and health administration: Building partnerships. American Association of Occupational Health Nurses Journal, 44(10), 493-499.

Stanhope, M., & Lancaster, J. (Eds.). (1996). Community health nursing: Promoting health of aggregates, families, and individuals (4th ed.). St. Louis: Mosby.

Stevens, P.E., & Hall, J.M. (1993). Environmental health. In J.M. Swanson & M. Abrech (Eds.), Community health nursing: Promoting the health of aggregates. Philadelphia: Saunders.

E

Examination Assistance

7680

Definition: Providing assistance to the patient and another health care provider during a procedure or exam

Activities:

Ensure consent is completed, as appropriate

Explain the rationale for the procedure

Provide sensory preparation information, as appropriate

Use developmentally appropriate language when explaining procedures to children

Ensure availability of emergency equipment and medications before procedure

Assemble appropriate equipment

Keep threatening equipment out of view, as appropriate

Provide a private environment

Include parent/significant other, as appropriate

Position and drape patient, as appropriate

Restrain patient, as appropriate

Explain need for restraints, as appropriate

Prepare procedure site, as appropriate

Maintain universal precautions

Maintain strict aseptic technique, as appropriate

Explain each step of the procedure to patient

Monitor patient status during procedure

Provide patient with emotional support, as indicated

Provide distraction during procedure, as appropriate

Assist patient to maintain positioning during procedure

Reinforce expected behavior during examination of a child

Facilitate use of equipment, as appropriate

Note amount and appearance of fluids removed, as appropriate

Collect, label, and arrange for transport of specimens, as appropriate

Provide site care and dressing, as appropriate

Ensure that follow-up tests (e.g., x-ray examinations) are done

Instruct patient on postprocedure care

Monitor patient after procedure, as appropriate

Background Readings:

Manion, J. (1990). Preparing children for hospitalization, procedures or surgery. In M.J. Craft & J.A. Denehy (Eds.), Nursing interventions for infants and children (pp. 74-92). Philadelphia: W.B. Saunders.

Millar, S., Sampson, L.K., & Soukup, S.M. (1985). AACN procedure manual for critical care. Philadelphia: W.B. Saunders.

Exercise Promotion   0200

> **Definition:** Facilitation of regular physical activity to maintain or advance to a higher level of fitness and health

Activities:

Appraise individual's health beliefs about physical exercise

Explore prior exercise experiences

Determine individual's motivation to begin/continue exercise program

Explore barriers to exercise

Encourage verbalization of feelings about exercise or need for exercise

Encourage individual to begin or continue exercise

Assist in identifying a positive role model for maintaining the exercise program

Assist individual to develop an appropriate exercise program to meet needs

Assist individual to set short-term and long-term goals for the exercise program

Assist individual to schedule regular periods for the exercise program into weekly routine

Perform exercise activities with individual, as appropriate

Include family/caregivers in planning and maintaining the exercise program

Inform individual about health benefits and physiological effects of exercise

Instruct individual about appropriate type of exercise for level of health, in collaboration with physician and/or exercise physiologist

Instruct individual about desired frequency, duration, and intensity of the exercise program

Monitor individual's adherence to exercise program/activity

Assist individual to prepare and maintain a progress graph/chart to motivate adherence to the exercise program

Instruct individual about conditions warranting cessation of or alteration in the exercise program

Instruct individual on proper warm-up and cool-down exercises

Instruct individual in techniques to avoid injury while exercising

Instruct individual in proper breathing techniques to maximize oxygen uptake during physical exercise

Provide reinforcement schedule to enhance individual's motivation (e.g., increased endurance estimation; weekly weigh-in)

Monitor individual's response to exercise program

Provide positive feedback for individual's efforts

Background Readings:

Allan, J.D., & Tyler, D.O. (1999). Exercise promotion. In G.M. Bulechek & J.C. McCloskey (Eds.), Nursing interventions: Effective nursing treatments (3rd ed.) (pp. 130-148). Philadelphia: W.B. Saunders.

Glick, O.J. (1992). Interventions related to activity and movement. In G.M. Bulechek & J.C. McCloskey (Eds.), Symposium on Nursing Interventions. Nursing Clinics of North America, 27(2), 541-568.

NIH Consensus Development Panel on Physical Activity and Cardiovascular Health. (1996). Physical activity and cardiovascular health. Journal of the American Medical Association, 276 (3), 241-246.

Rippe, J., Ward, A., Porcari, J. et al. (1989). The cardiovascular benefits of walking. Practical Cardiology. 15(1)

Sorenson, S., & Poh, A. (1989). Physical fitness. In P. Swinford & J. Webster (Eds.), Promoting wellness: A nurse's handbook (pp. 101-140). Rockville, MD: Aspen.

Timmermans, H., & Martin, M. (1987). Top ten potentially dangerous exercises. Journal of Physical Education, Recreation and Dance, 58, 29.

Topp, R. (1991). Development of an exercise program for older adults: Pre-exercise testing, exercise prescription and program maintenance. Nurse Practitioner, 16(10), 16-28.

E

Exercise Promotion: Strength Training   0201

Definition: Facilitating regular resistive muscle training to maintain or increase muscle strength

Activities:

Conduct pre-exercise health screening to identify risks for exercise using standardized physical activity readiness scales and/or complete history and physical exam

Obtain medical clearance for initiating a strength training program, as appropriate

Assist patient to express own beliefs, values, and goals for muscle fitness and health

Provide information about muscle function, exercise physiology, and consequences of disuse

Determine muscle fitness levels using exercise field or laboratory tests (e.g., maximum lift, number of lifts per unit of time)

Provide information about types of muscle resistance that can be used (e.g., free weights, weight machines, rubberized stretch bands, weighted objects, aquatic)

Assist to set realistic short- and long-term goals and to take ownership of the exercise plan

Assist to develop ways to minimize effects of procedural, emotional, attitudinal, financial, or comfort barriers to resistance muscle training

Assist to obtain resources needed to engage in progressive muscle training

Assist to develop a home/work environment that facilitates engaging in the exercise plan

Instruct to wear clothing that prevents overheating or cooling

Assist to develop a strength training program consistent with muscle fitness level, musculoskeletal constraints, functional health goals, exercise equipment resources, personal preference, and social support

Specify level of resistance, number of repetitions, number of sets, and frequency of "training" sessions according to fitness level and presence/absence of exercise risk factors

Instruct to rest briefly after each set, as needed

Specify type and duration of warm-up/cool-down activity (e.g. stretches, walking, calisthenics)

Demonstrate proper body alignment (posture) and lift form for exercising each major muscle group

Use reciprocal movements to avoid injury in selected exercises

Assist to talk through/perform the prescribed movement patterns without weights until correct form is learned

Modify movements and methods of applying resistance for chair- or bed-bound patients

Instruct to recognize signs/symptoms of exercise tolerance/intolerance during and after exercise sessions (e.g., light-headedness; SOB; more than usual muscle, skeletal, or joint pain; weakness; extreme fatigue; angina; profuse sweating; palpitations)

Instruct to conduct exercise sessions for specific muscle groups every other day to facilitate muscle adaptation to training

Instruct to perform three training sessions with each muscle group each week until training goals are achieved and then start on a maintenance program

Instruct to avoid strength training exercise during temperature extremes

Assist to determine rate of progressively increasing muscle work (i.e., amount of resistance and number of repetitions and sets)

Provide illustrated, take-home, written instructions for general guidelines and movement form for each muscle group

Activities:—cont'd

Assist to develop a record-keeping system that includes amount of resistance, number of repetitions and sets to monitor progress in muscle fitness

Reevaluate muscle fitness levels monthly

Establish a follow-up schedule to maintain motivation, assist in problem solving, and monitor progress

Assist to alter programs or develop other strategies to prevent boredom and dropout

Collaborate with family and other health professionals (e.g., activity therapist, exercise physiologist, occupational therapist, recreational therapist, physical therapist) in planning, teaching, and monitoring a muscle training program

E

Background Readings:

Hyatt, G. (1996). Strength training for the aging adult. In J. Clark (Ed.), Exercise programming for older adults (pp. 27-36). New York: Haworth Press, Inc.

Mobily, K., & Mobily, P. (1996). Progressive resistive training. In M. Titler (Ed.), Gerontological Nursing Interventions Research Center research development and dissemination core. Iowa City: The University of Iowa.

Robbins, G., Fowers, D., & Burgess, S. (1997). A wellness way of life. Madison, WI: Brown-Benchmark.

Roberts, S. (1997). Principles of prescribing exercise. In S. Roberts, P. Hanson, & R. Robergs (Eds.), Clinical exercise testing and prescription, theory and application (pp. 235-261). Boca Raton, FL: CRC Press.

Sharpe, F., & McConnell, C. (1992). Exercise beliefs and behaviors among older employees: A health promotion trial. The Gerontologist, 32(4), 444-449.

Southard, D., & Lonbard, D. (1997). Principles of health behavior change. In S. Roberts, P. Hanson, & R. Robergs (Eds.). Clinical exercise testing and prescription, theory and application. Boca Raton, New York: CRC Press.

E

Exercise Promotion: Stretching   0202

Definition: Facilitation of systematic slow-stretch-hold muscle exercises to induce relaxation, to prepare muscles/joints for more vigorous exercise, or to increase or maintain body flexibility

Activities:

Obtain medical clearance for instituting a stretching exercise plan, as needed

Assist patient to explore own beliefs, motivation, and level of neuromusculoskeletal fitness

Assist to develop realistic short- and long-term goal(s), based on current fitness level and lifestyle

Provide information about aging-related changes in neuromusculoskeletal structure and the effects of disuse

Provide information about options for sequence, specific stretching activities, place, and time

Assist to develop a schedule for exercise consistent with age, physical status, goals, motivation, and lifestyle

Assist to develop an exercise plan that incorporates an orderly sequence of stretching movements, increments in the duration of the hold phase of the movement, and increments in number of repetitions for each slow-stretch-hold movement, consistent with level of musculoskeletal fitness or presence of pathology

Instruct to begin exercise routine in muscle/joint groups that are least stiff or sore and gradually move to more restricted muscle/joint groups

Instruct to slowly extend muscle/joint to point of full stretch (or reasonable discomfort) and hold for specified time and slowly release the stretched muscles

Instruct to avoid quick, forceful, or bouncing movement to prevent overstimulation of the myostatic reflex or excessive muscle soreness

Instruct in ways to monitor own adherence to schedule and progress toward goal(s) (e.g., increments in joint range of motion, awareness of releasing muscle tension, increasing duration of "hold" phase and number of repetitions without pain and fatigue, and increases in tolerance for vigorous exercise)

Provide illustrated, take-home, written instructions for each movement component

Coach return demonstrations of exercises, as needed

Monitor adherence to technique and schedule at specified follow-up time and place

Monitor exercise tolerance (e.g., presence of such symptoms as breathlessness, rapid pulse, pallor, lightheadedness, and joint/muscle pain or swelling) during exercise

Reevaluate exercise plan if symptoms of low exercise tolerance persist after cessation of exercise

Collaborate with family members in planning, teaching, and monitoring an exercise plan

Background Readings:

Allan, J.D., & Tyler, D.O. (1999). Exercise promotion. In G.M. Bulechek & J.C. McCloskey (Eds.), Nursing interventions: Effective nursing treatments (3rd ed.) (pp. 130-148). Philadelphia: W.B. Saunders.

Burke, E.J., & Humphreys, J.H.L. (1992). Fit to exercise. (pp. 90-96). London: Pelham Books.

Maas, M. (1991). Impaired physical mobility. In M. Maas, K. Buckwalter, & M. Hardy (Eds.), Nursing diagnoses and interventions for the elderly (pp. 274-277). Redwood City, CA: Addison-Wesley.

Piscopo, J. (1985). Fitness and aging (pp. 169-189). New York: Wiley & Sons.

Pollock, M.L., & Wilmore, J.H. (1990). Exercise in health and disease: Evaluation and prescription for prevention and rehabilitation (2nd ed.). Philadelphia: W.B. Saunders.

Sharkey, B.J. (1990). Physiology of fitness (3rd ed.) (pp. 66, 78, 331-335). Champaign, IL: Human Kinetics Books.

Sorenson, A.J., & Poh, A.E. (1989). Physical fitness. In P. Swinford & J. Webster (Eds.), Promoting wellness: A nurse's handbook (pp. 108-109, 122-125). Rockville, MD: Aspen.

Exercise Therapy: Ambulation 0221

Definition: Promotion and assistance with walking to maintain or restore autonomic and voluntary body functions during treatment and recovery from illness or injury

Activities:

Dress patient in nonrestrictive clothing

Assist patient to use footwear that facilitates walking and prevents injury

Provide low-height bed, as appropriate

Place bed-positioning switch within easy reach

Encourage patient to sit in bed, on side of bed ("dangle"), or in chair, as tolerated

Assist patient to sit on side of bed to facilitate postural adjustments

Consult physical therapist about ambulation plan, as needed

Instruct in availability of assistive devices, if appropriate

Instruct patient how to position self throughout the transfer process

Use a gait belt to assist with transfer and ambulation, as needed

Assist patient to transfer, as needed

Provide cuing card(s) at head of bed to facilitate learning to transfer

Apply/provide assistive device (cane, walker, or wheelchair) for ambulation, if the patient is unsteady

Assist patient with initial ambulation and as needed

Instruct patient/caregiver about safe transfer and ambulation techniques

Monitor patient's use of crutches or other walking aids

Assist patient to stand and ambulate specified distance and with specified number of staff

Assist patient to establish realistic increments in distance for ambulation

Encourage independent ambulation within safe limits

Encourage patient to be "up ad lib," if appropriate

Background Readings:

Alora, J. (1981). Exercise and skeletal health. Journal of the American Geriatric Society, 29(3), 104-107.

Donohue, K., Miller, C., & Craig, B. (1988). Chronic alterations in mobility. In P.H. Mitchell, L.C. Hodges, M. Muwaswes, et al. (Eds.), AANN's neuroscience nursing. Phenomena and practice (pp. 319-343). Norwalk, CT: Appleton & Lange.

Glick, O.J. (1992). Interventions related to activity and movement. In G.M. Bulechek & J.C. McCloskey (Eds.), Symposium on Nursing Interventions. Nursing Clinics of North America, 27(2), 541-568.

Lubkin, I. (1990). Chronic illness: Impact and interventions (2nd ed.). Boston: Jones & Bartlett.

McFarland, G.K., & McFarlane, E.A. (1997). Nursing diagnosis and intervention. (3rd ed.). St. Louis: Mosby.

Moorhouse, M., Geissler, A., & Doenges, M. (1987). Critical care plans, guidelines for patient care. Philadelphia: F.A. Davis.

Smith, E.L., & Gillian, C. (1983). Physical activity prescription for the older adult. The Physician & Sports Medicine, 11(8), 91-182.

Snyder, M. (1992). Exercise. In M. Snyder (Ed.), Independent nursing interventions. (2nd ed.) (pp. 67-77). Albany, NY: Delmar Publishers.

E

E

Exercise Therapy: Balance   0222

Definition: Use of specific activities, postures, and movements to maintain, enhance, or restore balance

Activities:

Determine patient's ability to participate in activities requiring balance

Collaborate with physical, occupational, and recreational therapists in developing and executing exercise program, as appropriate

Consult physical therapy for type, number, and sequence of movement patterns required to enhance balance

Evaluate sensory functions (e.g., vision, hearing, and proprioception)

Dress patient in nonrestrictive clothing

Provide safe environment for practice of exercises

Adjust environment to facilitate concentration

Provide assistive devices (e.g., cane, walker, pillows, or pads) to support patient in performing exercise

Assist patient to formulate realistic, measurable goals

Reinforce or provide instruction about how to position self and perform movements to maintain or improve balance during exercises or activities of daily living

Assist patient to participate in stretching exercises while lying, sitting, or standing

Assist patient to move to sitting position, stabilize trunk with arms placed at side on bed/chair, and rock trunk over supporting arms

Assist patient to rock trunk while in a sitting position without using extremities

Use a mirror to facilitate sitting and standing postural alignment, if appropriate

Assist to stand (or sit) and rock body from side to side to stimulate balance mechanisms

Encourage patient to maintain wide base of support, if needed

Assist patient to practice standing with eyes closed for short periods at regular intervals to stimulate proprioception

Monitor patient's response to balance exercises

Encourage patient to participate in a walking program, if appropriate

Assist patient to ambulate at regular intervals

Refer to physical and/or occupational therapy for vestibular habituation training exercises

Background Readings:

Glick, O.J. (1992). Interventions related to activity and movement. In G.M. Bulechek & J.C. McCloskey (Eds.), Symposium on Nursing Interventions. Nursing Clinics of North America, 27(2), 541-568.

Hickey, J. (1992). The clinical practice of neurological and neurosurgical nursing (3rd ed.). Philadelphia: J.B. Lippincott.

Lewis, C.B. (1989). Improving mobility in older persons. Rockville, MD: Aspen.

Norre, M., & Beckers, A. (1989). Vestibular habituation training for positional vertigo in elderly patients. Archives of Gerontology and Geriatrics, 8, 117.

Pender, N.J. (1987). Health promotion nursing practice (2nd ed.). Norwalk, CT: Appleton & Lange.

Roberts, B. (1989). Effects of walking on balance among elders. Nursing Research, 38(3), 180.

Roberts, B., & Fitzpatrick, J. (1983). Improving balance: Therapy of movement. Journal of Gerontological Nursing, 9(3), 151.

Roberts, B., & Mueller, M. (1987). The balance scale: Factor analysis and reliability. Perceptual & Motor Skills, 63, 367.

Shumway-Cook, A., Anson, D., & Haller, I. (1988). Postural sway biofeedback: Its effect on reestablishing stance stability in hemiplegic patients. Archives of Physical Medicine Rehabilitation, 69, 395.

Sullivan, P., & Markos, P. (1993). Clinical procedures in therapeutic exercise. Norwalk, CT: Appleton & Lange.

Vogt, G., Miller, M., & Esluer, M. (1985). Mosby's manual of neurological care. St. Louis: Mosby.

Exercise Therapy: Joint Mobility   0224

Defintion: Use of active or passive body movement to maintain or restore joint flexibility

Activities:

Determine limitations of joint movement and effect on function

Collaborate with physical therapy in developing and executing an exercise program

Determine patient motivation level for maintaining or restoring joint movement

Explain to patient/family the purpose and plan for joint exercises

Monitor location and nature of discomfort or pain during movement/activity

Initiate pain control measures before beginning joint exercise

Dress patient in nonrestrictive clothing

Protect patient from trauma during exercise

Assist patient to optimal body position for passive/active joint movement

Encourage active range-of-motion (ROM) exercises, according to regular, planned schedule

Perform passive or assisted ROM exercises, as indicated

Instruct patient/family how to systematically perform passive, assisted, or active ROM exercises

Provide written discharge instructions for exercise

Assist patient to develop a schedule for active ROM exercises

Encourage patient to visualize body motion before beginning movement

Assist with regular rhythmic joint motion within limits of pain, endurance, and joint mobility

Encourage patient to sit in bed, on side of bed ("dangle"), or in chair, as tolerated

Encourage ambulation, if appropriate

Determine progress toward goal achievement

Provide positive reinforcement for performing joint exercises

Background Readings:

Glick, O.J. (1992). Interventions related to activity and movement. In G.M. Bulechek & J.C. McCloskey (Eds.), Symposium on Nursing Interventions. Nursing Clinics of North America, 27(2), 541-568.

Hickey, J. (1992). The clinical practice of neurological and neurosurgical nursing (3rd ed.). Philadelphia: J.B. Lippincott.

Hogue, C. (1985). Mobility. In E.G. Schneider et al. (Eds.), The teaching nursing home. New York: Raven Press.

Lewis, C.B. (1989). Improving mobility in older persons. Rockville, MD: Aspen.

Lubkin, I. (1990). Chronic illness: Impact and interventions (2nd ed.). Boston: Jones & Bartlett.

McFarland, G.K., & McFarlane, E.A. (1997). Nursing diagnosis and intervention. (3rd ed.). St. Louis: Mosby.

Moorhouse, M., Geissler, A., & Doenges, M. (1987). Critical care plans, guidelines for patient care. Philadelphia: F.A. Davis.

Pender, N.J. (1987). Health promotion nursing practice (2nd ed.). Norwalk, CT: Appleton & Lange.

Snyder, M. (1992). Exercise. In M. Snyder (Ed.), Independent nursing interventions (2nd ed.) (pp. 67-77). Albany, NY: Delmar Publishers.

Sullivan, P., & Markos, P. (1993). Clinical procedures in therapeutic exercise. Norwalk, CT: Appleton & Lange.

Vogt, G., Miller, M., & Esluer, M. (1985). Mosby's manual of neurological care. St. Louis: Mosby.

Exercise Therapy: Muscle Control 0226

Definition: Use of specific activity or exercise protocols to enhance or restore controlled body movement

Activities:

Determine patient's readiness to engage in activity or exercise protocol

Collaborate with physical, occupational, and recreational therapists in developing and executing exercise program, as appropriate

Consult physical therapy to determine optimal position for patient during exercise and number of repetitions for each movement pattern

Evaluate sensory functions (e.g., vision, hearing, and proprioception)

Explain rationale for type of exercise and protocol to patient/family

Provide patient privacy for exercising, if desired

Adjust lighting, room temperature, and noise level to enhance patient's ability to concentrate on the exercise activity

Sequence daily care activities to enhance effects of specific exercise therapy

Initiate pain control measures before beginning exercise/activity

Dress patient in nonrestrictive clothing

Assist patient to maintain trunk and/or proximal joint stability during motor activity

Apply splints to achieve stability of proximal joints involved with fine motor skills, as prescribed

Reevaluate need for assistive devices at regular intervals in collaboration with PT, OT, or RT

Assist patient to sitting/standing position for exercise protocol, as appropriate

Reinforce instructions provided to patient about the proper way to perform exercises to minimize injury and maximize effectiveness

Determine accuracy of body image

Reorient patient to body awareness

Reorient patient to movement functions of the body

Coach patient to visually scan affected side of body when performing activities of daily living (ADLs) or exercises, if indicated

Provide step-by-step cues for each motor activity during exercise or ADLs

Instruct patient to "recite" each movement as it is being performed

Use visual aids to facilitate learning how to perform ADLs or exercise movements, as appropriate

Provide restful environment for patient after periods of exercise

Assist patient to develop exercise protocol for strength, endurance, and flexibility

Assist patient to formulate realistic, measurable goals

Use motor activities that require attention to and use of both sides of the body

Incorporate ADLs into exercise protocol, if appropriate

Encourage patient to practice exercises independently, as indicated

Assist patient with/encourage patient to use warm-up and cool-down activities before and after exercise protocol

Use tactile (and/or tapping) stimuli to minimize muscle spasm

Assist patient to prepare and maintain a progress graph/chart to motivate adherence to exercise protocol

Monitor patient's emotional, cardiovascular, and functional responses to exercise protocol

Activities:—cont'd

Monitor patient's self-exercise for correct performance

Evaluate patient's progress toward enhancement/restoration of body movement and function

Provide positive reinforcement for patient's efforts in exercise and physical activity

Collaborate with home caregivers regarding exercise protocol and ADLs

Assist patient/caregiver to make prescribed revisions in home exercise plan, as indicated

Background Readings:

Donohue, K., Miller, C., & Craig, B. (1988). Chronic alterations in mobility. In P.H. Mitchell, L.C. Hodges, M. Muwaswes, et al. (Eds.), AANN's neuroscience nursing: Phenomena and practice (pp. 319-343). Norwalk, CT: Appleton & Lange.

Glick, O.J. (1992). Interventions related to activity and movement. In G.M. Bulechek & J.C. McCloskey (Eds.), Symposium on Nursing Interventions. Nursing Clinics of North America, 27(2) 541-568.

Hickey, J. (1992). The clinical practice of neurological and neurosurgical nursing (3rd ed.). Philadelphia: J.B. Lippincott.

Hogue, C. (1985). Mobility. In E.G. Schneider et al. (Eds.), The teaching nursing home. New York: Raven Press.

Lewis, C.B. (1989). Improving mobility in older persons. Rockville, MD: Aspen.

Lubkin, I. (1990). Chronic illness. Impact and intervention (2nd ed.). Boston: Jones & Bartlett.

McFarland, G.K., & McFarlane, E.A. (1997). Nursing diagnosis and intervention. (3rd ed.). St. Louis: Mosby.

Moorhouse, M., Geissler, A., & Doenges, M. (1987). Critical care plans, guidelines for patient care. Philadelphia: F.A. Davis.

Pender, N.J. (1987). Health promotion nursing practice (2nd ed.). Norwalk, CT: Appleton & Lange.

Sullivan, P., & Markos, P. (1993). Clinical procedures in therapeutic exercise. Norwalk, CT: Appleton & Lange.

Vogt, G., Miller, M., & Esluer, M. (1985). Mosby's manual of neurological care. St. Louis: Mosby.

E

Eye Care

1650

Definition: Prevention or minimization of threats to eye or visual integrity

Activities:

Monitor for redness, exudate, or ulceration

Instruct patient not to touch eye

Monitor corneal reflex

Remove contact lenses, as appropriate

Apply eye shield, as appropriate

Patch the eyes, as needed

Alternate eye patch for diplopia

Apply lubricating eyedrops, as appropriate

Apply lubricating ointment, as appropriate

Tape eyelids shut, as appropriate

Apply moisture chamber, as appropriate

Background Readings:

Ackerman, L.L. (1992). Interventions related to neurological care. In G.M. Bulechek & J.C. McCloskey (Eds.), Symposium on Nursing Interventions. Nursing Clinics of North America, 27(2), 325-346.

Hickey, J.V. (1992). The clinical practice of neurological and neurosurgical nursing (3rd ed.). Philadelphia: J.B. Lippincott.

Martin, E.M., & Hummilgard, A.B. (1987). Detachable balloon occlusion of carotid-cavernous sinus fistula. Journal of Neuroscience Nursing, 19(3), 132-140.

Wincek, J., & Turrnam, M.S. (1989). Exposure keratitis in comatose children. Journal of Neuroscience Nursing, 21(4), 241-244.

Fall Prevention   6490

Definition: Instituting special precautions with patient at risk for injury from falling

Activities:

Identify cognitive or physical deficits of the patient that may increase potential falls in a particular environment

Identify behaviors and factors that affect risk of falls

Review history of falls with patient and family

Identify characteristics of environment that may increase potential for falls (e.g., slippery floors and open stairways)

Monitor gait, balance, and fatigue level with ambulation

Ask patient for perception of balance, as appropriate

Share with patient observations about gait and movement

Suggest changes in gait to patient

Coach patient to adapt to suggested gait modifications

Assist unsteady individual with ambulation

Provide assistive devices (e.g., cane and walker) to steady gait

Encourage patient to use cane or walker, as appropriate

Instruct patient about use of cane or walker, as appropriate

Maintain assistive devices in good working order

Lock wheels of wheelchair, bed, or gurney during transfer of patient

Place articles within easy reach of the patient

Instruct patient to call for assistance with movement, as appropriate

Teach patient how to fall so as to minimize injury

Post signs to remind patient to call for help when getting out of bed, as appropriate

Monitor ability to transfer from bed to chair and vice versa

Use proper technique to transfer patient to and from wheelchair, bed, toilet, and so on

Provide elevated toilet seat for easy transfer

Provide chairs of proper height, with backrests and armrests for easy transfer

Provide bed mattress with firm edges for easy transfer

Use side rails of appropriate length and height to prevent falls from bed, as needed

Place a mechanical bed in lowest position

Provide a sleeping surface close to the floor, as needed

Provide seating on bean bag chair to limit mobility, as appropriate

Place a foam wedge in seat of chair to prevent patient from arising without assistance, as appropriate

Use partially filled water mattress on bed to limit mobility, as appropriate

Provide the dependent patient with a means of summoning help (e.g., bell or call light) when caregiver is not present

Answer call light immediately

Assist with toileting at frequent, scheduled intervals

Use a bed alarm to alert caretaker that individual is getting out of bed, as appropriate

Continued

Activities:—cont'd

Mark doorway thresholds and edges of steps, as needed

Remove low-lying furniture (e.g., footstools and tables) that present a tripping hazard

Avoid clutter on floor surface

Provide adequate lighting for increased visibility

Provide nightlight at bedside

Provide visible handrails and grab bars

Place gates in open doorways leading to stairways

Provide nonslip, nontrip floor surfaces

Provide a nonslip surface in bathtub or shower

Provide sturdy, nonslip step stools to facilitate easy reaches

Provide storage areas that are within easy reach

Provide heavy furniture that will not tip if used for support

Orient patient to physical "setup" of room

Avoid unnecessary rearrangement of physical environment

Ensure that patient wears shoes that fit properly, fasten securely, and have nonskid soles

Instruct patient to wear prescription glasses, as appropriate, when out of bed

Educate family members about risk factors that contribute to falls and how they can decrease these risks

Suggest home adaptations to increase safety

Instruct family on importance of handrails for stairs, bathrooms, and walkways

Assist family in identifying hazards in the home and modifying them

Suggest safe footwear

Instruct patient to avoid walking on ice and other slippery outdoor surfaces

Develop ways for patient to participate safely in leisure activities

Institute a routine physical exercise program that includes walking

Post signs to alert staff that patient is at high risk for falls

Collaborate with other health care team members to minimize side effects of medications that contribute to falling (e.g., orthostatic hypotension and unsteady gait)

Provide close supervision and/or a restraining device (e.g., infant seat with seat belt) when placing infants/young children on elevated surfaces (e.g., table and highchair)

Remove objects that provide young child with climbing access to elevated surfaces

Maintain crib side rails in elevated position when caregiver is not present, as appropriate

Provide a "bubble top" on hospital cribs of pediatric patients who may climb over elevated side rails, as appropriate

Fasten the latches securely on access panel of incubator when leaving bedside of infant in incubator, as appropriate

Background Readings:

Foley, G. (1999). The multidisciplinary team: Partners in patient safety. Cancer Practice: A Multidisciplinary Journal of Cancer Care, 7(3), 108.

Kanak, M.F. (1992). Interventions related to safety. In G.M. Bulechek & J.C. McCloskey (Eds.), Symposium on Nursing Interventions. Nursing Clinics of North America, 27(2), 371-396.

Maciorowski, L.F., Monro, B.H., Dietrick-Gallagher, M., et al. (1989). A review of the patient fall literature. Journal of Nursing Quality Assurance, 3(1), 18-27.

Stolley, J.M., Lewis, A., Moore, L., & Harvey, P. (2001). Risk for injury: Falls. In M. Maas, K. Buckwalter, M. Hardy, T. Tripp-Reimer, M. Titler, & J. Specht (Eds.), Nursing care of older adults: Diagnoses, outcomes, and interventions (pp. 23-33). St. Louis: Mosby.

Sullivan, R.P. (1999). Recognize factors to prevent patient falls. Nursing Management, 30(5), 37-40.

Tack, K.A., Ulrich, B., & Kehr, C. (1987). Patient falls: Profiles for prevention. Journal of Neuroscience Nursing, 19(2), 83-89.

Tideiksaar, R. (1997). Falling in old age: Prevention and management. New York: Springer.

F

Family Integrity Promotion   7100

Definition: Promotion of family cohesion and unity

Activities:

Be a listener for the family members

Establish trusting relationship with family members

Determine family understanding of causes of illness

Determine guilt family may feel

Assist family to resolve feelings of guilt

Determine typical family relationships

Monitor current family relationships

Identify typical family coping mechanisms

Identify conflicting priorities among family members

Assist family with conflict resolution

Counsel family members on additional effective coping skills for their own use

Respect privacy of individual family members

Provide for family privacy

Tell family members it is safe and acceptable to use typical expressions of affection

Facilitate a tone of togetherness within/among the family

Provide family members with information about the patient's condition regularly, according to patient's preference

Collaborate with family in problem solving

Encourage family to maintain positive relationships

Facilitate open communication among family members

Provide for care of patient by family members, as appropriate

Provide for family visitation

Refer family to support group of other families dealing with similar problems

Refer for family therapy, as indicated

Background Readings:

Craft, M.J., & Denehy, J.A. (1990). Nursing interventions for infants and children. Philadelphia: W.B. Saunders.

Craft, M.J., & Willadsen, J.A. (1992). Interventions related to family. In G.M. Bulechek & J.C. McCloskey (Eds.), Symposium on Nursing Interventions. Nursing Clinics of North America, 27(2), 517-540.

Dixon, M. (1991). Altered family processes: Caring for the dependent elderly family member. In M. Maas, K. Buckwalter, & M. Hardy (Eds.), Nursing diagnoses and interventions for the elderly (pp. 542-550). Redwood City, CA: Addison-Wesley.

Family Integrity Promotion: Childbearing Family   7104

Definition: Facilitation of the growth of individuals or families who are adding an infant to the family unit

Activities:

Create an atmosphere to facilitate trust

Provide atmosphere of acceptance

Convey accepting attitude (one that creates a nonthreatening environment for the patient and family to express feelings)

Establish trusting relationship with parent(s)

Offer to be a listener

Offer to be a listener for significant other

Spend time with parent(s) to convey acceptance

Spend time with parent(s) to contribute to feelings of self-worth

Provide step-by-step verbal support in a calm, strong voice

Monitor current family situation

Monitor psychosocial status of family

Monitor effects of newborn on family structure

Analyze role adaptations of family to newborn

Monitor couple's relationship to one another after birth of infant, as appropriate

Monitor relationships among family members

Determine strength of intrafamily bonds

Identify family interaction system

Monitor family's ability to perform tasks appropriate to family developmental stage

Identify normal family coping mechanisms

Identify coping mechanisms of individual family members

Assist family in identifying support systems used by the family

Determine family's relationship to support systems

Assist family in developing new support network

Offer to be an advocate for the family

Offer to be an advocate for the child

Prepare parent(s) for expected role changes involved in becoming a parent(s)

Prepare parent(s) for responsibilities of parenthood

Monitor parent's adaptation to parenthood

Determine parent's self-esteem

Reinforce positive parenting behaviors

Monitor parent's self-perception as a parent

Appraise parent's perceptions of self as individual

Encourage parent(s) to maintain individual hobbies or outside interests

Provide parent(s) an opportunity to express their feelings about parenthood

Continued

Activities:—cont'd

Encourage verbalization of feelings, perceptions, and concerns about prenatal experience

Encourage verbalization of feelings, perceptions, and concerns about the birth experience

Discuss the grieving process associated with the loss of "being pregnant"

Explain causes and manifestations of postpartum depression

Provide for family and sibling visitation during postpartum period

Make sibling(s) feel special when visiting unit, as appropriate

Provide toys for siblings in waiting room, as needed

Determine how parent(s) prepared sibling(s) for coming of new baby, as appropriate

Provide information about sibling preparation, as appropriate

Provide family with information about measures to assist sibling(s) to feel important to the family, as appropriate

Encourage family to attend sibling preparation classes, as appropriate

Discuss reaction of sibling(s) to newborn, as appropriate

Determine sibling reaction to newborn, as appropriate

Encourage parent(s) to observe sibling reaction to newborn, as appropriate

Give family information on how to prevent sibling rivalry, as appropriate

Give family information on how to deal with sibling rivalry, as appropriate

Develop policies that permit presence of family members as much as desired

Background Readings:

Denehy, J.A. (1992). Interventions related to parent-infant attachment. In G.M. Bulechek & J.C. McCloskey (Eds.), Symposium on Nursing Interventions. Nursing Clinics of North America, 27(2), 425-444.

Tulman, L., Fawcett, J., Groblewski, L., & Silverman, L. (1990). Changes in functional status after childbirth. Nursing Research, 39(2), 425-444.

F

Family Involvement Promotion　7110

Definition: Facilitating family participation in the emotional and physical care of the patient

Activities:

Establish a personal relationship with the patient and family members who will be involved in care

Identify family members' capabilities for involvement in care of the patient

Determine physical, emotional, and educational resources of primary caregiver

Identify patient's self-care deficits

Identify family members' preferences for involvement with patient

Identify family members' expectations for the patient

Encourage family members and patient to assist in the development of a plan of care, including expected outcomes and implementation of the plan of care

Encourage family members and patient to be assertive in interactions with health care professionals.

Monitor family structure and roles

Monitor involvement by family members in patient's care

Encourage care by family members during hospitalization or stay in a long-term care facility

Provide crucial information to family members about the patient in accordance with patient's preference

Facilitate understanding of the medical aspects of the patient's condition for family members

Identify family members' perceptions of the situation, precipitating events, patient's feelings, and patient's behaviors

Identify other situational stressors for family members

Identify individual family members' physical symptoms related to stress (e.g., tearfulness, nausea, vomiting, distractibility)

Determine level of patient dependence on family members as appropriate for age or illness

Encourage focus on any positive aspects of the patient's situation

Identify and respect coping mechanisms used by family members

Identify with family members the patient's coping difficulties

Identify with family members the patient's strengths and abilities

Inform family members of factors that may improve patient's condition

Encourage family members to keep or maintain family relationships, as appropriate

Discuss options for type of home care, such as group living, residential care, or respite care, as appropriate

Facilitate management of the medical aspects of illness by family members

Background Readings:

Aldous, J. (1996). Family careers: Rethinking the developmental perspective (pp. 70-92). Thousand Oaks, CA: Sage Publications.

Cohen, M.S. (1999). Families coping with childhood chronic illness: A research review. Families, Systems, & Health, 17(2) 149-164.

Faux, S.A., & Seideman, R.T. (1996). Heatlh care professionals and their relationships with families who have members with developmental disabilities. Journal of Family Nursing, 2(2), 217-238.

Family Mobilization   7120

Definition: Utilization of family strengths to influence patient's health in a positive direction

Activities:

Be a listener for family members

Establish trusting relationships with family members

View family members as potential experts in the care of the patient

Identify strengths and resources within the family, in family members, and in their support system and community

Determine the readiness and ability of family members to learn

Provide information frequently to the family to assist them in identifying the patient's limitations, progress, and implications for care

Foster mutual decision making with family members related to the patient's care plan

Teach home caregivers about the patient's therapy, as appropriate

Explain to family members the need for continuing professional health care, as appropriate

Collaborate with family members in planning and implementing patient therapies and lifestyle changes

Support family activities in promoting patient health or management of condition, when appropriate

Assist family members to identify health services and community resources that can be used to enhance the health status of the patient

Monitor the current family situation

Refer family members to support groups of other families, as appropriate

Determine expected patient outcome achievement systematically

Background Readings:

Craft, M., Lakin, J., Opplinger, R., Clancy, G., & Vanderlinden, D. (1990). Siblings as change agents for promoting the functional status of children with cerebral palsy. Developmental Medicine & Child Neurology, 32, 1049-1057.

Judge, S. (1998). Parental coping strategies and strengths in families of young children with disabilities. Family Relations: Interdisciplinary Journal of Applied Family Studies, 47,(3), 263-269.

Kaslow, N.J, Collins, M., Rashid, F. Baskin, M., Griffith, J.R., Hollins, L., & Eckman, J.E. (2000). The efficacy of a pilot family psychoeducational intervention for pediatric sickle cell disease (SCD). Families, Systems, & Health, 18 (4), 381-404.

Family Planning: Contraception   6784

Definition: Facilitation of pregnancy prevention by providing information about the physiology of reproduction and methods to control conception

Activities:

Determine need for family planning

Explain reasons for most unplanned pregnancies

Determine ability and motivation of patient and partner to correctly and regularly use contraception

Appraise patient's knowledge of contraception and plans for selecting a contraceptive method

Explain female reproductive cycle to patient, as needed

Explain advantages and disadvantages of appropriate contraceptive methods

Assist female patient to determine ovulation through basal body temperature, changes in vaginal secretions, and other physiological indicators

Instruct patient in use of chemical, hormonal, or mechanical contraceptives

Refer patient to community resources for family planning services, as needed

Background Readings:

Bobak, I.M., Jensen, M., & Lowdermilk, D.L. (1993). Maternity & gynecologic care: The nurse and the family (5th ed.). St. Louis: Mosby.

Franklin, M. (1990). Recently approved and experimental methods of contraception. Journal of Nurse-Midwifery, 35(6), 365-375.

Jarrett, M.E., & Lethbridge, D.J. (1990). The contraceptive needs of midlife women. Nurse Practitioner, 15(12), 34-39.

F

F

Family Planning: Infertility   6786

Definition: Management, education, and support of the patient and significant other undergoing evaluation and treatment for infertility

Activities:

Explain female reproductive cycle to patient, as needed

Assist female patient to determine ovulation through basal body temperature, changes in vaginal secretions, and other physiological indicators

Prepare patient physically and psychologically for gynecological examination

Explain purpose of procedure and sensations the patient might experience during the procedure

Determine patient's understanding of test results and recommended therapy

Support patient through infertility history and evaluation, acknowledging stress often experienced in providing detailed history and during lengthy evaluation and treatment process

Assist with expressions of grief and disappointment and feelings of failure

Encourage expressions of feelings about sexuality, self-image, and self-esteem

Determine extent to which patient (and significant other) are engaging in magical thinking

Assist individuals to redefine concepts of success and failure, as needed

Refer patient to support group for infertile couples, as appropriate

Assist with problem solving to help couple evaluate alternatives to biological parenthood

Determine effect of infertility on couple's relationship

Background Readings:

Bernstein, J., Brill, M., Levin, S. & Seibel, M. (1992). Coping with infertility: A new nursing perspective. NAACOG's Clinical Issues in Perinatal & Women's Health Nursing, 3(2), 335-342.

Bobak, I.M., Jensen, M., & Lowdermilk, D.L. (1993). Maternity & gynecologic care: The nurse and the family (5th ed.). St. Louis: Mosby.

James, C.A. (1992). The nursing role in assisted reproductive technologies. NAACOG's Clinical Issues in Perinatal & Women's Health Nursing, 3(2), 328-334.

Olshansky, E.F., (1992). Redefining the concepts of success and failure in infertility treatment. NAACOG's Clinical Issues in Perinatal & Women's Health Nursing, 3(2), 343-346.

Family Planning: Unplanned Pregnancy   6788

Definition: Facilitation of decision making regarding pregnancy outcome

Activities:

Determine whether patient has made a choice about outcome of pregnancy

Encourage patient and significant other to explore options regarding outcomes of pregnancy, including termination, keeping the infant, or relinquishing the infant for adoption

Discuss alternatives to abortion with patient and significant other

Discuss factors related to unplanned pregnancy (e.g., multiple partners, drug and/or alcohol use, and likelihood of sexually transmitted disease)

Assist patient in identifying support system

Encourage patient to involve support system during decision-making process

Support patient and significant other in decision about pregnancy outcome

Clarify misinformation about contraceptive use

Refer to community agencies that have services that will support patient in acting on decision regarding pregnancy outcome, as well as other health concerns (e.g., sexually transmitted diseases and substance abuse)

Background Readings:

Bobak, I.M., Jensen, M., & Lowdermilk, D.L. (1993). Maternity & gynecologic care: The nurse and the family (5th ed.). St. Louis: Mosby.

O'Campo, P., Faden, R.R., Gielen, A.C., Kass, N., & Anderson, J. (1993). Contraceptive practices among single women with an unplanned pregnancy: Partner influences. Family Planning Perspectives, 25(5), 215-219.

Sulak, P.J., & Haney, A.F. (1993). Unwanted pregnancies: Understanding contraceptive use and benefits in adolescents and older women. American Journal of Obstetrics & Gynecology, 168(6), 2042-2048.

F

Family Presence Facilitation   7170

Definition: Facilitation of the family's presence in support of an individual undergoing resuscitation and/or invasive procedures

Activities:

Introduce yourself to the staff treating the patient and family

Determine suitability of the physical location for family presence

Obtain consensus from the staff for the family's presence and the timing of the family's presence

Apprise the treatment team of the family's emotional reaction to patient's condition, as appropriate

Obtain information concerning the patient's status, response to treatment, identified needs

Introduce yourself and other members of the support team to the family and patient

Communicate information concerning the patient's current status in a timely manner

Assure family that best care possible is being given to patient

Use the patient's name when speaking to the family

Determine the patient's and the family's emotional, physical, psychosocial, and spiritual support needs and initiate measures to meet those needs, as appropriate

Determine the psychological burden of prognosis for family

Foster realistic hope, as appropriate

Advocate for family, as appropriate

Prepare the family, ensuring that they have been informed about what to expect, what they will see, hear, and/or smell

Inform family of behavior expectations and limits

Provide a dedicated staff person to ensure that family members are never left unattended at the bedside

Accompany the family to and from the treatment or resuscitation area, announce their presence to the treatment staff each time the family enters the treatment area

Provide information about and explanations of the interventions, medical/nursing jargon, and expectations of the patient's response to treatment

Escort the family from the bedside if requested by the staff providing direct care

Provide the opportunity for the family to ask questions and to see, touch and speak to the patient prior to transfers

Assist the patient or family members in making telephone calls, as needed

Offer and provide comfort measures and support, including appropriate referrals, as needed

Participate in the evaluation of staff's and own emotional needs

Assist in identifying need for critical incident stress debriefing, individual defusing of events, etc., as appropriate

Participate, initiate, and/or coordinate family bereavement follow-up at established intervals, as appropriate

Background Readings:

American Heart Association. (2000). Part 2: Ethical aspects of CPR and ECC. Circulation, 102, I-12-I-21.

Eichhorn, D.J., Meyers, T.A., Guzzetta, C.E., Clark, A.P., Klein, J.D., & Calvin, A.O. (2001). During invasive procedures and resuscitation: Hearing the voice of the patient. American Journal of Nursing, 101, 48-55.

Emergency Nurses Association. (1998). Emergency Nurses Association position statement: Family presence at the bedside during invasive procedures and/or resuscitation. Journal of Emergency Nursing, 21, 26A.

Emergency Nurses Association. (2000). Presenting the option for family presence. (2nd ed.). Des Plaines, IL:Emergency Nurses Association.

Hampe, S.O. (1975). Needs of a grieving spouse in a hospital setting. Nursing Research, 24, 113-120.

McPhee, A.T. (1983). Let the family in. Nursing, 83, 2-120.

Meyers, T.A., Eichborn, D.J., & Guzzetta, C.E. (1998). Do families want to be present during CPR? A retrospective survey. Journal of Emergency Nursing, 24, 405.

Meyers, T.A., Eichborn, D.J., Guzzetta, C.E., Clark, A.P., Klein, J.D., Taliaferro, E., & Calvin, A. (2000). Family presence during invasive procedures and resuscitation. American Journal of Nursing, 100, 32-42.

F

F

Family Process Maintenance   7130

Definition: Minimization of family process disruption effects

Activities:

Determine typical family processes

Determine disruption in typical family processes

Identify effects of role changes on family processes

Encourage visitation of family members, as appropriate

Keep opportunities for visiting flexible to meet needs of family members and patient

Discuss strategies for normalizing family life with family members

Assist family members to implement normalizing strategies for their situation

Discuss existing social support mechanisms for the family

Assist family members to use existing support mechanisms

Minimize family routine disruption by facilitating family routines and rituals, such as private meals together or family discussions for communication and decision making

Provide mechanisms for family members staying at health care agency to communicate with other family members (e.g., telephones, tape recordings, open visiting, photographs, videotapes, and e-mail access)

Provide mechanisms for patient communication with family members, such as telephones, tape recordings, open visiting, videotapes, photographs, and letters

Provide opportunities for ongoing parental care of children, when the patient is a child

Provide opportunities for adult family members to maintain ongoing commitments to their jobs

Assist family members in finding child care when parent must be absent, as appropriate

Assist family members to facilitate home visits by patient, when appropriate

Identify patient home care needs and how these might be incorporated into family lifestyle

Design schedules of patient home care activities that minimize disruption of family routine

Teach family time management/organization skills when performing patient home care, as needed

Background Readings:

Craft, M.J., & Willadsen, J.A. (1992). Interventions related to family. In G.M. Bulechek & J.C. McCloskey (Eds.), Symposium on Nursing Interventions. Nursing Clinics of North America, 27(2), 517-540.

Friedman, M.M. (1992). Family nursing. Theory and practice. Norwalk, CT: Appleton & Lange.

Titler, M.G., Cohen, M.Z., & Craft, M.J. (1991). Impact of critical hospitalization: Perceptions of patients, spouses, children, and nurses. Heart & Lung, 20(2), 174-181.

Family Support   7140

Definition: Promotion of family values, interests and goals

Activities:

Assure family that best care possible is being given to patient

Appraise family's emotional reaction to patient's condition

Determine the psychological burden of prognosis for family

Foster realistic hope

Listen to family concerns, feelings, and questions

Facilitate communication of concerns/feelings between patient and family or between family members

Promote trusting relationship with family

Accept the family's values in a nonjudgmental manner

Answer all questions of family members or assist them to get answers

Orient family to the health care setting, such as hospital unit or clinic

Provide assistance in meeting basic needs for family, such as shelter, food, and clothing

Identify nature of spiritual support for family

Identify congruence between patient, family, and health professional expectations

Reduce discrepancies in patient, family, and health professional expectations through use of communication skills

Assist family members in identifying and resolving a conflict in values

Respect and support adaptive coping mechanisms used by family

Provide feedback for family regarding their coping

Counsel family members on additional effective coping skills for their own use

Provide spiritual resources for family, as appropriate

Provide family with information about patient's progress frequently, according to patient preference

Teach the medical and nursing plans of care to family

Provide necessary knowledge of options to family that will assist them to make decisions about patient care

Include family members with patient in decision making about care, when appropriate

Encourage family decision making in planning long-term patient care affecting family structure and finances

Acknowledge understanding of family decision about postdischarge care

Assist family to acquire necessary knowledge, skills, and equipment to sustain their decision about patient care

Advocate for family, as appropriate

Foster family assertiveness in information seeking, as appropriate

Provide opportunities for visitation by extended family members, as appropriate

Introduce family to other families undergoing similar experiences, as appropriate

Give care to patient in lieu of family to relieve them and/or when family is unable to give care

Arrange for ongoing respite care, when indicated and desired

Provide opportunities for peer group support

Continued

Activities:—cont'd

Refer for family therapy, as appropriate

Tell family members how to reach the nurse

Assist family members through the death and grief processes, as appropriate

Background Readings:

Craft, M.J. (1987). Health care preferences of rural teens. Journal of Pediatric Nursing, 2(1), 3-13.

Craft, M.J., & Craft, J. (1989). Perceived changes in siblings of hospitalized children: A comparison of parent and sibling report. Children's Health Care, 18(1), 42-49.

Craft, M.J., & Willadsen, J.A. (1992). Interventions related to family. In G.M. Bulechek & J.C. McCloskey (Eds.), Symposium on Nursing Interventions. Nursing Clinics of North America, 27(2), 517-540.

Gilliss, C., Highley, B., Roberts, B., & Martinson, I. (1989). Toward a science of family nursing. Menlo Park, CA: Addison-Wesley.

Goldenberg, I., & Goldenberg, H. (1985). Family therapy: An overview (2nd ed.). Monterey, CA: Brooks/Cole.

Leske, J.S. (1992). Needs of adult family members after critical illnesses: Prescriptions for interventions. Critical Care Nursing Clinics of North America, 4(4), 587-596.

Peirce, A.G., Wright, F., & Fulmer, T.T. (1992). Needs of family during critical illness of elderly patients. Critical Care Nursing Clinics of North America, 4(4), 597-606.

Titler, M.G., & Walsh, S.M. (1992). Visiting critically ill adults: Strategies for practice. Critical Care Nursing Clinics of North America, 4(4), 623-633.

F

Family Therapy   7150

Definition: Assisting family members to move their family toward a more productive way of living

Activities:

Share therapy plan with family

Determine patient's usual roles within the family system

Determine specific disabilities related to role expectations

Determine areas of dissatisfaction and/or conflict and see whether family members want to resolve them

Use family history taking to encourage family discussion

Use data tracking to monitor family

Monitor family boundaries as an attempt to change distance between family subsystems

Monitor for adverse therapeutic responses

Incorporate therapeutic use of self as nurse change agent

Plan termination and evaluation strategies

Progress discussion from least to most emotionally laden material

Ask family members to participate in homework assignments of experiential activities, such as eating some of their meals together

Facilitate family discussion, as members prioritize data and select the most immediate family issue to address

Help family members clarify what they need and expect from each other

Use therapeutic spontaneity in interactions with families

Give confirmation to family members to recognize and reward positives

Provide challenge within family discussion to break or expand contexts and to encourage new possibilities to emerge

Facilitate challenging or confronting family subsystems, as appropriate

Discuss hierarchical relationship of subsystem members

Assist family members to change by changing self as they relate to other family members

Facilitate restructuring family subsystems, as appropriate

Help family reset goals away from continuity of the same toward a more competent way of handling dysfunctional behavior

Background Readings:

Craft, M.J., & Willadsen, J.A. (1992). Interventions related to family. In G.M. Bulechek & J.C. McCloskey (Eds.), Symposium on Nursing Interventions. Nursing Clinics of North America, 27(2), 517-540.

Haber, J., McMahon, A.L., Price-Hoskins, P. & Sideleau, B.F. (1992). Comprehensive psychiatric nursing (4th ed.). St. Louis: Mosby.

Johnson, B.S. (1993). Psychiatric mental health nursing: Adaptation and growth (2nd ed.). Philadelphia: J.B. Lippincott.

Minuchen, S., & Fishmen, H.C. (1981). Family therapy techniques. Cambridge: Harvard University Press.

Wilson, H.S., & Kneisl, C.R. (1992). Psychiatric nursing (4th ed.). Menlo Park, CA: Addision-Wesley.

Feeding   1050

Definition: Providing nutritional intake for patient who is unable to feed self

Activities:

Identify prescribed diet

Set food tray and table attractively

Create a pleasant environment during mealtime (e.g., put bedpans, urinals, and suctioning equipment out of sight)

Provide for adequate pain relief before meals, as appropriate

Provide for oral hygiene before meals

Identify presence of swallowing reflex, if necessary

Sit down while feeding to convey pleasure and relaxation

Offer opportunity to smell foods to stimulate appetite

Ask patient preference for order of eating

Fix foods as patient prefers

Maintain patient in an upright position, with head and neck flexed slightly forward during feeding

Place food in the unaffected side of the mouth, as appropriate

Follow feedings with water, if needed

Protect patient's clothing with a bib, as appropriate

Ask the patient to indicate when finished, as appropriate

Record intake, if appropriate

Avoid disguising drugs in food

Provide a drinking straw, as needed or desired

Provide finger foods, as appropriate

Provide foods at most appetizing temperature

Avoid distracting patient during swallowing

Feed unhurriedly/slowly

Postpone feeding, if patient is fatigued

Encourage parents/family to feed patient

Background Readings:

Evans-Stoner, N.J. (1999). Feeding. In G.M. Bulechek & J.C. McCloskey (Eds.), Nursing interventions: Effective nursing treatments (3rd ed.) (pp. 31-46). Philadelphia: W.B. Saunders.

Styker, R. (1977). Rehabilitative aspects of acute and chronic nursing care. Philadelphia: W.B. Saunders.

Fertility Preservation   7160

Definition: Providing information, counseling, and treatment that facilitate reproductive health and the ability to conceive

Activities:

Discuss factors related to infertility (e.g., maternal age >35 and sexually transmitted diseases)

Encourage conception before age 35, as appropriate

Teach patient how to prevent sexually transmitted diseases

Inform patient of signs and symptoms of sexually transmitted diseases and importance of early, aggressive treatment

Perform pelvic examination, as appropriate

Obtain cervical cultures, as appropriate

Prescribe treatment, as indicated for sexually transmitted disease or vaginal infection

Advise patient to seek evaluation and treatment for sexually transmitted disease if partner exhibits any symptoms, even if patient experiences no symptoms

Advise patient to have partner treated for sexually transmitted disease, if culture is positive

Report positive sexually transmitted disease cultures, as required by law

Discuss effects of different contraceptive methods on future fertility

Counsel patient about contraceptive use

Advise patient to avoid use of intrauterine devices

Inform patients about occupational and environmental hazards to fertility (e.g., radiation, chemicals, stress, infections, other environmental factors, and shift rotation)

Inform patient about more conservative options that are likely to preserve fertility, when gynecological or abdominal surgery is indicated

Refer patient for thorough physical examination for health problems affecting fertility (e.g., amenorrhea, diabetes, endometriosis, and thyroid disease)

Encourage early, aggressive treatment for endometriosis

Review lifestyle habits that may alter fertility (e.g., smoking, substance use, alcohol consumption, nutrition, exercise, and sexual behavior)

Refer to wellness or lifestyle modification program, as appropriate

Inform patient about the effects of alcohol, tobacco, drugs, and other factors on sperm production and male sexual function

Refer patient with history indicative of possible fertility disorder for early diagnosis and treatment

Assist patient in receiving occupational support for fertility treatment

Inform patient about the potential or lack of potential reversibility of different methods of sterilization

Advise patient considering sterilization to consider procedure irreversible

Background Readings:

Keating, C.E. (1992). The role of the expanded function nurse in fertility preservation. NAACOG's Clinical Issues in Perinatal and Women's Health Nursing, 3(2), 293-300.

Keleher, K.C. (1991). Occupational health: How work environments can affect reproductive capacity and outcome. Nurse Practitioner, 16(9), 23-8, 33-34, 37.

Wilson, B. (1991). The effect of drugs on male sexual function and fertility. Nurse Practitioner, 16(9), 12-17, 21-22.

Fever Treatment 3740

Definition: Management of a patient with hyperpyrexia caused by nonenvironmental factors

Activities:

Monitor temperature as frequently as is appropriate

Monitor for insensible fluid loss

Institute a continuous core temperature–monitoring device, as appropriate

Monitor skin color and temperature

Monitor blood pressure, pulse, and respiration, as appropriate

Monitor for decreasing levels of consciousness

Monitor for seizure activity

Monitor WBC, hemoglobin, and hematocrit values

Monitor intake and output

Monitor for electrolyte abnormalities

Monitor for acid-base imbalance

Monitor for presence of cardiac arrhythmias

Administer antipyretic medication, as appropriate

Administer medications to treat the cause of fever, as appropriate

Cover the patient with a sheet, only as appropriate

Administer a tepid sponge bath, as appropriate

Encourage increased intake of oral fluids, as appropriate

Administer IV fluids, as appropriate

Apply ice bag covered with a towel to groin and axilla

Increase air circulation by using a fan

Encourage or administer oral hygiene, as appropriate

Give appropriate medication to prevent or control shivering

Administer oxygen, as appropriate

Place patient on hypothermia blanket, as appropriate

Monitor temperature closely to prevent treatment-induced hypothermia

Background Readings:

Beutler, B., & Beutler, S. (1992). Pathogenesis of fever. In J.B. Wyngaarden, L.H. Smith, Jr., & J.C. Bennett, Jr. (Eds.), Cecil textbook of medicine (19th ed.) (pp. 1568-1571). Philadelphia: W.B. Saunders.

Thompson, J.M., McFarland, G.K., Hirsch, J.E., & Tucker, S.M. (1993). Mosby's clinical nursing (3rd ed.). St. Louis: Mosby.

Financial Resource Assistance   7380

Definition: Assisting an individual/family to secure and manage finances to meet health care needs

Activities:

Determine patient's current use of health care system and the financial impact of this use

Assist patient to identify financial needs, including analysis of assets and liabilities

Determine patient's cognitive ability to read, fill out forms, balance checkbook, manage money

Determine patient's daily living expenses

Prioritize patient's daily living needs and assist patient to develop a plan to meet those needs

Devise a plan of care to encourage patient/family to access appropriate levels of care in the most cost-effective manner

Inform patient of services available through state and federal programs

Determine if patient is eligible for waiver programs

Refer patient who may be eligible for state or federally funded programs to appropriate individuals

Inform patient of available resources and assist in accessing resources (e.g., medication assistance program, county relief program)

Assist patient to develop a budget and/or make referral to appropriate financial resource person (e.g., financial planner, estate planner, consumer counselor), as needed

Assist patient to fill out applications for available resources, as needed

Assist patient in long-term care placement planning, as needed

Assist patient to ensure money is in secure place (i.e., bank), as needed

Assist patient in obtaining a burial fund, as appropriate

Encourage family to be involved in financial management, as appropriate

Represent economic needs of patients at multidisciplinary conferences, as needed

Collaborate with community agencies to provide needed services to patient

Background Readings:

Antonello, S.J. (1996). Social skills development: Practical strategies for adolescents and adults with developmental disabilities. Boston: Allyn & Bacon.

Bush, G.W. (1990). Calculating the cost of long-term living: A four-step process. Journal of Head Trauma Rehabilitation 5(1), 47-56.

Horner, M., Rawlins, P., & Giles, K. (1987). How parents of children with chronic conditions perceive their own needs. Maternal Child Nursing 12, 40-43.

Klug, R.M. (1991). Understanding private insurance for funding pediatric home care. Pediatric Nursing 17 (2), 197-198.

McDowell, I., & Newell, C. (1996). Measuring health: A guide to rating scales and questionnaires (2nd ed). New York: Oxford University Press.

Olen, D.R. (1984). Teaching life skills to children: A practical guide for parents and teachers. New York: Paulist Press.

Peterson, D.A. (1983). Facilitating education for older learners. San Francisco: Jossey Bass.

Pfeffer, R.I., Kurosaki, T.T., Harrah, C.H., et al. (1992). Measurement of functional activities in older adults in the community. Journal of Gerontology 37, 323-329.

Schmall, V.L. (1995). Family caregiver education and training: Enhancing self-efficacy. Journal of Case Management 4(4), 156-162.

Social Security Administration Office of Disability (1998). Disability evaluation under social security. SSA Publication No. 64-039. ICN 486600.

Fire-Setting Precautions   6500

Definition: Prevention of fire-setting behaviors

Activities:

Search patient for incendiary materials (e.g., matches/lighters) on admission and each time that patient returns to care environment (e.g., from a pass or a recreational activity)

Search patient environment on routine basis to remove fire-setting materials

Determine appropriate behavioral expectations and consequences, given the patient's level of cognitive functioning and capacity for self-control

Communicate rules, behavioral expectations, and consequences to patient

Communicate risk to other care providers

Provide ongoing surveillance in an environment that is free of fire-setting materials

Provide close supervision, if patient is allowed to smoke

Obtain verbal contract from patient to refrain from fire-setting activity

Encourage the expression of feelings in an appropriate manner

Assist patient, as appropriate, with impulse control training

Increase surveillance and security (e.g., area restriction or seclusion), if risk of fire-setting behavior increases

Background Reading:

Schultz, J.M., & Dark, S.L. (1990). Manual of psychiatric nursing care plans (3rd ed.). Philadelphia: J.B. Lippincott.

First Aid   6240

Definition: Providing initial care for a minor injury

Activities:

Control bleeding

Immobilize the affected body part, as appropriate

Elevate the affected body part

Apply a sling, if appropriate

Cover any open or exposed bony parts

Apply ice to the affected body part, as appropriate

Monitor vital signs, as appropriate

Cool the skin with water in cases of minor burns

Flood with water any tissue exposed to a chemical irritant

Remove the stinger from an insect bite, as appropriate

Remove the tick from the skin, as appropriate

Cleanse and remove secretions from the area around a nonpoisonous snake bite

Cover patient with a blanket, as appropriate

Administer tetanus antitoxin, as appropriate

Instruct to seek further medical care, as appropriate

Coordinate emergency transport, as needed

Background Readings:

Arnold, R.E. (1973). What to do about bites and stings from venomous animals. New York: Macmillan.

Bizjak, G., Elling, B., Gaull, E.S., & Linn, D. (1994). Emergency care (6th ed.). Englewood Cliffs, NJ: Prentice Hall.

Judd, R.L. (1982). The first responder: The critical first minutes. St. Louis: Mosby.

Phillips, C. (1986). Basic life support skills manual: For EMT-As and first responders. Bowie, MD: Brady.

Sorensen, K., & Luckmann, J. (1986). Basic nursing: A psychophysiologic approach (2nd ed.). Philadelphia: W.B. Saunders.

Fiscal Resource Management   8550

Definition: Procuring and directing the use of financial resources to ensure the development and continuation of programs and services

Activities:

Develop a business plan

Develop a cost-benefit analysis of programs and services

Maintain a budget appropriate to the services provided

Identify sources of financing services

Generate grant applications

Identify marketing efforts to enhance programs

Identify "in-kind" (contributed) resources that support programs and services

Analyze economic viability of program based on trends

Implement relevant policies and procedures to secure reimbursement

Maximize potential reimbursement (e.g., program certification, qualified providers)

Use appropriate accounting methods to ensure accurate and designated use of funds

Use appropriate methods to address fiduciary responsibility

Evaluate outcomes and cost-effectiveness of the program

Make appropriate changes in financial management in response to evaluation

Background Readings:

Branowiki, P.A., & Shermont, H. (1997). Maximizing resources: A microanalysis assessment tool. Nursing Management, 28(5), 65-70.

Grimaldi, P.L. (1996). Financial management: Unsettling times for public health care providers. Nursing Management, 27(9), 14, 16-17.

Klainberg, M., Holzemer, S., Leonard, M., & Arnold, J. (1998). Community health nursing: An alliance for health. New York: McGraw-Hill.

Stanhope, M., & Lancaster, J. (1996). Community health nursing: Promoting health of aggregates, families, and individuals. (4th ed.). St. Louis: Mosby.

Storfjell, J.L., & Jessup, S. (1996). Bridging the gap between finances and clinical operations with activity-based cost management. Journal of Nursing Administration, 26(12), 12-17.

Flatulence Reduction 0470

Definition: Prevention of flatus formation and facilitation of passage of excessive gas

Activities:

Teach patient how flatus is produced and methods for alleviation

Teach patient to avoid situations that cause excessive air swallowing, such as chewing gum, drinking carbonated beverages, eating rapidly, sucking through straws, chewing with mouth open, or talking with mouth full

Teach patient to avoid foods that cause flatulence, such as beans, cabbage, radishes, onions, cauliflower, and cucumbers

Discuss use of dairy products

Monitor for bloated feeling, abdominal distension, cramping pains, and excessive passage of gas from the mouth or anus

Monitor bowel sounds

Monitor vital signs

Provide for adequate exercise (e.g., ambulate)

Insert lubricated nasogastric tube or rectal tube into the rectum, as appropriate; tape in place; and insert distal end of tube into a receptacle

Administer a laxative, suppository, or enema, as appropriate

Monitor side effects of medication administration

Limit oral intake, if lower gastrointestinal system is inactive

Position on left side with knees flexed, as appropriate

Offer antiflatulence medications, as appropriate

Background Readings:

Craven, R.F. & Hirnle, C.J. (2000) Fundamentals of nursing: Human health and function (3rd ed.) (pp. 1086, 1098, 1102). Philadelphia: Lippincott.

Levy, D.J., & Rosenthal, W.S. (1985). Gastrointestinal gas. Hospital Medicine, 21(4), 13, 17-19, 22-25.

Ribakove, B.M. (1982). Gas . . . flatus. Health, 14(12), 48-49.

Sorensen, K., & Luckmann, J. (1986). Basic nursing: A psychophysiologic approach (2nd ed.). Philadelphia: W.B. Saunders.

Vaughn, J.B., & Nemcek, M.A. (1986). Postoperative flatulence: Causes and remedies. Today's OR Nurse, 8(10), 19-23.

F

Fluid/Electrolyte Management 2080

Definition: Regulation and prevention of complications from altered fluid and/or electrolyte levels

Activities:

Monitor for abnormal serum electrolyte levels, as available

Obtain laboratory specimens for monitoring of altered fluid or electrolyte levels (e.g., hematocrit, BUN, protein, sodium, and potassium levels), as appropriate

Weigh patient daily and monitor trends

Restrict free water intake in the presence of dilutional hyponatremia with serum sodium level below 130 mEq/L

Give fluids, as appropriate

Promote oral intake (e.g., provide oral fluids that are the patient's preference, place in easy reach, provide a straw, and provide fresh water), as appropriate

Administer prescribed nasogastric replacement based on output, as appropriate

Administer fiber as prescribed for the tube-fed patient to reduce fluid and electrolyte loss through diarrhea

Minimize the number of ice chips consumed or amount of oral intake by patients with gastric tubes connected to suction

Irrigate nasogastric tubes with normal saline

Provide free water with tube feedings, as appropriate

Set an appropriate intravenous infusion (or blood transfusion) flow rate

Monitor laboratory results relevant to fluid balance (e.g., hematocrit, BUN, albumin, total protein, serum osmolality, and urine specific gravity levels)

Monitor laboratory results relevant to fluid retention (e.g., increased specific gravity, increased BUN, decreased hematocrit, and increased urine osmolality levels)

Monitor hemodynamic status, including CVP, MAP, PAP, and PCWP levels, if available

Keep an accurate record of intake and output

Monitor for signs and symptoms of fluid retention

Institute fluid restriction, as appropriate

Monitor vital signs, as appropriate

Correct preoperative dehydration, as appropriate

Maintain intravenous solution containing electrolyte(s) at constant flow rate, as appropriate

Monitor patient's response to prescribed electrolyte therapy

Monitor for manifestations of electrolyte imbalance

Provide prescribed diet appropriate for specific fluid or electrolyte imbalance (e.g., low-sodium, fluid-restricted, renal, and no added salt)

Monitor for side effects of prescribed supplemental electrolytes (e.g., GI irritation)

Assess patient's buccal membranes, sclera, and skin for indications of altered fluid and electrolyte balance (e.g., dryness, cyanosis, and jaundice)

Consult physician if signs and symptoms of fluid and/or electrolyte imbalance persist or worsen

Administer prescribed supplemental electrolytes, as appropriate

Administer prescribed electrolyte binding/excreting resins, as appropriate

Institute measures to control excessive electrolyte loss (e.g., by resting the gut, changing type of diuretic, or administering antipyretics), as appropriate

Institute measures to rest the bowel (e.g., restrict food or fluid intake and decrease intake of milk products), if appropriate

Follow quick-acting glucose with long-acting carbohydrates and proteins for management of acute hypoglycemia, as appropriate

Prepare patient for dialysis (e.g., assist with catheter placement for dialysis), as appropriate

Monitor for fluid loss (e.g., bleeding, vomiting, diarrhea, perspiration, and tachypnea)

Promote a positive body image and self-esteem, if concerns are expressed as a result of excessive fluid retention, if appropriate

F

Background Readings:

Askanazi, J., Starker, P., & Wissman, C. (1986). Fluid and electrolyte management in critical care. Boston: Butterworths.

Baer, C.L. (1993). Fluid and electrolyte balance. In M.R. Kinney, D.R. Packa, & S.B. Dunbar (Eds.), AACN's clinical reference for critical-care nursing (pp. 173-208). St. Louis: Mosby.

Chan, J., & Gill, J. (1990). Kidney electrolyte disorders. New York: Churchill Livingstone.

Cullen, L.M. (1992). Interventions related to fluid and electrolyte balance. In G.M. Bulechek & J.C. McCloskey (Eds.), Symposium on Nursing Interventions. Nursing Clinics of North America, 27(2), 569-598.

Horne, M., & Swearingen, P. (1997). Pocket guide to fluids and electrolytes (3rd ed.). St. Louis: Mosby.

Kokko, J., & Tannen, R. (1990). Fluids and electrolytes (2nd ed.). Philadelphia: W.B. Saunders.

Melillo, K.D. (1993). Interpretation of laboratory values in older adults. Nurse Practitioner, 18(7), 59-67.

Stark, J. (1991). The renal system. In J. Alspach (Ed.), American Association of Critical-Care Nurses core curriculum for critical-care nursing (4th ed.) (pp. 472-608). Philadelphia: W.B. Saunders.

F

Fluid Management   4120

Definition: Promotion of fluid balance and prevention of complications resulting from abnormal or undesired fluid levels

Activities:

Weigh patient daily and monitor trends

Count or weigh diapers, as appropriate

Maintain accurate intake and output record

Insert urinary catheter, if appropriate

Monitor hydration status (e.g., moist mucous membranes, adequacy of pulses, and orthostatic blood pressure), as appropriate

Monitor laboratory results relevant to fluid retention (e.g., increased specific gravity, increased BUN, decreased hematocrit, and increased urine osmolality levels)

Monitor hemodynamic status, including CVP, MAP, PAP, and PCWP, if available

Monitor vital signs, as appropriate

Monitor for indications of fluid overload/retention (e.g., crackles, elevated CVP or pulmonary capillary wedge pressure, edema, neck vein distention, and ascites), as appropriate

Monitor patient's weight change before and after dialysis, if appropriate

Assess location and extent of edema, if present

Monitor food/fluid ingested and calculate daily caloric intake, as appropriate

Administer IV therapy, as prescribed

Monitor nutrition status

Give fluids, as appropriate

Administer prescribed diuretics, as appropriate

Administer IV fluids at room temperature

Promote oral intake (e.g., provide a drinking straw, offer fluids between meals, change ice water routinely, make freezer pops using child's favorite juice, cut gelatin into fun squares, use small medicine cups), as appropriate

Instruct patient on nothing by mouth (NPO) status, as appropriate

Administer prescribed nasogastric replacement based on output, as appropriate

Distribute the fluid intake over 24 hours, as appropriate

Encourage significant other to assist patient with feedings, as appropriate

Offer snacks (e.g., frequent drinks and fresh fruits/fruit juice), as appropriate

Restrict free water intake in the presence of dilutional hyponatremia with serum sodium level below 130 mEq/L

Monitor patient's response to prescribed electrolyte therapy

Consult physician, if signs and symptoms of fluid volume excess persist or worsen

Arrange availability of blood products for transfusion, if necessary

Prepare for administration of blood products (e.g., check blood with patient identification and prepare infusion setup), as appropriate

Administer blood products (e.g., platelets and fresh frozen plasma), as appropriate

Background Readings:

Askanazi, J., Starker, P., & Wissman, C. (1986). Fluid and electrolyte management in critical care. Boston: Butterworths.

Baer, C.L. (1993). Fluid and electrolyte balance. In M.R. Kinney, D.R. Packa, & S.B. Dunbar (Eds.), AACN's clinical reference for critical-care nursing (pp. 173-208). St. Louis: Mosby.

Cullen, L.M. (1992). Interventions related to fluid and electrolyte balance. In G.M. Bulechek & J.C. McCloskey (Eds.), Symposium on Nursing Interventions. Nursing Clinics of North America, 27(2), 569-598.

Horne, M., & Swearingen, P. (1997). Pocket guide to fluids and electrolytes (3rd ed.). St. Louis: Mosby.

Kokko, J., & Tannen, R. (1990). Fluids and electrolytes (2nd ed.). Philadelphia: W.B. Saunders.

Stark, J. (1991). The renal system. In J. Alspach (Ed.), American Association of Critical-Care Nurses core curriculum for critical-care nursing (4th ed.) (pp. 472-608). Philadelphia: W.B. Saunders.

Wong, D.L. (1995). Whaley and Wong's nursing care of infants and children (5th ed.). St. Louis: Mosby.

F

Fluid Monitoring 4130

Definition: Collection and analysis of patient data to regulate fluid balance

Activities:

Determine history of amount and type of fluid intake and elimination habits

Determine possible risk factors for fluid imbalance (e.g., hyperthermia, diuretic therapy, renal pathologies, cardiac failure, diaphoresis, liver dysfunction, strenuous exercise, heat exposure, infection, postoperative state, polyuria, vomiting, and diarrhea)

Monitor weight

Monitor intake and output

Monitor serum and urine electrolyte values, as appropriate

Monitor serum albumin and total protein levels

Monitor serum and urine osmolality levels

Monitor blood pressure, heart rate, and respiratory status

Monitor orthostatic blood pressure and change in cardiac rhythm, as appropriate

Monitor invasive hemodynamic parameters, as appropriate

Keep an accurate record of intake and output

Monitor mucous membranes, skin turgor, and thirst

Monitor color, quantity, and specific gravity of urine

Monitor for distended neck veins, crackles in the lungs, peripheral edema, and weight gain

Monitor venous access device, as appropriate

Monitor for signs and symptoms of ascites

Note presence or absence of vertigo on rising

Administer fluids, as appropriate

Restrict and allocate fluid intake, as appropriate

Maintain prescribed intravenous flow rate

Administer pharmacological agents to increase urinary output, as appropriate

Administer dialysis, as appropriate, noting patient's response

Background Readings:

Reed, G.M. & Sheppard, V.F. (1971). Regulation of fluid and electrolyte balance. Philadelphia: W.B. Saunders.

Titler, M.G. (1992). Interventions related to surveillance. In G.M. Bulechek & J.C. McCloskey (Eds.), Symposium on Nursing Interventions. Nursing Clinics of North America, 27(2), 495-516.

Fluid Resuscitation   **4140**

Definition: Administering prescribed intravenous fluids rapidly

Activities:

Obtain and maintain a large-bore IV

Collaborate with physicians to ensure administration of both crystalloids (e.g., normal saline and lactated Ringer's solution) and colloids (e.g., Hesban, and Plasmanate), as appropriate

Administer IV fluids, as prescribed

Obtain blood specimens for cross-matching, as appropriate

Administer blood products, as prescribed

Monitor hemodynamic response

Monitor oxygen status

Monitor for fluid overload

Monitor output of various body fluids (e.g., urine and nasogastric and chest tube drainage)

Monitor BUN, creatine, total protein, and albumin levels

Monitor for pulmonary edema and third spacing

Background Readings:

Thelan, L.A., & Urden, L.D. (1998). Critical care nursing: Diagnosis and management (3rd ed.). St. Louis: Mosby.

Thompson, J.M., McFarland, G.K., Hirsch, J.E., & Tucker, S.M. (1998). Mosby's clinical nursing (4th ed.). St. Louis: Mosby.

F

Foot Care 1660

Definition: Cleansing and inspecting the feet for the purposes of relaxation, cleanliness, and healthy skin

Activities:

Inspect skin for irritation, cracking, lesions, corns, calluses, deformities, or edema

Inspect patient's shoes for proper fit

Administer foot soaks, as needed

Dry carefully between toes

Apply lotion

Clean nails

Apply moisture-absorbing powder, as indicated

Discuss with patient usual foot care routine

Instruct patient/family on the importance of foot care

Offer positive feedback about self-care foot activities

Monitor patient's gait and weight distribution on feet

Monitor cleanliness and general condition of shoes and stockings

Instruct patient to inspect inside of shoes for rough areas

Monitor hydration level of feet

Monitor for arterial insufficiency in lower legs

Monitor legs and feet for edema

Instruct patient to monitor temperature of feet using the back of the hand

Instruct patient in the importance of inspection, especially when sensation is diminished

Cut normal-thickness toenails when soft, using a toenail clipper and using the curve of the toe as a guide

Refer to podiatrist for trimming of thickened nails, as appropriate

Inspect nails for thickness, discoloration

Teach patient how to prepare and trim nails

Background Readings:

Christensen, M.H., Funnell, M.M., Ehrlich, M.R., et al (1991). How to care for the diabetic foot. American Journal of Nursing, 91(3), 50-57.

Evanski, P.M. (1991). Easing the pain of common foot problems. Patient Care, 25(2), 38-44, 47-50, 52-54.

Harley, J.R. (1993). Preventing diabetic foot disease. Nurse Practitioner, 18(10), 37-44.

Maier, T. (1991). The foot and foot wear. Nursing Clinics of North America, 26(1), 223-231.

Perry, A.G., & Potter, P.A. (1998). Clinical nursing skills and techniques. (4th ed.) St. Louis: Mosby.

Smith, S., & Duell, D. (1992). Clinical nursing skills (3rd ed.). Los Altos, CA: National Nursing Review.

Forgiveness Facilitation   5280

Definition: Assisting an individual to forgive and/or experience forgiveness in relationship with self, others, and higher power

Activities:

Identify patient's beliefs that may hinder/help in "letting go" of an issue

Identify source of guilt and/or anger, when possible

Listen empathetically without moralizing or offering platitudes

Explore forgiveness as a process

Help the patient explore feelings of anger, bitterness, and resentment

Use presence, touch, and empathy, as appropriate, to facilitate the process

Explore possibilities of making amends and reconciliation with self, others, and/or higher power

Assist the patient to examine the health and healing dimension of forgiveness

Assist patient to overcome blocks to healing by using spiritual practices (e.g. prayers of praise, guidance, and discernment, and thanksgiving; healing touch; and visualization of healing), as appropriate.

Teach the art of emotional release and relaxation

Assist client to seek out arbitrator (objective party) to facilitate process of individual or group concern

Invite use of faith tradition rituals, as appropriate (e.g., anointing, confession, reconciliation)

Communicate God's/higher power's or inner self's forgiveness through prayer, scripture, other readings, as appropriate

Communicate acceptance for the individual's level of progress

Background Readings:

Bakken, K. L. (1986). The call to wholeness: Health as a spiritual journey. New York: Crossroad.

Fish, S., & Shelly, J. (1983). Spiritual care: The nurse's role. Downers Grove, IL: Intervarsity Press.

Hopkins, E., Woods, Z., Kelley, R., Bentley, K., & Murphy, J. (1995). Working with groups on spiritual themes: Structured exercise in healing. Volume 2, p. 123-125.

Augsburge, D. (1983). Caring enough to forgive. Ventura, CA: Regal Books, a division of GL Publications.

Gastrointestinal Intubation

Definition: Insertion of a tube into the gastrointestinal tract

Activities:

Select type and size of nasogastric tube to insert, considering use and rationale for insertion

Explain to the patient and family the rationale for using a gastrointestinal tube

Insert the tube according to agency protocol

Provide the patient with a glass of water or ice chips to swallow during insertion, as appropriate

Position patient on right side to facilitate movement of the tube into the duodenum, as appropriate

Administer medication to increase peristalsis, as appropriate

Determine correct placement of the tube by observing for signs and symptoms of tracheal entry, checking color and/or pH level of aspirate, inspecting oral cavity, and/or noting placement on x-ray film, if appropriate

Background Readings:

Boyes, R.J., & Kruse, J.A. (1992). Nasogastric and nasoenteric intubation. Critical Care Clinics, 8(4), 865-878.

Metheny, N. (1988). Measures to test placement of nasogastric and nasointestinal feeding tubes: A review. Nursing Research, 37, 324-329.

Metheny, N. (1993). Minimizing respiratory complications of nasoenteric tube feedings: State of the science. Heart & Lung 22(3), 213-223.

Rakel, B.A., Titler, M., Goode, C., et al. (1994). Nasogastric and nasointestinal feeding tube placement: An integrated review of research. AACN Clinical Issues in Critical Care Nursing, 5(2), 194-206.

Thelan, L.A., & Urden, L.D. (1993). Critical care nursing: Diagnosis and management (2nd ed.). St. Louis: Mosby.

Thompson, J.M., McFarland, G.K., Hirsch, J.E., et al. (1998). Mosby's clinical nursing (4th ed.). St. Louis: Mosby.

G

Genetic Counseling   5242

Definition: Use of an interactive helping process focusing on assisting an individual, family, or group, manifesting or at risk for developing or transmitting a birth defect or genetic condition, to cope

Activities:

Provide privacy and ensure confidentiality

Establish a therapeutic relationship based on trust and respect

Determine the patient's purpose, goals, and agenda for the genetic counseling session

Determine knowledge base, myths, perceptions, and misperceptions related to a birth defect or genetic condition

Determine presence and quality of family support, other support systems, and previous coping skills

Provide estimates of patient's risk based upon phenotype (patient characteristics), family history (pedigree analysis), calculated risk information, or genotype (genetic testing results)

Provide estimates of occurrence or recurrence risk for patient and at-risk family members

Provide information on the natural history of the disease or condition, treatment and/or management strategies, and prevention strategies, if known

Provide information about the risks, benefits, and limitations of treatment/management options, as well as options for dealing with recurrence risk in a nondirective manner

Provide decision-making support as patients consider their options

Prioritize areas of risk reduction in collaboration with the individual, family, or group

Monitor response when patient learns about own genetic risk factors

Allow expression of feelings

Support patient's coping process

Institute crisis support measures as needed

Provide referral to genetic health care specialists, as necessary

Provide referral to community resources, including genetic support groups, as needed

Provide patient a written summary of genetic counseling session, as indicated

Background Readings:

Cohen, F.L. (1984). Clinical genetics in nursing practice. Philadelphia: J.B. Lippincott.

Forsman, I. (1994). Evolution of the nursing role in genetics. Journal of Obstetric, Gynecologic, and Neonatal Nursing, 23(6), 481-486.

Scanlon, C., & Fibison, W. (1995). Managing genetic information: Implications for nursing practice. Washington, DC: American Nurses Association.

Williams, J.K. (1993). New genetic discoveries increase counseling opportunities. American Journal of Maternal Child Nursing, 18(4), 218-222.

G

Grief Work Facilitation   5290

Definition: Assistance with the resolution of a significant loss

Activities:

Identify the loss

Assist the patient to identify the nature of the attachment to the lost object or person

Assist the patient to identify the initial reaction to the loss

Encourage expression of feelings about the loss

Listen to expressions of grief

Encourage discussion of previous loss experiences

Encourage the patient to verbalize memories of the loss, both past and current

Make empathetic statements about grief

Encourage identification of greatest fears concerning the loss

Instruct in phases of the grieving process, as appropriate

Support progression through personal grieving stages

Include significant others in discussions and decisions, as appropriate

Assist patient to identify personal coping strategies

Encourage patient to implement cultural, religious, and social customs associated with the loss

Communicate acceptance of discussing loss

Answer children's questions associated with the loss

Use clear words, such as *dead* or *died*, rather than euphemisms

Encourage children to discuss feelings

Encourage expression of feelings in ways comfortable to the child, such as writing, drawing, or playing

Assist the child to clarify misconceptions

Identify sources of community support

Support efforts to resolve previous conflict, as appropriate

Reinforce progress made in the grieving process

Assist in identifying modifications needed in lifestyle

Background Readings:

Beck, C.K., Rawlins, R.P., & Williams, S.R. (1988). Mental health-psychiatric nursing. St. Louis: Mosby.

Craven, R.F., & Hirnle, C.J. (2000) Fundamentals of nursing: Human health and function (3rd ed.) (pp. 1275-1291). Philadelphia: Lippincott.

Collison, C., & Miller, S. (1987). Using images of the future in grief work. Image: Journal of Nursing Scholarship, 19(1), 9-11.

Gifford, B.J., & Cleary, B.B. (1990). Supporting the bereaved. American Journal of Nursing, 90(2), 48-53.

Hampe, S.D. (1975). Needs of a grieving spouse in a hospital setting. Nursing Research, 24(2), 113-119.

Smith, S., & Duell, D. (1992). Clinical nursing skills (3rd ed.). Los Altos, CA: National Nursing Review.

Sorensen, K., & Luckmann, J. (1986). Basic nursing: A psychophysiologic approach (2nd ed.). Philadelphia: W.B. Saunders.

Whiting, G., & Buckwalter, K. (1991). Dysfunctional grieving. In M. Maas, K. Buckwalter, & M. Hardy (Eds.), Nursing diagnoses and interventions for the elderly (pp. 505-518). Redwood City, CA: Addison-Wesley.

Grief Work Facilitation: Perinatal Death 5294

Definition: Assistance with the resolution of a perinatal loss

Activities:

Encourage participation in decisions about discontinuing life support

Assist in keeping infant alive until parents arrive

Baptize the infant, as appropriate

Encourage parents in holding infant while infant dies, as appropriate

Determine how and when the fetal or infant death was diagnosed

Discuss plans that have been made (e.g., burial, funeral, and infant name)

Discuss decisions that will need to be made about funeral arrangements, autopsy, genetic counseling, and family participation

Describe mementos that will be obtained, including footprints, handprints, pictures, caps, gowns, blankets, diapers, and blood pressure cuffs, as appropriate

Discuss available support groups, as appropriate

Discuss differences between male and female patterns of grieving, as appropriate

Obtain infant footprints, handprints, length, and weight, as needed

Prepare infant for viewing by bathing and dressing, including parents in activities as appropriate

Encourage family members to view and hold infant for as long as desired

Discuss appearance of infant based on gestational age and length of demise

Focus on normal features of infant, while sensitively discussing anomalies

Encourage family time alone with infant, as desired

Provide referrals to chaplain, social service, grief counselor, and genetic counselor, as appropriate

Create keepsakes and present to family before discharge, as appropriate

Discuss characteristics of normal and abnormal grieving, including triggers that precipitate feelings of sadness

Notify laboratory or funeral home, as appropriate, for disposition of body

Transfer infant to morgue or prepare body to be transported by family to funeral home

Background Readings:

Carr, D., & Knupp, S.F. (1985). Grief and perinatal loss. A community hospital approach to support. Journal of Obstetric, Gynecologic, and Neonatal Nursing, 14(2), 130-139.

Davis, D.L., Stewart, M., & Harmon, R.J. (1988). Perinatal loss: Providing emotional support for bereaved parents. Birth, 15(4), 242-246.

Gilbert, E.S., & Harmon, J.S. (1998). Manual of high risk pregnancy and delivery. (2nd ed.). St. Louis: Mosby.

Klingbeil, C.G. (1986). Extended nursing care after a perinatal loss: Theoretical implications. Neonatal Network, 5(3), 21-28.

Page-Lieberman, J., & Hughes, C.B. (1990). How fathers perceive perinatal death. MCN, American Journal of Maternal Child Nursing, 15, 320-323.

Primeau, M.R., & Recht, C.K. (1994). Professional bereavement photographs: One aspect of a perinatal bereavement program. Journal of Obstetric, Gynecologic, and Neonatal Nursing, 23(1), 22-25.

York, C.R., & Stichler, J.F. (1985). Cultural grief expressions following infant death. Dimensions of Critical Care Nursing, 4(2), 120-127.

Guilt Work Facilitation

5300

Definition: Helping another to cope with painful feelings of responsibility, actual or perceived

Activities:

Guide patient/family in identifying painful feelings of guilt

Help patient/family identify and examine the situations in which these feelings are experienced or generated

Assist patient/family members to identify their behaviors in the guilt situation

Help family accept that guilt is a universal reaction to catastrophic illness in children

Use reality testing to help the patient/family identify possible irrational beliefs

Help patient/family to identify destructive displacement of feelings onto other individuals sharing responsibility in the situation

Facilitate discussion of the impact of the situation on family relationships

Facilitate genetic counseling, as appropriate

Facilitate spiritual support, as appropriate

Background Readings:

Beck, C.K., Rawlins, R.P., & Williams, S.R. (1988). Mental health-psychiatric nursing. St. Louis: Mosby.
Grainger, R.D. (1991). Dealing with feelings: Guilt and shame. American Journal of Nursing, 91(6), 12.
Solursh, D.S. (1990). The family of the trauma victim. Nursing Clinics of North America, 25(1), 155-162.
Stuart, G.W., & Sundeen, S.J. (1998). Principles and practice of psychiatric nursing (6th ed.). St. Louis: Mosby.
Whaley, L.F., & Wong, D.L. (1998). Nursing care of infants and children (6th ed.). St. Louis: Mosby.

Hair Care   1670

Definition: Promotion of neat, clean, attractive hair

Activities:

Wash hair, as needed and desired

Dry hair with hair dryer

Brush/comb hair daily or more frequently, as needed

Inspect hair daily

Monitor scalp daily

Apply mineral oil to scalp, as needed

Braid or otherwise arrange hair as patient wishes

Arrange for barber/hair dresser to cut hair, as needed

Use hair care products of patient's preference, as available

H

Background Readings:

Patrick, M.L., Woods, S.L., Craven, R.F., Rokosky, J.S., & Bruno, P.M. (1991). Medical surgical nursing pathophysiological concepts (2nd ed.). Philadelphia: J.B. Lippincott.

Titler, M.G., Pettit, D., Bulechek, G.M., McCloskey, J.C., Craft, M.J., Cohen, M.Z., Crossley, J.D., Denehy, J.A., Glick, O.J., Kruckeberg, T.W., Maas, M.L., Prophet, C.M., & Tripp-Reimer, T. (1991). Classification of nursing interventions for care of the integument. Nursing Diagnosis, 2(2), 45-56.

Hallucination Management 6510

Definition: Promoting the safety, comfort, and reality orientation of a patient experiencing hallucinations

Activities:

Establish a trusting, interpersonal relationship with the patient

Monitor and regulate the level of activity and stimulation in the environment

Maintain a safe environment

Provide appropriate level of surveillance/supervision to monitor patient

Record patient behaviors that indicate hallucinations

Maintain a consistent routine

Assign consistent caregivers on a daily basis

Promote clear and open communication

Provide patient with opportunities to discuss hallucinations

Encourage patient to express feelings appropriately

Refocus patient to topic, if patient's communication is inappropriate to circumstances

Monitor hallucinations for presence of content that is violent or self-harmful

Encourage patient to develop control/responsibility over own behavior, if ability allows

Encourage patient to discuss feelings and impulses, rather than acting on them

Encourage patient to validate hallucinations with trusted others (e.g., reality testing)

Point out, if asked, that you are not experiencing the same stimuli

Avoid arguing with patient about the validity of the hallucinations

Focus discussion upon the underlying feelings, rather than the content of the hallucinations (e.g., "It appears as if you are feeling frightened.")

Provide antipsychotic and antianxiety medications on a routine and PRN basis

Provide medication teaching to patient and significant others

Monitor patient for medication side effects and desired therapeutic effects

Provide for safety and comfort of patient and others when patient is unable to control behavior (e.g., limit setting, area restriction, physical restraint, and seclusion)

Discontinue or decrease medications (after consulting with prescribing caregiver) that may be causing hallucinations

Provide illness teaching to patient/significant others if hallucinations are illness based (e.g., delirium, schizophrenia, and depression)

Educate family and significant others about ways to deal with patient who is experiencing hallucinations

Monitor self-care ability

Assist with self-care, as needed

Monitor physical status of patient (e.g., body weight, hydration, and soles of feet in patient who paces)

Provide for adequate rest and nutrition

Involve patient in reality-based activities that may distract from the hallucinations (e.g., listening to music)

Background Readings:

Eklund, E.S. (1991). Perception/cognition, altered. In G.K. McFarland & M.D. Thomas (Eds.), Psychiatric mental health nursing. Application to the nursing process (pp. 332-357). Philadelphia: J.B. Lippincott.

Moller, M.D. (1989). Understanding and communicating with a person who is hallucinating. [Videotape]. Omaha, NE: NurSeminars.

Norris, J. (1987). Schizophrenia and schizophreniform disorders. In J. Norris, M. Kunes-Cornell, S. Stockard, P.M. Ehrhart, & G.R. Newton (Eds.), Mental health-psychiatric nursing. A continuum of care (pp. 785-811). New York: John Wiley & Sons.

Varcarolis, E.M. (2000) Psychiatric nursing clinical guide (pp. 230-232). Philadelphia: W.B. Saunders Company.

H

Health Care Information Exchange 7960

Definition: Providing patient care information to other health professionals

Activities:

Identify referring nurse and location

Identify essential demographic data

Describe pertinent health history

Identify current nursing and medical diagnoses

Identify resolved nursing and medical diagnoses, as appropriate

Describe plan of care, including diet, medications, and exercise

Describe nursing interventions being implemented

Identify equipment and supplies necessary for care

Summarize progress of patient toward goals

Identify anticipated date of discharge or transfer

Identify planned return appointment for follow-up care

Describe role of family in continuing care

Identify capabilities of patient and family in implementing care after discharge

Identify other agencies providing care

Request information from health professionals in other agencies

Coordinate care with other health professionals

Discuss patient's strengths and resources

Share concerns of patient or family with other health care providers

Share information from other health professionals with patient and family, as appropriate

Background Readings:

Jenkins, C.A., Schullz, M., Hanson, J., Bruera. E. (2000). Demographic, symptom and medication profiles of cancer patients seen by a palliative care consult team in a tertiary referral hospital. Journal of Pain & Symptom Management 19(3), 174-184.

Job, T. (1999). A system for determining the priority of referrals within a multidisciplinary community mental health team. British Journal of Occupation Therapy 62(11), 486-490.

Kron, T., & Gray, A. (1987). The management of patient care. Putting leadership skills to work (6th ed.). Philadelphia: W.B. Saunders.

Smith, F.A. (2000). The function of consumer health information centers in hospitals. Medical Library Association News 327(Jun-Jul), 23.

Summerton, H. (1998). Clinical management. Discharge planning: Establishing an effective coordination team. British Journal of Nursing 7(20), 1263-7.

Health Education   5510

Definition: Developing and providing instruction and learning experiences to facilitate voluntary adaptation of behavior conducive to health in individuals, families, groups, or communities

Activities:

Target high-risk groups and age ranges that would benefit most from health education

Target needs identified in Healthy People 2000: National Health Promotion and Disease Prevention Objectives or other local, state, and national needs

Identify internal or external factors that may enhance or reduce motivation for healthy behavior

Determine personal context and social-cultural history of individual, family, or community health behavior

Determine current health knowledge and lifestyle behaviors of individual, family, or target group

Assist individuals, families, and communities in clarifying health beliefs and values

Identify characteristics of target population that affect selection of learning strategies

Prioritize identified learner needs based on client preference, skills of nurse, resources available, and likelihood of successful goal attainment

Formulate objectives for health education program

Identify resources (e.g., personnel, space, equipment, money) needed to conduct program

Consider accessibility, consumer preference, and cost in program planning

Strategically place attractive advertising to capture attention of target audience

Avoid use of fear or scare techniques as strategy to motivate people to change health or lifestyle behaviors

Emphasize immediate or short-term positive health benefits to be received by positive lifestyle behaviors rather than long-term benefits or negative effects of noncompliance

Incorporate strategies to enhance the self-esteem of target audience

Develop educational materials written at a reading level appropriate to target audience

Teach strategies that can be used to resist unhealthy behavior or risk taking rather than give advice to avoid or change behavior

Keep presentation focused, short, and beginning and ending on main point

Use group presentations to provide support and lessen threat to learners experiencing similar problems or concerns, as appropriate

Use peer leaders, teachers, and support groups in implementing programs to groups less likely to listen to health professionals or adults (e.g., adolescents), as appropriate

Use lectures to convey the maximum amount of information when appropriate

Use group discussions and role-playing to influence health beliefs, attitudes, and values

Use demonstrations/return demonstrations, learner participation, and manipulation of materials when teaching psychomotor skills

Use computer-assisted instruction, television, interactive video, and other technologies to convey information

Use teleconferencing, telecommunications, and computer technologies for distance learning

Involve individuals, families, and groups in planning and implementing plans for lifestyle or health behavior modification

Determine family, peer, and community support for behavior conducive to health

Continued

Activities:—cont'd

Utilize social and family support systems to enhance effectiveness of lifestyle or heath behavior modification

Emphasize importance of healthy patterns of eating, sleeping, exercising, etc. to individuals, families, and groups who model these values and behaviors to others, particularly children

Use variety of strategies and intervention points in educational program

Plan long-term follow-up to reinforce health behavior or lifestyle adaptations

Design and implement strategies to measure client outcomes at regular intervals during and after completion of program

Design and implement strategies to measure program and cost-effectiveness of education, using these data to improve the effectiveness of subsequent programs

Influence development of policy that guarantees health education as an employee benefit

Encourage policy whereby insurance companies give consideration for premium reductions or benefits for healthful lifestyle practices

H

Background Readings:

APHA Technical Report. (1987). Criteria for the development of health promotion and education programs. American Journal of Public Health, 77 (1), 89-92.

Bastable, S.B. (2003). Nurse as educator: Principles of teaching and learning for nursing practice. Boston: Jones and Bartlett Publishers.

Clark, M.J. (1992). Nursing in the community. The health education process (pp. 126-141). Norfolk, CT: Appleton & Lange.

Damrosch, S. (1991). General strategies for motivating people to change their behavior. Nursing Clinics of North America, 26(4), 833-843.

Department of Health and Human Services. (1991). Healthy People 2000: National health promotion and disease prevention objectives (DHHS Publication No. PHS 91-50213). Washington, DC. U.S. Government Printing Office.

Green, L.W., & Johnson, K.W. (1983). Health education and health promotion. In D. Mechanic (Ed.), Handbook of health, health care, and the health professional (pp. 744-765). New York: The Free Press, Macmillan Publishing Co.

Somas Job, R.F. (1988). Effective and ineffective use of fear in health promotion campaigns. American Journal of Public Health, 78(2), 163-167.

Pahnos, M.L. (1992). The continuing challenge of multicultural health education. Journal of School Health 62(1), 24-26.

Health Policy Monitoring   7970

Definition: Surveillance and influence of government and organization regulations, rules, and standards that affect nursing systems and practices to ensure quality care of patients

Activities:

Review proposed policies and standards in organizational, professional, and governmental literature and in the popular media

Assess implications and requirements of proposed policies and standards for quality patient care

Compare requirements of policies and standards with current practices

Assess negative and positive effects of health policies and standards on nursing practice, patient, and cost outcomes

Identify and resolve discrepancies between health policies and standards and current nursing practice

Acquaint policy makers with implications of current and proposed policies and standards for patient welfare

Lobby policy makers to make changes in health policies and standards to benefit patients

Testify in organization, profession, and public forums to influence the formulation of health policies and standards that benefit patients

Assist consumers of health care to be informed of current and proposed changes in health policies and standards and the implications for health outcomes

Background Readings:

Dean-Barr, S.L. (1994). Standards and guidelines: How do they assure quality? In J. McCloskey & H.K. Grace (Eds.), Current issues in nursing (4th ed.). St. Louis: Mosby.

Donahue, M. (1985). Advocacy. In G.M. Bulechek & J.C. McCloskey (Eds.), Nursing interventions: Treatments for nursing diagnoses (pp. 338-351). Philadelphia: W.B. Saunders.

Maas, M., & Mulford, C. (1989). Structural adaptation of organizations: Issues and strategies for nurse executives (pp. 3-40). Redwood City, CA: Addison-Wesley.

Mason, D.J., Talbott, S.W., & Leavitt, J.K. (1993). Policy and politics for nurses. Philadelphia: W.B. Saunders.

Specht, J. (1992). Implications of the ethics and economics of health care rationing for nursing administration. In M. Johnson (Ed.), Economic myths and realities: Doing more with no more. Series on Nursing Administration, Vol. 4 (pp. 19-36).

Warner, D.M., Holloway, D.C., & Grazier, K.L. (1984). Decision making and control for health administration. Ann Arbor, MI: Health Administration Press.

H

Health Screening 6520

Definition: Detecting health risks or problems by means of history, examination, and other procedures

Activities:

Determine target population for health screening

Advertise health-screening services to increase public awareness

Provide easy access to screening services (e.g., time and place)

Schedule appointments to enhance efficiency and individualized care

Use valid, reliable health-screening instruments

Instruct on rationale and purpose of health screenings and self-monitoring

Obtain informed consent for health-screening procedures, as appropriate

Provide for privacy and confidentiality

Provide for comfort during screening procedures

Obtain health history, as appropriate, including description of health habits, risk factors, and medications

Obtain family health history, as appropriate

Perform physical assessment, as appropriate

Measure blood pressure, height, weight, percent body fat, cholesterol and blood sugar levels, and perform urinalysis, as appropriate

Perform (or refer for) Pap smear, mammography, prostate check, EKG, testicular examination, and vision check, as appropriate

Obtain specimens for analysis

Complete appropriate Department of Health or other records for monitoring abnormal results, such as high blood pressure

Provide appropriate self-monitoring information during screening

Provide results of health screenings to patient

Inform patient of limitations and margin of error of specific screening tests

Counsel patient who has abnormal findings about treatment alternatives or need for further evaluation

Refer patient to other health care providers, as necessary

Provide follow-up contact for patient with abnormal findings

Background Readings:

Ahlbom, A., & Norell, S. (1990). Introduction to modern epidemiology (2nd ed.). Chestnut Hill, MA: Epidemiology Resources.

Aspholm, D. (1991). Primary interventions: A rewarding challenge in nursing. Urologic Nursing, 11(4), 21-23.

Ferren-Carter, K. (1991). The health fair as an effective health promotion strategy. AAOHN Journal, 39(11), 513-516.

Goeppinger, J., & Labuhn, K.T. (1992). Self-health care through risk appraisal and reduction. In M. Stanhope & J. Lancaster (Eds.), Community health nursing (3rd ed.) (pp. 578-591). St. Louis: Mosby.

Hamwi, D.A. (1990). Screening mammography. Increasing the effort toward breast cancer detection. Nurse Practitioner, 15(12), 27-32.

Hornsey, J. (1991). Screening by program. Occupational Health, 43(5), 150-151.

Lange, B.A. (1991) Implementation of a screening program for carcinoma of the prostate. Urologic Nursing, 11(4), 24-27.

Leatherman, J., & Davidhizar, R. (1992). Health screening on a college campus by nursing students. Journal of Community Health Nursing, 9(1), 43-51.

May, A. (1992). Implementing an annual screening program. Health Visitor, 65(7), 240-241.

Summer, J. (1991). Screening the elderly. Nursing Times, 87(3), 60-82.

Health System Guidance   7400

Definition: Facilitating a patient's location and use of appropriate health services

Activities:

Explain the immediate health care system, how it works, and what the patient/family can expect

Assist patient or family to coordinate health care and communication

Assist patient or family to choose appropriate health care professionals

Instruct patient on what type of services to expect from each type of health care provider (e.g., nurse specialists, registered dietitians, registered nurses, licensed practical nurses, physical therapists, cardiologists, internists, optometrists, and psychologists)

Inform the patient about different types of health care facilities (e.g., general hospital, specialty hospital, teaching hospital, walk-in clinic, and outpatient surgical clinic), as appropriate

Inform the patient of accreditation and state health department requirements for judging the quality of a facility

Inform patient of appropriate community resources and contact persons

Advise use of second opinion

Inform patient of right to change health care provider

Inform the patient as to the meaning of signing a consent form

Provide patient with copy of Patient's Bill of Rights

Inform patient how to access emergency services by telephone and vehicle, as appropriate

Encourage patient to go to the emergency department, if appropriate

Identify and facilitate communication among health care providers and patient/family, as appropriate

Inform patient/family how to challenge decision made by a health care provider, as needed

Encourage consultation with other health care professionals, as appropriate

Request services from other health professionals for patient, as appropriate

Coordinate referrals to relevant health care providers, as appropriate

Review and reinforce information given by other health care professionals

Provide information on how to obtain equipment

Coordinate/schedule time needed by each service to deliver care, as appropriate

Inform patient of the cost, time, alternatives, and risks involved in a specific test or procedure

Give written instructions for purpose and location of post-hospitalization/outpatient activities, as appropriate

Give written instructions for purpose and location of health care activities, as appropriate

Discuss outcome of visit with other health care providers, as appropriate

Identify and facilitate transportation needs for obtaining health care services

Provide follow-up contact with patient, as appropriate

Monitor adequacy of current health care follow-up

Provide report to post-hospital caregivers, as appropriate

Encourage the patient/family to ask questions about services and charges

Comply with regulations for third-party reimbursement

Continued

Activities:—cont'd

Assist individual to complete forms for assistance, such as housing and financial aid, as needed

Notify patient of scheduled appointments, as appropriate

Background Readings:

Arnold, E., & Boggs, K. (1989). Interpersonal relationships: Professional communication skills for nurses. Philadelphia: W.B. Saunders.

Dunne, P.J. (1998). The emerging health care delivery system. American Association of Respiratory Care (AARC) Times 22(1), 24-8.

Matthews, P. (2000). Planning for successful outcomes in the new millennium. Topics in Health Information Management 20(3), 55-64.

Viscardis, L. (1998). The family-centered approach to providing services: A parent perspective. Physical & Occupation Therapy in Pediatrics 18(1), 41-53.

Zarbock, S.G. (1999). Sharing in all dimensions: Providing nourishment at home. Home Care Provider 4(3), 106-107.

H

Heat/Cold Application   1380

Definition: Stimulation of the skin and underlying tissues with heat or cold for the purpose of decreasing pain, muscle spasms, or inflammation

Activities:

Explain the use of heat or cold, the reason for the treatment, and how it will affect the patient's symptoms

Screen for contraindications to cold or heat, such as decreased or absent sensation, decreased circulation, and decreased ability to communicate

Select a method of stimulation that is convenient and readily available, such as waterproof plastic bags with melting ice; frozen gel packs; chemical ice envelope; ice immersion; cloth or towel in freezer for cold; hot water bottle; electric heating pad; hot, moist compresses; immersion in tub or whirlpool; paraffin wax; sitz bath; radiant bulb; or plastic wrap for heat

Determine availability and safe working condition of all equipment used for heat or cold application

Determine condition of skin and identify any alterations requiring a change in procedure or contraindications to stimulation

Select stimulation site, considering alternate sites when direct application is not possible (e.g., adjacent to, distal to, between affected areas and the brain, and contralateral)

Wrap the heat/cold application device with a protective cloth, if appropriate

Use a moist cloth next to the skin to increase the sensation of cold/heat, when appropriate

Instruct how to avoid tissue damage associated with heat/cold

Check the temperature of the application, especially when using heat

Determine duration of application based on individual verbal, behavioral, and biological responses

Time all applications carefully

Apply cold/heat directly on or near the affected site, if possible

Inspect the site carefully for signs of skin irritation or tissue damage throughout the first 5 minutes and then frequently during the treatment

Evaluate general condition, safety, and comfort throughout the treatment

Position to allow movement from the temperature source, if needed

Instruct not to adjust temperature settings independently without prior instruction

Change sites of cold/heat application or switch form of stimulation, if relief is not achieved

Instruct that cold application may be painful briefly, with numbness about 5 minutes after the initial stimulation

Instruct on indications for, frequency of, and procedure for application

Instruct to avoid injury to the skin after stimulation

Evaluate and document response to heat/cold application

Background Readings:

Herr, K.A., & Mobily, P.R. (1992). Interventions related to pain. In G.M. Bulechek & J.C. McCloskey (Eds.), Symposium on Nursing Interventions. Nursing Clinics of North America, 27(2), 347-370.

McCaffery, M., & Beebe, A. (1989). Pain. Clinical manual for nursing practice (pp. 145-154). St. Louis: Mosby.

Perry, A.G., & Potter, P.A. (1998). Clinical nursing skills and techniques (pp. 1113-1132). St. Louis: Mosby.

Ridgeway, S., Brauer, D., Cross, J., Daniels, J.S., & Steffes, M. (1998). Application of heat and cold. In M. Snyder & R. Lindquist. (Eds.), Complementary/alternative therapies in nursing (3rd ed.) (pp. 89-102). New York: Springer Publishing Company.

Sorensen, K., & Luckmann, J. (1986). Basic nursing: A psychophysiologic approach (2nd ed.) (pp. 966-981). Philadelphia: W.B. Saunders.

H

Heat Exposure Treatment 3780

Definition: Management of patient overcome by heat due to excessive environmental heat exposure

Activities:

Remove patient from direct sunlight and/or heat source

Loosen or remove clothing, as appropriate

Wet the body surface and fan the patient

Give cool oral fluids if patient is able to swallow

Administer IV fluids, as appropriate

Provide fluids rich in electrolytes, such as Gatorade

Transport to a cool environment, as appropriate

Determine the cause as exertional or nonexertional

Immerse in cool (11° C) water, as appropriate

Place on hypothermia blanket, as appropriate

Discontinue cooling when core body temperature reaches 39° C

Insert NG tube, as appropriate

Monitor level of consciousness

Monitor core body temperature, as appropriate

Monitor for electrolyte imbalances, particularly hypokalemia and hypophosphatemia

Monitor for hypoglycemia

Monitor for hypotension, cardiac arrhythmias, and signs of respiratory distress

Monitor for acid-base imbalance

Teach measures to prevent heat exhaustion and heat stroke

Teach early indications of heat exhaustion and appropriate actions to take

Background Readings:

Davis, L. (1997). Environmental heat-related illnesses. MEDSURG Nursing, 6 (3), 153-161.

Knochel, J.P. (1992). Disorders due to heat and cold. In J.B. Wyngaarden, L.H. Smith, Jr., & J.C. Bennett, Jr. (Eds.), Cecil textbook of medicine (19th ed.) (pp. 2358-2361). Philadelphia: W.B. Saunders.

Thompson, J.M., McFarland, G.K., Hirsch, J.E., & Tucker, S.M. (1998). Mosby's clinical nursing (4th ed.). St. Louis: Mosby–Year Book.

Hemodialysis Therapy   2100

Definition: Management of extracorporeal passage of the patient's blood through a dialyzer

Activities:

Draw blood sample and review blood chemistries (e.g., BUN, serum creatinine, serum sodium, potassium and PO_4 levels) before treatment

Record baseline vital signs: weight, temperature, pulse, respirations, and blood pressure

Explain hemodialysis procedure and its purpose

Check equipment and solutions, according to protocol

Use sterile technique to initiate hemodialysis and for needle insertions and catheter connections

Use gloves, eyeshield, and clothing to prevent direct contact with blood

Initiate hemodialysis, according to protocol

Anchor connections and tubing securely

Check system monitors (e.g., flow rate, pressure, temperature, pH level, conductivity, clots, air detector, negative pressure for ultrafiltration, and blood sensor) to ensure patient safety

Monitor blood pressure, pulse, respirations, temperature, and patient response during dialysis

Administer heparin, according to protocol

Monitor clotting times and adjust heparin administration appropriately

Adjust filtration pressures to remove an appropriate amount of fluid

Institute appropriate protocol, if patient becomes hypotensive

Discontinue hemodialysis according to protocol

Compare postdialysis vital signs and blood chemistries with predialysis values

Avoid taking blood pressure or doing intravenous punctures in arm with fistula

Provide catheter or fistula care, according to protocol

Work collaboratively with patient to adjust diet regulations, fluid limitations, and medications to regulate fluid and electrolyte shifts between treatments

Teach patient to self-monitor signs and symptoms that indicate need for medical treatment (e.g., fever, bleeding, clotted fistula, thrombophlebitis, and irregular pulse)

Work collaboratively with patient to relieve discomfort from side effects of the disease and treatment (e.g., cramping, fatigue, headaches, itching, anemia, bone demineralization, body image changes, and role disruption)

Work collaboratively with patient to adjust length of dialysis, diet regulations, and pain and diversion needs to achieve optimal benefit of the treatment

Background Readings:

Fearing, M.O., & Hart, L.K. (1992). Dialysis therapy. In G.M. Bulechek & J.C. McCloskey (Eds.), Nursing interventions: Essential nursing treatments (2nd ed.) (pp. 587-601). Philadelphia: W.B. Saunders.

Thompson, J.M., McFarland, G.K., Hirsch, J.E., & Tucker, S.M. (1998). Mosby's clinical nursing (4th ed.). St. Louis: Mosby.

H

Hemodynamic Regulation 4150

Definition: Optimization of heart rate, preload, afterload, and contractility

Activities:

Recognize presence of blood pressure alterations

Auscultate lung sounds for crackles or other adventitious sounds

Auscultate heart sounds

Monitor and document heart rate, rhythm, and pulses

Monitor electrolyte levels

Monitor systemic and pulmonary vascular resistance, as appropriate

Monitor cardiac output and/or cardiac index and left ventricular stroke work index, as appropriate

Administer positive inotropic/contractility medications

Evaluate side effects of negative inotropic medications

Monitor peripheral pulses, capillary refill, and temperature and color of extremities

Elevate the head of the bed, as appropriate

Place in Trendelenberg position, if appropriate

Monitor for peripheral edema, jugular vein distension, and S_3 and S_4 heart sounds

Monitor pulmonary capillary/artery wedge pressure and central venous/right-atrial pressure, if appropriate

Maintain fluid balance by administering IV fluids or diuretics, as appropriate

Administer vasodilator and/or vasoconstrictor medication, as appropriate

Monitor intake/output, urine output, and patient weight, as appropriate

Insert urinary catheter, if appropriate

Minimize/eliminate environmental stressors

Administer antiarrhythmic medications, as appropriate

Monitor effects of medications

Monitor pacemaker functioning, if appropriate

Evaluate effects of fluid therapy

Background Readings:

Cullen, L.M. (1992). Interventions related to circulatory care. In G.M. Bulechek & J.C. McCloskey (Eds.), Symposium on Nursing Interventions. Nursing Clinics of North America, 27(2), 445-476.

Johanson, B.C., Wells, S.J., Hoffmeister, D., & Dungca, C.U. (1988). Standards for critical care (3rd ed.). St. Louis: Mosby.

Wessel, S., & Kim, M. (1984). Nursing functions related to the nursing diagnosis: Decreased cardiac output. In M. Kim, G. McFarland, & A. McLane (Eds.), Classification of Nursing Diagnoses: Proceedings of the Fifth Conference (pp. 192-198). St. Louis: Mosby.

Hemofiltration Therapy   2110

Definition: Cleansing of acutely ill patient's blood via a hemofilter controlled by the patient's hydrostatic pressure

Activities:

Determine baseline vital signs and weight

Draw blood sample and review blood chemistries (e.g., BUN, serum creatinine, serum sodium, calcium, potassium and PO_4 levels) before therapy

Determine and record patient's hemodynamic function

Explain procedure to patient and significant others, as appropriate

Obtain written consent

Adjust technology to account for patient's multiple system pathologies (e.g., place patient on rotating air-flow bed)

Use sterile technique to flush and prime the arterial tubing, venous tubing, and hemofilter with heparinized saline, and to connect to other tubing as required

Remove all air bubbles from hemofiltration system

Administer heparin loading dose per protocol or physician's order

Use mask, gloves, and apron to prevent contact with blood

Use sterile technique to initiate venous and arterial access per protocol

Anchor connections and tubing securely

Apply restraints as appropriate

Monitor ultrafiltration rate, adjusting rate per protocol or physician's order

Monitor hemofiltration system for leaks at connections and clotting of filter or tubing

Monitor patient's multiple system parameters per protocol

Monitor and care for access sites and lines according to protocol

Monitor for signs and symptoms of infection

Instruct patient/family about precautions after treatment

Background Readings:

Gutch, C., Stoner, M., & Corea, A. (1993). Review of hemodialysis for nurses and dialysis personnel (5th ed.). St. Louis. Mosby.

Holloway, N. (1988). Nursing the critically ill adult (3rd ed.). Menlo Park, CA: Addison-Wesley Publishing Co.

Kinney, M., Packa, D., & Dunbar, S. (1998). AACN's reference for critical-care nursing (4th ed.). St. Louis: Mosby.

Lewis, S., & Collier, I. (1992). Medical-surgical nursing: Assessment and management of clinical problems (3rd ed.). St. Louis: Mosby.

H

Hemorrhage Control   **4160**

Definition: Reduction or elimination of rapid and excessive blood loss

Activities:

Apply a pressure dressing, as indicated

Identify the cause of the bleeding

Monitor the amount and nature of blood loss

Apply manual pressure over the bleeding or the potential bleeding area

Apply ice pack to affected area

Note hemoglobin/hematocrit level before and after blood loss, as indicated

Evaluate patient's psychological response to hemorrhage and perception of events

Inspect for bleeding from mucous membranes, bruising after minimal trauma, oozing from puncture sites, and presence of petechiae

Monitor for signs and symptoms of persistent bleeding (e.g., check all secretions for frank or occult blood)

Hematest all excretions and observe for blood in emesis, sputum, feces, urine, NG tube drainage, and wound drainage, as appropriate

Monitor neurological functioning

Background Readings:

Cullen, L.M. (1992). Interventions related to circulatory care. In G.M. Bulechek & J.C. McCloskey (Eds.), Symposium on Nursing Interventions. Nursing Clinics of North America, 27(2), 445-478.

Kitt, S., & Karser, J. (1990). Emergency nursing: A physiological and clinical perspective. Philadelphia: W.B. Saunders.

Thompson, J.M., McFarland, G.K., Hirsch, J.E., & Tucker, S.M. (1998). Mosby's clinical nursing (4th ed.). St. Louis: Mosby.

High-Risk Pregnancy Care   6800

Definition: Identification and management of a high-risk pregnancy to promote healthy outcomes for mother and baby

Activities:

Determine the presence of medical factors that are related to poor pregnancy outcome (e.g., diabetes, hypertension, lupus erythmatosus, herpes, hepatitis, HIV, and epilepsy)

Review obstetrical history for pregnancy-related risk factors (e.g., prematurity, postmaturity, preeclampsia, multifetal pregnancy, intrauterine growth retardation, abruption, previa, Rh sensitization, premature rupture of membranes, and family history of genetic disorder)

Recognize demographic and social factors related to poor pregnancy outcome (e.g., maternal age, race, poverty, late or no prenatal care, physical abuse, and substance abuse)

Determine client's knowledge of identified risk factors

Encourage expression of feelings and fears about lifestyle changes, fetal well-being, financial changes, family functioning, and personal safety

Provide educational materials that address the risk factors and usual surveillance tests and procedures

Instruct client in self-care techniques to increase the chance of a healthy outcome (e.g., hydration, diet, activity modifications, importance of regular prenatal check-ups, normalization of blood sugars, and sexual precautions, including abstinence)

Instruct about alternate methods of sexual gratification and intimacy

Refer as appropriate for specific programs (e.g., smoking cessation, substance abuse treatment, diabetes education, preterm birth prevention education, abuse shelter, and sexually transmitted disease clinic)

Instruct client on use of prescribed medication (e.g., insulin, tocolytics, antihypertensives, antibiotics, anticoagulants, and anticonvulsants)

Instruct client on self-monitoring skills, as appropriate (e.g., vital signs, blood glucose testing, uterine activity monitoring, and continuous subcutaneous medication delivery)

Write guidelines for signs and symptoms that require immediate medical attention (e.g., bright red vaginal bleeding, change in amniotic fluid, decreased fetal movement, four or more contractions/hour before 37 weeks of gestation, headache, visual disturbances, epigastic pain, and rapid weight gain with facial edema)

Discuss fetal risks associated with preterm birth at various gestational ages

Tour the neonatal intensive care unit if preterm birth is anticipated (e.g., multifetal pregnancy)

Teach fetal movement counts

Conduct tests to evaluate fetal status and placental function, such as nonstress, oxytocin challenge, biophysical profiles, and ultrasound tests

Obtain cervical cultures, as appropriate

Assist with fetal diagnostic procedures (e.g., amniocentesis, chorionic villus sampling, percutaneous umbilical blood sampling, and Doppler blood flow studies)

Assist with fetal therapy procedures (e.g., fetal transfusions, fetal surgery, selective reduction, and termination procedure)

Interpret medical explanations for test and procedure results

Administer $Rh_o(D)$ immune globulin (e.g., Rho-GAM or Gamulin Rh), as appropriate, to prevent Rh sensitization after invasive procedures

Establish plan for clinic follow-up

Provide anticipatory guidance for likely interventions during birth process (e.g., Electronic Fetal Monitoring: Intrapartum, Labor Suppression, Labor Induction, Medication Administration, Cesarean Section Care)

Continued

Activities:—cont'd

Encourage early enrollment in prenatal classes or provide childbirth education materials for patients on bed rest

Provide anticipatory guidance for common experiences that high-risk mothers have during the postpartum period (e.g., exhaustion, depression, chronic stress, disenchantment with childbearing, loss of income, partner discord, and sexual dysfunction)

Refer to high-risk mother support group, as needed

Refer to home care agencies (e.g., specialized perinatal nursing services, perinatal case management, and public health nursing)

Monitor physical and psychosocial status closely throughout pregnancy

Report deviations from normal in maternal and/or fetal status immediately to physician or nurse midwife

Document client education, lab results, fetal testing results, and client responses

Background Readings:

Association of Women's Health, Obstetric, and Neonatal Nurses. (1993). Didactic content and clinical skills verification for professional nurse providers of basic, high-risk and critical-care intrapartum nursing. Washington, DC: AWHONN.

Field, P.A., & Marck, P. (1994). Uncertain motherhood: Negotiating the risks of the childbearing years. Newbury Park, CA: Sage Publishing.

Gilbert, E.S., & Harmon, J.S. (1998). Manual of high risk pregnancy and delivery. (2nd ed.). St. Louis: Mosby.

Mandeville, L.K., & Troiano, N.H. (Eds.). (1992). High-risk intrapartum nursing. Philadelphia: J.B. Lippincott.

Mattson, S. & J.E. Smith (Eds.). (1993). Core curriculum for maternal-newborn nursing. Philadelphia: W.B. Saunders.

H

Home Maintenance Assistance   7180

Definition: Helping the patient/family to maintain the home as a clean, safe, and pleasant place to live

Activities:

Determine patient's home maintenance requirements

Involve patient/family in deciding home maintenance requirements

Suggest necessary structural alterations to make home accessible

Provide information on how to make home environment safe and clean

Assist family members to develop realistic expectations of themselves in performance of their roles

Advise the alleviation of all offensive odors

Suggest services for pest control, as needed

Facilitate cleaning of dirty laundry

Suggest services for home repair, as needed

Discuss cost of needed maintenance and available resources

Offer solutions to financial difficulties

Order homemaker services, as appropriate

Help family use social support network

Provide information on respite care, as needed

Coordinate use of community resources

Background Readings:

Dickerson, A.E. (1993). Age differences in functional performance. American Journal of Occupational Therapy, 47(8), 686-692.

Scott, E. (2001). The potential benefits of infection control measures in the home. American Journal of Infection Control, 29(4), 247-249.

H

Hope Instillation 5310

Definition: Facilitation of the development of a positive outlook in a given situation

Activities:

Assist patient/family to identify areas of hope in life

Inform the patient about whether the current situation is a temporary state

Demonstrate hope by recognizing the patient's intrinsic worth and viewing the patient's illness as only one facet of the individual

Expand the patient's repertoire of coping mechanisms

Teach reality recognition by surveying the situation and making contingency plans

Assist the patient to devise and revise goals related to the hope object

Help the patient expand spiritual self

Avoid masking the truth

Facilitate the patient's incorporating a personal loss into his/her body image

Facilitate the patient's/family's reliving and savoring past achievements and experiences

Emphasize sustaining relationships, such as mentioning the names of loved ones to the unresponsive patient

Employ guided life review and/or reminiscence, as appropriate

Involve the patient actively in own care

Develop a plan of care that involves degree of goal attainment, moving from simple to more complex goals

Encourage therapeutic relationships with significant others

Teach family about the positive aspects of hope (e.g., develop meaningful conversational themes that reflect love and need for the patient)

Provide patient/family opportunity to be involved with support groups

Create an environment that facilitates patient practicing religion, as appropriate

Background Readings:

Brown, P. (1989). The concept of hope: Implications for care of the critically ill. Critical Care Nurse, 9(5), 97-105.

Forbes, S.B. (1994). Hope: An essential human need in the elderly. Journal Gerontological Nursing, 20(6), 5-10.

Parse, R.R. (1990). Parse's research methodology with an illustration of the lived experience of hope. Nursing Science Quarterly, 3(1), 9-17.

Snyder, M. (1988). Nursing management strategies: An overview. In P.H. Mitchell, L.C. Hodges, M. MuWasews, & C. Nalleck (Eds.), AANN's neuroscience nursing, phenomena and practice. Norwalk, CT: Appleton & Lange.

H

Hormone Replacement Therapy   2280

Definition: Facilitation of safe and effective use of hormone replacement therapy

Activities:

Determine reason for choosing hormone replacement therapy

Review alternatives to hormone replacement therapy

Monitor patient for therapeutic effect

Monitor for adverse effects

Review information regarding beneficial and adverse effects of the different hormonal components (e.g., estrogen, progesterone, androgen)

Review information regarding interaction effects of adjunct therapies (e.g., calcium and vitamin D supplementation, exercise, thiazide use)

Review information regarding the different methods of administration (e.g., oral continuous combined, oral sequential, dermal, vaginal)

Facilitate the decision to continue/discontinue

Facilitate changes in hormone replacement therapy with primary care provider, as appropriate

Recommend patients make short-term annual decisions about continuation

Adjust medications or medication dose, as appropriate

H

Background Readings:

Blackwood, M., Creasman, W., Speroff, L. (2001, October). Postmenopausal hormone therapy: Informed patients, shared decisions. Women's Health in Primary Care, Supplement, 28-34.

Speroff, L., Glass, R., Kase, N. (1999). Clinical gynecologic endocrinology and infertility (6th ed.) (pp. 725-779). Baltimore: Lippincott Williams & Wilkins.

Wingo, P., McTiernam, A. (2000). The risks and benefits of hormone replacement therapy: Weighing the evidence. In M. Goldman & M. Hatch (Eds.), Women and health (pp. 1169-1187). San Diego: Academic Press.

Humor   5320

Definition: Facilitating the patient to perceive, appreciate, and express what is funny, amusing, or ludicrous in order to establish relationships, relieve tension, release anger, facilitate learning, or cope with painful feelings

Activities:

Determine the types of humor appreciated by the patient

Determine the patient's typical response to humor (e.g., laughter or smiles)

Determine the time of day that patient is most receptive

Avoid content areas about which patient is sensitive

Discuss advantages of laughter with patient

Select humorous materials that create moderate arousal for the individual

Make available a selection of humorous games, cartoons, jokes, videos, tapes, books, and so on

Point out humorous incongruity in a situation

Encourage visualization with humor (e.g., picture a forbidding authority figure dressed only in underwear)

Encourage silliness and playfulness

Remove environmental barriers that prevent or diminish the spontaneous occurrence of humor

Monitor patient response and discontinue humor strategy, if ineffective

Avoid use with patient who is cognitively impaired

Demonstrate an appreciative attitude about humor

Respond positively to humor attempts made by patient

Background Readings:

Buxman, K. (1991). Make room for laughter. American Journal of Nursing, 91(12), 46-51.

Kolkmeier, L.G. (1988). Play and laughter: Moving toward harmony. In B.M. Dosseyk, L. Keegan, C.E. Guzetta, & L.G. Kolkmeier (Eds.), Holistic nursing: A handbook for practice (pp. 289-304). Rockville, MD: Aspen.

Smith, K. (2001). Humor. In M. Snyder & R. Lindquist. (Eds.), Complementary/alternative therapies in nursing (3rd ed.) (pp. 269-284). New York: Springer Publishing Company.

Sullivan, J.L., & Deane, D.M. (1988). Humor and health. Journal of Gerontological Nursing, 14(1), 20-24.

Hyperglycemia Management   2120

Definition: Preventing and treating above normal blood glucose levels

Activities:

Monitor blood glucose levels, as indicated

Monitor for signs and symptoms of hyperglycemia: polyuria, polydipsia, polyphagia, weakness, lethargy, malaise, blurring of vision, or headache

Monitor urine ketones, as indicated

Monitor ABG, electrolyte, and betahydroxybutyrate levels, as available

Monitor orthostatic blood pressure and pulse, as indicated

Administer insulin, as prescribed

Encourage oral fluid intake

Monitor fluid status (including intake & output), as appropriate

Maintain IV access, as appropriate

Administer IV fluids, as needed

Administer potassium, as prescribed

Consult physician if signs and symptoms of hyperglycemia persist or worsen

Assist with ambulation if orthostatic hypotension is present

Provide oral hygiene, if necessary

Identify possible cause of hyperglycemia

Anticipate situations in which insulin requirements will increase (e.g., intercurrent illness)

Restrict exercise when blood glucose levels are >250 mg/dl, especially if urine ketones are present

Instruct patient and significant others on prevention, recognition, and management of hyperglycemia

Encourage self-monitoring of blood glucose levels

Assist patient to interpret blood glucose levels

Review blood glucose records with patient and/or family

Instruct on urine ketone testing, as appropriate

Instruct on indications for, and significance of, urine ketone testing, if appropriate

Instruct patient to report moderate or high urine ketone levels to the health professional

Instruct patient and significant others on diabetes management during illness, including use of insulin and/or oral agents; monitoring fluid intake; carbohydrate replacement; and when to seek health professional assistance, as appropriate

Provide assistance in adjusting regimen to prevent and treat hyperglycemia (e.g., increasing insulin or oral agent), as indicated

Facilitate adherence to diet and exercise regimen

Test blood glucose levels of family members

Background Readings:

Guthrie, D.W. (Ed.). (1988). Diabetes education: Core curriculum for health professionals. Chicago: American Association of Diabetes Educators.

Thompson, J.M., McFarland, G.K., Hirsch, J.E., & Tucker, S.M. (1998). Mosby's clinical nursing (4th ed.). St. Louis: Mosby.

H

Hypervolemia Management 4170

Definition: Reduction in extracellular and/or intracellular fluid volume and prevention of complications in a patient who is fluid overloaded

Activities:

Weigh patient daily and monitor trends

Monitor hemodynamic status, including CVP, MAP, PAP, and PCWP, if available

Monitor serum albumin and total protein levels, if available

Monitor respiratory pattern for symptoms of respiratory difficulty (e.g., dyspnea, tachypnea, and shortness of breath)

Monitor renal function (e.g., BUN and Cr levels), if appropriate

Monitor intake and output

Monitor vital signs, as appropriate

Monitor changes in peripheral edema, as appropriate

Monitor laboratory results relevant to fluid retention (e.g., increased specific gravity, increased BUN, decreased hematocrit, and increased urine osmolality levels)

Set an appropriate intravenous infusion (or blood transfusion) flow rate

Monitor prescribed IV fluids for appropriateness (e.g., avoid free water in patient with fluid overload and hyponatremia)

Administer prescribed diuretics, as appropriate

Monitor for therapeutic effect of diuretic (e.g., increased urine output, decreased CVP/PCWP, and decreased adventitious breath sounds)

Teach patient the rationale for use of diuretic therapy

Administer prescribed unloading agent(s) (e.g., morphine, furosemide, and nitroglycerine), as appropriate

Monitor potassium levels after diuresis

Prepare patient for dialysis (e.g., assist with catheter placement for dialysis), as appropriate

Monitor patient's weight change before and after dialysis, if appropriate

Monitor patient's hemodynamic response to dialysis, as appropriate

Monitor infused and returned volume of peritoneal dialysate, as appropriate

Monitor returned peritoneal dialysate for indications of complications (e.g. infection, excessive bleeding, and clots), as appropriate

Elevate head of bed to improve ventilation, as appropriate

Maintain PEEP for patient with pulmonary edema on mechanical ventilator, as appropriate

Use closed-system suction for patient with pulmonary edema on mechanical ventilation with PEEP, as appropriate

Turn the patient with dependent edema frequently

Promote skin integrity (e.g., monitor areas at risk for breakdown, provide frequent weight shifts, prevent shearing, and provide adequate nutrition), as appropriate

Monitor for excessive diuresis

Observe for indications of dehydration (e.g., poor skin turgor, delayed capillary refill, weak/thready pulse, severe thirst, dry mucous membranes, decreased urine output, and hypotension)

Instruct the patient/family on use of voiding record, as appropriate

Instruct patient and/or family on measures instituted to treat the hypervolemia

Provide appropriate diet, as indicated

Promote a positive body image and self-esteem if concerns are expressed as a result of excessive fluid retention, if appropriate

Background Readings:

American Association of Critical-Care Nurses. (1990). Outcome standards for nursing care of the critically ill. Laguna Niguel, CA: AACN.

Askanazi, J., Starker, P., & Wissman, C. (1986). Fluid and electrolyte management in critical care. Boston: Butterworths.

Cullen, L.M. (1992). Interventions related to fluid and electrolyte balance. In G.M. Bulechek & J.C. McCloskey (Eds.), Symposium on Nursing Interventions. Nursing Clinics of North America, 27(2), 569-598.

Horne, M., & Swearingen, P. (1992). Pocket guide to fluids and electrolytes (2nd ed.). St. Louis: Mosby.

Kinney, M., Packa, D., & Dunbar, S. (1993). AACN's clinical reference for critical-care nursing (pp. 193-236). New York: McGraw-Hill.

Kokko, J., & Tannen, R. (1990). Fluids and electrolytes (2nd ed.). Philadelphia: W.B. Saunders.

Stark, J. (1991). The renal system. In J. Alspach (Ed.), American Association of Critical-Care Nurses core curriculum for critical-care nursing (4th ed.) (pp. 472-608). Philadelphia: W.B. Saunders.

H

Hypnosis

Definition: Assisting a patient to induce an altered state of consciousness to create an acute awareness and a directed focus experience

Activities:

Select patient with positive attitudes about hypnosis

Select hypnosis as an early form of treatment

Establish trusting relationship with patient

Discuss patient's experiences with trance states, such as daydreaming and "highway hypnosis," as appropriate

Discuss myths of hypnosis with patient, as appropriate

Obtain history of the problem to be treated by hypnosis

Determine goals for hypnosis with patient

Instruct patient that he/she will induce the trance state and retain control

Sit comfortably, half facing the patient, when appropriate

Instruct patient to close eyes for induction to promote relaxation

Discuss with patient hypnotic suggestions to be used before induction

Use patient's language as much as possible

Give a small number of suggestions in an assertive manner

Combine suggestions with naturally occurring events

Convey permissive attitude to aid in trance induction

Use a rhythmical, soothing, monotone voice during hypnosis induction

Pace statements with patient's respirations

Encourage patient to take deep breaths to intensify the state of relaxation and decrease tension

Assist patient to select a method of instruction, such as progressive relaxation, visual imagery, or rhythmical talking

Assist patient to escape to a pleasant place, using guided imagery

Avoid guessing what the patient is thinking

Assist patient to use all senses during the process

Determine whether to use directive or nondirective imagery with the patient, as appropriate

Facilitate quick induction through a specific cue (verbal or visual) with experience

Instruct patient that the level of trance is not important to successful hypnosis

Provide a quiet environment to enhance the level of the trance

Facilitate patient's coming out of the trance by counting to a prearranged number, as appropriate

Assist patient to come out of the trance at own pace, as appropriate

Provide positive feedback to patient after each episode

Encourage patient to use self-induction independent of the nurse to manage problem under treatment

Identify situations, such as painful procedures, in which patient requires additional staff support for effective induction

Background Readings:

Emdon, T. (1989). Entrancing therapy. Nursing Times, 85(50), 54-56.

Graves, P., & Lancaster, J. (1992). Stress management and crisis intervention. In M. Stanhope & J. Lancaster (Eds.), Community health nursing (3rd ed.) (pp. 612-631). St. Louis: Mosby.

Puskar, K., & Mumford, K. (1990). The healing power. Nursing Times, 86(33), 50-52.

Woods, M. (1989). Pain control and hypnosis. Nursing Times, 85(7), 38-40.

Zahourek, R.P. (1982). Hypnosis in nursing practice: Emphasis on the "problem patient" who has pain. 1. Journal of Psychosocial Nursing and Mental Health Services, 20(3), 13-17.

Zahourek, R.P. (1982). Hypnosis in nursing practice: Emphasis on the "problem patient" who has pain. 2. Journal of Psychosocial Nursing and Mental Health Services, 20(4), 21-24.

H

Hypoglycemia Management   2130

Definition: Preventing and treating low blood glucose levels

Activities:

Identify patient at risk for hypoglycemia

Determine recognition of hypoglycemia signs and symptoms

Monitor blood glucose levels, as indicated

Monitor for signs and symptoms of hypoglycemia (e.g., shakiness, tremor, sweating, nervousness, anxiety, irritability, impatience, tachycardia, palpitations, chills, clamminess, light-headedness, pallor, hunger, nausea, headache, tiredness, drowsiness, weakness, warmth, dizziness, faintness, blurred vision, nightmares, crying out in sleep, paresthesias, difficulty concentrating, difficulty speaking, incoordination, behavior change, confusion, coma, seizure)

Provide simple carbohydrate, as indicated

Provide complex carbohydrate and protein, as indicated

Administer glucagon, as indicated

Contact emergency medical services, as necessary

Administer intravenous glucose, as indicated

Maintain IV access, as appropriate

Maintain patent airway, as necessary

Protect from injury, as necessary

Review events prior to hypoglycemia to determine probable cause

Provide feedback regarding appropriateness of self-management of hypoglycemia

Instruct patient and significant others on signs and symptoms, risk factors, and treatment of hypoglycemia

Instruct patient to have simple carbohydrate available at all times

Instruct patient to obtain and carry/wear appropriate emergency identification

Instruct significant others on the use and administration of glucagon, as appropriate

Instruct on interaction of diet, insulin/oral agents, and exercise

Provide assistance in making self-care decisions to prevent hypoglycemia, (e.g., reducing insulin/oral agents and/or increasing food intake for exercise)

Encourage self-monitoring of blood glucose levels

Encourage ongoing telephone contact with diabetes care team for consultation regarding adjustments in treatment regimen

Collaborate with patient and diabetes care team to make changes in insulin regimen (e.g., multiple daily injections), as indicated

Modify blood glucose goals to prevent hypoglycemia in the absence of hypoglycemia symptoms

Inform patient of increased risk of hypoglycemia with intensive therapy and normalization of blood glucose levels

Instruct patient regarding probable changes in hypoglycemia symptoms with intensive therapy and normalization of blood glucose levels

Background Readings:

American Diabetes Association. (1995). Intensive diabetes management. Alexandria, VA: Author.

American Diabetes Association. (1994). Medical management of insulin-dependent (type I) diabetes. (2nd ed.). Alexandria, VA: Author.

Ahern, J., & Tamborlane, W.V. (1997). Steps to reduce the risks of severe hypoglycemia. Diabetes Spectrum, 10(1), 39-41.

Cryer, P.E., Fisher J.N., & Shamoon, H (1994). Hypoglycemia. Diabetes Care,17(7), 734-755.

Havlin, C.E., & Cryer, P.E. (1988). Hypoglycemia: The limiting factor in the management of insulin-dependent diabetes mellitus. Diabetes Educator, 14(5), 407-411.

Levandoski, L.A. (1993). Hypoglycemia. In V. Peragallo-Dittko (Ed.), A core curriculum for diabetes education (pp. 351-372). Chicago: American Association of Diabetes Educators and AADE Education and Research Foundation.

H

Hypothermia Treatment 3800

Definition: Rewarming and surveillance of a patient whose core body temperature is below 35° C

Activities:

Remove the patient from the cold, and place in a warm environment

Remove cold, wet clothing and replace with warm, dry clothing

Monitor patient's temperature, using a low-recording thermometer if necessary

Institute a continuous core temperature monitoring device, as appropriate

Monitor for symptoms associated with hypothermia: fatigue, weakness, confusion, apathy, impaired coordination, slurred speech, shivering, and change in skin color

Determine factors leading to the hypothermic episode by questioning about recent activities, such as heavy activity in cold wet weather, elderly living alone in a cool environment, and poor nutritional state

Monitor for underlying medical conditions that may precipitate hypothermia (e.g., diabetes, myxedema, or anorexia nervosa)

Place on a cardiac monitor, as appropriate

Monitor for and treat ventricular defibrillation

Cover with warmed blankets, as appropriate

Minimize stimulation of the patient to avoid precipitating ventricular fibrillation

Administer warmed (37° to 40° C) IV fluids, as appropriate

Administer heated oxygen, as appropriate

Institute active external rewarming measures (e.g., immersion in warm water, application of hot water bottles, and placement on a heating blanket), as appropriate

Institute active core rewarming techniques (e.g., colonic lavage, hemodialysis, peritoneal dialysis, and extracorpeal blood rewarming), as appropriate

Monitor for rewarming shock

Administer plasma volume expanders, as appropriate

Monitor skin color and temperature

Monitor vital signs, as appropriate

Monitor for bradycardia

Monitor for electrolyte imbalance

Monitor for acid-base imbalance

Monitor intake and output

Monitor cardiac output, PCWP, SVR, and RAP, using invasive hemodynamic monitoring as appropriate

Avoid giving IM or subcutaneous medications during the hypothermic state

Monitor for increased actions of medications as rewarming occurs

Institute routine skin surveillance, as appropriate

Monitor respiratory status

Give patient warm oral fluids, if alert and able to swallow

Monitor nutritional status

Teach patient to consume a caloric intake sufficient to maintain a normal body temperature

Emphasize the importance of wearing warm, protective clothing when going into a cold environment

Teach early warning signs of hypothermia

Establish support systems for elderly patient to prevent isolation and residing in excessively cool environments, as appropriate

Background Readings:

Knochel, J.P. (1992). Disorders due to heat and cold. In J.B. Wyngaarden, L.H. Smith, Jr., & J.C. Bennett (Eds.), Cecil textbook of medicine (19th ed.) (pp. 2358-2361). Philadelphia: W.B. Saunders.

Summers, S. (1992). Hypothermia: One nursing diagnosis or three. Nursing Diagnosis, 3(1), 2-11.

Thompson, J.M., McFarland, G.K., Hirsch, J.E., & Tucker, S.M. (1998). Mosby's clinical nursing (4th ed.). St. Louis: Mosby.

H

Hypovolemia Management   4180

Definition: Expansion of intravascular fluid volume in a patient who is volume depleted

Activities:

Monitor fluid status, including intake and output, as appropriate

Maintain patent IV access

Monitor hemoglobin and hematocrit levels, if appropriate

Monitor for fluid loss (e.g., bleeding, vomiting, diarrhea, perspiration, and tachypnea)

Monitor vital signs, as appropriate

Calculate fluid needs based on body surface area and size of burn, as appropriate

Monitor patient response to fluid challenge

Administer hypotonic solutions (e.g., D_5W, D_5, or one half NS) for intracellular rehydration, if appropriate

Administer isotonic solutions (e.g., normal saline and lactated Ringer's solution) for extracellular rehydration, if appropriate

Combine crystalloid (e.g., normal saline and lactated Ringer's solution) and colloid (e.g., Hespan and Plasmanate) solutions for replacement of intravascular volume, as prescribed

Initiate prescribed fluid challenge, as appropriate

Monitor IV site for signs of infiltration or infection, if appropriate

Monitor for insensible fluid loss (e.g., diaphoresis and respiratory tract infection)

Promote skin integrity (e.g., monitor areas at risk for breakdown, provide frequent weight shifts, prevent shearing, and provide adequate nutrition), as appropriate

Assist patient with ambulation in case of postural hypotension

Instruct the patient to avoid rapid position changes, especially from supine to sitting or standing

Provide frequent oral hygiene

Monitor weight

Observe for indications of dehydration (e.g., poor skin turgor, delayed capillary refill, weak/thready pulse, severe thirst, dry mucous membranes, decreased urine output, and hypotension)

Encourage oral fluid intake (e.g., distribute fluids over 24 hours and give fluids with meals), if indicated

Monitor hemodynamic status, including CVP, MAP, PAP, and PCWP, if available

Administer IV fluids at room temperature

Maintain a steady IV infusion flow rate

Position for peripheral perfusion

Arrange availability of blood products for transfusion, if necessary

Institute autotransfusion of blood loss, if appropriate

Administer blood products (e.g., platelets and fresh frozen plasma), as appropriate

Monitor for blood reaction, if appropriate

Place patient in Trendelenburg position when hypotensive, if appropriate

Administer prescribed vasodilators with caution (e.g., nitroglycerine, nitroprusside, and calcium channel blockers) when rewarming a postoperative patient, as appropriate

Instruct the patient and/or family on measures instituted to treat the hypovolemia

Monitor for clinical signs and symptoms of overhydration/fluid excess

Monitor for signs of impending renal failure (e.g., increased BUN and creatinine levels, myoglobinemia, and decreased urine output), as appropriate

Background Readings:

American Association of Critical-Care Nurses. (1990). Outcome standards for nursing care of the critically ill. Laguna Niguel, CA: AACN.

Askanazi, J., Starker, P., & Wissman, C. (1986). Fluid and electrolyte management in critical care. Boston: Butterworths.

Baer, C.L. (1993). Fluid and electrolyte balance. In M.R. Kinney, D.R. Packa, & S.B. Dunbar (Eds.), AACN's clinical reference for critical-care nursing (pp. 173-208). St. Louis: Mosby.

Cullen, L.M. (1992). Interventions related to fluid and electrolyte balance. In G.M. Bulechek & J.C. McCloskey (Eds.), Symposium on Nursing Interventions. Nursing Clinics of North America, 27(2), 569-598.

Horne, M., & Swearingen, P. (1997). Pocket guide to fluids and electrolytes (3rd ed.). St. Louis: Mosby.

Kokko, J., & Tannen, R. (1990). Fluids and electrolytes (2nd ed.). Philadelphia: W.B. Saunders.

Stark, J. (1991). The renal system. In J. Alspach (Ed.), American Association of Critical-Care Nurses core curriculum for critical-care nursing (4th ed.) (pp. 472-608). Philadelphia: W.B. Saunders.

H

Immunization/Vaccination Management   6530

Definition: Monitoring immunization status, facilitating access to immunizations, and providing immunizations to prevent communicable disease

Activities:

Teach parent(s) recommended immunization necessary for children, their route of medication administration, reasons and benefits of use, adverse reactions, and side effects schedule (e.g., hepatitis B, diphtheria, tetanus, pertussis, *Haemophilus influenza*, polio, measles, mumps, rubella, and varicella)

Inform individuals of immunization protective against illness but not presently required by law (e.g. influenza, pneumonia, and hepatitis B vaccinations)

Teach individual/families about vaccinations available in the event of special incidence and/or exposure (e.g., cholera, influenza, plague, rabies, Rocky Mountain spotted fever, smallpox, typhoid fever, typhus, yellow fever, and tuberculosis)

Provide vaccine information statements prepared by CDC

Provide and update diary for recording date and type of immunizations

Identify proper administration techniques, including simultaneous administration

Identify latest recommendations regarding use of immunizations

Follow the 5 rights of medication administration

Note patient's medical history and history of allergies

Administer injections to infant in the anterolateral thigh, as appropriate

Document vaccination information per agency protocol (e.g., manufacturer, lot number, expiration date)

Inform families which immunizations are required by law for entering preschool, kindergarten, junior high, high school, and college

Audit school immunization records for completeness on a yearly basis

Notify individual/family when immunizations are not up-to-date

Follow the American Academy of Pediatrics, American Academy of Family Physicians, and U.S. Public Health Service guidelines for immunization administration

Inform travelers of vaccinations appropriate for travel to foreign countries

Identify true contraindications for administering immunizations (anaphylactic reaction to previous vaccine and moderate or severe illness with or without fever)

Recognize that a delay in series administration does not indicate restarting the schedule

Secure informed consent to administer vaccine

Help family with financial planning to pay for immunizations (e.g., insurance coverage and health department clinics)

Identify providers who participate in Federal "Vaccine for Children" program to provide free vaccines

Inform parent(s) of comfort measures helpful after medication administration to child

Observe patient for a specified period after medication administration

Schedule immunizations at appropriate time intervals

Determine immunization status at every health care visit (including emergency department and hospital admission), and provide immunizations as needed

Advocate for programs and policies that provide free or affordable immunizations to all populations

Support national registry to track immunization status

Background Readings:

Centers for Disease Control. (1997). Recommended childhood immunization schedule: United States 1997. Mortality and Morbidity Weekly Report, 46(2), 35-40.

Centers for Disease Control. (2002). Recommended adult immunization schedule: United States, 2002-2003. Mortality and Morbidity Weekly Report, 51(40), 904-908.

Lambert, J. (1995). Every child by two. A program of the American Nurses Foundation. American Nurse, 27(8), 12

Lerner-Durjava, L. (1998). Nurse's guide to immunizations. Nursing 28(7), 32hn10-12

Scudder, L. (1995). Child immunization initiative: Politics and health policy in action. Nursing Policy Forum, 1 (3), 20-29.

Scarbrough, M.L., & Landis, S.E. (1997). A pilot study for the development of a hospital-based immunization program. Clinical Nurse Specialist, 11(2), 70-75.

West, A.R., & Kopp, M. (1999). Making a difference: Immunizing infants and children. American Nurse Foundation, A1-A6.

I

Impulse Control Training 4370

Definition: Assisting the patient to mediate impulsive behavior through application of problem-solving strategies to social and interpersonal situations

Activities:

Select a problem-solving strategy that is appropriate to the patient's developmental level and cognitive functioning

Use a behavior modification plan, as appropriate, to reinforce the problem-solving strategy that is being taught

Assist patient to identify the problem or situation that requires thoughtful action

Teach patient to cue himself/herself to "stop and think" before acting impulsively

Assist patient to identify courses of possible action and their costs/benefits

Assist patient to choose the most beneficial course of action

Assist patient to evaluate the outcome of the chosen course of action

Provide positive reinforcement (e.g., praise and rewards) for successful outcomes

Encourage patient to self-reward for successful outcomes

Assist patient to evaluate how unsuccessful outcomes could have been avoided by different behavioral choices

Provide opportunities for patient to practice problem solving (role playing) within the therapeutic environment

Provide models who demonstrate the steps of the problem-solving strategy in the context of situations that are meaningful to the patient

Encourage patient to practice problem solving in social and interpersonal situations outside the therapeutic environment, followed by evaluation of outcome

Background Readings:

Alexander, D.I. (1991). Impulse control, altered. In G.K. McFarland, & M.D. Thomas (Eds.), Psychiatric mental health nursing. Application of the nursing process (pp. 282-285). Philadelphia: J.B. Lippincott.

Cipkala-Gaffin, J.A., & Cipkala-Gaffin, G.L. (1989). Developmental disabilities and nursing interventions. In L.M. Birckhead (Ed.), Psychiatric mental health nursing. The therapeutic use of self (pp. 349-379). Philadelphia: J.B. Lippincott.

Kendall, P.C. (1977). On the efficacious use of verbal self-instructional procedures with children. Cognitive Therapy and Research, 1, 331-334.

Kendall, P.C., & Braswell, L. (1985). Cognitive-behavioral therapy for impulsive children. New York: The Guilford Press.

Kendall, P.C., & Finch, A.J. (1979). Developing nonimpulsive behavior in children. Cognitive-behavioral strategies for self control. In P.C. Kendall & S.D. Hollon (Eds.), Cognitive behavioral interventions: Theory, research, & procedures. New York: Academic Press.

Meichenbaum, D., & Goodman, J. (1971). Training impulsive children to talk to themselves: A means of developing self control. Journal of Abnormal Psychology, 77, 115-126.

Incident Reporting 7980

Definition: Written and verbal reporting of any event in the process of patient care that is inconsistent with desired patient outcomes or routine operations of the health care facility

Activities:

Identify events (e.g., patient falls, blood transfusion reactions, and equipment malfunction) that require reporting, as defined in agency policy

Notify physician to evaluate patient, as appropriate

Notify nursing supervisor, as appropriate

Document in patient record that physician was notified

Complete incident report form(s) to include factual information, patient hospital number, medical diagnosis, and date of admission

Document factual information about the event in the patient record

Document nursing assessments and interventions after the event

Identify and report medical device failures leading to patient injury, as appropriate

Maintain confidentiality of incident report, according to agency policy

Initiate Medical Device Reporting System for deaths or serious injury resulting from medical devices

Discuss event with involved staff to determine what, if any, corrective action is necessary

Background Readings:

Benson-Flynn, J. (2001) Incident reporting: Clarifying occurrences, incidents, and sentinel events. Home Healthcare Nurse, 19(11), 701-706.

Feutz-Harper, S. (1989). Documentation principles and pitfalls. Journal of Nursing Administration, 19(12), 7-9.

Peters, G. (1991). Details are not incidental. Geriatric Nursing, 12(2), 90-93.

Understanding incident reporting systems. (1993). Minimally Invasive Surgical Nursing, 7(1), 5.

Incision Site Care   3440

> *Definition:* Cleansing, monitoring, and promotion of healing in a wound that is closed with sutures, clips, or staples

Activities:

Explain the procedure to the patient, using sensory preparation

Inspect the incision site for redness, swelling, or signs of dehiscence or evisceration

Note characteristics of any drainage

Monitor the healing process in the incision site

Cleanse the area around the incision with an appropriate cleansing solution

Swab from the clean area toward the less clean area

Monitor incision for signs and symptoms of infection

Use sterile, cotton-tipped applicators for efficient cleansing of tight-fitting wire sutures, deep and narrow wounds, or wounds with pockets

Cleanse the area around any drain site or drainage tube last

Maintain the position of any drainage tube

Apply closure strips, as appropriate

Apply antiseptic ointment, as ordered

Remove sutures, staples, or clips, as indicated

Change the dressing at appropriate intervals

Apply an appropriate dressing to protect the incision

Facilitate the patient's viewing of the incision

Instruct the patient on how to care for the incision during bathing or showering

Teach the patient how to minimize stress on the incision site

Teach the patient and/or the family how to care for the incision, including signs and symptoms of infection

Background Readings:

Perry, A.G., & Potter, P.A. (1998). Clinical nursing skills and techniques. (4th ed.) St. Louis: Mosby.

Sorensen, K., & Luckman, J. (1986). Basic nursing: A psychophysiologic approach (2nd ed.) (pp. 932-964). Philadelphia: W.B. Saunders.

Infant Care   6820

Definition: Provision of developmentally appropriate family-centered care to the child under 1 year of age

Activities:

Monitor infant's height and weight

Monitor intake and output, as appropriate

Change diapers, as appropriate

Feed infant foods that are developmentally appropriate

Provide opportunities for nonnutritive sucking, as appropriate

Keep side rails of crib up when not caring for infant

Monitor safety of infant's environment

Provide developmentally appropriate, safe toys for infant

Provide information to parents about child development and childrearing

Provide developmentally appropriate activities to stimulate cognitive development

Provide stimulation that appeals to all senses

Structure play and care around infant's behavioral style/temperament patterns

Talk to infant while giving care

Rock infant to promote security or sleep

Encourage parents to provide daily care of infant, as appropriate

Instruct parents to perform special care for infant, as appropriate

Reinforce parent's skill in performing special care for infant

Inform parents about infant's progress

Explain rationale for treatments, procedures, and so on, to parents

Restrain infant during procedures

Comfort infant after painful procedure

Explain to parents that regression is normal during times of stress, such as illness or hospitalization

Comfort infant when experiencing separation anxiety

Encourage family visitation

Maintain infant's daily routine during hospitalization

Provide quiet, uninterrupted environment during nap time and nighttime, as appropriate

Background Readings:

Dickinson-Hazard, N. (1992). The first through sixth years of life. In M. Stanhope & J. Lancaster (Eds.) Community health nursing (3rd ed.) (pp. 485-511). St. Louis: Mosby.

Mott, S.R., Fazekas, N.F., & James, S.R. (1985). Nursing care of children and families. Menlo Park, CA: Addison-Wesley.

I

Infection Control   6540

Definition: Minimizing the acquisition and transmission of infectious agents

Activities:

Allocate the appropriate square feet per patient, as indicated by CDC guidelines

Clean the environment appropriately after each patient use

Change patient care equipment per agency protocol

Isolate persons exposed to communicable disease

Institute designated isolation precautions, as appropriate

Maintain isolation techniques, as appropriate

Limit the number of visitors, as appropriate

Teach improved hand washing to health care personnel

Instruct patient on appropriate hand washing techniques

Instruct visitors to wash hands on entering and leaving the patient's room

Use antimicrobial soap for hand washing, as appropriate

Wash hands before and after each patient care activity

Institute universal precautions

Wear gloves as mandated by universal precaution policy

Wear scrub clothes or gown when handling infectious material

Wear sterile gloves, as appropriate

Scrub the patient's skin with an antibacterial agent, as appropriate

Shave and prep the area, as indicated, in preparation for invasive procedures and/or surgery

Maintain an optimal aseptic environment during bedside insertion of central lines

Maintain an aseptic environment while changing TPN tubing and bottles

Maintain a closed system while doing invasive hemodynamic monitoring

Change peripheral IV and central line sites and dressings according to current CDC guidelines

Ensure aseptic handling of all IV lines

Ensure appropriate wound care technique

Use intermittent catheterization to reduce the incidence of bladder infection

Teach patient to obtain midstream urine specimens at first sign of return of symptoms, as appropriate

Encourage deep breathing and coughing, as appropriate

Promote appropriate nutritional intake

Encourage fluid intake, as appropriate

Encourage rest

Administer antibiotic therapy, as appropriate

Administer an immunizing agent, as appropriate

Instruct patient to take antibiotics, as prescribed

Teach patient and family about signs and symptoms of infection and when to report them to the health care provider

Teach patient and family members how to avoid infections

Promote safe food preservation and preparation

Background Readings:

Degroot-Kosolcharoen, J., & Jones, J.M. (1989). Permeability of latex and vinyl gloves to water and blood. American Journal of Infection Control, 17, 196-201.

Ehrenkranz, J.J., Eckert, D.G., & Phillips, P.M. (1989). Sporadic bacteremia complicating central venous catheter use in a community hospital. American Journal of Infection Control, 17(2), 69-76.

Larsen, E., Mayur, K., & Laughon, B.A. (1989). Influence of two handwashing frequencies on reduction in colonizing flora with three handwashing products used by health care personnel. American Journal of Infection Control, 17(2), 83-88.

Pottinger, J., Burns, S., & Manske, C. (1989). Bacterial carriage by artificial versus natural nails. American Journal of Infection Control, 17, 340-344.

Pugliese, G., & Lampinen, T. (1989). Prevention of human immunodeficiency virus infection: Our responsibilities as health care professionals. American Journal of Infection Control, 17(1), 1-22.

Thompson, J.M., McFarland, G.K., Hirsch, J.E., & Tucker, S.M. (1998). Mosby's clinical nursing (4th ed.). St. Louis: Mosby.

Turner, J., & Lovvorn, M. (1992). Communicable diseases and infection control practices in community health nursing. In M. Stanhope & J. Lancaster (Eds.), Community health nursing (3rd ed.) (pp. 312-331). St. Louis: Mosby.

I

I

Infection Control: Intraoperative   **6545**

Definition: Preventing nosocomial infection in the operating room

Activities:

Damp dust flat surfaces and lights in operating room

Monitor and maintain room temperature between 20° and 24° C

Monitor and maintain relative humidity between 40% and 60%

Monitor and maintain laminar airflow

Limit and control traffic

Verify that prophylactic antibiotics have been administered, as appropriate

Use universal precautions

Ensure that operating personnel are wearing appropriate attire

Use designated isolation precautions, as appropriate

Monitor isolation techniques, as appropriate

Verify integrity of sterile packaging

Verify sterilization indicators

Open sterile supplies and instruments using aseptic technique

Scrub, gown, and glove, as per agency policy

Assist with gowning and gloving of team members

Assist with draping the patient, ensuring protection of eyes and minimizing pressure to body parts

Separate sterile from nonsterile supplies

Monitor sterile field for break-in sterility and correct breaks, as indicated

Maintain integrity of catheters and intravascular lines

Inspect skin/tissue around surgical site

Apply drip towels to prevent pooling of antimicrobial prep solution

Apply antimicrobial solution to surgical site, as per agency policy

Remove drip towels

Obtain cultures, as needed

Contain contamination when it occurs

Administer antibiotic therapy, as appropriate

Maintain a neat and orderly room to limit contamination

Apply and secure surgical dressings

Remove drapes and supplies to limit contamination

Clean and sterilize instruments, as appropriate

Coordinate cleaning and preparation of the operating room for the next patient

Background Readings:

Association of Operating Room Nurses. (1993). Standards and recommended practices. Denver: Association of Operating Room Nurses.

Classen, D., Evans, S., Pestohnic, S., Horn, S., Menlove, R., & Burke, J. (1992). The timing of prophylactic administration of antibiotics and the risk of surgical wound infection. The New England Journal of Medicine, 326(5), 281-286.

Fairchild, S. (1993). Perioperative nursing: Principles and practice. Boston: Jones & Bartlett Publishers.

Kneedler, J., & Dodge, G. (1994). Perioperative patient care: The nursing perspective (3rd ed.). Boston: Jones & Bartlett Publishers.

Infection Protection 6550

Definition: Prevention and early detection of infection in a patient at risk

Activities:

Monitor for systemic and localized signs and symptoms of infection

Monitor vulnerability to infection

Monitor absolute granulocyte count, WBC count, and differential results

Follow neutropenic precautions, as appropriate

Limit the number of visitors, as appropriate

Screen all visitors for communicable disease

Maintain asepsis for patient at risk

Maintain isolation techniques, as appropriate

Provide appropriate skin care to edematous areas

Inspect skin and mucous membranes for redness, extreme warmth, or drainage

Inspect condition of any surgical incision/wound

Obtain cultures, as needed

Promote sufficient nutritional intake

Encourage fluid intake, as appropriate

Encourage rest

Monitor for change in energy level/malaise

Encourage increased mobility and exercise, as appropriate

Encourage deep breathing and coughing, as appropriate

Administer an immunizing agent, as appropriate

Instruct patient to take antibiotics as prescribed

Teach the patient and family about signs and symptoms of infection and when to report them to the health care provider

Teach patient and family members how to avoid infections

Eliminate fresh fruits, vegetables, and pepper from the diet of patients with neutropenia

Remove fresh flowers and plants from patient areas, as appropriate

Provide private room, as needed

Ensure water safety by instituting hyperchlorination and hyperheating, as appropriate

Report suspected infections to infection control personnel

Report positive cultures to infection control personnel

Background Readings:

Degroot-Kosolcharoen, J., & Jones, J.M. (1989). Permeability of latex and vinyl gloves to water and blood. American Journal of Infection Control, 17, 196-201.

Ehrenkranz, J.J., Eckert, D.G., & Phillips, P.M. (1989). Sporadic bacteremia complicating central venous catheter use in a community hospital. American Journal of Infection Control, 17(2), 69-76.

Larsen, E., Mayur, K., & Laughon, B.A. (1989). Influence of two handwashing frequencies on reduction in colonizing flora with three handwashing products used by health care personnel. American Journal of Infection Control, 17(2), 83-88.

Pottinger, J., Burns, S., & Manske, C. (1989). Bacterial carriage by artificial versus natural nails. American Journal of Infection Control, 17, 340-344.

Pugliese, G., & Lampinen, T. (1989). Prevention of human immunodeficiency virus infection: Our responsibilities as health care professionals. American Journal of Infection Control, 17(1), 1-22.

Thompson, J.M., McFarland, G.K., Hirsch, J.E., & Tucker, S.M. (1998). Mosby's clinical nursing (4th ed.). St. Louis: Mosby.

Insurance Authorization 7410

Definition: Assisting the patient and provider to secure payment for health services or equipment from a third party

Activities:

Explain reasons for obtaining preapproval for health services or equipment

Explain consent for release of information

Obtain signature of patient or responsible adult on release of information form

Obtain information and signature of patient or responsible adult on assignment of benefits form, as needed

Provide information to third-party payer about the necessity of the health service or equipment

Obtain or write a prescription for equipment, as appropriate

Submit prescription for equipment to the third-party payer

Record evidence of preapproval (e.g., validation number) on the patient's chart, as necessary

Inform patient or responsible adult of the status of the preapproval request

Discuss financial responsibilities of client (e.g., out-of-pocket expenses), as appropriate

Notify appropriate health professional if approval is refused by the third-party payer

Negotiate alternative modalities of care, as appropriate, if approval is refused (e.g., outpatient status or change in care/acuity level)

Provide preapproval information to other departments, as necessary

Document care provided, as required

Assist with the completion of claim forms, as needed

Facilitate communication with third-party payers, as needed

Collaborate with other health professionals about continued need for health services, as appropriate

Document continued need for health services, as required

Provide necessary information (e.g., name, Social Security number, and provider) to third-party payer for billing, as needed

Assist client to access needed health services or equipment

Background Readings:

Grossman, J. (1987). The psychiatric, alcohol and drug algorithm: A decision model for the nurse reviewer. Quality Review Bulletin, 13(9), 302-308.

Kozier, B., Erb, G., & Olivieri, R. (1991). Fundamentals of nursing: concepts, process, and practice (pp. 107-121). Redwood City, CA: Addison-Wesley.

LeNoble, E. (1991). Pre-admission possible. The Canadian Nurse, 14(2), 18-20.

Pechansky, R., & Macnee, C.L. (1993). Ensuring excellence: Reconceptualizing quality assurance, risk management, and utilization review. Quality Review Bulletin, 19(6), 182-189.

Stone, C.L., & Krebs, K. (1990). The use of utilization review nurses to decrease reimbursement denials. Home Healthcare Nurse, 8(3), 13-17.

Intracranial Pressure (ICP) Monitoring   2590

Definition: Measurement and interpretation of patient data to regulate intracranial pressure

Activities:

Assist with ICP monitoring device insertion

Provide information to family/significant others

Calibrate and level the transducer

Irrigate flush system

Set alarms

Obtain cerebrospinal fluid (CSF) drainage samples, as appropriate

Record ICP pressure readings and analyze waveforms

Monitor cerebral perfusion pressure

Note patient's change in response to stimuli

Monitor patient's ICP and neurological responses to care activities

Monitor amount/rate of CSF drainage

Monitor intake and output

Restrain patient, as needed

Monitor pressure tubing for bubbles

Change transducer/flush system

Change and/or reinforce insertion site dressing, as necessary

Monitor insertion site for infection

Monitor temperature and WBC count

Check patient for nuchal rigidity

Administer antibiotics

Position the patient with head elevated 30 to 45 degrees and with neck in a neutral position

Minimize environmental stimuli

Space nursing care to minimize ICP elevation

Alter suctioning procedure to minimize increase in ICP with catheter introduction (e.g., give lidocaine and limit number of suction passes)

Maintain controlled hyperventilation, as ordered

Maintain systemic arterial pressure within specified range

Administer pharmacological agents to maintain ICP within specified range

Notify physician of elevated ICP that does not respond to treatment protocols

Background Readings:

Ackerman, L.L. (1992). Interventions related to neurological care. In G.M. Bulechek & J.C. McCloskey (Eds.), Symposium on Nursing Interventions. Nursing Clinics of North America, 27(2), 325-346.

Alspach, J.G. (Ed.). (1991). Core curriculum for critical care nursing (4th ed.). Philadelphia: W.B. Saunders.

Cammermeyer, M., & Appledorn, C. (Eds.). (1990). Core curriculum for neuroscience nursing (3rd ed.) (pp. Id1-Id11). Chicago: American Association of Neuroscience Nurses.

German, K. (1988). Interpretation of ICP pulse waves to determine intracerebral compliance. Journal of Neuroscience Nursing, 20(6), 344-349.

Hichman, K.M., & Muwaswes, M. (1990). Intracranial pressure monitoring: Review of risk factors associated with infection. Heart & Lung, 19(1), 84-90.

Continued

Background Readings:—cont'd

Hollingsworth-Fridlund, P., Vos, H., & Daily, E.K. (1988). Use of fiber-optic pressure transducers for intracranial pressure measurements: A preliminary report. Heart & Lung, 17(2), 111-118.

Johanson, B.C., Wells, S.J., Hoffmeister, D., & Dungca, C.U. (1988). Standards for critical care (3rd ed.). St. Louis: Mosby.

Titler, M.G. (1992). Interventions related to surveillance. In G.M. Bulechek & J.C. McCloskey (Eds.), Symposium on Nursing Interventions. Nursing Clinics of North America, 27(2), 495-516.

I

Intrapartal Care   6830

Definition: Monitoring and management of stages one and two of the birth process

Activities:

Determine whether patient is in labor

Determine whether membranes are ruptured

Admit to birthing area

Determine patient's childbirth preparation and goals

Encourage family participation in the birth process consistent with patient goals

Prepare patient for labor per protocol, practitioner request, and patient preference

Drape patient to ensure privacy during examination

Perform Leopold maneuver to determine fetal position

Perform vaginal exams, as appropriate

Monitor maternal vital signs between contractions, per protocol or as needed

Auscultate the fetal heart every 30 to 60 minutes in early labor, every 15 to 30 minutes during active labor, and every 5 to 10 minutes in second stage, depending on risk status

Auscultate fetal heart rate between contractions to establish baseline

Monitor fetal heart rate during and after contractions to detect decelerations or accelerations

Apply electronic fetal monitor, per protocol or as appropriate, to obtain additional information

Report abnormal fetal heart rate changes to primary practitioner

Palpate contractions to determine frequency, duration, intensity, and resting tone

Encourage ambulation during early labor

Monitor pain level during labor

Explore positions that improve maternal comfort and maintain placental perfusion

Teach breathing, relaxation, and visualization techniques

Provide alternative methods of pain relief consistent with patient's goals (e.g., simple massage, effleurage, aromatherapy, hypnosis, and transcutaneous electrical nerve stimulation [TENS])

Provide ice chips, wet washcloth, or hard candy

Encourage patient to empty bladder every 2 hours

Assist labor coach or family in providing comfort and support during labor

Administer analgesics to promote comfort and relaxation during labor

Observe effects of medication on mother and fetus

Advise patients of options for anesthesia that would require referral to another practitioner

Assist with regional analgesia/anesthesia, as appropriate

Perform or assist with amniotomy, as appropriate

Auscultate fetal heart rate before and after amniotomy

Reevaluate position of fetus and cord after amniotomy

Document characteristics of fluid, fetal heart rate, and contraction pattern after spontaneous or artificial rupture of membranes

Cleanse perineum and change absorbent pads regularly

Continued

Activities:—cont'd

Monitor progress of labor, including vaginal discharge, cervical dilation, effacement, position, and fetal descent

Keep patient and labor coach informed of progress

Explain purpose of required labor interventions

Obtain informed consent before invasive procedures

Monitor family coping during labor

Perform vaginal exam to determine complete cervical dilation, fetal position, and station

Teach pushing techniques for second stage labor, based on the woman's birth preparation and preference

Coach during second-stage labor

Monitor pushing progress, fetal descent, fetal heart rate, and maternal vital signs, per protocol

Encourage spontaneous bearing-down efforts during the second stage

Evaluate pushing efforts and length of time in second stage

Recommend pushing changes to enhance fetal descent

Massage perineum to stretch and relax tissue

Apply warm compresses, as appropriate

Assist coach to continue supportive activities

Prepare delivery supplies

Document events of labor

Notify primary practitioner at the appropriate time to scrub for attending delivery

Background Readings:

Martin, E.J. (1990). Intrapartum management modules. Baltimore: Williams & Wilkins.

Malinowski, J.S., Pedigo, C.G., & Phillips, C.R. (1989). Nursing care during the labor process (3rd ed.). Philadelphia: F.A. Davis.

May, K.A., & Mahlmeister, L.R. (1994). Maternal and neonatal nursing: Family-centered care (3rd ed.). Philadelphia: Lippincott.

NAACOG. (1990). Fetal heart rate auscultation. OGN nursing practice resource. Washington, DC: NAACOG.

Olds, S.B., London, M.L., & Ladewig, P.A. (1988). Maternal-newborn nursing: A family centered approach (3rd ed.). Menlo Park, CA: Addison-Wesley.

Varney, H. (1987). Nurse-midwifery (2nd ed.). St. Louis: Mosby.

Intrapartal Care: High-Risk Delivery   6834

Definition: Assisting with vaginal delivery of multiple or malpositioned fetuses

Activities:

Inform patient and support person of extra procedures and personnel to anticipate during birth process

Communicate changes in maternal or fetal status to primary practitioner, as appropriate

Prepare appropriate equipment, including electronic fetal monitor, ultrasound, anesthesia machine, neonatal resuscitation supplies, forceps (e.g., Piper), and extra infant warmers

Notify extra assistants to attend birth (e.g., neonatologist, neonatal intensive care nurses, and anesthesiologist)

Provide assistance for gowning and gloving obstetrical team

Continue intervention for Electronic Fetal Monitoring: Intrapartum

Coach during second-stage pushing

Alert primary practitioner to abnormalities in maternal vital signs or fetal heart tracing(s)

Encourage support person to assist with comfort measures

Use universal precautions

Perform perineal scrub

Perform or assist with manual rotation of fetal head from occiput posterior to anterior position, as appropriate

Record time of delivery of first twin or of breech to the level of the umbilicus

Assist with amniotomy of additional amniotic membranes, as needed

Continue to monitor heart rate(s) of second or third fetus

Perform ultrasound exam to locate fetal position, as appropriate

Follow fetal head with hand to promote flexion during breech delivery, as directed by primary practitioner

Support body as primary practitioner delivers aftercoming head

Assist with application of forceps or vacuum extractor, as needed

Assist with administration of maternal anesthesic, as needed (e.g., intubation)

Record time of birth(s)

Assist with neonatal resuscitation, as needed

Document procedures (e.g., anesthesia, forceps, vacuum extraction, suprapubic pressure, McRobert maneuver, and neonatal resuscitation) used to facilitate birth

Explain newborn characteristics related to high-risk birth (e.g., bruising and forceps marks)

Observe closely for postpartum hemorrhage

Assist mother to recover from anesthesic, as appropriate

Encourage parental interaction with newborn(s) soon after delivery

Background Readings:

Eganhouse, D.J. (1992). Fetal monitoring of twins. Journal of Obstetric, Gynecologic, and Neonatal Nursing, 21(1), 16-22.

Gilbert, E.S., & Harmon, J.S. (1993). Manual of high risk pregnancy and delivery. St. Louis: Mosby.

Mattson, S., & Smith, J.E. (Eds.). (1993). Core curriculum for maternal-newborn nursing. Philadelphia: W.B. Saunders.

I

Intravenous (IV) Insertion   4190

Definition: Insertion of a needle into a peripheral vein for the purpose of administering fluids, blood, or medications

Activities:

Verify order for IV therapy

Instruct patient about procedure

Maintain strict aseptic technique

Identify whether patient is allergic to any medications, iodine, or tape

Identify whether patient has a clotting problem or is taking any medications that would affect clotting

Ask patient to hold still while performing venipuncture

Provide emotional support, as appropriate

Ask parents to hold and comfort a child, as appropriate

Select an appropriate vein for venipuncture

Start IVs in the opposite arm for patients with arteriovenous fistulas or shunts

Choose an appropriate type of needle, based on purpose and length of expected use

Choose an 18-gauge needle, if possible, for blood administration in adults

Apply a tourniquet 3 to 4 inches above the anticipated puncture site, as appropriate

Instruct patient to hold the extremity lower than the heart

Massage patient's arm from proximal to distal end, as appropriate

Lightly tap the puncture area after applying the tourniquet, as appropriate

Cleanse area with an appropriate solution, based on agency protocol

Administer 1% lidocaine at the insertion site, as appropriate

Insert needle according to manufacturer's instructions

Determine correct placement by observing for blood in flash chamber or in tubing

Remove tourniquet as soon as possible

Tape needle securely in place

Connect needle to IV tubing or heplock, as appropriate

Apply a small transparent dressing over IV insertion site

Label IV site dressing

Apply arm board, being careful not to compromise circulation, as appropriate

Maintain universal precautions

Background Readings:

Channell, S.R. (1985). Manual for IV therapy procedures. Oradell, NJ: Medical Economics Books.

Craven, R.F., & Hirnle, C.J. (2000) Fundamentals of nursing: Human health and function (3rd ed.) (pp. 566-568). Philadelphia: Lippincott.

McGill, S.L., & Smith, J.R. (1983). IV therapy. Bowie, MD: Brady Communications.

Plumer, A.L. (1987). Principles and practice of intravenous therapy. Boston: Little, Brown & Co.

Intravenous (IV) Therapy   4200

Definition: Administration and monitoring of intravenous fluids and medications

Activities:

Verify order for IV therapy

Instruct patient about procedure

Maintain strict aseptic technique

Examine the solution for type, amount, expiration date, character of the solution, and lack of damage to container

Perform the 5 rights prior to starting infusion or administering medications (right drug, dose, patient, route, & frequency)

Select and prepare an IV infusion pump, as indicated

Spike container with appropriate tubing

Administer IV fluids at room temperature, unless otherwise ordered

Identify whether patient is taking medication that is incompatible with medication ordered

Administer IV medications, as prescribed, and monitor for results

Monitor IV flow rate and IV site during infusion

Monitor for fluid overload and physical reactions

Monitor for IV patency before administration of IV medication

Replace IV cannula, apparatus, and infusate every 48 to 72 hours, according to agency protocol

Maintain occlusive dressing

Perform IV site checks according to agency protocol

Perform IV site care according to agency protocol

Monitor vital signs

Monitor amount of IV potassium to not exceed 200 mEq per 24 hours for adults, as appropriate

Flush IV lines between administration of incompatible solutions

Record intake and output as appropriate

Monitor for signs and symptoms associated with infusion phlebitis and local infection

Document prescribed therapy per agency protocol

Maintain universal precautions

Background Readings:

Hadaway, L.C. (2000). Managing IV therapy "high-alert" drugs keep nurse managers ever watchful. Nursing Management. 31(10), 38-40.

Perry, A.G., & Potter, P.A. (2002). Clinical nursing skills and techniques (5th ed.) (pp. 559-616). St. Louis: Mosby.

Revised intravenous nursing standards of practice (2000). Journal of Intravenous Nursing 21(1S), S1-S95, Nov-Dec.(Is-suppl).

I

Invasive Hemodynamic Monitoring   4210

Definition: Measurement and interpretation of invasive hemodynamic parameters to determine cardiovascular function and regulate therapy as appropriate

Activities:

Assist with insertion and removal of invasive hemodynamic lines

Assist with Allen test for evaluation of collateral ulnar circulation before radial artery cannulation, if appropriate

Assist with chest x-ray examination after insertion of pulmonary artery catheter

Monitor heart rate and rhythm

Zero and calibrate equipment every 4 to 12 hours, as appropriate, with transducer at the level of the right atrium

Monitor blood pressure (systolic, diastolic, and mean), central venous/right atrial pressure, pulmonary artery pressure (systolic, diastolic, and mean), and pulmonary capillary/artery wedge pressure

Monitor hemodynamic waveforms for changes in cardiovascular function

Compare hemodynamic parameters with other clinical signs and symptoms

Use closed-system cardiac output setup

Obtain cardiac output by administering cardiac output injectate within 4 seconds, and average three injections that are within less than 1 L of each other

Monitor pulmonary artery and systemic arterial waveforms; if dampening occurs, check tubing for kinks or air bubbles, check connections, aspirate clot from tip of catheter, gently flush system, or assist with repositioning of catheter

Document pulmonary artery and systemic arterial waveforms

Monitor peripheral perfusion distal to catheter insertion site every 4 hours or as appropriate

Monitor for dyspnea, fatigue, tachypnea, and orthopnea

Monitor for forward progression of pulmonary catheter resulting in spontaneous wedge, and notify physician if it occurs

Refrain from inflating balloon more frequently than every 1 to 2 hours, or as appropriate

Monitor for balloon rupture (e.g., assess for resistance when inflating balloon and allow balloon to passively deflate after obtaining pulmonary capillary/artery wedge pressure)

Prevent air emboli (e.g., remove air bubbles from tubing; if balloon rupture is suspected, refrain from attempts to reinflate balloon and clamp balloon port)

Maintain sterility of ports

Maintain closed-pressure system to ports, as appropriate

Perform sterile dressing changes and site care, as appropriate

Inspect insertion site for signs of bleeding or infection

Change IV solution and tubing every 24 to 72 hours, based on protocol

Monitor laboratory results to detect possible catheter-induced infection

Administer fluid and/or volume expanders to maintain hemodynamic parameters within specified range

Administer pharmacological agents to maintain hemodynamic parameters within specifiied range

Instruct patient and family on therapeutic use of hemodynamic monitoring catheters

Instruct patient on activity restriction while catheters remain in place

Background Readings:

Barcelona, M., Patague, L., Bunoy, M., et al. (1985). Cardiac output determination by the thermodilution method: Comparison of ice temperature injectate versus room temperature injectate contained in prefilled syringes or closed injectate delivery system. Heart & Lung, 14(3), 232-235.

Chulay, M., & Miller, T. (1984). The effect of backrest elevation on pulmonary capillary wedge pressure in patients after cardiac surgery. Heart & Lung, 16(3), 294-300.

Cullen, L.M. (1992). Interventions related to circulatory care. In G.M. Bulechek & J.C. McCloskey (Eds.), Symposium on Nursing Interventions. Nursing Clinics of North America, 27(2), 445-476.

Daily, E., & Mersch, J. (1987). Thermodilution cardiac output using room and ice temperature injectate: Comparison with the Fick method. Heart & Lung, 16(3), 294-300.

Daily, J.S., & Schroeder, J.S. (1989). Techniques in bedside hemodynamic monitoring (4th ed.). St. Louis: Mosby.

Doering, L., & Dracup, K. (1988). Comparison of cardiac output in supine and lateral position. Nursing Research, 37(2), 114-118.

Groom, L., Frisch, S., & Elliot, M. (1990). Reproducibility and accuracy of pulmonary artery pressure measurement in supine and lateral positions. Heart & Lung, 19(2), 147-151.

Harvey, C. (1991). Critical care obstetrics. Rockville, MD: Aspen.

Johanson, B.C., Wells, S.J., Hoffmeister, D., & Dungca, C.U. (1988). Standards for critical care (3rd ed.). St. Louis: Mosby.

Kennedy, B., Bryant, A., & Crawford, M. (1984). The effects of lateral body positioning on measurements of pulmonary artery and pulmonary artery wedge pressure. Heart & Lung, 13(2), 155-158.

Lipp-Ziff, E., & Kawanishi, D. (1991). A technique for improving accuracy of the pulmonary artery diastolic pressure as an estimate of left ventricular end-diastolic pressure. Heart & Lung, 20(2), 107-115.

Titler, M.G. (1992). Interventions related to surveillance. In G.M. Bulechek & J.C. McCloskey (Eds.), Symposium on Nursing Interventions. Nursing Clinics of North America, 27(2), 495-516.

I

Kangaroo Care 6840

Definition: Promoting closeness between parent and physiologically stable preterm infant by preparing the parent and providing the environment for skin-to-skin contact

Activities:

Discuss parent reaction to premature birth of infant

Determine image parent has of premature infant

Determine and monitor parent's level of confidence in caring for infant

Encourage parent to initiate infant care

Explain kangaroo care and its benefits to parent

Determine whether infant's physiological status meets guidelines for participation in kangaroo care

Prepare a quiet, private, draft-free environment

Provide parent with a reclining or rocking chair

Have parent wear comfortable, open-front clothing

Instruct parent how to transfer infant from incubator, warmer bed, or bassinet and how to manage equipment and tubing, as appropriate

Position diaper-clad infant in prone upright position on parent's chest

Wrap parent's clothing around or place blanket over infant to maintain infant's position and temperature

Encourage parent to focus on infant, rather than high-tech setting and equipment

Encourage parent to gently stroke infant in prone upright position, as appropriate

Encourage parent to gently rock infant in prone upright position, as appropriate

Encourage auditory stimulation of infant, as appropriate

Reinforce eye contact with infant, as appropriate

Support parent in nurturing and providing hands-on care for infant

Encourage parent to hold infant with full, encompassing hands

Encourage parent to identify infant's behavioral cues

Point out infant state changes to parent

Instruct parent to decrease activity when infant shows signs of overstimulation, distress, or avoidance

Encourage parent to let the infant sleep during kangaroo care

Encourage breastfeeding during kangaroo care, as appropriate

Encourage parent to provide kangaroo care from 20 minutes to 3 hours at a time on a consistent basis, as appropriate

Encourage postpartum mothers to change position and get up every 90 minutes to prevent thrombolytic disease

Monitor parent's emotional reaction to kangaroo care

Monitor infant's physiological status (e.g., color, temperature, heart rate, and apnea), and discontinue kangaroo care if infant becomes physiologically compromised or agitated

Background Readings:

Anderson, G.C. (1989). Skin to skin: Kangaroo care in western Europe. American Journal of Nursing, 89, 662-666.

Anderson, G.C. (1991). Current knowledge about skin-to-skin (kangaroo) care for preterm infants. Journal of Perinatology, 11(3), 216-226.

Breitbach, K.M. (1994). Development and validation of nursing activities in kangaroo care. Master's thesis, Iowa City: University of Iowa.

Ludington-Hoe, S. (1990). Energy conservation during skin-to-skin contact between premature infants and their mothers. Heart & Lung, 19(5), 445-451.

Ludington-Hoe, S., & Golant, S. (1993). Kangaroo care: The best you can do to help your preterm infant. New York: Bantam Books.

Ludington-Hoe, S.M., Thompson, C., Swinth, J., Hadeed, A.J., & Anderson, G.C. (1994). Kangaroo care: Research results, and practice implication and guidelines. Neonatal Network, 13(1), 19-27.

Whitelaw, A. (1990). Kangaroo baby care: Just a nice experience or an important advance for preterm infants? Pediatrics, 85(4), 604-605.

K

Labor Induction 6850

Definition: Initiation or augmentation of labor by mechanical or pharmacological methods

Activities:

Determine medical and/or obstetrical indication for induction

Review obstetrical history for pertinent information that may influence induction, such as gestational age and length of prior labor and such contraindications as complete placenta previa, classical uterine incision, and pelvic structural deformities

Monitor maternal and fetal vital signs before induction

Perform or assist with application of mechanical or pharmacological agents (e.g., laminaria and prostaglandin gel) at the appropriate intervals, as needed, to enhance cervical readiness

Monitor for side effects of procedures used to ready cervix

Reevaluate cervical status and verify presentation before initiating further induction measures

Perform or assist with amniotomy, if cervical dilatation is adequate and vertex is well engaged

Determine fetal heart rate by auscultation or electronic fetal monitoring after amniotomy and per protocol

Encourage ambulation, if no contraindications are present for both mother and fetus

Observe for onset or change in uterine activity

Initiate IV medication (e.g., oxytocin) to stimulate uterine activity, as needed, after physician consultation

Monitor labor progress closely, being alert to signs of abnormal labor progress

Avoid uterine hyperstimulation by infusing oxytocin to achieve adequate contraction frequency, duration, and relaxation

Observe for signs of uteroplacental insufficiency (e.g., late decelerations) during the process of induction

Reduce or increase uterine stimulant (e.g., oxytocin), as needed or per protocol, until birth is imminent

Background Readings:

Day, M.L., & Snell, B.J. (1993). Use of prostaglandins for induction of labor. Journal of Nurse-Midwifery, 38(2), 42S-48S.

Gilbert, E.S., & Harmon, J.S. (1998). Manual of high risk pregnancy & delivery. (2nd ed.). St. Louis: Mosby.

Nurses Association of the American College of Obstetricians and Gynecologists. (1988). OGN nursing practice resource. The nurse's role in the induction/augmentation of labor. Washington, DC: NAACOG.

Nurses Association of the American College of Obstetricians and Gynecologists, Mattson, S., & Smith, J.E. (Eds.). (1993). Core curriculum for maternal-newborn nursing. Philadelphia: W.B. Saunders.

Pozaic, S. (1992). Induction and augmentation of labor. In L.K. Mandeville & N.H. Troiano (Eds.), High-risk intrapartum nursing. Philadelphia: J.B. Lippincott.

Labor Suppression   6860

Definition: Controlling uterine contractions prior to 37 weeks of gestation to prevent preterm birth

Activities:

Review history for risk factors commonly related to preterm labor (e.g., multifetal pregnancy, uterine anomalies, prior history of preterm birth, early cervical change, and uterine irritability)

Determine fetal age, based on last menstrual period, early sonogram, fundal height measurements, date of quickening, and date of audible fetal heart tones

Interview about onset and duration of preterm labor symptoms

Ask about activities preceding onset of preterm labor symptoms

Determine status of amniotic membranes

Perform cervical exam for dilation, effacement, softening, and position

Palpate fetal position, station, and presentation

Obtain urine and cervical cultures

Document uterine activity, using palpation, as well as electronic fetal monitoring

Obtain baseline maternal weight

Position mother laterally to optimize placental perfusion

Discuss bed rest and activity limits during acute phase of labor suppression

Initiate oral or IV hydration

Note contraindications to use of tocolytics (e.g., chorioamnionitis, preeclampsia, hemorrhage, fetal demise, or severe intrauterine growth retardation)

Initiate subcutaneous or IV tocolytics, per physician order or protocol, if hydration does not reduce uterine activity

Monitor maternal vital signs, fetal heart rate, and uterine activity every 15 minutes during initiation of IV tocolysis

Monitor for side effects of tocolytic therapy, including loss of deep tendon reflexes, if magnesium sulfate is administered

Educate the patient and family about normal tocolytic side effects (e.g., tremors, headache, palpitations, anxiety, nausea, vomiting, flushing, and warmth)

Provide interventions to reduce discomforts of normal side effects (e.g., relaxation therapy, anxiety reduction, and therapeutic touch)

Educate patient and family about abnormal tocolytic side effects (e.g., chest pain, shortness of breath, tachycardia, or recurrent contractions) to report to physician

Obtain baseline EKG, as appropriate

Monitor intake and output

Auscultate lungs

Begin oral or subcutaneous tocolysis, per physician order, after achieving adequate uterine quiescence

Determine patient and family knowledge of fetal development and preterm birth, as well as motivation to prolong pregnancy

Involve patient and family in plan for home care

Begin discharge teaching for home care, including medication regimens, activity restrictions, diet and hydration, sexual abstinence, and ways to avoid constipation

Teach contraction palpation techniques

Continued

Activities:—cont'd

Provide written patient education material for family

Provide referrals to assist family with child care, home maintenance, and diversionary activities, as appropriate

Discuss signs of recurrent preterm labor and reinforce the need to seek care immediately, if symptoms return and continue for 1 hour

Provide written discharge instructions, including explicit directions for seeking medical care

Background Readings:

Eganhouse, D.J. (1994). Development of a nursing program for preterm birth prevention. Journal of Obstetric, Gynecologic, and Neonatal Nursing, 23(9), 756-766.

Gilbert, E.S., & Harmon, J.S. (1998). Manual of high risk pregnancy & delivery. (2nd ed.). St. Louis: Mosby.

Nance, N. (1990). Module 8: Caring for the woman at risk for preterm labor or with premature rupture of membranes. In E.J. Martin (Ed.), Intrapartum management modules (pp. 259-284). Baltimore: Williams & Wilkins.

Wheeler, D.G. (1994). Preterm birth prevention. Journal of Nurse-Midwifery, 39(2), 665-805.

L

Laboratory Data Interpretation   7690

Definition: Critical analysis of patient laboratory data in order to assist with clinical decision making

Activities:

Be familiar with accepted abbreviations for particular institution

Use the reference ranges from the laboratory that is performing the particular test(s)

Recognize physiological factors that can affect laboratory values, including gender, age, pregnancy, diet (especially hydration), time of day, activity level, and stress

Recognize the effect of drugs on laboratory values, including prescription drugs, as well as over-the-counter medications

Note time and site of specimen collection, as applicable

Use peak drug levels when testing for toxicity

Recognize that trough drug levels are useful for demonstrating satisfactory therapeutic level

Consider influences of pharmacokinetics (e.g., half-life, peak, protein binding, and excretion) when evaluating toxic and therapeutic levels of drugs

Consider that multiple test abnormalities are more likely to be significant than single test abnormalities

Compare test results with other related laboratory and/or diagnostic test results

Compare results with previous values obtained when the patient was not ill (if available) to determine baseline values

Monitor sequential test results for trends or gross changes

Consult appropriate references/texts for clinical implication of unfamiliar tests

Recognize that incorrect test results most often result from clerical errors

Perform confirmation of grossly abnormal test results with close attention to patient and specimen identification, condition of specimen, and prompt delivery to the laboratory

Report results of lab tests to patient, as appropriate

Send split samples to the laboratory for verification of results, if appropriate

Report sudden changes in laboratory values to physician immediately

Report critical values (as determined by institution) to physician immediately

Analyze whether results obtained are consistent with patient behavior and clinical status

Background Readings:

Call-Schmidt, T. (2001). Interpreting lab results: A primer. MEDSURG Nursing, 10(4), 179-184.

Corbett, J.V. (2000). Laboratory tests and diagnostic procedures with nursing diagnoses (5th ed.). Upper Saddle River, NJ: Prentice Hall Health.

Kee, J.F. (2001). Handbook of laboratory and diagnostic tests with nursing implications (4th ed.). Upper Saddle River, NJ: Prentice Hall.

Pagana, K.D., & Pagana, T.J. (2001). Mosby's diagnostic and laboratory test reference (5th ed.). St. Louis: Mosby.

Perry, A.C., & Potter, P.A. (2002). Clinical nursing skills & techniques (5th ed.) (pp. 1148-1149). St. Louis: Mosby.

Titler, M.G. (1992). Interventions related to surveillance. In G.M. Bulechek & J.C. McCloskey (Eds.), Symposium on Nursing Interventions. Nursing Clinics of North America, 27(2), 495-516.

Lactation Counseling 5244

Definition: Use of an interactive helping process to assist in maintenance of successful breastfeeding

Activities:

Determine knowledge base about breastfeeding

Educate parent(s) about infant feeding for informed decision making

Provide information about advantages and disadvantages of breastfeeding

Correct misconceptions, misinformation, and inaccuracies about breastfeeding

Determine mother's desire and motivation to breastfeed

Provide support of mother's decisions

Give parent(s) recommended education material as needed

Refer parents to appropriate classes or support groups for breastfeeding

Evaluate mother's understanding of infant's feeding cues (e.g., rooting, sucking, alertness)

Determine frequency of feedings in relationship to baby's needs

Monitor maternal skill with latching infant to the nipple

Evaluate newborn suck/swallow pattern

Demonstrate suck training, as appropriate

Instruct on relaxation techniques, including breast massage

Encourage ways of increasing rest, including delegation of household tasks and ways of requesting help

Instruct on record keeping of length and frequency of nursing sessions

Instruct about infant stool and urination patterns, as appropriate

Instruct mother about infant growth spurts to identify normal patterns of breastfeeding infants

Evaluate adequacy of breast emptying with feeding

Evaluate quality and use of breastfeeding aids

Encourage mother to offer both breasts at each feeding

Determine appropriateness of breast pump use

Provide formula information for temporary low supply problems

Demonstrate breast massage and discuss its advantages to increasing milk supply

Instruct parents on how to differentiate between perceived and actual insufficient milk supply

Encourage breast pumping between feedings if low milk supply is suspected

Monitor skin integrity of nipples

Recommend nipple care as needed

Monitor ability to correctly relieve breast congestion

Evaluate understanding of plugged milk ducts and mastitis

Instruct mothers on the importance of monitoring hemoglobin/hematocrit levels and thyroid function while breastfeeding

Instruct on signs of problems to report to health care practitioner

Demonstrate equipment available to assist with breastfeeding following breast surgery, such as a breast pump, warm packs, and nursing supplementer

Instruct on how to relactate as appropriate

Encourage continued lactation upon return to work or school

Discuss signs of readiness to wean

Discuss options for weaning

Discuss alternative methods of feeding

Instruct mother to consult her health care practitioner before taking any medications while breastfeeding, prescribed or over-the-counter

Encourage mother to avoid birth control pills while breastfeeding

Discuss alternative methods of contraception

Encourage mother to avoid cigarettes while breastfeeding

Encourage employers to provide opportunities for and private facilities for lactating mothers to pump and store breast milk during the workday

Background Readings:

Department of Health and Human Services. (1990). Healthy People 2000: National health promotion and disease prevention objectives. DHHS Publication No. PHS 90-50213. Washington, DC: DHHS.

Denehy, J.A. (1992). Interventions related to parent-infant attachment. In G.M. Bulechek & J.C. McCloskey (Eds.), Symposium on Nursing Interventions. Nursing Clinics of North America. 27(2).

Isabella, P., & Isabella, R. (1994). Correlates of successful breastfeeding: A study on social and personal factors. Journal of Human Lactation, 10(4), 257-264.

Littleton, L.Y., & Engbertson, J.C. (2002). Maternal, neonatal, & women's health nursing (pp. 985-997). Albany, NY: Delmar

Olds, S.B., London, M.L., & Ladewig, P.A. (1988). Maternal-newborn nursing: A family centered approach (3rd ed.). Menlo Park, CA: Addison-Wesley.

Riordan, J., & Auerbach, L. (1993). Breastfeeding and human lactation. Boston: Jones & Bartlett Publishers.

Walker, M. (1989). Management of selected early breastfeeding problems seen in clinical practice. Birth, 16(3), 148-157.

L

Lactation Suppression 6870

Definition: Facilitating the cessation of milk production and minimizing breast engorgement after giving birth

Activities:

Administer lactation suppression drug, if appropriate

Monitor blood pressure during drug therapy for lactation suppression

Monitor breast engorgement and discomfort

Apply ice packs to axillary area of breasts for 20 minutes qid and at home, as needed

Inform patient that engorgement may occur after discharge

Administer analgesics, as needed

Encourage patient to wear supportive, well-fitting bra continuously until lactation is suppressed

Apply breast binder, as appropriate

Instruct patient to avoid breast stimulation

Inform patient about early return of ovulation

Instruct patient about appropriate contraceptive measures

Background Readings:

Olds, S.B., London, M.L., & Ladewig, P.A. (1992). Maternal-newborn nursing: A family-centered approach (4th ed.). Menlo Park, CA: Addison-Wesley.

Radestad, I., Nordin, C., Steineck, G. (1998), A comparison of women's memories of care during pregnancy, labour, and delivery after stillbirth or live birth. Midwifery, 14, 111-117.

L

Laser Precautions   6560

Definition: Limiting the risk of laser-related injury to the patient

Activities:

Provide appropriate laser, fiber(s), filters, lenses, and attachments

Provide appropriate eye protection

Verify that instruments and supplies are laser-safe

Verify that ointments and solutions are nonflammable

Provide a rectal pack, as appropriate

Cover windows, as appropriate

Set up and connect plume evacuator, as appropriate

Provide high-filtration masks, as appropriate

Place laser use sign(s) on entrance(s) to room

Check fire-extinguishing supplies/equipment

Set up laser, per protocol

Inspect electrical cords

Inspect laser fibers for breaks

Activate area entryway control system, as appropriate

Test-fire laser

Instruct patient about importance of not moving during laser use, as appropriate

Instruct patient about importance of eyewear, as appropriate

Immobilize patient's body part, as appropriate

Protect tissue around laser site with moistened towels or sponges

Remove other pedals from the area

Adjust laser settings, per physician or agency protocol

Monitor patient for potential injury

Monitor environment for possible fire

Monitor environment for flammable substance or breaks in precautions

Return laser key to designated secure location

Sterilize laser lenses, as appropriate

Record information, per protocol

Background Readings:

Association of Operating Room Nurses. (1993). Standards and recommended practices. Denver: Association of Operating Room Nurses.

Ball, K. (1995). Lasers: The perioperative challenge. (2nd ed.). St. Louis: Mosby.

Fairchild, S. (1993). Perioperative nursing: Principles and practice (3rd ed.). Boston: Jones & Bartlett.

Kneedler, J., & Dodge, G. (1994). Perioperative patient care: The nursing perspective. Boston: Jones & Bartlett.

L

Latex Precautions   6570

Definition: Reducing the risk of a systemic reaction to latex

Activities:

Question patient or appropriate other about history of neural tube defect (e.g., spina bifida) or congenital urological condition (e.g., exstrophy of the bladder)

Question patient or appropriate other about history of systemic reactions to natural rubber latex (e.g., facial or scleral edema, tearing eyes, urticaria, rhinitis, and wheezing)

Question patient or appropriate other about allergies to foods such as bananas, kiwi, avocado, mango, and chestnuts

Refer patient to allergist for allergy testing, as appropriate

Record allergy or risk in patient's medical record

Place allergy band on patient

Post sign indicating latex precautions

Survey environment and remove latex products

Monitor latex-free environment

Monitor patient for signs and symptoms of a systemic reaction

Report information to physician, pharmacist, and other care providers, as indicated

Administer medications, as appropriate

Instruct patient and family about risk factors for developing a latex allergy

Instruct patient and family about signs and symptoms of a reaction

Instruct patient and family about latex content in household products and substitution with nonlatex products, as appropriate

Instruct patient to wear a medical alert tag

Instruct patient and family about emergency treatment (e.g., epinephrine), as appropriate

Instruct visitors about latex-free environment (e.g., latex balloons not allowed)

Background Readings:

Floyd, P.T. (2000). Latex allergy update. Journal of Peri Anesthesia Nursing, 15(1), 26-30.

Kelly, K.J., & Walsh-Kelly, C.M. (1998). Latex allergy: A patient and healthcare system emergency. Annals of Emergency Medicine, 32(6), 723-729.

Kim, K.T., Graves, P.B., Safadi, G.S., Alhadeff, G., Metcalfe, J. (1998). Implementation recommendations for making health care facilities latex safe. AORN, 67(3), 615-632.

Miller, K.K., & Weed, P. (1998). The latex allergy trigger admission tool: An algorithm to identify which patient would benefit from latex safe precautions. Journal of Emergency Nursing, 24(2), 145-152.

Tarlo, S.M. (1998). Latex allergy: A problem for both healthcare professionals and patients. Ostomy/Wound Management, 44(8), 80-88.

Learning Facilitation   5520

Definition: Promoting the ability to process and comprehend information

Activities:

Begin the instruction only after the patient demonstrates readiness to learn

Set mutual, realistic learning goals with the patient

Identify learning objectives clearly and in measurable/observable terms

Adjust the instruction to the patient's level of knowledge and understanding

Tailor the content to the patient's cognitive, psychomotor, and/or affective abilities/disabilities

Provide information appropriate to developmental level

Provide an environment conducive to learning

Arrange the information in a logical sequence

Arrange the information from simple to complex, known to unknown, or concrete to abstract, as appropriate

Differentiate "critical" content from "desirable" content

Adapt the information to comply with the patient's lifestyle/routines

Relate the information to the patient's personal desires/needs

Provide information that is consistent with the patient's values/beliefs

Provide information that is compatible with the patient's locus of control

Ensure that the material is current and up-to-date

Provide educational materials to illustrate important and/or complex information

Use multiple teaching modalities, as appropriate

Use familiar language

Define unfamiliar terminology

Relate new content to previous knowledge, as appropriate

Present the information in a stimulating manner

Introduce the patient to persons who have undergone similar experiences

Encourage the patient's active participation

Use self-paced instruction, when possible

Avoid setting time limits

Provide adequate time for mastery of content, as appropriate

Keep teaching sessions short, as appropriate

Simplify instructions, as appropriate

Repeat important information

Provide verbal prompts/reminders, as appropriate

Provide memory aids, as appropriate

Avoid demands for abstract thinking, if patient can think only in concrete terms

Ensure that consistent information is being provided by various members of the health care team

Use demonstration and return demonstration, as appropriate

Provide opportunities for practice, as appropriate

Continued

Activities:—cont'd

Provide frequent feedback about learning progress

Correct information misinterpretations, as appropriate

Reinforce behavior, as appropriate

Provide time for the patient to ask questions and discuss concerns

Answer questions in a clear, concise manner

Background Readings:

Bastable, S.B. (2003). Nurse as educator: Principles of teaching and learning for nursing practice. Boston: Jones and Bartlett Publishers.

Burke, L.E. (1981). Learning and retention in the acute care setting. Critical Care Quarterly, December, 67.

Lindeman, C.A. (1988). Patient education. In J.J. Fitzpatrick, R.L. Taunton, & J.Q. Benoliel (Eds.), Annual Review of Nursing Research, 6, 29-60.

Miller, V. (1979). Helping the patient learn. Nursing Times, June 14, 1016.

Rakel, B.A. (1992). Interventions related to patient teaching. In G.M. Bulechek & J.C. McCloskey (Eds.), Symposium on Nursing Interventions. Nursing Clinics of North America, 27(2), 397-424.

Roy, S.C. (1988). Human information processing. In J.J. Fitzpatrick, R.L. Taunton, & J.Q. Benoliel (Eds.), Annual Review of Nursing Research, 6, 237-262.

Springhouse. (1987). Understanding basic concepts. In Patient teaching (nurse's reference library): Learning needs, discharge preparation, tips and checklists (pp. 1-17). Springhouse, PA: Springhouse.

L

Learning Readiness Enhancement   5540

Definition: Improving the ability and willingness to receive information

Activities:

Provide a nonthreatening environment

Establish rapport

Establish teacher credibility, as appropriate

Maximize the patient's hemodynamic status to facilitate brain oxygenation (e.g., positioning and medication adjustments), as appropriate

Fulfill the patient's basic physiological needs (e.g., hunger, thirst, warmth, and oxygen)

Decrease the patient's level of fatigue, as appropriate

Control the patient's pain, as appropriate

Avoid the use of medications that may alter the patient's perception (e.g., narcotics and hypnotics), as appropriate

Monitor the patient's level of orientation/confusion

Increase the patient's orientation to reality, as appropriate

Maximize sensory input by use of eyeglasses, hearing aids, and so on, as appropriate

Minimize the degree of sensory overload/underload, as appropriate

Satisfy the patient's safety needs (e.g., security, control, and familiarity), as appropriate

Monitor the patient's emotional state

Assist the patient to deal with intense emotions (e.g., anxiety, grief, and anger), as appropriate

Encourage verbalization of feelings, perceptions, and concerns

Provide time for the patient to ask questions and discuss concerns

Address the patient's specific concerns, as appropriate

Establish a learning environment as early in contact with patient as possible

Facilitate the patient's acceptance of the situation, as appropriate

Assist the patient to develop confidence in ability, as appropriate

Enlist participation of family/significant others, as appropriate

Explain how the information will help the patient meet goals, as appropriate

Explain how the patient's past unpleasant experiences with health care differ from the current situation, as appropriate

Assist the patient to realize the severity of the illness, as appropriate

Assist the patient to realize that treatment options exist, as appropriate

Assist the patient to realize susceptibility to complications, as appropriate

Assist the patient to realize the ability to prevent illness or condition, as appropriate

Assist the patient to realize ability to control the progression of the illness, as appropriate

Assist the patient to realize that current situation differs from past stressful situation, as appropriate

Assist the patient to see alternative actions that are less risky to lifestyle, as appropriate

Provide a trigger or cue (e.g., motivating comments/rationale and new information) toward appropriate action, as appropriate

Continued

Background Readings:

Bastable, S.B. (2003). Nurse as educator: Principles of teaching and learning for nursing practice. Boston: Jones and Bartlett Publishers.

Jenny, J. (1978). A strategy for patient teaching. Journal of Advanced Nursing, 3, 341.

Murdaugh, C.L. (1982). Barriers to patient education in the coronary care unit. Cardiovascular Nursing, 18, 31.

Rakel, B.A. (1992). Interventions related to patient teaching. In G.M. Bulechek & J.C. McCloskey (Eds.), Symposium on Nursing Interventions. Nursing Clinics of North America, 27(2), 397-424.

Redman, B.K. (1993). Assessment of motivation to learn & the need for patient education. In B.K. Redman (Ed.), The process of patient education (7th ed.) (pp. 16-43). St. Louis: Mosby.

Smith, C.E. (1987). Using the teaching process to determine what to teach and how to evaluate learning. In C.E. Smith (Ed.), Patient education: Nurses in partnership with other health professionals (pp. 61-95). Philadelphia: W.B. Saunders.

Springhouse. (1987). Assessing learning needs. In Patient teaching (nurse's reference library): Learning needs, discharge preparation, tips and checklists (pp. 19-43). Springhouse, PA: Springhouse.

L

Leech Therapy 3460

Definition: Application of medicinal leeches to help drain replanted or transplanted tissue engorged with venous blood

Activities:

Use leeches only if patient has an intact arterial blood supply to prevent infection from the endosymbiotic bacterium present in gut of the leech

Instruct patient that the leech's salivary glands secrete a local anesthetic that helps mask the sensation of the bite

Instruct patient that a local anesthetic will not be needed in replanted tissue because the nerves are newly reanastomosed

Instruct patient that leeches secrete hirudin, an anticoagulant, so site will ooze up to 50 ml of blood for 24 to 48 hours after removal

Reassure the patient that leech therapy is an accepted medical treatment

Use universal precautions

Use each leech for only one patient to prevent transfer of infection from another patient

Cleanse the flap or digit with sterile water and dry it with a sterile cloth

Instruct the patient to not touch leech or remove the leeches manually once applied

Surround the site with towels and/or gauze to prevent the leech from migrating

Enhance the leech's interest in attaching by placing a drop of 5% dextrose and water on the site

Gently apply leech to site, using forceps

Ensure that both the anterior and posterior ends of the leech attach to the affected area

Continuously monitor leech until it is fully distended (10 to 15 minutes after attachment) and drops off patient

Remove leeches that do not drop off by gently stroking with an alcohol pad

Refrigerate unused leeches in a container filled with salt solution (spring or distilled water) covered with netting

Handle leeches carefully after feeding to prevent regurgitation of gut contents

Place leeches in a small container of alcohol for incineration

Cleanse the treated area every 1 to 2 hours with a half-and-half solution of hydrogen peroxide and sterile water to prevent bloody drainage from hardening and constricting blood flow

Administer antibiotics as appropriate to prevent iatrogenic *A. hydrophilia* infection

Monitor hemoglobin and hematrocrit at least once a day, as appropriate

Document the patient's response to treatment

Background Readings:

Kocent, L.S., & Spinner, S.S. (1992). Leech therapy: New procedures for an old treatment. Pediatric Nursing, 18(5), 481-483, 542.
Peel, K. (1993). Making sense of leeches. Nursing Times, 89(27), 34-35.
Shinnkman, R. (2000). Worms and squirms: Maggots, leeches making a comeback in modern medicine. Modern Healthcare, 30(43), 54.
Voge, C., & Lehnherr, S.M. (1999). Getting attached to leeches. Nursing 99, 29(11), 46-47.

Limit Setting 4380

Definition: Establishing the parameters of desirable and acceptable patient behavior

Activities:

Discuss concerns about behavior with patient

Identify (with patient input, when appropriate) undesirable patient behavior

Discuss with patient, when appropriate, what is desirable behavior in a given situation or setting

Establish reasonable expectations for patient behavior, based on the situation and the patient

Establish consequences (with patient input, when appropriate) for occurrence/nonoccurrence of desired behaviors

Communicate the established behavioral expectations and consequences to the patient in language that is easily understood and nonpunitive

Communicate established behavioral expectations and consequences with other staff who are caring for patient

Refrain from arguing or bargaining about the established behavioral expectations and consequences with the patient

Assist patient, when necessary and appropriate, to show the desired behaviors

Monitor patient for occurrence/nonoccurrence of the desired behaviors

Modify behavioral expectations and consequences, as needed, to accommodate reasonable changes in the patient's situation

Initiate the established consequences for the occurrence/nonoccurrence of the desired behaviors

Decrease limit setting, as patient behavior approximates the desired behaviors

Background Readings:

Davidhizar, R. (1989). The art of setting limits. Advancing Clinical Care, November/December, 26-27.

Kanak, M.F. (1992). Interventions related to safety. In G.M. Bulechek & J.C. McCloskey (Eds.), Symposium on Nursing Interventions. Nursing Clinics of North America, 27(2), 371-396.

Kunes-Connell, M. (1987). Adolescent disorders. In J. Norris, M. Kunes-Connell, S. Stockard, P.M. Eckhart, & G.R. Newton (Eds.), Mental health-psychiatric nursing: A continuum of care (pp. 693-720). New York: John Wiley & Sons.

Stockard, S. (1987). Disorders of childhood. In J. Norris, M. Kunes-Connell, S. Stockard, P.M. Ehrhart, & G.R. Newton (Eds.), Mental health-psychiatric nursing: A continuum of care (pp. 657-691). New York: John Wiley & Sons.

Stockard, S., & Cullen, S. (1987). Personality disorders. In J. Norris, M. Kunes-Connell, S. Stockard, P.M. Ehrhart, & G.R. Newton (Eds.), Mental health-psychiatric nursing: A continuum of care (pp. 571-603). New York: John Wiley & Sons.

Thackrey, M. (1987). Therapeutics for aggression: Psychological/physical crisis intervention. New York: Human Sciences Press.

Lower Extremity Monitoring   3480

Definition: Collection, analysis, and use of patient data to categorize risk and prevent injury to the lower extremities

Activities:

Inspect skin for evidence of poor hygiene

Inspect lower extremities for presence of edema

Inspect toenails for changes (e.g., thickening, fungal infection, ingrown, and evidence of improper trimming)

Inspect skin for color, temperature, hydration, hair growth, texture, and cracking or fissuring

Inspect between the toes for maceration, cracking, or fissuring

Inquire about changes in feet and recent or remote history of foot ulcers or amputation

Determine mobility status (i.e., walks without assistance, walks with an assistive device, or does not walk/uses a wheelchair)

Inspect foot for deformities including cocked-up toes, prominent metatarsal heads, and high or low arch or Charcot changes

Monitor muscle strength in ankle and foot

Inspect foot for evidence of pressure (i.e., the presence of localized redness, increased temperatures, blisters, corns, or callus formation)

Inquire about the presence of paresthesias (e.g., numbness, tingling, or burning)

Palpate thickness of fat pads over metatarsal heads

Palpate dorsalis pedis and posterior tibial pulses

Determine ankle pressure index, as indicated

Inquire about the presence of intermittent claudication, rest pain, or night pain

Determine capillary refill time

Monitor level of protective sensation using Semmes-Weinstein nylon monofilament

Determine vibration perception threshold

Determine proprioceptive responses

Elicit deep tendon reflexes (i.e., ankle and knee) as indicated

Monitor gait and weight distribution on feet (e.g., observe walking and determine wear pattern on shoes)

Monitor condition of shoes and socks (i.e., clean and in good repair)

Monitor appropriateness of shoes (i.e., low-heeled with a shoe shape that matches foot shape; adequate depth of toe box; soles made of material that will absorb shock; adjustable fit by lace or straps; uppers made of breathable, soft, and flexible materials; changes made for gait and limb length disorders; and potential for modification if necessary)

Monitor appropriateness of socks (i.e., absorbent material and nonconstricting)

Monitor joint mobility (e.g., ankle dorsiflexion and subtalar joint motion)

Perform ongoing surveillance of the lower extremities to determine need for referral at least four times per year

Use level of risk for injury as a guide for determining appropriate referrals

Identify specialty foot care services required (e.g., orthotics or prescription footwear, callus trimming, toenail trimming, mobility evaluation and exercises, foot deformity evaluation and management, treatment of skin or nail deformities/infection, correction of abnormal gait or weight-bearing, and/or evaluation and management of impaired arterial circulation)

Continued

Activities:—cont'd

Consult with physician regarding recommendation for further evaluation and therapy (e.g., x-ray), as needed

Provide patient/family/significant others with information about recommended specialty foot care services

Identify patient/family/significant others' preference for referral health professional or agency, as appropriate

Determine patient's financial resources for payment for specialty foot care services

Provide assistance in obtaining necessary financial resources (e.g., contact social services), as appropriate

Contact health professional/agency as appropriate to arrange for specialty foot care services (i.e., schedule an appointment)

Complete written referral, as appropriate

Background Readings:

American Diabetes Association. (1998). Preventive foot care in people with diabetes. Diabetes, 21(12), 2178-2179.

Collier, J.H., & Brodbeck, C.A. (1993). Assessing the diabetic foot: Plantar callus and pressure sensation. The Diabetes Educatior, 19(6), 503-508.

Culleton, J.L. (1999) Preventing diabetic foot complications. Postgraduate Medicine, 106 (1), 78-84.

Halpin-Landry, J.E., & Goldsmith, S. (1999). Feet first, diabetic care. American Journal of Nursing, 99 (2), 26-33.

Jacobs, A.M., & Appleman, K.K. (1999). Foot-ulcer prevention in the elderly patient. Clinics in Geriatric Medicine, 15(2), 351-369.

McNeely, M.J., Boyko, E.J., Ahroni, J.H., Stensel, V.L., Reiber, G.E., Smith, D.G., & Pecararo, R.E. (1995). The independent contributions of diabetic neuropathy and vasculopathy in foot ulceration. Diabetes Care, 18 (2), 216-219.

Mayfield, J.A., Reiber, G.E., Sanders, L.J., Janise, D., & Pogach, L.M. (1998). Preventive foot care in people with diabetes. Diabetes Care, 21(12), 2161-2177.

Spollett, G.R. (1998). Preventing amputations in the diabetic population. Nursing Clinics of North America, 33 (4), 629-641.

L

Malignant Hyperthermia Precautions   3840

Definition: Prevention or reduction of hypermetabolic response to pharmacological agents used during surgery

Activities:

Maintain emergency equipment for malignant hyperthermia, per protocol, in operative areas

Review malignant hyperthermia emergency care with staff, per protocol

Ask patient about personal or family history of malignant hyperthermia, unexpected deaths from anesthetic, muscle disorder, or unexplained postoperative fever

Notify anesthesiologist and surgeon of patient history

Provide anesthesia machine free of precipitating anesthetic agents

Check patient's hospital record for elevation of enzymes

Provide emergency management supplies

Provide a cooling blanket

Prepare dantrolene sodium for administration

Administer dantrolene sodium, as appropriate

Use nontriggering anesthetic agents for surgical patients with susceptibility to malignant hyperthermia (e.g., spinal, epidural, regional blocks; nitrous oxide; narcotics; barbiturates; droperidol; diazepam and midazolam; and nondepolarizing muscle relaxants)

Monitor for signs of malignant hyperthermia (e g , hypercarbia, rise in temperature, tachycardia, tachypnea, arrhythmias, cyanosis, mottled skin, rigidity, profuse sweating, and unstable blood pressure)

Discontinue use of triggering agents

Switch to neurolept anesthesics

Provide sterile ice and cold IV solutions

Provide malignant hyperthermia tub

Irrigate wound with cold solutions

Pack patient in ice

Apply a hypothermia blanket

Insert NG tube and Foley catheter with a urometer

Lavage stomach, bladder, and rectum with iced saline

Assist with intubation or intubate patient

Initiate second IV line

Assist with arterial and central venous pressure line insertion

Monitor vital signs, including temperature, blood pressure, EKG, and arterial blood gas end-tidal carbon dioxide levels

Obtain blood and urine samples

Monitor electrolyte, enzyme, and blood sugar levels

Administer medications to maintain urine output

Avoid use of drugs, including calcium chloride or gluconate, cardiac glycosides, adrenergics, atropine, and lactated Ringer's solutions

Administer medications, as appropriate (e.g., chlorpromazine and steroids)

Decrease environmental stimuli

Continued

Activities:—cont'd

Observe for signs of late complications (e.g., consumption coagulopathy, renal failure, hypothermia, pulmonary edema, hyperkalemia, neurological sequelae, muscle necrosis, and reoccurrence of symptoms after treatment of initial episode)

Provide patient and family education about needed precautions for future anesthetic administration

Connect family with the North American Malignant Hyperthermia Registry and the Medic Alert Hotline

Background Readings:

Beck, C.F. (1994). Malignant hyperthermia: Are you prepared? AORN Journal, 59(2), 367-390.

Corkill, M.S. (1990). Not too hot to handle: Malignant hyperthermia (Film study guide). Denver: Association of Operating Room Nurses.

Donnelly, A.J. (1994). Malignant hyperthermia: Epidemiology, pathophysiology, treatment. AORN Journal, 59(2), 393-405.

Malignant Hyperthermia Association of the United States (MHAUS). (1990). Understanding malignant hyperthermia. Westport, CT: MHAUS.

Waugaman, W.R., Foster, S.D., & Rigor, B.M. (1992). Principles and practice of nurse anesthesia. Norwalk, CT: Appleton & Lange.

M

Mechanical Ventilation   3300

Definition: Use of an artificial device to assist a patient to breathe

Activities:

Monitor for respiratory muscle fatigue

Monitor for impending respiratory failure

Consult with other health care personnel in selection of a ventilator mode

Initiate setup and application of the ventilator

Instruct the patient and family about the rationale and expected sensations associated with use of mechanical ventilators

Routinely monitor ventilator settings

Monitor for decrease in exhaled volume and increase in inspiratory pressure

Ensure that ventilator alarms are on

Administer muscle-paralyzing agents, sedatives, and narcotic analgesics as appropriate

Monitor the effectiveness of mechanical ventilation on patient's physiological and psychological status

Initiate relaxation techniques, as appropriate

Provide patient with a means for communication (e.g., paper and pencil, alphabet board)

Check all ventilator connections regularly

Empty condensed water from water traps, as appropriate

Ensure change of ventilator circuits every 24 hours, as appropriate

Use aseptic technique, as appropriate

Monitor ventilator pressure readings and breath sounds

Stop NG tube feedings during suctioning and 30 to 60 minutes before chest physiotherapy

Silence ventilator alarms during suctioning to decrease frequency of false alarms

Monitor patient's progress on current ventilator settings and make appropriate changes as ordered

Monitor for adverse effects of mechanical ventilation: infection, barotrauma, reduced cardiac output

Position to facilitate ventilation/perfusion matching ("good lung down"), as appropriate

Collaborate with physician to use pressure support or PEEP to minimize alveolar hypoventilation, as appropriate

Perform chest physiotherapy, as appropriate

Perform suctioning based on presence of adventitious breath sounds and/or increased inspiratory pressure

Promote adequate fluid and nutritional intake

Provide routine oral care

Monitor effects of ventilator changes on oxygenation: ABG, SaO_2, SvO_2, end-tidal CO_2, Q_{sp}/Q_t, $A\text{-}aDO_2$, patient's subjective response

Monitor degree of shunt, vital capacity, V_d/V_t, MVV, inspiratory force, and FEV_1 for readiness to wean from mechanical ventilation based on agency protocol

Background Readings:

Bolton, P.J., & Kline, K.A. (1994). Understanding modes of mechanical ventilation. American Journal of Nursing, 94(6), 36-43.

Knipper, J.S., & Alpen, M.A. (1992). Ventilatory support. In G.M. Bulechek & J.C. McCloskey (Eds.), Nursing interventions: Essential nursing treatments (2nd ed.) (pp. 531-543). Philadelphia: W.B. Saunders.

Thelan, L.A., & Urden, L.D. (1998). Critical care nursing: Diagnosis and management (3rd ed.). St. Louis: Mosby–Year Book.

Thompson, K.S., Caddick, K., Mathie, J., Newton, B., & Abraham, J. (1991). Building a critical path for ventilator dependency. American Journal of Nursing, 91(7), 28-31.

Turner, P., Glass, C., & Grap, M.J. (1997). Care of the patient requiring mechanical ventilation. MEDSURG Nursing, 6 (2), 68-75.

M

Mechanical Ventilatory Weaning 3310

Definition: Assisting the patient to breathe without the aid of a mechanical ventilator

Activities:

Monitor degree of shunt, vital capacity, V_d/V_t, MVV, inspiratory force, and FEV_1 for readiness to wean from mechanical ventilation based on agency protocol

Monitor to ensure patient is free of significant infection prior to weaning

Monitor for optimal fluid and electrolyte status

Collaborate with other health team members to optimize patient's nutritional status, ensuring that 50% of the diet's nonprotein caloric source is fat rather than carbohydrate

Position patient for best use of ventilatory muscles and to optimize diaphragmatic descent

Suction the airway, as needed

Administer chest physiotherapy, as appropriate

Consult with other health care personnel in selecting a method for weaning

Alternate periods of weaning trials with sufficient periods of rest and sleep

Avoid delaying return of patient with fatigued respiratory muscles to mechanical ventilation

Set a schedule to coordinate other patient care activities with weaning trials

Promote the best use of the patient's energy by initiating weaning trials after the patient is well rested

Monitor for signs of respiratory muscle fatigue (e.g., abrubt rise in $PaCO_2$; rapid, shallow ventilation; paradoxical abdominal wall motion), hypoxemia, and tissue hypoxia while weaning is in process

Administer medications that promote airway patency and gas exchange

Set discrete, attainable goals with the patient for weaning

Use relaxation techniques, as appropriate

Coach the patient during difficult weaning trials

Assist the patient to distinguish spontaneous breaths from mechanically delivered breaths

Minimize excessive work of breathing that is nontherapeutic by eliminating extra dead space, adding pressure support, administering bronchodilators, and maintaining airway patency, as appropriate

Avoid pharmacological sedation during weaning trials, as appropriate

Provide some means of patient control during weaning

Stay with the patient and provide support during initial weaning attempts

Tell patient about ventilator setting changes that increase the work of breathing, as appropriate

Provide the patient with positive reinforcement and frequent progress reports

Consider using alternate methods of weaning as determined by patient's response to the current method

Instruct the patient and family about what to expect during various stages of weaning

Prepare discharge arrangements through multidisciplinary involvement with patient and family

Background Readings:

A Collective Task Force Facilitated by the American College of Chest Physicians, the American Association of Respiratory Care, and the American College of Critical Care Medicine. (2002). Evidenced-based guidelines for weaning and discontinuing ventilatory support. Respiratory Care, 47(1), 69-90.

Criteria for Weaning from Mechanical Ventilation. (June 2000). Summary, Evidence report/Technology Assessment: Number 23, AHRQ Publication No. 00-E028. Rockville, MD: Agency for Healthcare Research and Quality. Retrieved December 5, 2001, from http://www.ahrq.gov/clinic/mechsumm.htm

Phelan, B.A., Cooper, D.A., & Sangkachand, P. (2002). Prolonged mechanical ventilation and tracheotomy in the elderly. AACN Clinical Issue, 13(1), 84-93.

Thelan, L.A., & Urden, L.D. (1998). Critical care nursing: Diagnosis and management (3rd ed.). St. Louis: Mosby–Year Book.

M

Medication Administration   2300

Definition: Preparing, giving, and evaluating the effectiveness of prescription and nonprescription drugs

Activities:

Develop agency policies and procedures for accurate and safe administration of medications

Develop and use an environment that maximizes safe and efficient administration of medications

Follow the five rights of medication administration

Verify the prescription or medication order before administering the drug

Prescribe and/or recommend medications, as appropriate, according to prescriptive authority

Monitor for possible medication allergies, interactions, and contraindications

Note patient's allergies before delivery of each medication and hold medications, as appropriate

Ensure that hypnotics, narcotics, and antibiotics are either discontinued or reordered on their renewal date

Note expiration date on medication container

Prepare medications using appropriate equipment and techniques for the drug administration modality

Restrict administration of medications not properly labeled

Dispose of unused or expired drugs, according to agency guidelines

Monitor vital signs and laboratory values before medication administration, as appropriate

Assist patient in taking medication

Give medication using appropriate technique and route

Use orders, agency policies, and procedures to guide appropriate method of medication administration

Instruct patient and family about expected actions and adverse effects of the medication

Monitor patient to determine need for PRN medications, as appropriate

Monitor patient for the therapeutic effect of the medication

Monitor patient for adverse effects, toxicity, and interactions of the administered medications

Sign out narcotics and other restricted drugs, according to agency protocol

Verify all questioned medication orders with the appropriate health care personnel

Document medication administration and patient responsiveness, according to agency protocol

Background Readings:

Deglin, J.H., & Vallerand, A.H. (2001). Davis's drug guide for nurses (7th ed.). Philadelphia: F.A. Davis Co.

Lehne, R.A. (2001). Pharmacology for nursing care (4th ed.). Philadelphia: Saunders.

Naegle, M.A. (1999). Medication management. In G.M. Bulechek & J.C. McCloskey (Eds.), Nursing interventions: Effective nursing treatments (3rd ed.) (pp. 234-242). Philadelphia: W.B. Saunders.

Perry, A.G., & Potter, P.A. (2002). Clinical nursing skills & techniques (5th ed.) (pp. 435-557). St. Louis: Mosby.

Strome, T., & Howell, T. (1991). How antipsychotics affect the elderly. American Journal of Nursing, 91(5), 46-49.

Medication Administration: Ear 2308

Definition: Preparing and instilling otic medications

Activities:

Follow the five rights of medication administration

Note patient's medical history and history of allergies

Determine patient's knowledge of medication and understanding of method of administration

Position patient in a side-lying position with ear to be treated facing up, or have patient sit in chair

Straighten ear canal by pulling auricle down and back (child) or upward and outward (adult)

Instill medication holding dropper 1 cm above ear canal

Instruct patient to remain in side-lying position for 5 to 10 minutes

Apply gentle pressure or massage to tragus of ear with finger

Teach and monitor self-administration technique, as appropriate

Document medication administration and patient responsiveness according to agency protocol

Background Readings:

Naegle, M.A. (1999). Medication management. In G.M. Bulechek & J.C. McCloskey (Eds.) Nursing interventions: Effective nursing treatments (3rd ed.) (pp. 234-242). Philadelphia: W.B. Saunders.

Perry, A.G., & Potter, P.A. (2002). Clinical nursing skills and techniques (5th ed.) (pp. 436-452, 475-479). St. Louis: Mosby.

Rice, J. (2002). Medications and mathematics for the nurse (9th ed.). Albany, NY: Delmar/Thomson Learning.

M

Medication Administration: Enteral   2301

Definition: Delivering medications through a tube inserted into the gastrointestinal system

Activities:

Follow the five rights of medication administration

Note patient's medical history and history of allergies

Determine patient's knowledge of medication and understanding of method of administration (e.g., nasogastric tube, orogastric tube, gastrostomy tube)

Determine any contraindications to patient receiving oral medication via tube (e.g., bowel inflammation, reduced peristalsis, recent gastrointestinal surgery, attached to gastric suction)

Prepare medication (e.g., crush or mix with fluids as appropriate)

Inform patient of expected actions and possible adverse effects of medications

Check placement of the tube by aspirating gastrointestinal contents, checking the pH level of the aspirate, or obtaining x-ray film, as appropriate

Schedule medication to be in accord with formula feeding

Place patient in high Fowler's position, if not contraindicated

Aspirate stomach contents, return aspirate by flushing with 30 ml of air or appropriate amount for age, and flush tube with 30 ml of water, as appropriate

Remove plunger from syringe and pour medication into syringe

Administer medication by allowing medication to flow freely from barrel of syringe, using plunger only as needed to facilitate flow

Flush tube with 30 ml of warm water, or appropriate amount for age, after medication administration

Monitor patient for therapeutic effects, adverse effects, drug toxicity, and drug interactions

Document medication administration and patient responsiveness according to agency protocol

Background Readings:

Bozzetti, F., Braga, M., Gianotti, L., Gavazzi, C., & Mariani, L. (2001). Postoperative enteral versus parenteral nutrition in malnourished patients with gastrointestinal cancer: A randomised multicentre trial. Lancet, 358, 1487-1492.

Keidan, I., & Gallagher, T.J. (2000). Electrocardiogram-guided placement of enteral feeding tubes. Critical Care Medicine, 28(7), 2631-2633.

Miller, D., & Miller, H. (2000). To crush or not to crush: What to consider before giving medications to a patient with a tube or who has trouble swallowing. Nursing, 30(2), 50-52.

Naegle, M.A. (1999). Medication management. In G.M. Bulechek & J.C. McCloskey (Eds.), Nursing interventions: Effective nursing treatments (3rd ed.) (pp. 234-242). Philadelphia: W.B. Saunders.

Perry, A.G., & Potter, P.A. (2002). Clinical nursing skills & techniques (5th ed.) (pp. 436-452, 461-465, 756-762). St. Louis: Mosby.

Rumalla, A., & Baron, T.H. (2000). Results of direct percutaneous endoscopic jejunostomy, an alternative method for providing jejunal feeding. Mayo Clinic Proceedings, 75, 807-810.

Spalding, H.K., Sullivan, K.J., Soremi, O., Gonzalez, F., & Goodwin, S.R. (2000). Bedside placement of transpyloric feeding tubes in the pediatric intensive care unit using gastric insufflation. Critical Care Medicine, 28(6), 2041-2044.

Trujillo, E.B., Robinson, M.K., & Jacobs, D.O. (2001). Feeding critically ill patients: Current concepts. Critical Care Nurse, 21(4), 60-69.

M

Medication Administration: Eye   2310

Definition: Preparing and instilling ophthalmic medications

Activities:

Follow the five rights of medication administration

Note patient's medical history and history of allergies

Determine patient's knowledge of medication and understanding of method of administration

Position patient supine or sitting in a chair with neck slightly hyperextended; ask patient to look at ceiling

Instill medication onto the conjunctival sac using aseptic technique

Apply gentle pressure to nasolacrimal duct if medication has systemic effects

Instruct patient to close eye gently to help distribute medication

Monitor for local, systemic, and adverse effects of medication

Teach and monitor self-administration technique, as appropriate

Document medication administration and patient responsiveness according to agency protocol

Background Readings:

Naegle, M.A. (1999). Medication management. In G.M. Bulechek & J.C. McCloskey (Eds.), Nursing interventions: Effective nursing treatments (3rd ed.) (pp. 234-242). Philadelphia: W.B. Saunders.

Perry, A.G., & Potter, P.A. (2002). Clinical nursing skills & techniques (5th ed.) (pp. 436-452, 470-475). St. Louis: Mosby.

Rice, J. (2002). Medications and mathematics for the nurse (9th ed.). Albany, NY: Delmar/Thomson Learning.

M

Medication Administration: Inhalation   2311

Definition: Preparing and administering inhaled medications

Activities:

Follow the five rights of medication administration

Note patient's medical history and history of allergies

Determine patient's knowledge of medication and understanding of method of administration

Determine patient's ability to manipulate and administer medication

Assist patient to use inhaler as prescribed

Instruct patient on use of aerochamber (spacer) with the inhaler, as appropriate

Shake inhaler

Remove inhaler cap and hold inhaler upside down

Assist patient to position inhaler in mouth or nose

Instruct patient to tilt head back slightly and exhale completely

Instruct patient to press down on inhaler to release medication while inhaling slowly

Have patient take slow, deep breaths, with a brief end-inspiratory pause, and passive exhalation while using a nebulizer

Have patient hold breath for 10 seconds, as appropriate

Have patient exhale slowly through nose or pursed lips

Instruct patient to repeat inhalations as ordered, waiting at least 1 minute between inhalations

Instruct patient to wait between inhalations if two metered-dose inhalers are prescribed per agency protocol

Instruct patient in removing medication canister and cleaning inhaler in warm water

Monitor patient's respirations and auscultate lungs, as appropriate

Monitor for effects of medication and instruct patient and caregivers on desired effects and possible side effects of medication

Teach and monitor self-administration technique, as appropriate

Document medication administration and patient responsiveness according to agency protocol

Background Readings:

Naegle, M.A. (1999). Medication management. In G.M. Bulechek & J.C. McCloskey (Eds.), Nursing interventions: Effective nursing treatments (3rd ed.) (pp. 234-242). Philadelphia: W.B. Saunders.

Perry, A.G., & Potter, P.A. (2002). Clinical nursing skills & techniques (5th ed.) (pp. 436-452, 485-493). St. Louis: Mosby.

Rice, J. (2002). Medications and mathematics for the nurse (9th ed.). Albany, NY: Delmar/Thomson Learning.

University of Michigan Health System. (2000). Asthma. Ann Arbor, MI: Regents of the University of Michigan. Available on-line: http://cme.med.umich.edu/pdf/guideline/asthma.pdf

M

Medication Administration: Interpleural   2302

Definition: Administration of medication through an interpleural catheter for reduction of pain

Activities:

Obtain written consent for insertion of interpleural catheter

Assemble equipment and assist with insertion of interpleural catheter, as appropriate

Teach patient purpose, benefits, and rationale for use of the interpleural catheter

Affirm correct catheter placement with chest x-ray examination, as appropriate

Monitor patient's pain before and after catheter insertion, as appropriate

Check for absence of blood return before medication administration

Administer pain medication through interpleural catheter intermittently or by continuous drip

Withhold medication if more than 2 cc of fluid returns when checking interpleural catheter

Position patient to avoid pressure on interpleural catheter

Monitor for shortness of breath or unequal/abnormal breath sounds

Note any leakage that may occur from interpleural catheter

Observe for pain relief, side effects, or adverse reactions from medication administered

Connect catheter to medication administration pump, as appropriate

Encourage early ambulation if possible with the use of the interpleural catheter, as appropriate

Change dressing, as appropriate

Observe for signs and symptoms of infection at interpleural catheter insertion site

Remove interpleural catheter as ordered

Background Readings:

El-Naggar, M., Schaberg, F., Jr., & Phillips, M. (1989). Intrapleural regional analgesia for pain management of cholecystectomy. Archives of Surgery, 124(5), 568-570.

Kralheim, L., & Reiestad, F. (1984). Interpleural catheter in the management of postoperative pain. Anesthesiology, 61(3A), 231.

Martin, B., & Meherg, D. (1994). Interpleural analgesia: A new technique. Critical Care Nurse, October, 31-35.

Naegle, M.A. (1999). Medication management. In G. M. Bulechek & J. C. McCloskey (Eds.), Nursing interventions: Effective nursing treatments (3rd ed.) (pp. 234-242). Philadelphia: W.B. Saunders.

Reiestad, F., & Stromskag, K. (1986). Interpleural catheter in the management of postoperative pain: A preliminary report. Regional Anesthesia, 11, 89-91.

Reiestad, F., Stromskag, K., & Holmquist, E. (1986). Intrapleural administration of bupivacaine in postoperative management of pain. Anesthesiology, 65(3A), 204.

Medication Administration: Intradermal   2312

Definition: Preparing and giving medications via the intradermal route

Activities:

Follow the five rights of medication administration

Note patient's medical history and history of allergies

Determine patient's understanding of purpose of injection and skin testing

Select correct needle and syringe based on type of injection

Note expiration date of drug

Prepare dose correctly from ampule or vial

Select appropriate injection site and inspect skin for bruises, inflammation, edema, lesions, or discoloration

Use aseptic technique

Insert needle at a 5- to 15-degree angle

Inject medication slowly while watching for small bleb on skin surface

Monitor patient for allergic reaction

Mark injection site and read site at the appropriate interval after the injection (e.g., 48-72 hours)

Monitor for expected effects of specific allergen or medication

Document area of injection and appearance of skin at injection site

Document appearance of injection site after the appropriate interval

Background Readings:

Naegle, M.A. (1999). Medication management. In G.M. Bulechek & J.C. McCloskey (Eds.), Nursing interventions: Effective nursing treatments (3rd ed.) (pp. 234-242). Philadelphia: W.B. Saunders.

Perry, A.G., & Potter, P.A. (2002). Clinical nursing skills & techniques (5th ed.) (pp. 436-452, 519-522). St. Louis: Mosby.

Rice, J. (2002). Medications and mathematics for the nurse (9th ed.). Albany, NY: Delmar/Thomson Learning.

M

Medication Administration: Intramuscular (IM)   2313

Definition: Preparing and giving medications via the intramuscular route

Activities:

Follow the five rights of medication administration

Note patient's medical history and history of allergies

Consider indications and contraindications for intramuscular injection

Determine patient's knowledge of medication and understanding of method of administration

Select correct needle and syringe based on patient and medication information

Note expiration dates of drugs

Prepare dose correctly from ampule, vial, or prefilled syringe

Select appropriate injection site; palpate site for edema, masses, or tenderness; avoid areas of scarring, bruising, abrasion, or infection

Position nondominant hand at proper anatomical landmark; spread skin tightly

Administer injection using aseptic technique and proper protocol

Inject needle quickly at a 90-degree angle

Aspirate prior to injection; if no blood is aspirated, inject medication slowly, wait 10 seconds after injecting medication, then smoothly withdraw needle and release skin

Apply gentle pressure at injection site; avoid massaging site

Monitor patient for acute pain at injection site

Monitor patient for sensory or motor alteration at or distal to injection site

Monitor for expected and unexpected medication effects

Discard mixed medications that are not properly labeled

Document medication administration and patient responsiveness, according to agency protocol

Background Readings:
Naegle, M.A. (1999). Medication management. In G.M. Bulechek & J.C. McCloskey (Eds.), Nursing interventions: Effective nursing treatments (3rd ed.) (pp. 234-242). Philadelphia: W.B. Saunders.

Perry, A.G., & Potter, P.A. (2002). Clinical nursing skills & techniques (5th ed.) (pp. 436-452, 528-534). St. Louis: Mosby.

M

Medication Administration: Intraosseous   2303

Definition: Insertion of a needle through the bone cortex into the medullary cavity for the purpose of short-term, emergency administration of fluid, blood, or medication

Activities:

Follow the five rights of medication administration

Note patient's medical history and history of allergies

Determine patient's comfort level

Determine patient's knowledge of medication and understanding of method of administration

Immobilize the extremity

Select an appropriate site for insertion by assessing landmarks to ensure proper needle placement away from the epiphyseal growth plate

Assist with insertion of intraosseous lines

Prepare the site with solution using aseptic technique

Administer 1% lidocaine at insertion point, as appropriate

Choose an appropriate size needle with a stylet (bone marrow biopsy/aspiration needle or 13- to 20-gauge rigid needle with stylet)

Insert needle with stylet at 60- to 90-degree angle directed inferiorly

Remove inner stylet, as necessary

Aspirate for bone marrow content to confirm needle placement, according to agency protocol

Flush needle with solution, according to agency protocol

Secure needle in place with tape and apply appropriate dressing, according to agency protocol

Connect tubing to needle and allow fluids to run by gravity or under pressure, as required by flow rate

Anchor IV lines to extremity

Identify compatibility of medications and fluids in infusion

Determine flow rate, and adjust accordingly

Monitor for signs and symptoms of extravasation of fluids or medications, infection, or fat embolism

Document site, needle type and size, type of fluid and medication, flow rate, and patient response, according to agency protocol

Report patient's response to therapy, according to agency protocol

Establish IV access and discontinue intraosseous line after patient's condition stabilizes

M

Background Readings:

Calkins, M.D., Fitzgerald, G., Bentley, T.B., & Burris, D. (2000). Intraosseous infusion devices: A comparison for potential use in special operations. The Journal of Trauma: Injury, Infection, and Critical Care, 48(6), 1068-1074.

Hurren, J.S. (2000). Can blood taken from intraosseous cannulations be used for blood analysis? Burns, 26, 727-730.

Dubick, M.A., & Holcomb, J.B. (2000). A review of intraosseous vascular access: Current status and military application. Military Medicine, 165, 552-559.

Miccolo, M. (1990). Intraosseous infusion. Critical Care Nurse, 10(10), 35-47.

Naegle, M.A. (1999). Medication management. In G.M. Bulechek & J.C. McCloskey (Eds.), Nursing interventions: Effective nursing treatments (3rd ed.) (pp. 234-242). Philadelphia: W.B. Saunders.

Medication Administration: Intraspinal 2319

Definition: Administration and monitoring of medication via an established epidural or intrathecal route

Activities:

Follow the five rights of medication administration

Note patient's medical history and history of allergies

Determine patient's comfort level

Determine patient's knowledge of medication and understanding of method of administration

Monitor patient's vital signs

Monitor neurological status

Maintain aseptic technique

Monitor patient's mobility and motor and sensory functions, as appropriate

Aspirate cerebral spinal fluid before injection of medication and evaluate for blood or cloudy returns prior to administering an intrathecal bolus injection

Aspirate epidural catheter gently with an empty syringe, checking for a return of air only, prior to administering an epidural bolus injection

Aseptically prepare preservative-free medication through filter needle

Observe aspirate for amount and color of return

Inject medication slowly per physician order, according to agency protocol

Monitor epidural or intrathecal catheter insertion site for signs of infection

Monitor dressing on epidural or intrathecal catheter insertion site for presence of clear drainage

Notify physician if epidural or intrathecal dressing is wet

Ensure that catheter is secured to patient's skin

Tape all tubing connections, as appropriate

Mark tubing as either intrathecal or epidural, as appropriate

Check infusion pump for proper calibration and operation, per agency protocol

Monitor IV setup, flow rate, and solution at regular intervals

Monitor for central nervous system infection (i.e., fever, change in level of consciousness, nausea and vomiting)

Document medication administration and patient response according to agency protocol

Background Readings:

Alpen, M.A., & Morse, C. (2001). Managing the pain of traumatic injury. Critical Care Nursing Clinics of North America, 13(2), 243-257.

Crul, B.J.P. (no date). Continuous spinal (intrathecal) technique: Is it better than epidural technique for cancer pain in home care? Retrieved May 9, 2002, from http://www.esraeurope.org/abstracts/abstracts98/

Francois, B., Vacher, P., Roustan, J., Salle, J-Y., Vidal, J., Moreau, J-J., & Vignon, P. (2001). Intrathecal Baclofen after traumatic brain injury: Early treatment using a new technique to prevent spasticity. The Journal of Trauma Injury, Infection, and Critical Care, 50(1), 158-161.

Larson, R.M. (no date). Intrathecal and epidural pumps for pain control. Retrieved May 9, 2002, from http://www.nursing.uiowa.edu/sites/PedsPain/Routes/Impumtt.htm

Lehne, R.A. (2001). Pharmacology for nursing care (4th ed.) (p. 236). Philadelphia: Saunders.

Naegle, M. A. (1999). Medication management. In G. M. Bulechek & J. C. McCloskey (Eds.), Nursing interventions: Effective nursing treatments (3rd ed.) (pp. 234-242). Philadelphia: W.B. Saunders.

National Institutes of Health. (2001). Living with cancer chemotherapy. Available on-line: http://www.cc.nih.gov/ccc/patient_education/CaTxeng/intrathec.pdf

Smith S.F., & Duell D.J. (1996). Clinical nursing skills: Basic to advanced skills (4th ed.) (pp. 426-427). Stamford, CT: Appleton & Lange.

Medication Administration: Intravenous (IV)   2314

Definition: Preparing and giving medications via the intravenous route

Activities:

Follow the five rights of medication administration

Note patient's medical history and history of allergies

Determine patient's knowledge of medication and understanding of method of administration

Check for IV drug incompatibilities

Note expiration dates of drugs and solutions

Set up proper equipment for medication administration

Prepare the appropriate concentration of IV medication from ampule or vial

Verify placement and patency of IV catheter within vein

Maintain sterility of patent IV system

Administer IV medication at the appropriate rate

Mix solution gently if adding medication to IV fluid container

Select injection port of IV tubing closest to patient, occlude IV line above port, and aspirate prior to injecting IV bolus into an existing line

Flush IV lock with appropriate solution before and after medication administration, per agency protocol

Complete medication additive label and apply to IV fluid container, as appropriate

Maintain IV access, as appropriate

Monitor patient to determine response to medication

Monitor IV setup, flow rate, and solution at regular intervals, per agency protocol

Monitor for infiltration and phlebitis at infusion site

Document medication administration and patient responsiveness according to agency protocol

Background Readings:

Naegle, M.A. (1999). Medication management. In G.M. Bulechek & J.C. McCloskey (Eds.), Nursing interventions: Effective nursing treatments (3rd ed.) (pp. 234-242). Philadelphia: W.B. Saunders.

Perry, A.G., & Potter, P.A. (2002). Clinical nursing skills & techniques (5th ed.) (pp. 436-452, 534-551). St. Louis: Mosby.

Rice, J. (2002). Medications and mathematics for the nurse (9th ed.). Albany, NY: Delmar/Thomson Learning.

M

Medication Administration: Nasal   2320

Definition: Preparing and giving medications via nasal passages

Activities:

Follow the five rights of medication administration

Note patient's medical history and history of allergies

Determine patient's knowledge of medication and understanding of method of administration

Instruct patient to blow nose gently prior to administration of nasal medication, unless contraindicated

Assist patient to supine position and position head appropriately, depending on which sinuses are to be medicated when nose drops are administered

Instruct patient to breathe through mouth during administration of nose drops

Hold dropper 1 cm above nares and instill prescribed number of drops

Instruct patient to remain supine for 5 minutes after administration of nose drops

Instruct patient to remain upright and to not tilt head backward when nasal spray is administer

Insert nozzle into nostril and squeeze bottle quickly and firmly when nasal spray is administered

Instruct patient not to blow nose for several minutes after administration

Monitor patient to determine response to medication

Document medication administration and patient response according to agency protocol

Background Readings:

Naegle, M.A. (1999). Medication management. In G.M. Bulechek & J.C. McCloskey (Eds.), Nursing interventions: Effective nursing treatments (3rd ed.) (pp. 234-242). Philadelphia: W.B. Saunders.

Perry, A.G., & Potter, P.A. (2002). Clinical nursing skills & techniques (5th ed.) (pp. 436-452, 482-485). St. Louis: Mosby.

M

Medication Administration: Oral 2304

Definition: Preparing and giving medications by mouth

Activities:

Follow the five rights of medication administration

Note patient's medical history and history of allergies

Determine patient's knowledge of medication and understanding of method of administration

Determine any contraindications to patient receiving oral medication (e.g., difficulty swallowing, nausea/vomiting, bowel inflammation, reduced peristalsis, recent gastrointestinal surgery, attached to gastric suction, NPO status, decreased level of consciousness)

Check for possible drug interactions and contraindications

Ensure that hypnotics, narcotics, and antibiotics are either discontinued or reordered on their renewal date

Note the expiration date on the medication container

Give medications on an empty stomach or with food, as appropriate

Mix offensive-tasting medications with food or fluids, as appropriate

Mix medication with flavored syrup from the pharmacy, as appropriate

Crush medication and mix with small amount of soft food (e.g., applesauce), as appropriate

Inform patient of expected actions and possible adverse effects of medications

Instruct patient on proper administration of sublingual medication

Place sublingual medications under the patient's tongue and instruct not to swallow the pill

Have patient place buccal medication in mouth against mucous membranes of the cheek until it dissolves

Instruct the patient not to eat or drink until the sublingual or buccal medication is completely dissolved

Assist patient with ingestion of medications, as appropriate

Monitor patient for possible aspiration, as appropriate

Perform mouth checks after delivery of medications, as appropriate

Instruct the patient or family member on how to administer the medication

Monitor patient for therapeutic effects, adverse effects, drug toxicity, and drug interactions

Document medications administered and patient responsiveness, according to agency protocol

Background Readings:

Naegle, M.A. (1999). Medication management. In G.M. Bulechek & J.C. McCloskey (Eds.), Nursing interventions: Effective nursing treatments (3rd ed.) (pp. 234-242). Philadelphia: W.B. Saunders.

Perry, A.G., & Potter, P.A. (2002). Clinical nursing skills & techniques (5th ed.) (pp. 436-452, 455-461). St. Louis: Mosby.

Rice, J. (2002). Medications and mathematics for the nurse (9th ed.). Albany, NY: Delmar/Thomson Learning.

Medication Administration: Rectal   2315

Definition: Preparing and inserting rectal suppositories

Activities:

Follow the five rights of medication administration

Note patient's medical history and history of allergies

Determine patient's knowledge of medication and understanding of method of administration

Review medical record for history of rectal surgery or bleeding

Check for any presenting signs and symptoms of gastrointestinal alterations (e.g., constipation or diarrhea)

Determine patient's ability to retain suppository

Assist patient to left side-lying Sim's position with upper leg flexed upward

Lubricate gloved index finger of dominant hand and rounded end of suppository

Instruct patient to take slow deep breaths through mouth and to relax anal sphincter

Insert suppository gently through anus, past internal anal sphincter and against rectal wall

Instruct patient to remain flat or on side for 5 minutes

Monitor for effects of medication

Teach and monitor self-administration technique as appropriate

Document medication administration and patient responsiveness according to agency protocol

M

Background Readings:

Naegle, M.A. (1999). Medication management. In G.M. Bulechek & J.C. McCloskey (Eds.), Nursing interventions: Effective nursing treatments (3rd ed.) (pp. 234-242). Philadelphia: W.B. Saunders.
Perry, A.G., & Potter, P.A. (2002). Clinical nursing skills & techniques (5th ed.) (pp. 436-452, 498-501). St. Louis: Mosby.
Rice, J. (2002). Medications and mathematics for the nurse (9th ed.). Albany, NY: Delmar/Thomson Learning.

Medication Administration: Skin   2316

Definition: Preparing and applying medications to the skin

Activities:

Follow the five rights of medication administration

Note patient's medical history and history of allergies

Determine patient's knowledge of medication and understanding of method of administration

Determine patient's skin condition over area to which medication will be applied

Remove previous dose of medication and cleanse skin

Measure the correct amount of topically applied systemic medications, using standardized measurement devices

Apply topical agent as prescribed

Apply transdermal patches and topical medications to nonhairy areas of the skin, as appropriate

Spread the medication evenly over the skin, as appropriate

Rotate application sites of topical systemic medications

Monitor for local, systemic, and adverse effects of the medication

Teach and monitor self-administration techniques, as appropriate

Document medication administration and patient responsiveness according to agency protocol

Background Readings:

Naegle, M.A. (1999). Medication management. In G.M. Bulechek & J.C. McCloskey (Eds.), Nursing interventions: Effective nursing treatments (3rd ed.) (pp. 234-242). Philadelphia: W.B. Saunders.

Perry, A.G., & Potter, P.A. (2002). Clinical nursing skills & techniques (5th ed.) (pp. 436-452, 465-469). St. Louis: Mosby.

M

Medication Administration: Subcutaneous   2317

Definition: Preparing and giving medications via the subcutaneous route

Activities:

Follow the five rights of medication administration

Note patient's medical history and history of allergies

Determine patient's knowledge of medication and understanding of method of administration

Consider indications and contraindications for subcutaneous injection

Note expiration dates of drugs

Select correct needle and syringe based on patient and medication information

Prepare dose correctly from ampule or vial

Select appropriate injection site

Rotate insulin injection sites systematically within one anatomical region

Palpate injection site for edema, masses, or tenderness; avoid areas of scarring, bruising, abrasion, or infection

Use abdominal sites when administering heparin subcutaneously

Administer injection using aseptic technique

Inject needle quickly at a 45- to 90-degree angle, depending on size of patient

Apply gentle pressure to site; avoid massaging site

Monitor for expected and unexpected medication effects

Educate patient, family member, and/or significant other regarding injection technique

Document medication administration and patient responsiveness, according to agency protocol

M

Background Readings:

Naegle, M.A. (1999). Medication management. In G.M. Bulechek & J.C. McCloskey (Eds.), Nursing interventions: Effective nursing treatments (3rd ed.) (pp. 234-242). Philadelphia: W.B. Saunders.

Perry, A.G., & Potter, P.A. (2002). Clinical nursing skills & techniques (5th ed.) (pp. 436-452, 523-528). St. Louis: Mosby.

Rice, J. (2002). Medications and mathematics for the nurse (9th ed.). Albany, NY: Delmar/Thomson Learning.

Medication Administration: Vaginal   2318

Definition: Preparing and inserting vaginal medications

Activities:

Follow the five rights of medication administration

Note patient's medical history and history of allergies

Determine patient's knowledge of medication and understanding of method of administration

Have client void prior to administration

Apply water-soluble lubricant to rounded end of suppository; lubricate gloved index finger of dominant hand

Insert rounded end of suppository along posterior wall of vaginal canal 3 to 4 inches, or insert applicator approximately 2 to 3 inches

Instruct patient to remain on her back for at least 10 minutes

Maintain good perineal hygiene

Monitor for effects of medication

Teach and monitor self-administration technique as appropriate

Document medication administration and patient responsiveness, according to agency protocol

Background Readings:

Naegle, M.A. (1999). Medication management. In G.M. Bulechek & J.C. McCloskey (Eds.), Nursing interventions: Effective nursing treatments (3rd ed.) (pp. 234-242). Philadelphia: W.B. Saunders.
Perry, A.G., & Potter, P.A. (2002). Clinical nursing skills & techniques (5th ed.) (pp. 436-452, 494-498). St. Louis: Mosby.

M

Medication Administration: Ventricular Reservoir   2307

Definition: Administration and monitoring of medication through an indwelling catheter into the lateral ventricle of the brain

Activities:

Follow the five rights of medication administration

Note patient's medical history and history of allergies

Determine patient's comfort level

Determine patient's knowledge of medication and understanding of method of administration

Monitor neurological status

Monitor vital signs

Maintain aseptic technique

Shave hair over reservoir, per agency protocol

Fill reservoir with cerebral spinal fluid by applying pressure gently with index finger

Collect cerebral spinal fluid specimen, as appropriate per order or agency protocol

Aspirate cerebral spinal fluid before injection of medication and evaluate for blood or cloudy returns

Inject medication slowly per physician order and according to agency protocol

Apply pressure with index finger to reservoir to ensure mixing of medication with cerebral spinal fluid

Apply dressing to site, as appropriate

Monitor for central nervous system infection (i.e., fever, change in level of consciousness, nausea and vomiting)

Document medication administration and patient response according to agency protocol

M

Background Readings:

Cummings, R. (1992). Understanding external ventricular drainage. Journal of Neuroscience Nursing, 24(2), 84-87.

Naegle, M.A. (1999). Medication management. In G.M. Bulechek & J.C. McCloskey (Eds.), Nursing interventions: Effective nursing treatments (3rd ed.) (pp. 234-242). Philadelphia: W.B. Saunders.

National Institutes of Health. (2001). NIH Clinical Center Nursing Department: Procedure: Accessing the Ommaya reservoir. Retrieved April 15, 2002, from http://www.cc.nih.gov/nursing/omayapro.html.

National Institutes of Health. (2001). NIH Clinical Center Nursing Department: SOP: Care of the patient with an Ommaya reservoir. Retrieved April 15, 2002, from http://www.cc.nih.gov/nursing/ommayasp.html

The Ohio State University Medical Center Department of Critical Care Nursing. (2000). Health for life: Ommaya reservoir access. Retrieved April 15, 2002, from http://www.acs.ohio-state.edu/units/osuhosp/patedu/homedocs.pdf/procedur.pdf/invas-pr.pdf/ommaya.pdf

Medication Management   2380

Definition: Facilitation of safe and effective use of prescription and over-the-counter drugs

Activities:

Determine what drugs are needed, and administer according to prescriptive authority and/or protocol

Discuss financial concerns related to medication regimen

Determine patient's ability to self-medicate, as appropriate

Monitor effectiveness of the medication administration modality

Monitor patient for the therapeutic effect of the medication

Monitor for signs and symptoms of drug toxicity

Monitor for adverse effects of the drug

Monitor serum blood levels (e.g., electrolytes, prothrombin, medications), as appropriate

Monitor for nontherapeutic drug interactions

Review periodically with the patient and/or family types and amounts of medications taken

Discard old, discontinued, or contraindicated medications, as appropriate

Facilitate changes in medication with physician, as appropriate

Monitor for response to changes in medication regimen, as appropriate

Determine the patient's knowledge about medication

Monitor adherence with medication regimen

Determine factors that may preclude the patient from taking drugs as prescribed

Develop strategies with the patient to enhance compliance with prescribed medication regimen

Consult with other health care professionals to minimize the number of drugs and frequency of doses needed for a therapeutic effect

Teach patient and/or family members the method of drug administration, as appropriate

Teach patient and/or family members the expected action and side effects of the medication

Provide patient and family members with written and illustrated information to enhance self-administration of medications, as appropriate

Develop strategies to manage side effects of drugs

Obtain physician order for patient self-medication, as appropriate

Establish a protocol for the storage, restocking, and monitoring of medications left at the bedside for self-medication purposes

Investigate possible financial resources for acquisition of prescribed drugs, as appropriate

Determine impact of medication use on patient's lifestyle

Provide alternatives for timing and modality of self-administered medications to minimize lifestyle effects

Assist the patient and family members in making necessary lifestyle adjustments associated with certain medications, as appropriate

Instruct patient when to seek medical attention

Identify types and amounts of over-the-counter drugs used

Provide information about the use of over-the-counter drugs and how they may influence the existing condition

Determine whether the patient is using culturally based home health remedies and the possible effects on use of over-the-counter and prescribed medications

Continued

Activities:—cont'd
Review with the patient strategies for managing medication regimen

Provide patient with a list of resources to contact for further information about the medication regimen

Contact patient and family after discharge, as appropriate, to answer questions and discuss concerns associated with the medication regimen

Encourage the patient to have screening tests to determine medication effects

Background Readings:

Le Sage, J. (1991). Polypharmacy in geriatric patients. Nursing Clinics of North America, 26(2), 273-290.

Malseed, R.T. (1990). Pharmacology drug therapy and nursing considerations (3rd ed.). Philadelphia: J.B. Lippincott.

Mathewson, M.J. (1986). Pharmacotherapeutics: A nursing approach. Philadelphia: F.A. Davis.

Weitzel, E.A. (1992). Medication management. In G.M. Bulechek & J.C. McCloskey (Eds.), Nursing interventions: Essential nursing treatments (2nd ed.) (pp. 213-220). Philadelphia: W.B. Saunders.

M

Medication Prescribing   2390

Definition: Prescribing medication for a health problem

Activities:

Evaluate signs and symptoms of current health problem

Determine health history and previous medication use

Identify known allergies

Determine patient/family's ability to administer medication

Identify medications that are indicated for current problems

Prescribe medications according to prescriptive authority and/or protocol

Write prescription, using name of medication and including dose and directions for administration

Spell out problematic abbreviations that are easily misunderstood (e.g., micrograms, milligrams, units)

Verify that decimal points used in dosages are clearly seen by using leading zeros (e.g., 0.2 vs. .2)

Avoid the use of trailing zeros (e.g., 2 vs. 2.0)

Use electronic prescribing methods, as available

Use standardized abbreviations, acronyms, and symbols

Verify that all medication orders are written accurately, completely, and with the necessary discrimination for their intended use

Follow recommendations for starting doses of medication (e.g., milligrams per kilogram body weight, body surface area, or lowest effective dose)

Consult with physician or pharmacist, as appropriate

Consult *Physician's Desk Reference* and other references, as necessary

Consult with representatives from drug companies, as appropriate

Teach patient and/or family members the method of drug administration, as appropriate

Teach patient and/or family members the expected action and side effects of the medication

Provide alternatives for timing and modality of self-administered medications to minimize lifestyle effects

Instruct patient and family about how to fill prescription, as necessary

Instruct patient/family when to seek additional assistance

Monitor for the therapeutic and adverse effects of the medication, as appropriate

Maintain knowledge of medications used in practice, including indications for use, precautions, adverse effects, toxic effects, and dosing information, as required by prescriptive authority rules and regulations

M

Background Readings:

Anonymous. (2001). Issue: Nurses impact 2001: Recognizing, nursing's independent license: Prescriptive authority for APNs. Michigan Nurse, 74(3 Suppl). Retrieved May 10, 2002, from http://80-gateway1.ovid.com.proxy. lib.uiowa.edu/ovid-web.cgi.

Anonymous. (2001). ARNP prescriptive authority rules approved at joint meeting. Washington Nurse, 31(2). Retrieved May 10, 2002, from http://80-gateway1.ovid.com.proxy.lib. uiowa.edu/ovidweb.cgi

Freeman, G. (Ed.). (2002). Medication errors related to poor communications. Healthcare Risk Management, 24(1), 9-10.

Talley, S., & Richens, S. (2001). Prescribing practices of advanced practice psychiatric nurses: Part 1—demographic, educational, and practice characteristics. Archives of Psychiatric Nursing, 15(5), 205-213.

Meditation Facilitation

5960

Definition: Facilitating a person to alter his/her level of awareness by focusing specifically on an image or thought

Activities:

Prepare a quiet environment

Instruct patient to sit quietly in a comfortable position

Instruct patient to close eyes, if desired

Instruct patient to relax all muscles and remain relaxed

Assist patient to select a mental device for repetition during procedure (e.g., repeating a word such as "one")

Instruct patient to say the mental device silently to self while breathing out through the nose

Continue with the breathing exercise focusing on the mental device chosen (e.g., "one") as long as needed or desired

When finished, instruct patient to sit quietly for several minutes with eyes open

Inform patient to ignore distracting thoughts by returning to the mental device being used

Inform patient to perform the procedure once or twice daily, but not within 2 hours after meals

Background Readings:

Graves, P., & Lancaster, J. (1992). Stress management and crisis intervention. In M. Stanhope & J. Lancaster (Eds.), Community health nursing (3rd ed.) (pp. 612-631). St. Louis: Mosby–Year Book.

McCaffery, M., & Beebe, A. (1989). Pain. Clinical manual for nursing practice (pp. 194, 202-203). St. Louis: Mosby–Year Book.

Kreitzer, M.J. Meditation. In M. Snyder & R. Lindquist. (Eds.), Complementary/alternative therapies in nursing (3rd ed.) (pp. 123-128). New York: Springer Publishing Company.

M

Memory Training   4760

Definition: Facilitation of memory

Activities:

Discuss with patient/family any practical memory problems experienced

Stimulate memory by repeating patient's last expressed thought, as appropriate

Reminisce about past experiences with patient, as appropriate

Implement appropriate memory techniques, such as visual imagery, mnemonic devices, memory games, memory cues, association techniques, making lists, using computers, using name tags, or rehearsing information

Assist in associated learning tasks, such as practice learning and recalling verbal and pictorial information presented, as appropriate

Provide for orientation training, such as patient rehearsing personal information and dates, as appropriate

Provide opportunity for concentration, such as a game matching pairs of cards, as appropriate

Provide opportunity to use memory for recent events, such as questioning patient about a recent outing

Guide new learning, such as locating geographical features on a map, as appropriate

Provide for picture recognition memory, as appropriate

Structure the teaching methods according to patient's organization of information

Refer to occupational therapy, as appropriate

Encourage patient to participate in group memory training programs, as appropriate

Monitor patient's behavior during therapy

Identify and correct with the patient errors in orientation

Monitor changes in memory with training

Background Readings:

Drofman, D.R., & Ager, C.L. (1989). Memory and memory training: Some treatment implications for use with the well elderly. Physical and Occupational Therapy in Geriatrics, 7(3), 21-41.

Godfrey, H.P.D., & Knight, R.G. (1988). Memory training and behavioral rehabilitation of a severely head-injured adult. Archives of Physical and Medical Rehabilitation, 69, 458-460.

Schmidt, I.W., Dijkstra, H.T., Berg, I.J., Deelman, B.G. (1999) Memory training for remembering names in older adults. Clinical Gerontologist, 20(2), 57-73.

Schmidt, I.W., Berg, I.J., Deelman, B.G. (2000) Memory training for remembering texts in older adults. Clinical Gerontologist, 21(4), 67-90.

M

Milieu Therapy   4390

Definition: Use of people, resources, and events in the patient's immediate environment to promote optimal psychosocial functioning

Activities:

Determine factors in environment that contribute to patient's behavior

Consider needs of others in addition to needs of particular individual

Make resources necessary for self-care available

Enhance the normality of the environment through use of clocks, calendars, railings, furniture, and so on

Facilitate open communication between patient, nurses, and other staff

Include patient in decisions about own care

Write behavioral expectations and agreements for the patient's and others' reference, when appropriate

Provide one-on-one nursing care, as appropriate

Support formal and informal group activities to promote sharing, cooperation, compromise, and leadership

Examine own attitudes toward issues of patients' rights, self-determination, social control, and deviancy

Ensure staff presence and supervision

Minimize restrictions that diminish privacy or self-control (autonomy)

Encourage use of personal property

Minimize as much as possible the use of locked doors, medications, and strict regulations of activity or property

Provide a telephone in a private space

Provide attractively furnished areas for private conversations with other patients, family, and friends

Provide books, magazines, and arts and crafts materials in accordance with patient's recreational, cultural, and educational background and needs

Monitor individual behavior that may be disruptive or detrimental to overall well-being of others

Limit the number of unmedicated psychotic patients at any time through controlled admissions and varying lengths of medication-free trials, as appropriate

Background Readings:

Love, C.C., & Buckwalter, K. (1991). Reactive depression. In M. Maas, K. Buckwalter, & M. Hardy (Eds.), Nursing diagnoses and interventions for the elderly (pp. 419-432). Redwood City, CA: Addison-Wesley.
Wilson, H.S., & Kneisl, C.R. (1992). Psychiatric nursing (4th ed.). Menlo Park, CA: Addison-Wesley.

Mood Management   5330

Definition: Providing for safety, stabilization, recovery, and maintenance of a patient who is experiencing dysfunctionally depressed or elevated mood

Activities:

Evaluate mood (e.g., signs, symptoms, personal history) initially, and on a regular basis, as treatment progresses

Administer self-report questionnaires (e.g., Beck Depression Inventory, functional status scales), as appropriate

Determine whether patient presents safety risk to self or others

Consider hospitalization of the mood-disordered patient who poses a safety risk, is unable to meet his or her self-care needs, and/or lacks social support

Initiate necessary precautions to safeguard the patient or others at risk for physical harm (e.g., suicide, self-harm, elopement, violence)

Provide or refer a patient for substance abuse treatment, if substance abuse is a factor contributing to the mood disorder

Adjust or discontinue medications that may be contributing to mood disorders (e.g., per appropriately licensed advanced practice nurses)

Refer patient for evaluation and/or treatment of any underlying medical illness that may be contributing to a dysfunctional mood (e.g., thyroid disorders)

Monitor self-care ability (e.g., grooming, hygiene, food/fluid intake, elimination)

Assist with self-care, as needed

Monitor physical status of patient (e.g., body weight and hydration)

Monitor and regulate level of activity and stimulation in environment in accord with patient's needs

Assist patient to maintain a normal cycle of sleep/wakefulness (e.g., scheduled rest times, relaxation techniques, sedating medications, and limited intake of caffeine)

Assist patient to assume increasing responsibility for self-care as he or she is able to do so

Provide opportunity for physical activity (e.g., walking or riding the exercise bike)

Monitor cognitive functioning (e.g., concentration, attention, memory, ability to process information, and decision-making ability)

Use simple, concrete, here-and-now language during interactions with the cognitively compromised patient

Use memory aids and visual cues to assist the cognitively compromised patient

Limit decision-making opportunities for the cognitively compromised patient

Teach patient decision-making skills, as needed

Encourage patient to engage in increasingly more complex decision making as he or she is able

Encourage patient to take an active role in treatment and rehabilitation, as appropriate

Provide or refer for psychotherapy (e.g., cognitive behavioral, interpersonal, marital, family, group), when appropriate

Interact with the patient at regular intervals to convey caring and/or to provide an opportunity for patient to talk about feelings

Assist patient to consciously monitor mood (e.g., 1 to 10 rating scale and journaling)

Assist patient to identify thoughts and feelings underlying the dysfunctional mood

Limit amount of time that patient is allowed to express negative feelings and/or accounts of past failures

M

Continued

Activities:—cont'd

Assist patient to ventilate feelings in an appropriate manner (e.g., punching bag, art therapy, and vigorous physical activity)

Assist patient to identify precipitants of dysfunctional mood (e.g., chemical imbalances, situational stressors, grief/loss, and physical problems)

Assist patient to identify aspects of precipitants that can/cannot be changed

Assist in identification of available resources and personal strengths/abilities that can be used in modifying the precipitants of dysfunctional mood

Teach new coping and problem-solving skills

Encourage the patient, as he/she can tolerate, to engage in social interactions and activities with others

Provide social skills and/or assertiveness training, as needed

Provide the patient with feedback regarding the appropriateness of his or her social behaviors

Utilize limit setting and behavioral management strategies to assist the manic patient to refrain from intrusive and disruptive behavior

Utilize restrictive interventions (e.g., area restriction, seclusion, physical restraint, chemical restraint) to manage unsafe or inappropriate behavior that is not responsive to less restrictive behavior management interventions

Manage and treat hallucinations and/or delusions that may accompany the mood disorder

Prescribe, adjust, and discontinue medications used to treat the dysfunctional mood (e.g., per appropriately licensed advanced practice nurse)

Administer mood-stabilizing medications (e.g., antidepressants, lithium, anticonvulsants, antipsychotics, anxiolytics, hormones, and vitamins)

Monitor patient for medication side effects and impact on mood

Treat and/or manage medication side effects or adverse drug reactions from medications used to treat mood disorders

Draw blood and monitor serum blood levels of medications (e.g., tricyclic antidepressants, lithium, anticonvulsants), as appropriate

Monitor and promote the patient's medication compliance

Assist physician with the provision of electroconvulsive therapy (ECT) treatments, when they are indicated

Monitor the physiological and mental status of the patient immediately after ECT

Assist with the provision of "phototherapy" to elevate mood

Provide procedural teaching to patient and significant others of patient who is receiving ECT or phototherapy

Monitor patient's mood for response to ECT or phototherapy

Provide medication teaching to patient/significant others

Provide illness teaching to patient/significant others, if dysfunctional mood is illness based (e.g., depression, mania, or premenstrual syndrome)

Provide guidance about development and maintenance of support systems (e.g., family, friends, spiritual resources, support groups, and counseling)

Assist patient to anticipate and cope with life changes (e.g., new job, leave of absence from work, new peer group)

Provide outpatient follow-up at appropriate intervals, as needed

Background Readings:

Chitty, C. K. (1996). Clients with mood disorders. In H. S. Wilson & C. R. Kneisel (Eds.), Psychiatric nursing (pp. 323-359). Menlo Park, CA: Addison-Wesley.

Depression Guideline Panel. (1993a). Depression in primary care: Volume 1. Detection and diagnosis. Clinical practice guideline. AHCPR Pub. No. 93-0550. Rockville, MD: Agency for Health Care Policy and Research, Public Health Service, U.S. Department of Health and Human Services.

Depression Guideline Panel. (1993b). Depression in primary care: Volume 2. Treatment of major depression. Clinical practice guideline. AHCPR Pub. No. 93-0551. Rockville, MD: Agency for Health Care Policy and Research, Public Health Service, U.S. Department of Health and Human Services.

Fortinash, K. M., & Holoday-Worret, P. A. (1995). Mood disorders. In K. M. Fortinash & P. A. Holoday-Worret (Eds.), Psychiatric nursing care plans (pp. 48-73). St. Louis: Mosby.

Hagerty, B. (1996). Mood disorders: Depression and mania. In K. M. Fortinash & P. A. Holoday-Worret (Eds.), Psychiatric mental health nursing (pp. 251-283). St. Louis: Mosby.

McFarland, G. K., Wasli, E., & Gerety, E. K. (1997). Mood disorders. In G. K. McFarland, E. Wasli, & E. K. Gerety (Eds.), Nursing diagnoses and processes in psychiatric mental health nursing. Philadelphia: Lippincott.

Schultz, J. M., & Videbeck, S. D. (1998). Lippincott's manual of psychiatric nursing care plans. Philadelphia: Lippincott.

Stuart, G. (1998). Emotional responses and mood disorders. In G. W. Stuart & S. J. Sundeen (Eds.), Principles and practice of psychiatric nursing (6th ed.) (pp. 413-451). St. Louis: Mosby.

Tommasini, N. R. (1995). The client with a mood disorder (depression). In D. Antai-Otong & G. Kongable (Eds.), Psychiatric nursing: Biological and behavioral concepts (pp. 157-189). Philadelphia: W.B. Saunders.

M

Multidisciplinary Care Conference   8020

Definition: Planning and evaluating patient care with health professionals from other disciplines

Activities:

Summarize health status data pertinent to patient care planning

Identify current nursing diagnoses

Describe nursing interventions being implemented

Describe patient and family responses to nursing interventions

Seek input about effectiveness of nursing interventions

Discuss progress toward goals

Revise patient care plan, as necessary

Solicit input for patient care planning

Establish mutually agreeable goals

Review discharge plans

Discuss referrals, as appropriate

Recommend changes in treatment plan, as necessary

Provide data to facilitate evaluation of patient care plan

Clarify responsibilities related to implementation of patient care plan

M

Background Readings:

Mariano, C. (1989). The case for interdisciplinary collaboration. Nursing Outlook, 37(6), 285-288.

Richardson, A.T. (1986). Nurses interfacing with other members of the team. In D.A. England (Ed.), Collaboration in nursing (pp. 163-185). Rockville, MD: Aspen.

Music Therapy   4400

Definition: Using music to help achieve a specific change in behavior, feeling, or physiology

Activities:

Define the specific change in behavior and/or physiology that is desired (e.g., relaxation, stimulation, concentration, pain reduction)

Determine the individual's interest in music

Identify the individual's musical preferences

Inform the individual as to the purpose of the music experience

Choose particular music selections representative of the individual's preferences

Assist the individual in assuming a comfortable position

Limit extraneous stimuli (e.g., lights, sounds, visitors, telephone calls) during the listening experience

Make music tapes/compact discs and equipment available to the individual

Ensure that tapes/compact discs and equipment are in good working order

Provide headphones, as indicated

Ensure that the volume is adequate but not too high

Avoid turning music on and leaving it on for long periods

Facilitate the individual's active participation (e.g., playing an instrument or singing), if this is desired and feasible within the setting

Avoid stimulating music after an acute head injury

M

Background Readings:

Chlan, L. (1998). Music therapy. In M. Snyder & R. Lindquist (Eds.), Complementary/alternative therapies in nursing (3rd ed.) (pp. 243-257). New York: Springer Publishing Company.

Gerdner, L.A., & Buckwalter, K.C. (1999). Music therapy. In G.M. Bulechek & J.C. McCloskey (Eds.), Nursing interventions: Effective nursing treatments (3rd ed) (pp. 451-468). Philadelphia: W.B. Saunders.

Tanabe, P., Thomas, R., Paice, J., Spiller, M., & Marcantonio, R. (2001). The effect of standard care, ibuprofen, and music on pain relief and patient satisfaction in adults with musculoskeletal trauma. Journal of Emergency Nursing, 27(2), 124-131.

White, J.M. (2001). Music as intervention: A notable endeavor to improve patient outcomes. Nursing Clinics of North America, 36(1), 83-92.

Mutual Goal Setting 4410

Definition: Collaborating with patient to identify and prioritize care goals, then developing a plan for achieving those goals

Activities:

Encourage the identification of specific life values

Assist patient and significant other to develop realistic expectations of themselves in performance of their roles

Determine patient's recognition of own problem

Encourage the patient to identify own strengths and abilities

Assist the patient in identifying realistic, attainable goals

Construct and use goal attainment scaling, as appropriate

Identify with patient the goals of care

State goals in positive terms

Assist the patient in breaking down complex goals into small, manageable steps

Recognize the patient's value and belief system when establishing goals

Encourage the patient to state goals clearly, avoiding the use of alternatives

Avoid imposing personal values on patient during goal setting

Explain to the patient that only one behavior should be modified at a time

Assist the patient in prioritizing (weighting) identified goals

Clarify with the patient roles of the health care provider and the patient, respectively

Explore with the patient ways to best achieve the goals

Assist the patient in examining available resources to meet the goals

Assist the patient in developing a plan to meet the goals

Assist the patient in setting realistic time limits

Assist the patient in prioritizing activities used for goal achievement

Appraise the patient's current level of functioning with regard to each goal

Facilitate the patient's identification of individualized expected outcomes for each goal

Assist the patient in identifying a specific measurement indicator (e.g., behavior, social event) for each goal

Prepare behavioral outcomes for use in goal attainment scaling

Help the patient focus on expected rather than desired outcomes

Encourage the acceptance of partial goal satisfaction

Develop a scale of upper and lower levels related to expected outcomes for each goal

Identify scale levels that are defined by behavioral or social events for each goal

Assist the patient in specifying the period of time in which each indicator will be measured

Explore with the patient methods of measuring progress toward goals

Coordinate with the patient periodic review dates for assessment of progress toward goals

Review the scale (as developed with the patient) during review dates for assessment of progress

Calculate a goal attainment score

Reevaluate goals and plan as appropriate

Background Readings:

Hefferin, E.A. (1979). Health goal setting: Patient-nurse collaboration at Veterans Administration facilities. Military Medicine, 144(12), 814-822.

Horsley, J.A., Crane, J., Haller, K.B., & Reynolds, M.A. (1982). Mutual goal setting in patient care. CURN Project. New York: Grune & Stratton.

Simons, M.R. (1992). Interventions related to compliance. In G.M. Bulechek & J.C. McCloskey (Eds.), Symposium on Nursing Interventions. Nursing Clinics of North America, 27(2) 477-494.

Stanley, B. (1984). Evaluation of treatment goals: The use of goal attainment scaling. Journal of Advanced Nursing, 9, 351-356.

Webster, J. (2002) Client-centered goal planning, Nursing Times, 98(6), 36-37.

M

Nail Care   1680

Definition: Promotion of clean, neat, attractive nails and prevention of skin lesions related to improper care of nails

Activities:

Monitor or assist with cleaning of nails, according to individual's self-care ability

Monitor or assist with trimming of nails, according to individual's self-care ability

Soak nails in warm water, clean under nails with orange stick, and push back cuticles with a cuticle stick

Moisturize area around nails to prevent dryness

Monitor nails for any changes

Remove nail polish before taking patient to surgery, as appropriate

Assist patient to apply nail polish, as desired

Background Readings:

Perry, A.G., & Potter, P.A. (2002). Clinical nursing skills & techniques (5th ed.) (pp. 145-150). St. Louis: Mosby.

Titler, M.G., Pettit, D., Bulechek, G.M., McCloskey, J.C., Craft, M.J., Cohen, M.Z., Crossley, J.D., Denehy, J.A., Glick, O.J., Kruckeberg, T.W., Maas, M.L., Prophet, C.M., & Tripp-Reimer, T. (1991). Classification of nursing interventions for care of the integument. Nursing Diagnosis, 2(2), 45-56.

N

Nausea Management   1450

Definition: Prevention and alleviation of nausea

Activities:

Encourage patient to monitor own nausea experience

Encourage patient to learn strategies for managing own nausea

Perform complete assessment of nausea including frequency, duration, severity, and precipitating factors, using such tools as Self-Care Journal, Visual Analog Scales, Duke Descriptive Scales, and Rhodes Index of Nausea and Vomiting (INV) Form 2

Observe for nonverbal cues of discomfort, especially for infants, children, and those unable to communicate effectively, such as individuals with Alzheimer's disease

Evaluate past experiences with nausea (e.g., pregnancy and car sickness)

Obtain a complete pretreatment history

Obtain dietary history including the person's likes, dislikes, and cultural food preferences

Evaluate the impact of nausea experience on quality of life (e.g., appetite, activity, job performance, role responsibility, and sleep)

Identify factors (e.g., medication and procedures) that may cause or contribute to nausea

Ensure that effective antiemetic drugs are given to prevent nausea when possible (except for nausea related to pregnancy)

Control environmental factors that may evoke nausea (e.g., aversive smells, sound, and unpleasant visual stimulation)

Reduce or eliminate personal factors that precipitate or increase the nausea (anxiety, fear, fatigue, and lack of knowledge)

Identify strategies that have been successful in relieving nausea

Demonstrate acceptance of nausea and collaborate with the patient when selecting a nausea control strategy

Consider the cultural influence on nausea response while implementing intervention

Encourage not to tolerate nausea but to be assertive with health care providers in obtaining pharmacological and nonpharmacological relief

Teach the use of nonpharmacological techniques (e.g., biofeedback, hypnosis, relaxation, guided imagery, music therapy, distraction, acupressure) to manage nausea

Encourage the use of nonpharmacological techniques before, during, and after chemotherapy; before nausea occurs or increases; and along with other nausea control measures

Inform other health care professionals and family members of any nonpharmacological strategies being used by the nauseated person

Promote adequate rest and sleep to facilitate nausea relief

Use frequent oral hygiene to promote comfort, unless it stimulates nausea

Encourage eating small amounts of food that are appealing to the nauseated person

Instruct on high-carbohydrate and low-fat food, as appropriate

Give cold, clear liquid and odorless and colorless food, as appropriate

Monitor recorded intake for nutritional content and calories

Weigh patient regularly

Provide information about the nausea, such as causes of the nausea and how long it will last

Continued

Activities:—cont'd

Assist to seek and provide emotional support

Monitor effects of nausea management throughout

Background Readings:

Fessele, K. S. (1996). Managing the multiple causes of nausea and vomiting in the patient with cancer. Oncology Nursing Forum, 23(9), 1409-1417.

Grant, M. (1987). Nausea, vomiting, and anorexia. Seminars in Oncology Nursing, 3(4), 227-286.

Hogan, C., M. (1990). Advances in the management of nausea and vomiting. Nursing Clinics of North America, 25(2), 475-497.

Hablonski, R. S. (1993). Nausea: The forgotten symptom. Holistic Nursing Practice, 7(2), 64-72.

Larson, P., Halliburton, P., & Di Julio, J. (1993). Nausea, vomiting, and retching. In V. Carrier-Kohlman, A.M. Lindsey, & C.M. West (Eds.), Pathophysiological phenomena in nursing human responses to illness. Philadelphia: W.B. Saunders Company.

Rhodes, V.A. (1990). Nausea, vomiting, and retching. Nursing Clinics of North America, 25(4), 885-900.

N

Neurologic Monitoring 2620

Definition: Collection and analysis of patient data to prevent or minimize neurologic complications

Activities:

Monitor pupillary size, shape, symmetry, and reactivity

Monitor level of consciousness

Monitor level of orientation

Monitor trend of Glascow Coma Scale

Monitor recent memory, attention span, past memory, mood, affect, and behaviors

Monitor vital signs: temperature, blood pressure, pulse, and respirations

Monitor respiratory status: ABG levels, pulse oximetry, depth, pattern, rate, and effort

Monitor invasive hemodynamic parameters, as appropriate

Monitor ICP and CPP

Monitor corneal reflex

Monitor cough and gag reflex

Monitor muscle tone, motor movement, gait, and proprioception

Monitor for pronator drift

Monitor grip strength

Monitor for tremor

Monitor facial symmetry

Monitor tongue protrusion

Monitor for tracking response

Monitor EOMs and gaze characteristics

Monitor for visual disturbance: diplopia, nystagmus, visual field cuts, blurred vision, and visual acuity

Note complaint of headache

Monitor speech characteristics: fluency, presence of aphasias, or word-finding difficulty

Monitor response to stimuli: verbal, tactile, and noxious

Monitor sharp/dull and hot/cold discrimination

Monitor for paresthesia: numbness and tingling

Monitor sense of smell

Monitor sweating patterns

Monitor Babinski response

Monitor for Cushing response

Monitor craniotomy/laminectomy dressing for drainage

Monitor response to medications

Consult with co-workers to confirm data, as appropriate

Identify emerging patterns in data

Increase frequency of neurologic monitoring, as appropriate

Avoid activities that increase intracranial pressure

N

Continued

Activities:—cont'd
Space required nursing activities that increase intracranial pressure

Notify physician of change in patient's condition

Institute emergency protocols, as needed

Background Readings:

Ackerman, L.L. (1992). Interventions related to neurological care. In G.M. Bulechek & J.C. McCloskey (Eds.), Symposium on Nursing Interventions. Nursing Clinics of North America, 27(2), 325-346.

Allan, D. (1986). Management of the head injured patient. Nursing Times, 82(25), 36-39.

Alspach, J.G. (Ed.). (1991). Core curriculum for critical care nursing (4th ed.). Philadelphia: W.B. Saunders.

Ammons, A.M. (1990). Cerebral injuries and intracranial hemorrhages as a result of trauma. Nursing Clinics of North America, 25(1), 23-34.

Cammermeyer, M., & Appeldorn, C. (Eds.). (1990). Core curriculum for neuroscience nursing (3rd ed.) (pp. Val-Val8 & Vbl-Vb5). Chicago: American Association of Neuroscience Nurses.

Crosby, L., & Parsons, L.C. (1989). Clinical neurologic assessment tool: Development and testing of an instrument to index neurologic status. Heart & Lung, 18(2), 121-125.

Hickey, J.V. (1992). The clinical practice of neurological and neurosurgical nursing (3rd ed.). Philadelphia: J.B. Lippincott.

Mitchell, P.H., & Ackerman, L.L. (1992). Secondary brain injury reduction. In G.M. Bulechek & J.C. McCloskey (Eds.), Nursing interventions: Essential nursing treatments (2nd ed.) (pp. 558-573). Philadelphia: W.B. Saunders.

Price, M.B., & Vroom, H.L. (1985). A quick and easy guide to neurological assessment. Journal of Neurosurgical Nursing, 17(5), 313-320.

Titler, M.G. (1992). Interventions related to surveillance. In G.M. Bulechek & J.C. McCloskey (Eds.), Symposium on Nursing Interventions. Nursing Clinics of North America, 27(2), 495-516.

N

Newborn Care   6880

Definition: Management of neonate during the transition to extrauterine life and subsequent period of stabilization

Activities:

Clear airway of mucus immediately after birth

Weigh and measure newborn

Determine gestational age

Compare newborn's weight with estimated gestational age

Monitor newborn's body temperature

Maintain warm body temperature of newborn

Dry infant immediately after birth to prevent heat loss

Wrap infant in blanket immediately after birth to maintain body temperature, if not to be placed in warmer

Apply stockinette cap to prevent heat loss

Place newborn in isolette or under warmer as needed

Elevate head of mattress of bassinet or isolette to promote respiratory function

Put infant to the mother's breast immediately after birth, as appropriate

Monitor/evaluate suck reflex during feeding

Give newborn initial bath after temperature is stabilized

Regularly hold or touch newborn in isolette, as appropriate

Provide prophylactic eye care

Measure head circumference

Determine maternal/infant blood group and type

Swaddle infant to promote sleep and provide a sense of security

Use blanket roll at newborn's back to position on side

Position newborn on back or side after feeding

Position the infant with the head elevated for burping

Reinforce or provide information about newborn's nutritional needs

Determine condition of infant's cord prior to transfusion using umbilical vein

Cleanse umbilical cord with prescribed preparation

Keep umbilical cord dry and exposed to air by diapering newborn below cord

Cleanse and apply petroleum jelly dressing to circumcision

Apply diapers loosely after circumcision

Remove infant from restraints immediately when procedures are needed

Protect newborn from sources of infection in hospital environment

Determine newborn's readiness state before providing care

Provide a quiet, soothing environment

Respond to newborn's cues for care to facilitate the development of trust

Make eye contact and talk to newborn while giving care

N

Continued

Background Readings:

Betz, C.L, Hussberger, M.M., & Wright, S. (1994). Family centered nursing of children. Philadelphia: W.B. Saunders.

Bobak, I.M., Jensen, M., & Lowdermilk, D.L. (1993). Maternity & gynecologic care: The nurse and the family (5th ed.). St. Louis: Mosby–Year Book.

Olds, S.B., London, M.L., & Ladewig, P.A. (1992). Maternal-newborn nursing: A family centered approach (4th ed.). Menlo Park, CA: Addison-Wesley.

Wong, D. (1997). Whaley & Wong's essentials of pediatric nursing. (5th ed.). St. Louis: Mosby.

N

Newborn Monitoring   6890

Definition: Measurement and interpretation of physiologic status of the neonate the first 24 hours after delivery

Activities:

Perform Apgar evaluation at 1 and 5 minutes after birth

Monitor newborn's temperature until stabilized

Monitor respiratory rate and breathing pattern

Monitor respiratory status, noting signs of respiratory distress: tachypnea, nasal flaring, grunting, retractions, rhonchi, or rales

Monitor for respiratory distress, hypoglycemia, and anomalies, if mother has diabetes

Monitor newborn's heart rate

Monitor newborn's color

Monitor for signs of hyperbilirubinemia

Monitor infant's ability to suck

Monitor newborn's first feeding

Monitor newborn's weight

Keep an accurate record of intake and output

Record newborn's first voiding and bowel movement

Monitor umbilical cord

Monitor male newborn's response to circumcision

N

Background Readings:

Bobak, I.M., Jensen, M., & Lowdermilk, D.L. (1993). Maternity & gynecologic care: The nurse and the family (5th ed.). St. Louis: Mosby–Year Book.

Olds, S.B., London, M.L., & Ladewig, P.A. (1992). Maternal-newborn nursing: A family centered approach (4th ed.). Menlo Park, CA: Addison-Wesley.

Nonnutritive Sucking   6900

Definition: Provision of sucking opportunities for the infant

Activities:

Select a smooth pacifier or pacifier substitute that meets standards to prevent airway obstruction

Use a pacifier that has been cleaned or sterilized daily, is used with only one patient, and has had no contact with contaminated areas

Place largest soft pacifier the infant can tolerate on top of the infant's tongue

Position infant to allow tongue to drop to floor of mouth

Position thumb and index finger under infant's mandible to support sucking reflex, if needed

Move infant's tongue rhythmically with the pacifier if needed to encourage sucking

Rub infant's cheek gently to stimulate the suck reflex

Provide pacifier to encourage sucking during tube feeding and for 5 minutes following the tube feeding

Provide pacifier to encourage sucking at least every 4 hours for infants receiving long-term hyperalimentation

Use pacifier after feedings if infant demonstrates continual need to suck

Rock and hold baby while he or she sucks on pacifier when possible

Play soft, appropriate music

Position infant to prevent loss of pacifier

Inform parent(s) about importance of meeting infant sucking needs

Encourage breastfeeding mother to allow nonnutritive sucking at breast after feeding is complete

Inform parents of alternatives to nipple sucking (e.g. thumb, parent's finger, pacifier)

Instruct parent(s) on the use of nonnutritive sucking

Background Readings:

Hill, A.S., Kurkowski, T.B., & Garcia, J. (2000). Oral support measures used in feeding the preterm infant. Nursing Research, 49(1), 2-9.

Standley, J.M. (2000). The effect of contingent music to increase nonnutritive sucking of premature infants. Pediatric Nursing, 26(5), 493-499.

Normalization Promotion 7200

Definition: Assisting parents and other family members of children with chronic illnesses or disabilities in providing normal life experiences for their children and families

Activities:

Promote development of membership of child into family system without letting child become central focus of family

Assist family to view affected child as a child first, rather than a chronically ill or disabled individual

Provide opportunities for child to have normal childhood experiences

Encourage interaction with normal peers

Deemphasize uniqueness of child's condition

Encourage parents to make child appear as normal as possible

Assist family in avoiding potentially embarrassing situations with child

Assist family in making changes in home environment that decrease reminders of child's special needs

Determine accessibility of activity and child's ability to participate in activity

Identify adaptations needed to accommodate child's limitations, so child can participate in normal activities

Communicate information about child's condition to those who need this information to provide safe supervision or appropriate educational opportunities for child

Assist family in altering prescribed therapeutic regimen in to fit normal schedule, when appropriate

Assist family in advocating for child in school system to ensure access to appropriate education programs

Encourage child to participate in school and community activities appropriate for developmental and ability level

Encourage parents to have same parenting expectations and techniques for affected child as for other children in family, as appropriate

Encourage parents to spend time with all children in family

Involve siblings in care and activities of child, as appropriate

Determine need for respite care for parents or other care providers

Identify resources for respite care in community

Encourage parents to take time to care for their personal needs

Provide information to family about child's condition, treatment, and associated support groups for families

Encourage parents to balance involvement in special programs for child's special needs and normal family and community activities

Encourage family to maintain usual social network and support system

Encourage family to maintain usual family habits, rituals, and routines

N

Background Readings:

Bossert, E., Holaday, B., Harkins, A., & Turner-Henson, A. (1990). Strategies of normalization used by parents of chronically ill school age children. Journal of Child and Adolescent Psychiatric and Mental Health Nursing, 3(2), 57-61.

Knafl, K.A., & Deatrick, J.A. (1986). How families manage chronic conditions. An analysis of the concept of normalization. Research in Nursing & Health, 9, 215-222.

Wong, D.L. (1997) Waley & Wong's essentials of pediatric nursing, (5th ed.) (p. 527). St. Louis: Mosby.

Nutrition Management   1100

Definition: Assisting with or providing a balanced dietary intake of foods and fluids

Activities:

Inquire if patient has any food allergies

Ascertain patient's food preferences

Determine, in collaboration with dietician as appropriate, number of calories and type of nutrients needed to meet nutrition requirements

Encourage calorie intake appropriate for body type and lifestyle

Encourage increased intake of protein, iron, and vitamin C, as appropriate

Offer snacks, (e.g., frequent drinks, fresh fruits/fruit juice), as appropriate

Give light, pureed, and bland foods, as appropriate

Provide a sugar substitute, as appropriate

Ensure that diet includes foods high in fiber content to prevent constipation

Offer herbs and spices as an alternative to salt

Provide patient with high-protein, high-calorie, nutritious finger foods and drinks that can be readily consumed, as appropriate

Provide food selection

Adjust diet to patient's lifestyle, as appropriate

Teach patient how to keep a food diary, as needed

Monitor recorded intake for nutritional content and calories

Weigh patient at appropriate intervals

Encourage patient to wear properly fitted dentures and/or obtain dental care

Provide appropriate information about nutritional needs and how to meet them

Encourage safe food preparation and preservation techniques

Determine patient's ability to meet nutritional needs

Assist patient in receiving help from appropriate community nutritional programs, as needed

Background Readings:

Mahan, L. K. (1996). Krause's food nutrition and diet therapy (pp. 403-423). Philadelphia: Saunders.
Thelan, L.A., & Urden, L.D. (1998). Critical care nursing: Diagnosis and management (3rd ed.). St. Louis: Mosby–Year Book.
Whitney, E.N., & Cataldo, C.B. (1991). Understanding normal and clinical nutrition (3rd ed.). St. Paul, MN: West Publishing.

Nutrition Therapy   1120

Definition: Administration of food and fluids to support metabolic processes of a patient who is malnourished or at high risk for becoming malnourished

Activities:

Complete a nutritional assessment, as appropriate

Monitor food/fluid ingested and calculate daily caloric intake, as appropriate

Monitor appropriateness of diet orders to meet daily nutritional needs, as appropriate

Determine—in collaboration with the dietitian, as appropriate—the number of calories and type of nutrients needed to meet nutrition requirements

Determine food preferences with consideration of cultural and religious preferences

Select nutritional supplements, as appropriate

Encourage patient to select semisoft food, if lack of saliva hinders swallowing

Encourage intake of high-calcium foods, as appropriate

Encourage intake of foods and fluids high in potassium, as appropriate

Ensure that diet includes foods high in fiber content to prevent constipation

Provide patient with high-protein, high-calorie, nutritious finger foods and drinks that can be readily consumed, as appropriate

Assist patient to select soft, bland, and nonacidic foods, as appropriate

Determine need for enteral tube feedings

Administer enteral feedings, as appropriate

Discontinue use of tube feedings, as oral intake is tolerated

Administer hyperalimentation fluids, as appropriate

Ensure availability of progressive therapeutic diet

Provide needed nourishment within limits of prescribed diet

Encourage bringing home-cooked food to the institution, as appropriate

Suggest trial elimination of foods containing lactose, as appropriate

Offer herbs and spices as an alternative to salt

Structure the environment to create a pleasant and relaxing atmosphere

Present food in an attractive, pleasing manner, giving consideration to color, texture, and variety

Provide oral care before meals, as needed

Assist patient to a sitting position before eating or feeding

Monitor lab values, as appropriate

Instruct patient and family about prescribed diet

Refer for diet teaching and planning, as needed

Give patient and family written examples of prescribed diet

Background Readings:

American Society for Parenteral and Enteral Nutrition, Board of Directors. (2001). Standards of practice for nutrition support nurses (pp. 56-62). Nutrition Support Nurses Standards, 16(1).

Bowers, S. (1999). Nutrition support for malnourished, acutely ill adults (pp. 145-146). MEDSURG Nursing, 8(3).

Cluskey, M., & Kim, Y.K. (2001). Use and perceived effectiveness of strategies for enhancing food and nutrient intakes among elderly persons in long-term care. Journal of the American Dietetic Association, 101(1), 111-114.

Creamer, K.M., Schotik Chan, D., Sutton, C., DeLeon, C., Moreno, C., Shoupe, B.A. (2001). A comprehensive pediatric inpatient nutrition support package: A multi-disciplinary approach. Nutrition in Clinical Practice, 16(4), 246-257.

Nutritional Counseling   5246

Definition: Use of an interactive helping process focusing on the need for diet modification

Activities:

Establish a therapeutic relationship based on trust and respect

Establish the length of the counseling relationship

Determine patient's food intake and eating habits

Facilitate identification of eating behaviors to be changed

Establish realistic short- and long-term goals for change in the nutritional status

Use accepted nutritional standards to assist client in evaluating adequacy of dietary intake

Provide information, as necessary, about the health need for diet modification: weight loss, weight gain, sodium restriction, cholesterol reduction, fluid restriction, and so on

Post attractive food guide material in the patient's room (e.g., The Food Guide Pyramid)

Help patient to consider factors of age, stage of growth and development, past eating experiences, injury, disease, culture, and finances in planning ways to meet nutritional requirements

Discuss patient's knowledge of the four basic food groups, as well as perceptions of the needed diet modification

Discuss nutritional requirements and patient's perceptions of prescribed/recommended diet

Discuss patient's food likes and dislikes

Assist patient to record what is usually eaten in a 24-hour period

Review with patient measurements of fluid intake and output, hemoglobin values, blood pressure readings, or weight gains and losses, as appropriate

Discuss food buying habits and budget constraints

Discuss the meaning of food to patient

Determine attitudes and beliefs of significant others about food, eating, and the patient's needed nutritional change

Evaluate progress of dietary modification goals at regular intervals

Assist patient in stating feelings and concerns about achievement of goals

Praise efforts to achieve goals

Provide referral/consultation with other members of the health care team, as appropriate

Background Readings:

Busse, G. (1985). Nutritional counseling. In G.M. Bulechek & J.C. McCloskey (Eds.), Nursing interventions: Treatments for nursing diagnoses (pp. 113-126). Philadelphia: W.B. Saunders.

Gabello, W.J. (1993). Dietary counseling. Patient Care, 27(5), 168-174, 177, 181-184.

N

Nutritional Monitoring   1160

Definition: Collection and analysis of patient data to prevent or minimize malnourishment

Activities:

Weigh patient at specified intervals

Monitor trends in weight loss and gain

Monitor type and amount of usual exercise

Monitor patient's emotional response when placed in situations that involve food and eating

Monitor parent/child interactions during feeding, as appropriate

Monitor environment where eating occurs

Schedule treatment and procedures at times other than feeding times

Monitor for dry, flaky skin with depigmentation

Monitor skin turgor, as appropriate

Monitor for dry, thin hair that is easy to pluck

Monitor gums for swelling, sponginess, receding, and increased bleeding

Monitor for nausea and vomiting

Monitor skinfold measurements: triceps skinfold, midarm muscle circumference, and midarm circumference

Monitor albumin, total protein, hemoglobin, and hematocrit levels

Monitor lymphocyte and electrolyte levels

Monitor food preferences and choices

Monitor growth and development

Monitor energy level, malaise, fatigue, and weakness

Monitor for pale, reddened, and dry conjunctival tissue

Monitor caloric and nutrient intake

Monitor for spoon-shaped, brittle, ridged nails

Monitor for redness, swelling, and cracking of mouth/lips

Note any sores, edema, and hyperemic and hypertrophic papillae of the tongue and oral cavity

Note if tongue is scarlet, magenta, or raw

Note significant changes in nutritional status and initiate treatments, as appropriate

Initiate a dietary consult, as appropriate

Determine whether the patient needs a special diet

Provide optimal environmental conditions at mealtime

Provide nutritional food and fluid, as appropriate

N

Background Readings:

Thelan, L.A., & Urden, L.D. (1998). Critical care nursing: Diagnosis and management (3rd ed.). St. Louis: Mosby.

Whitney, E.N., & Cataldo, C.B. (1991). Understanding normal and clinical nutrition (3rd ed.). St. Paul, MN: West Publishing.

Oral Health Maintenance 1710

Definition: Maintenance and promotion of oral hygiene and dental health for the patient at risk for developing oral or dental lesions

Activities:

Establish a mouth care routine

Apply lubricant to moisten lips and oral mucosa, as needed

Monitor teeth for color, shine, and presence of debris

Identify the risk for development of stomatitis secondary to drug therapy

Encourage and assist patient to rinse mouth

Monitor for therapeutic effects of topical anesthetics, oral protective pastes, and topical or systemic analgesics, as appropriate

Instruct and assist patient to perform oral hygiene after eating and as often as needed

Monitor for signs and symptoms of glossitis and stomatitis

Consult physician or dentist about readjustment of wires/appliances and alternative methods of oral care, if irritation of oral mucous membranes occurs from these devices

Consult physician if oral dryness, irritation, and discomfort persist

Facilitate toothbrushing and flossing at regular intervals

Recommend the use of a soft-bristle toothbrush

Instruct person to brush teeth, gums, and tongue

Recommend a healthy diet and adequate water intake

Arrange for dental checkups, as needed

Assist with denture care, as needed

Encourage denture wearers to brush gums and tongue and rinse the oral cavity daily

Discourage smoking and tobacco chewing

Instruct patient to chew sugarless gum to increase saliva and cleanse teeth

Background Readings:

Locker, D. (1992). Smoking and oral health in older adults. Canadian Journal of Public Health, 83(6), 429-432.

Payton, L. (2000). The winning smile. Arkansas Nursing News, 16(3), 27-30.

Perry, A.G., & Potter, P.A. (2002). Clinical nursing skills & techniques (5th ed.) (pp. 117-118, 132-140). St. Louis: Mosby.

Stiefel, K.A., Damron, S., Sowers, N.J., & Velez, L. (2000). Improving oral hygiene for the seriously ill patient: Implementing research-based practice. MEDSURG Nursing, 9(1), 40-46.

Titler, M.G., Pettit, D., Bulechek, G.M., McCloskey, J.C., Craft, M.J., Cohen, M.Z., Crossley, J.D., Denehy, J.A., Glick, O.J., Kruckeberg, T.W., Maas, M.L., Prophet, C.M., & Tripp-Reimer, T. (1991). Classification of nursing interventions for care of the integument. Nursing Diagnosis, 2(2), 45-56.

Walton, J.C., Miller, J., & Tordecilla, L. (2001). Elder oral assessment and care. MEDSURG Nursing, 10(1), 37-44.

Oral Health Promotion   1720

Definition: Promotion of oral hygiene and dental care for a patient with normal oral and dental health

Activities:

Instruct in necessity of daily oral care routine

Monitor oral mucosa on a regular basis

Discourage smoking and tobacco chewing

Promote regular dental checkups

Teach and encourage flossing

Instruct the patient to avoid excessive gum chewing

Assist with brushing teeth and rinsing mouth, according to patient's self-care ability

Remove, clean, and reinsert dentures, as needed

Apply lubricant to moisten lips and oral mucosa, as needed

Massage the gums, as appropriate

Background Readings:

Craven, R.F., & Hirnle, C.J. (2000) Fundamentals of nursing: Human health and function (3rd ed.) (pp. 686-687). Philadelphia: Lippincott.

Potter, P.A., & Perry, A.G. (1989). Fundamentals of nursing (2nd ed.) (pp. 836-845). St. Louis: Mosby.

Titler, M.G., Pettit, D., Bulechek, G.M., McCloskey, J.C., Craft, M.J., Cohen, M.Z., Crossley, J.D., Denehy, J.A., Glick, O.J., Kruckeberg, T.W., Maas, M.L., Prophet, C.M., & Tripp-Reimer, T. (1991). Classification of nursing interventions for care of the integument. Nursing Diagnosis, 2(2), 45-56.

O

Oral Health Restoration   1730

Definition: Promotion of healing for a patient who has an oral mucosa or dental lesion

Activities:

Remove dentures in case of severe stomatitis

Use a soft toothbrush for removal of dental debris

Use toothettes or disposable foam swabs to stimulate gums and clean oral cavity

Encourage flossing between teeth twice daily with unwaxed dental floss, if platelet levels are above 50,000/mm^3

Encourage frequent rinsing of the mouth with any of the following: sodium bicarbonate solution, warm saline, or hydrogen peroxide solution

Discourage smoking and alcohol consumption

Monitor lips, tongue, mucous membranes, tonsillar fossae, and gums for moisture, color, texture, presence of debris, and infection, using good lighting and a tongue blade

Determine the patient's perception of changes in taste, swallowing, quality of voice, and comfort

Reinforce oral hygiene regimen as part of discharge teaching

Instruct patient to avoid commercial mouthwashes

Instruct patient to report signs of infection to physician immediately

Monitor for therapeutic effects of topical anesthetics, oral protective pastes, and topical or systemic analgesics, as appropriate

Instruct and assist patient to perform oral hygiene after eating and as often as needed

Monitor patient every shift for dryness of the oral mucosa

Assist patient to select soft, bland, and nonacidic foods

Increase mouth care to every 2 hours and twice at night, if stomatitis is not controlled

Monitor for signs and symptoms of glossitis and stomatitis

Consult physician if signs and symptoms of glossitis and stomatitis persist or worsen

Plan small, frequent meals; select soft foods; and serve chilled or room-temperature foods

Avoid use of lemon-glycerin swabs

Increase liquids on the meal tray

Apply topical anesthetics, oral protective pastes, and topical or systemic analgesics, as needed

Background Readings:

Potter, P.A., & Perry, A.G. (1989). Fundamentals of nursing (2nd ed.) (pp. 836-845). St. Louis: Mosby.

Titler, M.G., Pettit, D., Bulechek, G.M., McCloskey, J.C., Craft, M.J., Cohen, M.Z., Crossley, J.D., Denehy, J.A., Glick, O.J., Kruckeberg, T.W., Maas, M.L., Prophet, C.M., & Tripp-Reimer, T. (1991). Classification of nursing interventions for care of the integument. Nursing Diagnosis, 2(2), 45-56.

Order Transcription   8060

Definition: Transferring information from order sheets to the nursing patient care planning and documentation system

Activities:

Ensure that order sheet is stamped with patient identification

Ensure that order sheet is in correct patient chart

Ensure that orders are written or cosigned by a licensed health care provider with clinical privileges

Repeat verbal order back to the physician to ensure accuracy

Avoid taking verbal orders by or through other providers

Ensure that verbal orders are documented per agency policy before noting

Clarify confusing or illegible orders

Evaluate appropriateness of orders and ensure that all needed information is provided

Consult with a pharmacist whenever you have doubts about an unfamiliar drug or dose that is prescribed

Document any disagreement with a physician's order after discussion of the order with the physician and a supervisor

Sign name, title, date, and time to each order noted

Transfer order to appropriate Kardex, worksheet, medication form, lab slip, or care plan

Schedule appointments, as appropriate

Note start and stop dates on medications, per agency policy

Note patient allergies when transcribing medication orders

Inform team members to initiate treatment

Background Readings:

Carson, W. (1994). What you should know about physician verbal orders. American Nurse, 26(3), 30-31.

Davis, N.M. (1994). Clarifying questionable orders. American Journal of Nursing, 26(3), 30-31.

Festa, J. (1983). The law and liability: A guide for nurses. New York: John Wiley & Sons.

O

Organ Procurement

Definition: Guiding families through the donation process to ensure timely retrieval of vital organs and tissue for transplant

Activities:

Review institutional policy and procedures for organ donation

Review potential donor medical history for contraindications to donation

Anticipate organ suitability for donation, depending on criteria of death

Determine whether patient has an organ donation card

Provide emotional support for families when donation is desired but contraindicated

Alert organ procurement team of potential donor

Participate in obtaining specimens to verify donor suitability

Prepare to articulate current criteria for brain death in terms that family members can understand

Obtain consent for organ donation from family, as appropriate

Collaborate with the family to complete separate consent forms that specifically name the organs and tissues authorized for removal

Allow family time for grieving

Provide emotional support for family

Answer commonly asked questions about financial responsibility for procurement, criteria for transplant, and length of procedure

Take actions to preserve viability of organ (e.g., intravenous fluids and ventilation)

Participate in organ procurement procedures, as appropriate

Provide postmortem care

Offer family postmortem viewing of body, when possible

Participate in postprocedure conference

Background Readings:

Adams, E.F., Just, G., De Young, S., & Temmler, L. (1993). Organ donation: Comparison of nurses' participation in two states. American Journal of Critical Care, 2(4), 310-316.

Chabalewski, F., & Norris, M.K.G. (1994). The gift of life: Talking to families about organ and tissue donation. American Journal of Nursing, 94(6), 28-33.

Goodell, A.S. (1993). Anencephalic tissue transplantation. The Canadian Nurse, 89(5), 36-38.

Grover, L.E.K. (1993). The potential role of accident and emergency departments in cadaveric organ donation. Accident and Emergency Nursing, 1(1), 8-13.

Kawamoto, K.L. (1992). Organ procurement in the operating room: Implications for perioperative nurses. AORN Journal, 55(6), 1541-1546.

Smith, K.A. (1992). Demystifying organ procurement: Initiating the protocols, understanding the sequence of events. AORN Journal, 55(6), 1530-1540.

Ostomy Care   0480

Definition: Maintenance of elimination through a stoma and care of surrounding tissue

Activities:

Instruct patient/significant other in the use of ostomy equipment/care

Have patient/significant other demonstrate use of equipment

Assist patient in obtaining needed equipment

Apply appropriately fitting ostomy appliance, as needed

Monitor for incision/stoma healing

Monitor for postop complications, such as intestinal obstruction, paralytic ileus, anastomotic leaks, mucocutaneous separation, as appropriate

Monitor stoma/surrounding tissue healing and adaptation to ostomy equipment

Change/empty ostomy bag, as appropriate

Irrigate ostomy, as appropriate

Assist patient in providing self-care

Encourage patient/significant other to express feelings and concerns about changes in body image

Explore patient's care of ostomy

Explain to the patient what the ostomy care will mean to his/her day-to-day routine

Assist patient to plan time for care routine

Instruct patient how to monitor for complications (e.g., mechanical breakdown, chemical breakdown, rash, leaks, dehydration, infection)

Instruct patient on mechanisms to reduce odor

Monitor elimination patterns

Assist patient to identify factors that affect elimination pattern

Instruct patient/significant other in appropriate diet and expected changes in elimination function

Provide support and assistance while patient develops skill in caring for stoma/surrounding tissue

Teach patient to chew thoroughly, avoid foods that caused digestive upset in the past, add new foods one at a time, and drink plenty of fluids

Instruct in Kegel exercises if patient has ileoanal reservoir

Instruct patient to intubate and drain Indiana pouch whenever it feels full (every 4-6 hours)

Discuss concerns about sexual functioning, as appropriate

Encourage visitation by persons from support group who have same condition

Express confidence that patient can resume normal life with ostomy

Encourage participation in ostomy support groups after discharge

Background Readings:

Bradley, M., & Pupiales, M. (1997). Essential elements of ostomy care. American Journal of Nursing, 97(7), 38-46.

Craven, R.F., & Hirnle, C.J. (2000) Fundamentals of nursing: Human health and function (3rd ed.) (pp. 1109-1112). Philadelphia: Lippincott.

Innes, B.S. (1986). Meeting bowel elimination needs. In K.C. Sorenson & J. Luckmann (Eds.), Basic nursing (pp 827-851) Philadelphia: W.B. Saunders.

O'Shea, H.S. (2001). Teaching the adult ostomy patient. Journal of Wound Ostomy and Continence Nurses Society, 28(1), 47-54.

O

Oxygen Therapy 3320

Definition: Administration of oxygen and monitoring of its effectiveness

Activities:

Clear oral, nasal, and tracheal secretions, as appropriate

Restrict smoking

Maintain airway patency

Set up oxygen equipment and administer through a heated, humidified system

Administer supplemental oxygen as ordered

Monitor the oxygen liter flow

Monitor position of oxygen delivery device

Instruct patient about importance of leaving oxygen delivery device on

Periodically check oxygen delivery device to ensure that the prescribed concentration is being delivered

Monitor the effectiveness of oxygen therapy (e.g., pulse oximetry, ABGs), as appropriate

Ensure replacement of oxygen mask/cannula whenever the device is removed

Monitor patient's ability to tolerate removal of oxygen while eating

Change oxygen delivery device from mask to nasal prongs during meals, as tolerated

Observe for signs of oxygen-induced hypoventilation

Monitor for signs of oxygen toxicity and absorption atelectasis

Monitor oxygen equipment to ensure that it is not interfering with the patient's attempts to breathe

Monitor patient's anxiety related to need for oxygen therapy

Monitor for skin breakdown from friction of oxygen device

Provide for oxygen when patient is transported

Instruct patient to obtain a supplementary oxygen prescription before air travel or trips to high altitude, as appropriate

Consult with other health care personnel regarding use of supplemental oxygen during activity and/or sleep

Instruct patient and family about use of oxygen at home

Arrange for use of oxygen devices that facilitate mobility and teach patient accordingly

Convert to alternate oxygen delivery device to promote comfort, as appropriate

Background Readings:

Alspach, J.G. (Ed.). (1991). Core curriculum for critical care nursing (4th ed.). Philadelphia: W.B. Saunders.

Gottlie, B.J. (1988). Breathing and gas exchange. In M. Kinney, D. Packa, & S. Dunbar (Eds.), AACN's clinical reference for critical-care nursing (2nd ed.) (pp. 160-192). St. Louis: Mosby–Year Book.

Lewis, S.M., & Collies, I.C. (1996). Medical-surgical nursing: Assessment and management of clinical problems (4th ed.). St. Louis: Mosby–Year Book.

Nelson, D.M. (1992). Interventions related to respiratory care. In G.M. Bulechek & J.C. McCloskey (Eds.), Symposium on Nursing Interventions. Nursing Clinics of North America, 27(2), 301-323.

Suddarth, D. (1991). The Lippincott manual of nursing practice (5th ed.) (pp. 210-226). Philadelphia: J.B. Lippincott.

Thelan, L.A., & Urden, L.D. (1998). Critical care nursing: Diagnosis and management (3rd ed.). St. Louis: Mosby–Year Book.

U.S. Department of Health and Human Services. (1994). Unstable angina: Diagnosis and management. Rockville, MD: Agency for Health Care Policy and Research.

Pain Management 1400

Definition: Alleviation of pain or a reduction in pain to a level of comfort that is acceptable to the patient

Activities:

Perform a comprehensive assessment of pain to include location, characteristics, onset/duration, frequency, quality, intensity or severity of pain, and precipitating factors

Observe for nonverbal cues of discomfort, especially in those unable to communicate effectively

Ensure that patient receives attentive analgesic care

Use therapeutic communication strategies to acknowledge the pain experience and convey acceptance of the patient's response to pain

Explore patient's knowledge and beliefs about pain

Consider cultural influences on pain response

Determine the impact of the pain experience on quality of life (e.g., sleep, appetite, activity, cognition, mood, relationships, performance of job, and role responsibilities)

Explore with patient factors that relieve/worsen pain

Evaluate past experiences with pain to include individual or family history of chronic pain or resulting disability, as appropriate

Evaluate, with the patient and the health care team, the effectiveness of past pain control measures that have been used

Assist patient and family to seek and obtain support

Utilize a developmentally appropriate assessment method that allows for monitoring of change in pain and that will assist in identifying actual and potential precipitating factors (e.g., flow sheet, daily diary)

Determine the needed frequency of making an assessment of patient comfort and implement monitoring plan

Provide information about the pain, such as causes of the pain, how long it will last, and anticipated discomforts from procedures

Control environmental factors that may influence the patient's response to discomfort (e.g., room temperature, lighting, noise)

Reduce or eliminate factors that precipitate or increase the pain experience (e.g., fear, fatigue, monotony, and lack of knowledge)

Consider the patient's willingness to participate, ability to participate, preference, support of significant others for method, and contraindications when selecting a pain relief strategy

Select and implement a variety of measures (e.g., pharmacological, nonpharmacological, interpersonal) to facilitate pain relief, as appropriate

Teach principles of pain management

Consider type and source of pain when selecting pain relief strategy

Encourage patient to monitor own pain and to intervene appropriately

Teach the use of nonpharmacological techniques (e.g., biofeedback, TENS, hypnosis, relaxation, guided imagery, music therapy, distraction, play therapy, activity therapy, acupressure, hot/cold application, and massage) before, after, and, if possible, during painful activities; before pain occurs or increases; and along with other pain relief measures

Explore patient's current use of pharmacological methods of pain relief

Teach about pharmacological methods of pain relief

Encourage patient to use adequate pain medication

Continued

Collaborate with the patient, significant other, and other health professionals to select and implement nonpharmacological pain relief measures, as appropriate

Provide the person optimal pain relief with prescribed analgesics

Implement the use of patient-controlled analgesia (PCA), if appropriate

Use pain control measures before pain becomes severe

Medicate prior to an activity to increase participation, but evaluate the hazard of sedation

Ensure pretreatment analgesia and/or nonpharmacological strategies prior to painful procedures

Verify level of discomfort with patient, note changes in the medical record, inform other health professionals working with the patient

Evaluate the effectiveness of the pain control measures used through ongoing assessment of the pain experience

Institute and modify pain control measures on the basis of the patient's response

Promote adequate rest/sleep to facilitate pain relief

Encourage patient to discuss his/her pain experience, as appropriate

Notify physician if measures are unsuccessful or if current complaint is a significant change from patient's past experience of pain

Inform other health care professionals/family members of nonpharmacological strategies being used by the patient to encourage preventive approaches to pain management

Utilize a multidisciplinary approach to pain management, when appropriate

Consider referrals for patient, family, and significant others to support groups, and other resources, as appropriate

Provide accurate information to promote family's knowledge of and response to the pain experience

Incorporate the family in the pain relief modality, if possible

Monitor patient satisfaction with pain management at specified intervals

Background Readings:

Acute Pain Management Guideline Panel. (1992). Acute pain management: Operative or medical procedures and trauma. Clinical practice guideline. AHCPR Pub. No. 92-0032. Rockville, MD: Agency for Health Care Policy and Research, Public Health Service, U.S. Department of Health and Human Services.

Herr, K.A., & Mobily, P.R. (1992). Interventions related to pain. In G.M. Bulechek & J.C. McCloskey (Eds.), Symposium on Nursing Interventions. Nursing Clinics of North America, 27(2), 347-370.

McCaffery, M., & Pasero, C. (1999). Pain. Clinical manual for nursing practice (2nd ed.). St. Louis: Mosby–Year Book.

McGuire, L. (1994). The nurse's role in pain relief. MEDSURG Nursing, 3(2), 94-107.

Mobily, P.R., & Herr, K.A. (2000). Pain. In M. Maas, K. Buckwalter, M. Hardy, T. Tripp-Reimer, M. Titler, & J. Specht (Eds.), Nursing diagnosis, interventions, and outcomes for elders (2nd ed.). Thousand Oaks, CA: Sage Publications.

Perry, A.G., & Potter, P.A. (2000). Clinical nursing skills and techniques (pp. 84-101). St. Louis: Mosby–Year Book.

Rhiner, M. (1999), Managing breakthrough pain: A new approach. American Journal of Nursing, March Suppl., 3-12.

Titler, M.G., & Rakel, B.A. (2001). Nonpharmacologic treatment of pain. Critical Care Nursing Clinics of North America, 13(2), 221-232.

Victor, K. (2001). Properly assessing pain in the elderly. RN, 64(5), 45-49.

P

Parent Education: Adolescent   5562

Definition: Assisting parents to understand and help their adolescent children

Activities:

Ask parents to describe the characteristics of their adolescent child

Discuss parent-child relationship during earlier, school-age years

Discuss disciplining of parents, themselves, when they were adolescents

Teach normal physiological, emotional, and cognitive characteristics of adolescents

Identify developmental tasks or goals of the adolescent period of life

Identify defense mechanisms used most commonly by adolescents, such as denial and intellectualization

Address the effects of adolescent cognitive development on information processing

Address the effects of adolescent cognitive development on decision making

Have parents describe methods of discipline used before adolescent years and their feelings of success with these measures

Describe the importance of power/control issues for both parents and adolescents during adolescent years

Teach parents essential communication skills that will increase their ability to empathize with their adolescent and assist their adolescent to problem solve

Teach parents methods of communicating their love to adolescents

Explore parallels between school-age dependency on parents and adolescent dependency on peer group

Reinforce normalcy of adolescent vacillation between desire for independence and regression to dependence

Discuss effects of adolescent separation from parents on spousal relationships

Share strategies for managing adolescent's perception of parental rejection

Facilitate expression of parental feelings

Assist parents to identify reasons for their responses to adolescents

Identify avenues to assist adolescent to manage anger

Teach parents how to use conflict for mutual understanding and family growth

Role play strategies for managing family conflict

Discuss with parents issues over which they will accept compromise and issues over which they cannot compromise

Discuss necessity and legitimacy of limit setting for adolescents

Address strategies for limit setting for adolescents

Teach parents to use reality and consequences to manage adolescent behavior

P

Background Readings:
Craft, M. (1981). Preference of hospitalized adolescents for information providers. Nursing Research, 30(4), 205-212.

Craft, M. (1983). Talking to adolescents about health. Children's Nurse, 1, 1-3.

Craft, M.J. (1987). Health care preferences of rural teens. Journal of Pediatric Nursing, 2(1), 3-13.

Craft, M.J., & Willadsen, J.A. (1992). Interventions related to family. In G.M. Bulechek & J.C. McCloskey (Eds.), Symposium on Nursing Interventions. Nursing Clinics of North America, 27(2), 517-540.

Wong, D.L. (1997). Waley & Wong's essentials of pediatric nursing (5th ed.) (pp. 165-188). St. Louis: Mosby.

Parent Education: Childrearing Family 5566

Definition: Assisting parents to understand and promote the physical, psychological, and social growth and development of their toddler, preschool, or school-age child/children

Activities:

Ask parent to describe behavioral characteristics of child/children

Discuss parent-child relationships

Teach normal physiological, emotional, and behavioral characteristics of child

Identify appropriate developmental task or goals for the child

Identify defense mechanisms used most by age group

Facilitate parents' discussion of methods of discipline available, selection, and results obtained

Teach importance of balanced diet, three meals/day, and nutritious snacks

Review nutritional requirements for specific age groups

Review dental hygiene facts with parents

Review grooming facts with parents

Review safety issues with parents, such as children meeting strangers and water and bicycle safety

Discuss avenues parents could use to assist children to manage anger

Discuss approaches parents could use to assist children to express feelings positively

Help parents identify evaluation criteria for day care and school settings

Inform parents of community resources

Give parents a variety of strategies to use in managing child's behavior

Encourage parents to try different childrearing strategies, as appropriate

Encourage parents to observe other parents interacting with children

Role play childrearing techniques and communication skills

Refer parents to support group or parenting classes, as appropriate

Provide parents with readings/other materials that will be helpful in performing parenting role

Background Readings:

Dickenson-Hazard, N. (1991). The second through sixth years of life. In M. Stanhope & J. Lancaster (Eds.), Community health nursing (3rd ed.) (pp. 428-441). St. Louis: Mosby.

Mott, S.R., Fazekas, N.F., & James, S.R. (1985). Nursing care of children and families. Menlo Park, CA: Addison-Wesley.

Wong, D.L. (1997) Waley & Wong's essentials of pediatric nursing (5th ed.) (pp. 399-464). St. Louis: Mosby.

P

Parent Education: Infant   5568

Definition: Instruction on nurturing and physical care needed during the first year of life

Activities:

Determine parent(s)' knowledge and readiness and ability to learn about infant care

Monitor learning needs of the family

Provide anticipatory guidance about developmental changes during the first year of life

Assist parent(s) in articulating ways to integrate infant into family system

Teach parent(s) skills to care for newborn

Instruct parent(s) on formula preparation and selection

Give parent(s) information about pacifiers

Give information about adding solid foods to diet during the first year

Instruct parent(s) on appropriate fluoride supplementation

Give information about developing dentition and oral hygiene during the first year

Discuss alternatives to a bedtime bottle to prevent bottle-feeding caries

Provide anticipatory guidance about changing elimination patterns during the first year

Instruct parent(s) on how to treat and prevent diaper rash

Provide anticipatory guidance about changing sleep patterns during the first year

Demonstrate ways in which parent(s) can stimulate infant's development

Encourage parent(s) to hold, cuddle, massage, and touch infant

Encourage parent(s) to talk and read to infant

Encourage parent(s) to provide pleasurable auditory and visual stimulation

Encourage parent(s) to play with infant

Give examples of safe toys or things available in home that can be used as toys

Encourage parent(s) to attend parenting classes

Provide parent(s) with written materials appropriate to identified knowledge needs

Reinforce parent(s)' ability to apply teaching to child care skills

Provide parent(s) with support when learning infant caretaking skills

Assist parent(s) in interpreting infant cues, including nonverbal cues, crying, and vocalizations

Provide information on newborn behavioral characteristics

Demonstrate reflexes to parent(s) and explain their significance to infant care

Discuss infant's capabilities for interaction

Assist parent(s) to identify behavioral characteristics of infant

Demonstrate infant's abilities and strengths to parent(s)

Explain and demonstrate infant states

Demonstrate quieting techniques

Monitor skill of parent(s) in recognizing the infant's physiological needs

Reinforce caregiver role behaviors

P

Continued

Activities:

Reinforce skills parent does well in caring for infant to promote confidence

Provide parent(s) information about making home environment safe for infant

Provide information about safety needs of infant while in a motor vehicle

Instruct parent(s) on how to reach health professionals

Place follow-up telephone call one to two weeks after encounter

Provide information about community resources

Background Readings:

American Academy of Pediatrics & American College of Obstetricians and Gynecologists. (1992). Guidelines for perinatal care (3rd ed.). Chapter 6: Postpartum and follow-up care (pp. 91-116). Evanston, IL: AAP/ACOG.

Barnes, L.P. (1994). Infant care: Teaching the basics. Maternal Child Nursing 19 (January/February):47.

Betz, C.L., Hunsberger, M.M., & Wright, S. (1994). Nursing care of children. Chapter 4: Families with neonates (pp. 107-142). Philadelphia: W.B. Saunders.

Denehy, J.A. (1990). Anticipatory guidance. In M.J. Craft & J.A. Denehy (Eds.), Nursing interventions for infants and children (pp. 53-68). Philadelphia: W.B. Saunders.

Denehy, J.A. (1992). Interventions related to parent-infant attachment. In G.M. Bulechek & J.C. McCloskey (Eds.), Symposium on Nursing Interventions. Nursing Clinics of North America, 27(2), 425-444.

Mott, S.R., James, S.R., & Sperhc, A.M. (1990). Nursing care of children and families (2nd ed.). Redwood City, CA: Addison-Wesley.

P

Parenting Promotion   8300

Definition: Providing parenting information, support, and coordination of comprehensive services to high-risk families

Activities:

Identify and enroll high-risk families in follow-up program

Encourage mothers to receive early and regular prenatal care

Visit mothers in the hospital before discharge to begin establishing trusting relationship and schedule follow-up visit

Make home visits as indicated by level of risk

Assist parents to have realistic expectations appropriate to developmental and ability level of child

Assist parents with role transition and expectations of parenthood

Make referrals to male home visitors to work with fathers, as appropriate

Provide anticipatory guidance needed at different developmental levels

Provide pamphlets, books, and other materials to develop parenting skills

Discuss age-appropriate behavior management strategies

Assist parents to identify unique temperament of infant

Teach parents to respond to behavior cues exhibited by their infant

Model and encourage parental interaction with children

Refer to parent support groups, as appropriate

Assist parents in developing, maintaining, and using social support systems

Listen to parents' problems and concerns nonjudgmentally

Provide positive feedback and structured successes at parenting skills to foster self-esteem

Assist parents to develop social skills

Teach and model coping skills

Enhance problem-solving skills through role modeling, practice, and reinforcement

Provide toys through toy lending library

Monitor child health status, well child checks, and immunization status

Monitor parental health status and health maintenance activities

Arrange transportation to well child visits or other services, as necessary

Refer to community resources, as appropriate

Coordinate community agencies working with family

Provide linkage to job training or employment, as needed

Inform parents where to receive family planning services

Monitor consistent and correct use of contraceptives, as appropriate

Assist in arranging day care, as needed

Refer for respite care, as appropriate

Refer to domestic violence center, as needed

Continued

Activities:—cont'd

Refer for substance abuse treatment, as needed

Collect and record data as indicated for follow-up and program evaluation

Background Readings:

Clarke, B.A., & Strauss, S.S. (1992). Nursing role supplementation for adolescent parents: Prescriptive nursing practice. Journal of Pediatric Nursing, 7(5), 312-318.

Denehy, J.A. (1998). Parenting promotion. In M.J. Craft-Rosenberg & J.A. Denehy (Eds.), Nursing interventions for childbearing and childrearing families. Thousand Oaks, CA: Sage Publishing Company.

Fuddy, L. (1989). A statewide system of family support for the prevention of child abuse and neglect. Family support for high risk infants: Prevention of child abuse. Honolulu: Maternal and Child Health Branch, Family Health Services Division, Department of Health, State of Hawaii.

Hardy, J.B., & Streett, R. (1989). Family support and parenting education in the home: An effective extension of clinic-based preventive health care services for poor children. Journal of Pediatrics, 115(6), 927-931.

Olds, D.L., & Kitzman, H. (1993). Review of research on home visiting for pregnant women and parents of young children. The Future of Children, 3(3), 53-92.

P

Pass Facilitation   7440

Definition: Arranging a leave for a patient from a health care facility

Activities:

Obtain physician order for pass, as appropriate

Establish objectives for the pass

Provide information about restrictions and length of time for pass

Provide information needed for emergency use on pass

Determine who is responsible for patient, as appropriate

Discuss pass with responsible person describing nursing care/self-care, as needed

Prepare medication to be taken on pass, and instruct responsible person

Provide assistive devices/equipment, as appropriate

Offer suggestions for appropriate pass activities, as needed

Help pack personal belongings for pass, as needed

Provide time for patient, family, and friends to ask questions and express concerns

Obtain signature of patient or responsible person on "sign-out" form

Instruct appropriate person that information will be needed about medication, food, and alcohol intake while patient is on leave

Evaluate whether objectives for pass were met on return

Background Readings:

March, C.S. (1992). The complete care plan manual for long-term care. Chicago: American Hospital Publishing.

Nurse's Reference Library. (1987). Patient teaching: Learning needs, discharge preparation, tips and checklists. Springhouse, PA: Springhouse.

Rakel, B.A. (1992). Interventions related to patient teaching. In G.M. Bulechek & J.C. McCloskey (Eds.), Symposium on Nursing Interventions. Nursing Clinics of North America, 27(2), 397-423.

P

Patient Contracting   4420

Definition: Negotiating an agreement with an individual that reinforces a specific behavior change

Activities:

Determine the individual's mental and cognitive ability to enter into a contract

Encourage the individual to identify own strengths and abilities

Assist the individual in identifying the health practices he/she wishes to change

Identify with individual the goals of care

Encourage the individual to identify own goals, not those he/she believes the health care provider expects

Avoid focusing on diagnosis or disease process alone when assisting the individual in identifying goals

Assist the individual in identifying realistic, attainable goals

Assist the individual in identifying appropriate short- and long-term goals

Encourage the individual to write down his/her own goals, if possible

State goals as easily observed behaviors

State goals in positive terms

Assist the individual in breaking down complex goals into small, manageable steps

Clarify with the individual roles of the health care provider and the individual, respectively

Explore with the individual ways to best achieve the goals

Assist the individual in examining available resources to meet the goals

Assist the individual in developing a plan to meet the goals

Assist the individual in identifying present circumstances in the environment that may interfere with the achievement of goals

Assist the individual in identifying methods of overcoming environmental circumstances that may interfere with goal achievement

Explore with the individual methods for evaluating accomplishment of the goals

Foster an open, accepting environment for the creation of the contract

Facilitate involvement of significant others in the contracting process, if desired by the individual

Facilitate the making of a written contract, including all agreed-upon elements

Assist the individual in setting time or frequency requirements for performance of behaviors/actions

Assist the individual in setting realistic time limits

Together with the individual, identify a target date for termination of the contract

Coordinate with the individual opportunities for review of the contract and goals

Facilitate renegotiation of contract terms, if necessary

Assist the individual in discussing his/her feelings about the contract

Observe individual for signs of incongruence that may indicate lack of commitment to fulfilling the contract

Identify with the individual consequences or sanctions for not fulfilling the contract, if desired

Have the contract signed by all involved parties

Provide the individual with a copy of the signed and dated contract

Encourage the individual to identify appropriate, meaningful reinforcers/rewards

Encourage the individual to choose a reinforcer/reward that is significant enough to sustain the behavior

Specify with the individual timing of delivery of reinforcers/rewards

Identify additional rewards with the individual if original goals are exceeded, if desired

Instruct the individual on various methods of observing and recording behaviors

Assist the individual in developing some form of flow chart to assist in tracking the progress toward goals

Assist the individual in identifying even small successes

Explore with the individual reasons for success, or lack of it

Background Readings:

McConnell, E.S. (2000). Health contract calendars: A tool for health professionals with older adults. The Gerontologist, 40(2), 235-239.

Newell, M. (1997). Patient contracting for improved outcomes. The Journal of Care Management, 3 (4), 76-87.

Sherman, J.M., Baumstein, S., & Hendeles, L. (2001). Intervention strategies for children poorly adherent with asthma med ications: one center's experience. Clinical Pediatrics, 40(5), 253-258.

Simons, M.R. (1999) Patient contracting. In G.M. Bulechek & J.C. McCloskey (Eds.), Nursing interventions. Effective nursing treatments (3rd ed.) (pp. 385-397). Philadelphia: W.B. Saunders.

Snyder, M. (1992). Contracting. In Independent nursing interventions (2nd ed.) (pp. 145-154). Albany: Delmar Publishers, Inc.

P

Patient-Controlled Analgesia (PCA) Assistance 2400

Definition: Facilitating patient control of analgesic administration and regulation

Activities:

Collaborate with physicians, patient, and family members in selecting the type of narcotic to be used

Recommend administration of aspirin and nonsteroidal antiinflammatory drugs in conjunction with narcotics, as appropriate

Avoid use of meperidine (Demerol)

Ensure that patient is not allergic to analgesic to be administered

Teach patient and family to monitor pain intensity, quality, and duration

Teach patient and family to monitor respiratory rate and blood pressure

Establish nasogastric, venous, subcutaneous, or spinal access, as appropriate

Validate that the patient can use a PCA device: is able to communicate, comprehend explanations, and follow directions

Collaborate with patient and family to select appropriate type of patient-controlled infusion device

Teach patient and family members how to use the PCA device

Assist patient and family to calculate appropriate concentration of drug to fluid, considering the amount of fluid delivered per hour via the PCA device

Assist patient or family member to administer an appropriate bolus loading dose of analgesic

Teach the patient and family to set an appropriate basal infusion rate on the PCA device

Assist the patient and family to set the appropriate lockout interval on the PCA device

Assist the patient and family in setting appropriate demand doses on the PCA device

Consult with patient, family members, and physician to adjust lockout interval, basal rate, and demand dosage, according to patient responsiveness

Teach patient how to titrate doses up or down, depending on respiratory rate, pain intensity, and pain quality

Teach patient and family members the action and side effects of pain-relieving agents

Document patient's pain, amount and frequency of drug dosing, and response to pain treatment in a pain flow sheet

Recommend a bowel regimen to avoid constipation

Consult with clinical pain experts for a patient who is having difficulty achieving pain control

Background Readings:

Craven, R.F., & Hirnle, C.J. (2000) Fundamentals of nursing: Human health and function (3rd ed.) (p. 1167). Philadelphia: Lippincott.

McCaffery, M., & Beebe, A. (1989). Pain. Clinical manual for nursing practice. St. Louis: Mosby.

The University of Iowa Hospitals and Clinics, Critical Care Nursing Division. (1990). Translating research into practice: Pain management in critical care. Research utilization project funded by AACN.

Patient Rights Protection   7460

Definition: Protection of health care rights of a patient, especially a minor, incapacitated, or incompetent patient unable to make decisions

Activities:

Provide patient with "Patient's Bill of Rights"

Provide environment conducive for private conversations between patient, family, and health care professionals

Protect patient's privacy during activities of hygiene, elimination, and grooming

Determine whether patient's wishes about health care are known in the form of advance directives (e.g., living will, durable power of attorney for health care)

Honor patient's right to receive appropriate pain management for acute, chronic, and terminal conditions

Determine who is legally empowered to give consent for treatment or research

Work with physician and hospital administration to honor patient and family wishes

Refrain from forcing the treatment

Note religious preference

Know the legal status of living wills in the state

Honor a patient's wishes expressed in a living will or durable power of attorney for health care, as appropriate

Honor written "Do Not Resuscitate" (DNR) orders

Assist the dying person with unfinished business

Note on medical record any observable facts bearing on the patient's mental competency to make a will

Intervene in situations involving unsafe or inadequate care

Be aware of mandatory reporting requirements in the state

Limit viewing of the patient's record to immediate health care providers

Maintain confidentiality of patient health information

Background Readings:

American Hospital Association Resource Center. (2001). A patient's bill of rights. Available on-line: http://www.aha.org/resource/pbillofrights.asp

American Hospital Association Resource Center. (2001). Ethical conduct for health care institutions. Available on-line: http://www.aha.org/resource/hethics.asp

Perry, A.G., & Potter, P.A. (2002). Clinical nursing skills and techniques (5th ed.) (pp. 4, 5-6). St. Louis: Mosby.

Weiler, K., & Moorhead, S. (1999). Patient rights protection. In G.M. Bulechek & J.C. McCloskey (Eds.), Nursing interventions: Effective nursing treatments (3rd ed.) (pp. 624-636) Philadelphia. W.B. Saunders.

Peer Review   7700

Definition: Systematic evaluation of a peer's performance compared with professional standards of practice

Activities:

Develop and use policies to guide function of the peer review committee and review process, as necessary

Participate in establishment of protocols and standards for professional practice

Participate in committee meetings, as appropriate

Coordinate evaluation process, as necessary

Observe peer during performance of service, as required for evaluation

Identify performance requiring support of peers

Perform evaluations of selected peers (including self when required)

Provide input in areas of strength and development needs, as indicated

Review credentials of selected peer, as necessary

Recommend promotion or clinical advancement, as appropriate

Provide supervision and counseling, as appropriate

Provide opportunity for feedback

Develop shared responsibility for change or improvement, as necessary

Coordinate appropriate continuing education and training, as necessary

Participate in grievance proceedings, as needed

Background Readings:

American Nurses Association. (1988). Peer review guidelines. Kansas City, MO: American Nurses Association.

Mann, L., Barton, C., Presti, M., & Hirsch, J. (1990). Peer review in performance appraisal. Nursing Administrative Quarterly, 14(4), 9-14.

Quigley, P., Hixon, A., & Janzen, S. (1991). Promoting autonomy and professional practice: A program of clinical privileging. Journal of Nursing Quality Assurance, 5(3), 27-32.

Supples, J. (1993). Self-regulation in the nursing profession: Response to substandard practice. Nursing Outlook, 41(1), 20-24.

Titlebaum, H., Hart, C., & Romano-Egan, J. (1992). Interagency psychiatric consultation liaison nursing peer review and peer board: Quality assurance and employment. Archives of Psychiatric Nursing, 7(2), 125-131.

P

Pelvic Muscle Exercise　　0560

Definition: Strengthening and training the levator ani and urogenital muscles through voluntary, repetitive contraction to decrease stress, urge, or mixed types of urinary incontinence

Activities:

Determine ability to recognize urge to void

Instruct individual to tighten, then relax, the ring of muscle around urethra and anus, as if trying to prevent urination or bowel movement

Instruct individual to avoid contracting the abdomen, thighs, and buttocks; holding breath, or straining down during the exercise

Ensure that the individual can differentiate between the desired drawing up-and-in muscle contraction and the nondesired bearing down effort

Instruct female individual to locate the levator ani and urogenital muscles by placing her finger in the vagina and squeezing

Instruct individual to perform muscle tightening exercises, working up to 300 contractions each day, holding the contractions for 10 seconds each and resting at least 10 seconds between each contraction, per agency protocol

Inform individual that it takes 6 to 12 weeks for exercises to be effective

Provide positive feedback for doing exercises as prescribed

Teach individual to monitor response to exercise by attempting to stop urine flow no more often than once a week

Incorporate biofeedback or electrical stimulation for selected individuals when assistance is indicated to identify correct muscles to contract and/or to elicit desired strength of muscle contraction

Provide written instructions describing the intervention and the recommended number of repetitions

Discuss daily record of continence with individual to provide reinforcement

P

Background Readings:

DeLancey, J.O.L. (1994). Structural support of the urethra as it relates to stress urinary incontinence: The hammock hypothesis. American Journal of Obstetrics & Gynecology, 170, 1713-1720.

Dougherty, M., Bishop, K., Mooney, R., Gimotty, P., & Williams, B. (1993). Graded pelvic muscle exercise. Effect on stress urinary incontinence. Journal of Reproductive Medicine, 39(9), 684-691.

Johnson, V.Y. (2001). How the principles of exercise physiology influence pelvic floor muscle training. Journal of Wound, Ostomy, and Continence Nursing, 28(3), 150-155.

Palmer, M.H. (2001). A long-term study of patient outcomes with pelvic muscle re-education for urinary incontinece. Journal of Wound, Ostomy, and Continence Nursing, 28(4), 199-205.

Sampselle, C. (1993). The urine stream interruption test: Using a stopwatch to assess pelvic muscle strength. The Nurse Practitioner: American Journal of Primary Health Care, 18, 14-20.

Perineal Care   1750

Definition: Maintenance of perineal skin integrity and relief of perineal discomfort

Activities:

Assist with hygiene

Keep the perineum dry

Provide cushion for chair, such as ring cushion, as appropriate

Inspect condition of incision or tear (e.g., episiotomy)

Apply cold pack, as appropriate

Apply a heat cradle/heat lamp, as appropriate

Instruct patient on rationale and use of sitz baths

Provide sitz baths

Clean the perineum thoroughly at regular intervals

Maintain patient in comfortable position

Apply absorbent pads to absorb drainage, as appropriate

Note characteristics of drainage, as appropriate

Provide scrotal support, as appropriate

Provide pain medications, as appropriate

Background Readings:
Potter, P.A., & Perry, A.G. (1998). Fundamentals of nursing: Concepts, process, and practice (4th ed.). St. Louis: Mosby.
Sorensen, K., & Luckmann, J. (1986). Basic nursing: A psychophysiologic approach (2nd ed.). Philadelphia: W.B. Saunders.
Taylor, C.M. (1987). Nursing diagnosis cards. Springhouse, PA: Springhouse.

P

Peripheral Sensation Management   2660

Definition: Prevention or minimization of injury or discomfort in the patient with altered sensation

Activities:

Monitor sharp/dull and/or hot/cold discrimination

Monitor for paresthesia: numbness, tingling, hyperesthesia, and hypoesthesia

Encourage patient to use the unaffected body part to determine temperature of food, liquids, bath water, and so on

Encourage patient to use the unaffected body part to identify location and texture of objects

Instruct patient or family to monitor position of body parts while patient is bathing, sitting, lying, or changing position

Instruct patient or family to examine skin daily for alteration in skin integrity

Monitor fit of bracing devices, prostheses, shoes, and clothing

Instruct patient or family to use thermometer to test water temperature

Encourage use of thermal insulated mitts when handling cooking utensils

Encourage use of gloves or other protective clothing over affected body part when body part is in contact with objects that—because of their thermal, textural, or other inherent characteristics—may be potentially hazardous

Avoid or carefully monitor use of heat or cold, such as heating pads, hot water bottles, and ice packs

Encourage patient to wear well-fitting, low-heeled, soft shoes

Place bed cradle over affected body parts to keep bed clothes off affected areas

Check shoes, pockets, and clothing for wrinkles or foreign objects

Instruct patient to use timed intervals, rather than presence of discomfort, as a signal to alter position

Use pressure-relieving devices, as appropriate

Protect body parts from extreme temperature changes

Immobilize the head, neck, and back, as appropriate

Monitor ability to void and defecate

Establish a means of voiding, as appropriate

Establish a means of bowel evacuation, as appropriate

Administer analgesics, as necessary

Monitor for thrombophlebitis and deep vein thrombosis

Discuss or identify causes of abnormal sensations or sensation changes

Instruct patient to visually monitor position of body parts, if proprioception is impaired

P

Background Readings:

Cammermeyer, M., & Appeldorn, C. (Eds.). (1990). Core curriculum for neuroscience nursing (3rd ed.). Chicago: American Association of Neuroscience Nurses.

Hickey, J.V. (1992). The clinical practice of neurological and neurosurgical nursing (3rd ed.). Philadelphia: J.B. Lippincott.

Johanson, B.C., Wells, S.J., Hoffmeister, D., & Dungca, C.U. (1988). Standards for critical care (3rd ed.). St. Louis: Mosby.

Mitchell, P.H., Hodges, L.C., Muwaswes, M., & Walleck, C.A. (Eds.). (1988). AANN's neuroscience nursing: Phenomena and practice. Norwalk, CT: Appleton & Lange.

Weitzel, E.A. (1991). Unilateral neglect. In M. Maas, K. Buckwalter, & M. Hardy (Eds.), Nursing diagnoses and interventions for the elderly (pp. 387-395). Redwood City, CA: Addison-Wesley.

Peripherally Inserted Central (PIC) Catheter Care 4220

Definition: Insertion and maintenance of a peripherally inserted catheter, either midline or centrally located

Activities:

Identify the intended use of the catheter to determine the type needed (e.g., vesicants or potentially irritating drugs should be run through a centrally inserted line)

Explain the purpose of the catheter, benefits, and risks associated with its use to patient/family

Obtain consent for the insertion procedure, as appropriate

Select an appropriate size and type of catheter to meet patient needs

Select most accessible and least used antecubital vein available (usually the basilic or cephalic vein of the dominant arm)

Determine desired placement of the catheter tip (e.g., superior vena cava or brachiocephalic and axillary or subclavian veins)

Instruct patient that the dominant arm is used when placement is in the superior vena cava to increase blood flow and prevent edema

Position patient supine for insertion with arm at a 90-degree angle to body

Measure the circumference of the upper arm

Measure the distance for catheter insertion

Prep the site for insertion, according to agency protocol

Instruct patient to turn head toward arm to be cannulated and drop chin to chest during insertion

Insert the catheter using sterile technique according to manufacturer's instructions and agency protocol

Connect extension tubing and aspirate for blood return

Flush with prepared heparin and saline, as appropriate

Secure the catheter and apply a sterile transparent dressing

Date and time the dressing

Verify catheter tip placement by x-ray examination, as appropriate

Avoid use of affected arm for blood pressure measurement and phlebotomy

Monitor for immediate complications, such as bleeding, nerve or tendon damage, cardiac decompression, respiratory distress, or catheter embolism

Monitor for signs of phlebitis (e.g., pain, redness, warm skin, edema)

Use sterile technique to change the insertion-site dressing, according to agency protocol

Instruct patient/family on dressing change technique, as appropriate

Flush the line after each use with an appropriate solution

Declot line according to agency protocol, as appropriate

Instruct patient/family about heparinization and medication administration techniques, as appropriate

Remove catheter according to manufacturer's instructions

Document reason for removal and condition of catheter tip

Instruct the patient to report signs of infection (e.g., fever, chills, drainage from insertion site)

Obtain a skin culture and blood culture (sample from the line and other arm), if purulent drainage is noted

Culture catheter tip, as appropriate

Maintain universal precautions

Background Readings:

Camara, D. (2001). Minimizing risks associated with peripherally inserted central catheters in the NICU. The American Journal of Maternal/Child Nursing, 26(1), 17.

Crawford, M., Soukup, M., Woods, S.S., Deisch, P. (2000). Peripherally inserted central catheter program. Nursing Clinics of North America, 35(2), 349-359.

Intravenous Nurses Society. (1998). Revised intravenous nursing standards of practice. Journal of Intravenous Nursing, 21(IS), S1-S9.

Klien, T. (2001). PICCs and midlines: Fine-tuning your care. RN, 64(8), 27-30.

Schmid, M.W. (2000). Risks & complications of peripherally and centrally inserted intravenous catheters. Perioperative Critical Care, 12(2), 165-74.

P

Peritoneal Dialysis Therapy   2150

Definition: Administration and monitoring of dialysis solution into and out of the peritoneal cavity

Activities:

Explain the selected peritoneal dialysis procedure and purpose

Warm the dialysis fluid before instillation

Assess patency of catheter, noting difficulty in inflow/outflow

Maintain record of inflow/outflow volumes and individual/cumulative fluid balance

Have patient empty bladder before peritoneal catheter insertion

Avoid excess mechanical stress on peritoneal dialysis catheters (e.g., coughing, dressing change, infusing large volumes)

Monitor blood pressure, pulse, respirations, temperature, and patient response during dialysis

Ensure aseptic handling of peritoneal catheter and connections

Draw blood samples and review blood chemistries (e.g.,BUN, serum Cr, and serum sodium, potassium, and PO_4 levels)

Obtain cell count cultures of peritoneal effluent, if indicated

Record baseline vital signs: weight, temperature, pulse, respirations, and blood pressure

Measure and record abdominal girth

Measure and record daily weight

Anchor connections and tubing securely

Check equipment and solutions, according to protocol

Administer dialysis exchanges (inflow, dwell, and outflow), according to protocol

Monitor for signs of infection (e.g., peritonitis and exit-site inflammation/drainage)

Monitor for signs of respiratory distress

Monitor for bowel perforation or fluid leaks

Work collaboratively with patient to adjust length of dialysis, diet regulations, and pain and diversion needs to achieve optimal benefit of the treatment

Teach patient to monitor self for signs and symptoms that indicate need for medical treatment (e.g., fever, bleeding, respiratory distress, irregular pulse, cloudy outflow, and abdominal pain)

Teach procedure to patient requiring home dialysis

Background Readings:

Fearing, M.O., & Hart, L.K. (1992). Dialysis therapy. In G.M. Bulechek & J.C. McCloskey (Eds.), Nursing interventions: Essential nursing treatments (2nd ed.) (pp. 587-601). Philadelphia: W.B. Saunders.

Thompson, J.M., McFarland, G.K., Hirsch, J.E., & Tucker, S.M. (1998). Mosby's clinical nursing (4th ed.). St. Louis: Mosby.

Pessary Management   0630

Definition: Placement and monitoring of a vaginal device for treating stress urinary incontinence, uterine retroversion, genital prolapse, or incompetent cervix

Activities:

Review patient history for contraindications for pessary therapy (e.g., pelvic infections, lacerations or space-occupying lesions; noncompliance; or endometriosis)

Determine estrogen requirements, as appropriate

Discuss maintenance regimen and cleaning procedures with patient prior to fitting pessary (e.g., fit is trial and error; frequent follow-up visits are required)

Discuss sexual activity needs prior to selecting pessary

Review manufacturer's directions regarding specific type of pessary

Select type of pessary, as appropriate

Instruct patient to empty bladder and rectum

Perform speculum exam to visualize status of vaginal mucosa

Perform pelvic examination

Insert pessary following manufacturer's instructions

Ask patient to change positions (e.g., stand, squat, walk, and bear down slightly)

Perform second exam in upright position to verify fit

Instruct on method for pessary removal, as appropriate

Instruct on contraindications for intercourse or douching based upon pessary type

Instruct to report discomfort; dysuria; changes in color, consistency, or frequency of vaginal discharge

Prescribe medication to reduce irritation, as appropriate

Determine ability to perform self-care of pessary

Schedule appointment to recheck pessary fit at 24 hours and 72 hours and then as appropriate

Recommend yearly Pap smears, as appropriate

Determine therapeutic response to pessary use

Observe for presence of vaginal discharge or odor

Palpate placement of pessary

Remove pessary, as appropriate

Inspect vagina for excoriation, laceration, or ulceration

Clean and inspect pessary per manufacturer's directions

Replace or refit pessary, as appropriate

Schedule ongoing practitioner follow-up at intervals of 1 to 3 months

Perform dilute vinegar or hydrogen peroxide douches, as needed

Apply topical estrogen to reduce inflammation, as needed

P

Background Readings:

Deger, R.B., Menzin, A.W., & Mikuta, J.J. (1993). The vaginal pessary: Past and present. Postgraduate Obstetrics & Gynecology, 13(18), 1-8.

Miller, D.S. (1992). Contemporary use of the pessary. In W. Droegemueller & J.J. Sciarra (Eds.), Gynecology & obstetrics (Vol. 1). Philadelphia: J.B. Lippincott.

Sulak, P.J., Kuehl, T.J., & Schull, B.L. (1993). Vaginal pessaries and their use in pelvic relaxation. The Journal of Reproductive Medicine, 38(12), 919-923.

Wood, N.J. (1992). The use of vaginal pessaries for uterine prolapse. Nurse Practitioner, 17(7), 31-38.

Zeitlin, M.P., & Lebherz, T.B. (1992). Pessaries in the geriatric patient. Journal of the American Geriatrics Society, 40(6), 635-639.

Phlebotomy: Arterial Blood Sample   4232

Definition: Obtaining a blood sample from an uncannulated artery to assess oxygen and carbon dioxide levels and acid-base balance

Activities:

Maintain universal precautions

Palpate brachial or radial artery for pulse

Perform Allen test before radial artery puncture

Cleanse area with an appropriate solution

Withdraw a small amount of heparin into syringe to coat the syringe barrel and needle lumen

Eject all air bubbles from syringe

Stabilize artery by pulling skin taut

Insert needle directly over pulse at 45- to 60-degree angle

Obtain 3- to 5-cc specimen of blood

Withdraw needle when sample is obtained

Apply pressure over site for 5 to 15 minutes

Cap syringe and place in ice immediately

Label specimen, according to agency protocol

Arrange for immediate transport of specimen to lab

Apply pressure bandage over site, as appropriate

Record temperature, oxygen percent, delivery method, site of puncture, and circulatory assessment after puncture

Interpret results and adjust treatment, as appropriate

P

Background Readings:

Garza, D., & Becan-McBride, K. (1984). Phlebotomy handbook (pp. 105-107). Norwalk, CT: Appleton-Century-Crofts.
Miller, K. (1985). Arterial puncture. In S. Millar, L. Sampson, & S. Soukup (Eds.), AACN procedure manual for critical care (pp. 54-61). Philadelphia: W.B. Saunders.

Phlebotomy: Blood Unit Acquisition   4234

Definition: Procuring blood and blood products from donors

Activities:

Maintain standard precautions

Adhere to agency protocol for donor screening and acceptance (e.g., drug abuse and HIV status)

Obtain demographic information from donor

Obtain written consent from donor authorizing collection and use of blood

Ensure that donor has eaten 4 to 6 hours before donating blood

Determine hemoglobin and hematocrit levels

Measure weight and vital signs before donation

Ensure availability of emergency equipment

Ensure that skin at site of venipuncture is free of lesions

Maintain strict aseptic technique

Assemble equipment

Place donor in semirecumbent position during donation process

Cleanse skin with an iodine preparation prior to venipuncture, according to agency protocol

Perform venipuncture

Connect blood-collecting tubing and bag

Ensure that blood collected in bag mixes with anticoagulant

Instruct individual to elevate arm and apply firm pressure for two to three minutes after completion of blood or blood product donation process

Place pressure bandage or dressing over venipuncture site, as appropriate

Instruct individual to remain recumbent for another one to two minutes, or longer if faintness or weakness is experienced

Encourage donor to remain seated for 10 to 15 minutes after donation

Instruct individual to eat food and drink fluids immediately after donation

Label and store blood, according to agency protocol

Stay with donor during and immediately after collection of blood

Instruction individual to leave the pressure bandage on for several hours after donation

Instruct individual to avoid heavy lifting for several hours after donation

Instruct individual to avoid smoking for 1 hour and alcoholic beverages for 3 hours after donation

Instruct individual to increase fluid intake for 2 days after donation

Instruct individual to eat well-balanced meals for 2 weeks after donation

P

Background Readings:

Beekmann, S.E., Vaughn, T.E., McCoy, K.D., Ferguson, K.J., Torner, J.C., Woolson, R.F., & Doebbeling, B.N. (2001). Hospital bloodborne pathogens programs: Program characteristics and blood and body fluid exposure rates. Infection Control and Hospital Epidemiology, 22(2), 73-82.

Ernst, D.J., & Ernst, C. (2001). Phlebotomy for nurses and nursing personnel. Ramsey, IN.: HealthStar Press.

Garza, D., & Becan-McBride, K. (1999). Phlebotomy handbook: Blood collection essentials (5th ed.) (pp. 227-252). Stamford, CT: Appleton & Lange.

Perry, A.G., & Potter, P.A. (2002). Clinical nursing skills and techniques (5th ed.) (pp. 1188-1196). St. Louis: Mosby.

Phlebotomy: Cannulated Vessel 4235

Definition: Aspirating a blood sample through an indwelling vascular catheter for laboratory tests

Activities:

Assemble equipment, wash hands, and don gloves

Stop any IV infusion that could contaminate the blood sample

Remove cap or tubing to access port; cleanse port with alcohol and allow to dry

Follow manufacturer's instructions to obtain a sample from an indwelling catheter

Apply tourniquet central to peripheral IV site, only if necessary

Connect needleless adapter and vacutainer, or syringe, to vascular access port; open pathway to patient by adjusting stopcocks or opening clamps

Gently aspirate blood into appropriate specimen tube or syringe; discard the first amount determined by catheter used, laboratory tests ordered, and agency policy; collect blood needed for laboratory tests

Remove tourniquet, if applicable

Flush port and catheter with appropriate solution, monitoring closely to prevent introducing air bubbles or clots into the line

Place clean cap on access port and resume any interrupted infusions

Fill specimen tubes from vacutainer syringe in appropriate order (e.g., heparinized tube last)

Label and package specimens according to agency policy; send to appropriate laboratory

Place all sharps and contaminated items in appropriate receptacle

Background Readings:

Darovic, G., & Vanriper, S. (1995). Arterial pressure monitoring. In G. Darovic (Ed.), Hemodynamic monitoring: Invasive and noninvasive clinical applications (2nd ed., pp. 205-207). Philadelphia: W.B. Saunders Co.

Kennedy, C., Angermuller, S., King, R., Noviello, S., Walker, J., Warden, J., & Vang, S. (1996). A comparison of hemolysis rates using intravenous catheters versus venipuncture tubes for obtaining blood samples. Journal of Emergency Nursing, 22(6), 566-569.

Laxson, C., & Titler, M. (1994). Drawing coagulation studies from arterial lines: An integrative literature review. American Journal of Critical Care, 3(1), 16-24.

Mohler, M., Sato, Y., Bobick, K., & Wise, L. (1988). The reliability of blood sampling from peripheral intravenous infusion lines: Complete blood cell counts, electrolyte panels, and survey panels. Journal of Intravenous Nursing, 21(4), 209-214.

NIH Clinical Center Nursing Department Procedure. Care and maintenance of central and peripheral venous access devices. Revised 5/99. Retrieved July 1, 2000, from http://www.cc.nih.gov/nursingcpvadpro.html

NIH Clinical Center Nursing Department Policy. Obtaining blood samples. Reviewed/revised 4/00. Retrieved July 1, 2000, from http://www.cc.nih.gov/nursing/blodsamp.html

P

Phlebotomy: Venous Blood Sample   4238

Definition: Removal of a sample of venous blood from an uncannulated vein

Activities:

Review physician's order for sample to be drawn

Verify correct patient identification

Minimize anxiety for the patient by explaining the procedure and rationale, as appropriate

Provide a private environment

Select vein, considering amount of blood needed, mental status, comfort, age, availability and condition of blood vessels, and presence of arteriovenous fistulas or shunts

Select appropriate size and type of needle

Select appropriate blood specimen tube

Promote vessel dilation through the use of a tourniquet, gravity, application of heat, milking the vein, or fist clenching and relaxation

Cleanse area with an appropriate solution

Cleanse site with circular motion, starting at the point of anticipated venipuncture and moving in an outward circle

Maintain strict aseptic technique

Maintain universal precautions

Ask patient to hold still while venipuncture is performed

Insert needle at a 20- to 30-degree angle in the direction of venous blood return

Observe for blood return in the needle

Withdraw sample of blood

Remove needle from the vein and immediately apply pressure to the site with dry gauze

Apply dressing, as appropriate

Label specimen(s) with patient name, date and time of collection, and other information, as appropriate

Send labeled specimen to appropriate laboratory

Place all sharps (needles) in sharps container

Background Readings:

Brown, B. (1984). Hematology: Principles and procedures (4th ed.) (pp. 1-8). Philadelphia: Lea & Febiger.

Cudworth, K.L. (1985). When you have to draw blood from a femoral vein. RN, 48(3), 47-49.

Wahid, S.R. (1993). New technique for starting IV lines (Wahid's maneuver) (Letter to the editor). Journal of Emergency Nursing, 19(3), 186-187.

P

Phototherapy: Mood/Sleep Regulation   6926

Definition: Administration of doses of bright light in order to elevate mood and/or normalize the body's internal clock.

Activities:

Obtain a physician's order for phototherapy (i.e., frequency, distance, intensity and duration of phototherapy), as appropriate

Instruct the patient/significant other about the treatment (i.e., indications for use, treatment procedure)

Assist the patient to obtain the appropriate light source for the treatment

Assist patient to set up the light source, as prescribed, in preparation for the treatment

Support the patient's use of the treatment

Supervise the patient, as needed, during the treatment

Monitor for side effects of the treatment (e.g., headache, eyestrain, nausea, insomnia, hyperactivity)

Terminate the treatment if patient experiences side effects

Notify the treating physician of side effects

Modify the treatment, as ordered, to decrease/eliminate side effects

Document the treatment and patient's response

Background Readings:

Elmore, S.K. (1991). Seasonal affective disorder, part II: Phototherapy, an expanded role of the psychosocial nurse. Archives of Psychiatric Nursing, 5(6), 365-372.

Frisch, N.C. (2001). Complimentary and somatic therapies. In N.C. Frisch & L.E. Frisch (Eds.), Psychiatric mental health nursing (2nd ed.) (pp. 743-757). Albany, NY: Delmar.

Haber, J. (1997) In J. Huber, B. Krainovich-Miller, A. Leach McMahon, P. Price-Hoskins (Eds.), Comprehensive psychiatric nursing (5th ed.) (pp. 607-651). St. Louis: Mosby.

Hagerty, B. (2000). Mood disorders: Depression and mania. In K.M. Fortinash & P.A. Holoday-Worret, (Eds.), Psychiatric mental health nursing (pp. 258-262). St. Louis: Mosby.

Society for Light Treatment and Biological Rhythms. (2000). Questions and answers about seasonal affective disorder and light therapy [Online]. Available: http://www.websciences.org/sltbr/sadfaq.htm [2002, March, 28].

Stuart, G. (1998). Somatic therapies. In G.W. Stuart & M.T. Laraia (Eds.), Principles and practice of psychiatric nursing (6th ed.) (pp. 604-617). St. Louis: Mosby.

Terman, M., & Terman, J. S. (1999). Bright light therapy: Side effects and benefits across the symptoms spectrum. Journal of Clinical Psychiatry, 60(11), 799-808.

Townsend, M. (2000). Psychiatric/mental health concepts of care (3rd ed.). Philadelphia: F.A. Davis.

University of Iowa Hospitals & Clinics Department of Nursing. (2001). Light therapy. In: Standards manual. Behavioral Health Service (BHS)—Psychiatric. Section II (16). Iowa City, IA: University of Iowa Hospitals and Clinics.

P

Phototherapy: Neonate   6924

Definition: Use of light therapy to reduce bilirubin levels in newborn infants

Activities:

Review maternal and infant history for risk factors for hyperbilirubinemia (e.g., Rh or ABO incompatibility, polycythemia, sepsis, prematurity, malpresentation)

Observe infant for signs of jaundice

Order serum bilirubin levels as appropriate per protocol or primary practitioner request

Report lab values to primary practitioner

Place infant in isolette

Instruct family on phototherapy procedures and care

Apply patches to cover both eyes, avoiding excessive pressure

Remove eye patches every 4 hours or when lights are off for parental contact and feeding

Monitor eyes for edema, drainage, and color

Place phototherapy lights above infant at appropriate height

Check intensity of lights daily

Monitor vital signs per protocol or as needed

Change infant position every 4 hours or per protocol

Monitor serum bilirubin levels per protocol or practitioner request

Evaluate neurological status every 4 hours or per protocol

Observe for signs of dehydration (e.g., depressed fontanels, poor skin turgor, loss of weight)

Weigh daily

Encourage eight feedings per day

Encourage family to participate in light therapy

Instruct family on home phototherapy as appropriate

P

Background Readings:

Merenstien, G., & Gardner, S. (1993). Handbook of neonatal intensive care. St. Louis: Mosby–Year Book.
Wong, D. L. (1997). Whaley & Wong's essentials of pediatric nursing. (5th ed.) St. Louis: Mosby–Year Book.

Physical Restraint   6580

Definition: Application, monitoring, and removal of mechanical restraining devices or manual restraints which are used to limit physical mobility of patient

Activities:

Obtain a physician's order, if required by institutional policy, to use a physically restrictive intervention or to reduce use

Provide patient with a private, yet adequately supervised, environment in situations in which a patient's sense of dignity may be diminished by the use of physical restraints

Provide sufficient staff to assist with safe application of physical restraining devices or manual restraints

Designate one nursing staff member to direct staff and communicate with the patient during the application of physical restraints

Use appropriate hold when manually restraining patient in emergency situations or during transport

Identify for patient and significant others those behaviors that necessitated the intervention

Explain procedure, purpose, and time period of the intervention to patient and significant others in understandable and nonpunitive terms

Explain to patient and significant others the behaviors necessary for termination of the intervention

Monitor the patient's response to procedure

Avoid tying restraints to side rails of bed

Secure restraints out of patient's reach

Provide appropriate level of supervision/surveillance to monitor patient and to allow for therapeutic actions, as needed

Provide for patient's psychological comfort, as needed

Provide diversional activities, (e.g., television, reading to patient, visitors, mobiles), when appropriate, to facilitate patient cooperation with the intervention

Administer PRN medications for anxiety or agitation

Monitor skin condition at restraint site(s)

Monitor color, temperature, and sensation frequently in restrained extremities

Provide for movement and exercise, according to patient's level of self-control, condition, and abilities

Position patient to facilitate comfort and prevent aspiration and skin breakdown

Provide for movement of extremities in patient with multiple restraints by rotating the removal/reapplication of one restraint at a time (as safety permits)

Assist with periodic changes in body position

Provide the dependent patient with a means of summoning help (e.g., bell or call light) when caregiver is not present

Assist with needs related to nutrition, elimination, hydration, and personal hygiene

Evaluate, at regular intervals, patient's need for continued restrictive intervention

Involve patient in activities to improve strength, coordination, judgment, and orientation

Involve patient, when appropriate, in making decisions to move to a more/less restrictive form of intervention

Remove restraints gradually (i.e., one at a time if in four-point restraints), as self-control increases

Monitor patient's response to removal of restraints

Process with the patient and staff, on termination of the restrictive intervention, the circumstances that led to the use of the intervention, as well as any patient concerns about the intervention itself

Provide the next appropriate level of restrictive action (e.g., area restriction or seclusion), as needed

Implement alternatives to restraints, such as sitting in chair with table over lap, self-releasing waist belt, geri-chair without tray table, or close observation, as appropriate

Teach family the risks and benefits of restraints and restraint reduction

Document the rationale for use of restrictive intervention, patient's response to the intervention, patient's physical condition, nursing care provided throughout the intervention, and rationale for terminating the intervention

Background Readings:

Craig, C., Ray, F., & Hix, C. (1989). Seclusion and restraint: Decreasing the discomfort. Journal of Psychosocial Nursing and Mental Health Services, 27(7), 16-19.

Craven, R.F., & Hirnle, C.J. (2000) Fundamentals of nursing: Human health and function (3rd ed.) (p. 645). Philadelphia: Lippincott.

Evans, L.K., & Strumpf, N.E. (1989). Tying down the elderly: A review of the literature on physical restraint. Journal of the American Geriatric Society, 37, 65-74.

Kanak, M.F. (1992). Interventions related to safety. In G.M. Bulechek & J.C. McCloskey (Eds.), Symposium on Nursing Interventions. Nursing Clinics of North America, 27(2), 371-396.

Munns, D., & Nolan, L. (1990). Potential for violence: Self-directed or directed at others. In M. Maas, K.C. Buckwalter, & M. Hardy (Eds.), Nursing diagnoses and interventions for the elderly (pp. 551-560). Menlo Park, CA: Addison-Wesley.

Thackrey, M. (1987). Therapeutics for aggression: Psychological/physical crisis intervention. New York: Human Sciences Press.

Yorker, B.C. (1988). The nurse's use of restraint with a neurologically impaired patient. Journal of Neuroscience Nursing, 20(6), 390-392.

P

Physician Support

7710

Definition: Collaborating with physicians to provide quality patient care

Activities:

Establish a professional working relationship with the medical staff

Participate in orientation of medical staff

Help physicians to learn routines of the patient care unit

Participate in educational programs for the medical staff

Encourage open, direct communication between physicians and nurses

Coach residents and physicians through unfamiliar routines

Alert physicians to changes in scheduled procedures

Discuss patient care concerns or practice-related issues directly with physician(s) involved

Assist patient to voice concerns to physician

Report changes in patient status, as appropriate

Report variation in physician practice within the quality assurance or risk management system, as appropriate

Participate on multidisciplinary committees to address clinical issues

Provide information to appropriate physician groups to encourage practice changes or innovations, as needed

Follow up physician requests for new equipment or supplies

Process practice changes through the appropriate administrative channels once physician groups have been educated about the need for change

Provide feedback to physicians about changes in practice, equipment, and staffing

Include physicians in in-services for new equipment or practice changes

Encourage physicians to participate in collaborative education programs

Use multidisciplinary projects and committees as forums to educate physicians about related nursing issues

Support collaborative research and quality assurance activities

Background Readings:

Alpert, H.B., Goldman, L.D., Kilroy, C.M., & Pike, A.W. (1992). 7 Gryzmish: Toward an understanding of collaboration. Nursing Clinics of North America, 27(1), 47-59.

Baggs, J., & Schmitt, M. (1988). Collaboration between nurses and physicians. Image: Journal of Nursing Scholarship, 20(3), 145-149.

Pike, A.W. (1991). Moral outrage and moral discourse in nurse-physician collaboration. Journal of Professional Nursing, 7(6), 351-363.

Pike, A., McHugh, M., Cannery, K.C., et al. (1993). A new architecture for quality assurance: Nurse-physician collaboration. Journal of Nursing Quality, 7(3), 1-8.

P

Pneumatic Tourniquet Precautions   6590

Definition: Applying a pneumatic tourniquet, while minimizing the potential for patient injury from use of the device

Activities:

Verify correct functioning of pneumatic tourniquet by checking the regulator against a calibrated gauge

Select a tourniquet cuff of appropriate width and length for extremity

Verify the correct functioning of the cuff by inflating the cuff and checking for leaks in the cuff and tubing

Instruct patient about purpose of tourniquet and sensations expected, as appropriate (e.g., tingling, numbness, and dull ache)

Inspect skin at the site of tourniquet cuff

Evaluate baseline peripheral pulses, sensation, and ability to move digits of involved extremity

Wrap cotton roll around extremity under site of tourniquet cuff, ensuring that cotton is wrinkle-free

Apply and secure tourniquet cuff around the extremity, avoiding neurovascular sites and ensuring that skin is not pinched

Protect the skin and cuff from prep and irrigation solutions, as appropriate

Adjust the tourniquet pressure, as instructed by physician or by agency policy

Exsanguinate extremity by elevating and wrapping with an elastic bandage before cuff inflation

Inflate the cuff, as instructed by physician

Monitor patient continuously during use and on deflation of tourniquet

Verify tourniquet pressure and cuff inflation periodically during use

Monitor tourniquet equipment and pressure continuously when used for an IV block

Notify physician of tourniquet times at regular intervals, per agency policy

Deflate the tourniquet cuff, as instructed by physician or by agency policy

Deflate the tourniquet cuff used for an IV block incrementally

Remove the tourniquet cuff

Inspect skin under the tourniquet cuff after removal of cuff

Evaluate the strength of peripheral pulses, sensation, and ability to move digits after deflation or removal of the cuff

Document tourniquet identification number, cuff site, pressure, inflation and deflation times, condition of skin under cuff, and results of peripheral circulatory and neurological evaluation, as per agency policy

Background Readings:

Association of Operating Room Nurses. (2002). Recommended practices for use of the pneumatic tourniquet. AORN Journal 75(2), 379-386.

Fairchild, S. (1993). Perioperative nursing: Principles and practice. Boston: Jones & Bartlett.

Kneedler, J., & Dodge, G. (1994). Perioperative patient care: The nursing perspective. Boston: Jones & Bartlett.

P

Positioning 0840

Definition: Deliberative placement of the patient or a body part to promote physiological and-or psychological well-being

Activities:

Place on an appropriate therapeutic mattress/bed

Provide a firm mattress

Explain to the patient that he/she is going to be turned, as appropriate

Encourage the patient to get involved in positioning changes, as appropriate

Monitor oxygenation status before and after position change

Premedicate patient before turning, as appropriate

Place in the designated therapeutic position

Incorporate preferred sleeping position into the plan of care, if not contraindicated

Position in proper body alignment

Immobilize or support the affected body part, as appropriate

Elevate the affected body part, as appropriate

Position to alleviate dyspnea (e.g., semi-Fowler position), as appropriate

Provide support to edematous areas (e.g., pillow under arms and scrotal support), as appropriate

Position to facilitate ventilation/perfusion matching ("good lung down"), as appropriate

Encourage active or passive range-of-motion exercises, as appropriate

Provide appropriate support for the neck

Avoid placing a patient in a position that increases pain

Avoid placing an amputation stump in the flexion position

Minimize friction and shearing forces when positioning and turning the patient

Apply a footboard to the bed

Turn using the log roll technique

Position to promote urinary drainage, as appropriate

Position to avoid placing tension on the wound, as appropriate

Prop with a backrest, as appropriate

Elevate affected limb 20 degrees or greater, above the level of the heart, to improve venous return, as appropriate

Instruct the patient how to use good posture and good body mechanics while performing any activity

Monitor traction devices for proper setup

Maintain position and integrity of traction

Elevate head of the bed, as appropriate

Turn as indicated by skin condition

Develop a written schedule for repositioning, as appropriate

Turn the immobilized patient at least every 2 hours, according to a specific schedule, as appropriate

Use appropriate devices to support limbs (e.g., hand roll and trochanter roll)

Place frequently used objects within reach

Place bed-positioning switch within easy reach

Place the call light within reach

Background Readings:

Metzler, D., & Finesilver, C. (1999). Positioning. In G.M. Bulechek & J.C. McCloskey, (Eds.), Nursing interventions: Effective nursing treatments (3rd ed.). Philadelphia: W.B. Saunders.

Sundberg, M.C. (1989). Alterations in mobility. In M.C. Sundberg, (Ed.), Fundamentals of nursing: With clinical procedures (2nd ed.) (pp. 767-807). Boston: Jones & Bartlett.

Titler, M.G., Pettit, D., Bulechek, G.M., McCloskey, J.C., Craft, M.J., Cohen, M.Z., Crossley, J.D., Denehy, J.A., Glick, O.J., Kruckeberg, T.W., Maas, M.L., Prophet, C.M., & Tripp-Reimer T. (1991). Classification of nursing interventions for care of the integument. Nursing Diagnosis, 2(2), 45-56.

P

Positioning: Intraoperative 0842

> **Definition:** Moving the patient or body part to promote surgical exposure while reducing the risk of discomfort and complications

Activities:
Determine patient's range of motion and stability of joints

Check peripheral circulation and neurological status

Check skin integrity

Use assistive devices for immobilization

Lock wheels of stretcher and operating room bed

Use an adequate number of personnel to transfer patient

Support the head and neck during transfer

Coordinate transfer and positioning with stage of anesthesia or level of consciousness

Protect IV lines, catheters, and breathing circuits

Protect the eyes, as appropriate

Use assistive devices to support extremities and head

Immobilize or support any body part, as appropriate

Maintain patient's proper body alignment

Place on an appropriate therapeutic mattress or pad

Place in the designated surgical position (e.g., supine, prone, lateral chest, or lithotomy)

Elevate extremities, as appropriate

Apply padding to bony prominences

Apply padding or avoid pressure to superficial nerves

Apply safety strap and arm restraint, as needed

Adjust operating bed, as appropriate

Monitor positioning and traction devices, as appropriate

Monitor patient's position intraoperatively

Record position and devices used

Background Readings:
Fairchild, S. (1993). Perioperative nursing: Principles and practice. Boston: Jones & Bartlett.

Gruendemann, B. (1987). Positioning plus: A clinical handbook on patient positioning for perioperative nurses. Chatsworth, CA: Devon Industries.

Positioning the Surgical Patient. (1993). In Standards and recommended practices. Denver: Association of Operating Room Nurses.

Ricker, L.E. (1998). Positioning the patient for surgery. In M.H. Meeker & J.C. Rothrock (Eds.), Alexander's care of the patient in surgery (10th ed.) (pp. 103-113). St. Louis: Mosby.

U.S. Department of Health and Human Services. (1992). Pressure ulcers in adults: Prediction and prevention. Rockville, MD: Agency for Health Care Policy and Research.

Positioning: Neurologic   0844

Definition: Achievement of optimal, appropriate body alignment for the patient experiencing or at risk for spinal cord injury or vertebral irritability

Activities:

Immobilize or support the affected body part, as appropriate

Place in the designated therapeutic position

Refrain from applying pressure to the affected body part

Support the affected body part

Provide appropriate support for the neck

Provide a firm mattress

Place on airflow bed, if possible

Maintain proper body alignment

Position with head and neck in alignment

Avoid positioning patient on bone flap removal site

Turn using the log roll technique

Apply an orthosis collar

Instruct on orthosis collar care, as needed

Monitor self-care ability while in orthosis collar/bracing device

Apply and maintain a splinting or bracing device

Monitor skin integrity under bracing device/orthosis collar

Instruct on bracing device care, as needed

Place a hand roll under the fingers

Instruct the patient how to use good posture and good body mechanics while performing any activity

Instruct on pin site care, as needed

Monitor traction pin insertion site

Perform traction/orthosis device pin insertion site care

Monitor traction device setup

Brace traction weights while moving patient

Background Readings:

Ackerman, L.L. (1992). Interventions related to neurological care. In G.M. Bulechek & J.C. McCloskey (Eds.), Symposium on Nursing Interventions. Nursing Clinics of North America, 27(2), 325-346.

Feride, T., & Habel, M. (1988). Spasticity in head trauma and CVA patients: Etiology and management. Journal of Neuroscience Nursing, 21(6), 348-352.

Fontaine, D.K., & McQuillan, K. (1989). Positioning as therapy in trauma care. In K.A. Gould (Ed.), Critical Care Nursing Clinics of North America, 1(1), 105-112.

Lee, S. (1989). Intracranial pressure changes during positioning of patients with severe head injury. Heart & Lung, 18(4), 411-414.

Ohman, K., & Spaniol, D. (1990). Halo immobilization: Discharge planning and patient education. Journal of Neuroscience Nursing, 22(6), 351-357.

Palmer, M., & Wyness, M.A. (1988). Positioning and handling: Important considerations in the care of the severely head-injured patient. Journal of Neuroscience Nursing, 20(1), 42-49.

P

Positioning: Wheelchair   0846

Definition: Placement of a patient in a properly selected wheelchair to enhance comfort, promote skin integrity, and foster independence

Activities:

Select the appropriate wheelchair for the patient: standard adult, semi-reclining, fully reclining, or amputee

Select a cushion tailored to the patient's needs

Check patient's position in the wheelchair while patient sits on selected pad and wears proper footwear

Position the pelvis in the middle and as far back on the seat as possible

Check that the iliac crests are level and aligned from side to side

Ensure that there is at least ½-inch clearance on each side of the chair

Ensure that wheelchair allows at least 2 to 3 inches of clearance from the back of knee to front of sling seat

Check that footrests have at least 2 inches of clearance from the floor

Maintain the angle of the hips at 100 degrees, the knees at 105 degrees, and the ankles at 90 degrees, with the heel(s) resting flat on the footrests

Measure the distance from the cushion to just under the elbow, add 1 inch, and adjust the armrests to this height

Adjust the backrest to provide the amount of support required, usually 10 to 15 degrees from vertical

Incline the seat 10 degrees toward the back

Position legs so they are 20 degrees from vertical

Monitor for patient's inability to maintain correct posture in wheelchair

Provide modifications or appliances to wheelchair to correct for patient problems or muscle weakness

Facilitate small shifts of body weight frequently

Determine appropriate time frame for patient to remain in wheelchair, based on health status

Instruct patient on how to transfer from bed to wheelchair, as appropriate

Provide trapeze to assist with transfer, as appropriate

Instruct patient on how to operate wheelchair, as appropriate

Instruct patient on exercises to increase upper body strength, as appropriate

Background Readings:

Loeper, J.M. (1992). Positioning. In G.M. Bulechek, & J.C. McCloskey (Eds.). Nursing interventions: Essential nursing treatments (2nd ed.) (pp. 86-93). Philadelphia: W.B. Saunders.

Mayall, J.K., & Desharnais, G. (1990). Positioning in a wheelchair. Thorofare, NJ: Slack.

P

Postanesthesia Care   2870

Definition: Monitoring and management of the patient who has recently undergone general or regional anesthesia

Activities:

Review patients allergies including allergy to latex

Administer oxygen, as appropriate

Monitor oxygenation

Ventilate, as appropriate

Monitor quality and number of respirations

Encourage patient to deep breathe and cough

Obtain a report from the operating room nurse and anesthetist/anesthesiologist

Monitor and record vital signs and perform pain assessment every 15 minutes or more often, as appropriate

Monitor temperature

Administer warming measures (warm blankets, convection blanket), as needed

Monitor urinary output

Provide nonpharmacological and pharmacological pain relief measures, as needed

Administer antiemetic, as ordered

Administer narcotic antagonists, as appropriate, per agency protocol

Contact physician, as appropriate

Monitor intrathecal anesthetic level

Monitor return of sensorium and motor function

Monitor neurological status

Monitor level of consciousness

Interpret diagnostic tests, as appropriate

Check patient's hospital record to determine baseline vital signs, as appropriate

Compare current status with previous status to detect improvements and deterioration in patient's condition

Provide verbal or tactile stimulation, as appropriate

Administer IV medication to control shivering, per agency protocol

Monitor surgical site, as appropriate

Restrain patient, as appropriate

Adjust the bed, as appropriate

Provide privacy, as appropriate

Provide emotional support to the patient and family, as appropriate

Determine patient's status for discharge

Provide patient report to the postoperative nursing unit

Discharge patient to next level of care

P

Continued

Background Readings:

American Society of Post-Anesthesia Nurses. (2002). The standards of perianesthesia nursing practice. Cherry Hill, NJ: ASPAN.

Brenner, A.R. (2000). Preventing postoperative complications: What's old, what's new, what's tried-and-true. Nursing Management, 31(12), 17-23.

Burdern, N. (Ed). (2000). Ambulatory surgical nursing (2nd ed.). Philadelphia: W.B. Saunders.

Litwack, K. (1999). Core curriculum for perianesthesia nursing practice (4th ed.). Philadelphia: W.B. Saunders.

Wilson, M. (2001). Giving postanesthesia care in the critical care unit. Dimensions in Critical Care Nursing, 19(2), 38-43.

P

Postmortem Care   1770

Definition: Providing physical care of the body of an expired patient and support for the family viewing the body

Activities:

Remove all tubes, as appropriate

Cleanse the body, as needed

Place incontinent pad securely under buttocks and between legs

Raise the head of the bed slightly to prevent pooling of fluids in head or face

Place dentures in mouth, if possible

Close the eyes

Maintain proper body alignment

Notify various departments and personnel, according to policy

Label personal belongings, and place in the appropriate place

Notify clergy, as requested by family

Facilitate and support the family's viewing of the body

Provide privacy and support for family members

Answer questions concerning organ donation

Label the body, according to policy, after the family has left

Transfer the body to the morgue

Notify mortician, as appropriate

Background Readings:

Luckmann, J., & Sorensen, K.C. (1987). Medical-surgical nursing (3rd ed.). Philadelphia: W.B. Saunders.
Perry, A.G., & Potter, P.A. (1998). Clinical nursing skills and techniques. (4th ed.). St. Louis: Mosby.
Smith, S., & Duell, D. (1992). Clinical nursing skills (3rd ed.). Los Altos, CA: National Nursing Review.

P

Postpartal Care

6930

Definition: Monitoring and management of the patient who has recently given birth

Activities:

Monitor vital signs

Monitor lochia for character, amount, odor, and presence of clots

Monitor for signs of infection

Have patient empty bladder before postpartum check

Monitor and record fundal height and firmness q15 min/1 hr; then q30 min/1 hr; then q1hr/4 hr; and then q4 hr/24 hr

Gently massage fundus until firm, as needed

Attempt to express clots until fundus is firm

Put infant to breast to stimulate oxytocin production

Monitor status of episiotomy for redness, edema, ecchymosis, discharge, and approximation

Encourage periodic sitz baths to promote perineal healing and comfort

Place ice bag/pack on perineum after delivery to minimize swelling

Reinforce appropriate perineal hygiene techniques to prevent infection

Encourage consumption of fluids and fiber to prevent constipation

Encourage early ambulation to promote bowel mobility and prevent thrombophlebitis

Administer analgesics PRN to promote comfort and sleep

Schedule nursing activities around daily rest period

Instruct patient on postpartal exercises

Encourage patient to begin postpartal exercises slowly and increase as tolerated

Instruct patient on resumption of ADLs

Encourage mother to discuss her labor and delivery experience

Assist patient in adjusting to loss of her fantasized child and accepting the child she has given birth to, as appropriate

Discuss feelings mother may have about infant, as appropriate

Demonstrate confidence in mother's ability to care for her newborn

Place newborn in nursery for the night to promote maternal rest, if desired

Inform mother of symptoms of postpartum depression that may occur after discharge

Monitor for symptoms of postpartum depression

Determine how patient feels about changes in body after delivery

Encourage patient to resume normal activities, as tolerated

Instruct patient on weight management program

Supplement discharge teaching with pamphlets and handouts

Provide anticipatory guidance regarding sexuality and family planning

Perform discharge teaching

Schedule newborn examination and postpartal examination before discharge

Schedule follow-up home visit, if appropriate

Background Readings:

Littleton, L.Y., & Engbretson, J.C. (2002). Maternal, neonatal, and women's health nursing (pp. 877-928). Albany, NY: Delmar.

Morten, A., Kohl, M., O'Mahoney, P., & Pelosi, K. (1991). Certified nurse-midwifery care of the postpartum client: A descriptive study. Journal of Nurse-Midwifery, 36(5), 276-288.

Olds, S.B., London, M.L., & Ladewig, P.A. (1992). Maternal-newborn nursing: A family-centered approach (4th ed.). Menlo Park, CA: Addison-Wesley.

P

Preceptor: Employee 7722

Definition: Assisting and supporting a new or transferred employee through a planned orientation to a specific clinical area

Activities:

Introduce new person to staff members

Describe clinical focus of the unit/agency

Communicate goals of the unit/agency

Display an accepting attitude to individual assigned to the unit/agency

Discuss the objectives of the orientation period

Provide orientation checklist, as appropriate

Tailor orientation to needs of new employee

Discuss clinical ladder and/or other types of care providers and their specific responsibilities

Review skills needed to fulfill clinical role

Review fire and disaster plans, as appropriate

Review code blue procedures, as appropriate

Discuss use of policy and procedure manuals, as appropriate

Instruct in use of clinical forms and other records, as appropriate

Provide information and standards for universal precautions, as appropriate

Discuss unit protocols, as appropriate

Share work responsibilities during orientation, as appropriate

Assist with locating needed supplies

Orient to computer system, as appropriate

Assist with new procedures, as appropriate

Answer questions and discuss concerns, as appropriate

Identify clinical specialists available for consultation, as appropriate

Provide feedback on performance at specific intervals

Include in unit social functions, as appropriate

Background Readings:

Bastable, S.B. (2003) Nurse as educator. Principles of teaching and learning for nursing practice. Boston: Jones and Bartlett Publishers.

Biancuzzo, M. (1994). Staff nurse preceptors: A program they "own." Clinical Nurse Specialist, 8(2), 97-102.

Davis, M.S., Savin, K.J., & Dunn, M. (1993). Teaching strategies used by expert nurse practitioner preceptors: A qualitative study. Journal of the American Academy of Nurse Practitioners, 5(1), 27-33.

Morrow, K.L. (1984). Preceptorships in nursing staff development. Rockville, MD: Aspen Systems.

Preceptor: Student   7726

Definition: Assisting and supporting learning experiences for a student

Activities:

Ensure patient's acceptance of students as caregivers

Introduce students to staff members and patients

Describe clinical focus of the unit/agency

Communicate goals of the unit/agency

Display an accepting attitude to student assigned to the unit/agency

Recognize the importance of your behavior as a role model

Discuss the objectives of the experience/program, as appropriate

Encourage open communication between the staff and students

Make recommendations for patient assignments or potential learning experiences available for students, considering course objectives, as appropriate

Assist students to use policy and procedure manuals, as appropriate

Orient students to the unit/agency

Ensure that students know and understand fire and disaster policies and code blue procedures

Assist students to locate needed supplies, as appropriate

Provide information and standards for universal precautions

Discuss care plan for assigned patient(s), as appropriate

Guide students in the application of the nursing process, as appropriate

Include students in care planning conferences, as appropriate

Discuss any problems with students with the clinical instructor as soon as possible, as appropriate

Provide observational experiences for activities beyond student's skill level

Provide feedback to clinical instructor about student performance, as appropriate

Provide constructive feedback to the student, when appropriate

Assist student with new procedures, as appropriate

Discuss issues in nursing practice with students based on specific patient situations, as appropriate

Cosign charting with students, as appropriate

Involve students in research activities, as appropriate

Support student leadership experiences, as appropriate

Serve as role model for developing collaborative relationships with other health care providers

Inform clinical instructor of any changes in policy, as appropriate

Orient to computer system, as appropriate

P

Background Readings:

Bastable, S.B. (2003) Nurse as educator. Principles of teaching and learning for nursing practice. Boston: Jones and Bartlett Publishers.

Reilly, D. (1992). Clinical teaching in nursing education. New York: National League for Nursing Press.

Shamian, J., & Inhaber, R. (1985). The concept and practice of preceptorships in nursing: A review of pertinent literature. International Journal of Nursing Studies, 22(2), 79-88.

Stuart-Siddal, S., & Haberlin, J. (Eds.). (1983). Preceptorships in nursing education. Rockville, MD: Aspen Systems.

Preconception Counseling 5247

Definition: Screening and providing information and support to individuals of childbearing age before pregnancy to promote health and reduce risks

Activities:

Establish a therapeutic, trusting relationship

Obtain client history

Develop a preconception, pregnancy-oriented health risk profile, based on history, prescription drug use, ethnic background, occupational and household exposures, diet, specific genetic disorders, and habits (e.g., smoking and alcohol and drug intake)

Explore readiness for pregnancy with both partners

Inquire about physical abuse

Obtain a thorough sexual history, including frequency and timing of intercourse, use of spermicidal lubricants, and postcoital habits, such as douching

Refer women with chronic medical conditions for a prepregnancy management plan

Provide information related to risk factors

Refer for genetic counseling for genetic risk factors

Refer for prenatal diagnostic tests as needed for genetic, medical, or obstetrical risk factors

Screen for or evaluate hemoglobin or hematocrit levels, Rh status, urine dipstick, toxoplasmosis, sexually transmitted diseases, rubella, and hepatitis

Counsel about avoiding pregnancy until appropriate treatment has been given (e.g., rubella vaccine, Rho(D) immune globulin, immune serum globulin, or antibiotics)

Screen individuals at risk or in populations at risk for tuberculosis, sexually transmitted diseases, hemoglobinopathies, Tay-Sachs disease, and genetic defects

Support decision making about advisability of pregnancy, based on identified risk factors

Evaluate the need for a screening mammogram, based on the woman's age and desire for prolonged breastfeeding

Encourage dental exam during preconception to minimize exposure to x-ray examinations and anesthetics

Instruct about the relationships among early fetal development and personal habits, medication use, teratogens, and self-care requisites (e.g., prenatal vitamins and folic acid)

Educate about ways to avoid teratogens (e.g., not handling cat litter, smoking cessation, and alcohol substitutes)

Refer to a teratogens information service to locate specific information about environmental agents

Discuss specific ways to prepare for pregnancy, including the social, financial, and psychological demands of childbearing and childrearing

Identify real or perceived barriers to family planning services and prenatal care and ways of overcoming barriers

Discuss available methods of reproductive assistance and technology, as appropriate

Encourage contraception until prepared for pregnancy

Discuss timing of cessation of contraception to maximize accurate pregnancy dating

Discuss methods of identifying fertility, signs of pregnancy, and ways to confirm pregnancy

Discuss the need for early registration and compliance with prenatal care, including specific high-risk programs that may be appropriate

Encourage attendance at early pregnancy and parenting classes

Encourage women to learn details of health insurance coverage, including waiting periods and available provider options

Recommend self-care needed during the preconception period

Provide education and referrals to appropriate community resources

Provide a copy of the written plan of care for the patients

Provide or recommend follow-up, as needed

Background Readings:

American College of Obstetricians and Gynecologists. (1990). ACOG guide to planning for pregnancy, birth, and beyond. Washington: ACOG.

Barron, M.L., Ganong, L.H., & Brown, M. (1987). An examination of preconception health teaching by nurse practitioners. Journal of Advanced Nursing, 12(5), 605-610.

Bushy, A. (1992). Preconception health promotion: Another approach to improve pregnancy outcomes. Public Health Nursing, 9(1), 10-14.

Cefalo, R.C., & Moos, M.K. (1988). Preconceptional health promotion: A practical guide. Rockville, MD: Aspen.

Chez, R. (1993). Preconception care. Resident and Staff Physician, 89(1), 49-51.

Department of Health and Human Services. (1990). Healthy People 2000: National health promotion and disease prevention objectives. Washington: DHHS.

Institute of Medicine. (1985). Preventing low birthweight (119-174). Washington, DC: National Academy Press.

Jack, B., & Culpepper, L. (1990). Preconception care. In I.R. Merkatz & J.E. Thompson (Eds.), New perspectives on prenatal care (pp. 69-81). New York: Elsevier Science Publications.

Littleton, L.Y., & Enbretson, J.C. (2002). Maternal, neonatal, & women's health nursing (pp. 384-388). Albany, NY: Delmar.

Summers, L., & Price, R.A. (1993). Preconception care: An opportunity to maximize health in pregnancy. Journal of Nurse-Midwifery, 38(4), 188-198.

P

Pregnancy Termination Care   6950

Definition: Management of the physical and psychological needs of the woman undergoing a spontaneous or elective abortion

Activities:

Prepare patient physically and psychologically for abortion procedure

Explain sensations patient might experience

Instruct on signs to report (e.g., increased bleeding, increased cramping, and passage of clots or tissue)

Provide analgesics or antiemetics, as appropriate

Administer medication to terminate pregnancy, as appropriate (e.g., prostaglandin suppositories; intraamniotic prostaglandin, saline, or potassium; or intravenous oxytocin)

Encourage significant other to support patient before, during, or after abortion, if desired

Monitor patient for bleeding and cramping

Initiate intravenous line, as appropriate

Observe for signs of spontaneous abortion (e.g., cessation of cramping, increased pelvic pressure, and loss of amniotic fluid)

Perform vaginal exam, as appropriate

Assist delivery, as appropriate, depending on gestational age of fetus

Weigh blood loss, as appropriate

Monitor vital signs

Observe for signs of shock

Save all passed tissue

Administer oxytocics after delivery, as appropriate

Provide teaching for procedures (e.g., suction curettage, dilation and curettage, and uterine evacuation)

Administer Rho(D) immune globulin for Rh-negative status

Instruct patient about postabortion self-care and monitoring of side effects

Provide anticipatory guidance about grief reaction to fetal death

Complete delivery record and report of death, as appropriate

Obtain specimens for genetic studies or autopsy, as appropriate

Background Readings:

Bobak, I.M., Jensen, M., & Lowdermilk, D.L. (1993). Maternity & gynecologic care: The nurse and the family (5th ed.). St. Louis: Mosby.

Gilbert, E.S., & Harmon, J.S. (1993). Manual of high risk pregnancy & delivery. St. Louis: Mosby.

Mattson, S., & Smith, J.E. (Eds.) (1993). Core curriculum for maternal-newborn nursing. Philadelphia: W.B. Saunders.

P

Premenstrual Syndrome (PMS) Management   1440

Definition: Alleviation/attenuation of physical and/or behavioral symptoms occurring during the luteal phase of the menstrual cycle.

Activities:

Instruct individual in the prospective identification of the major premenstrual symptoms (e.g., bloating, cramping, irritability), use of a prospective calendar checklist or symptom log, and recording of timing and severity of each symptom

Review symptom log/checklist

Collaborate with individual to identify most problematic symptoms

Discuss the complexity of management and need for stepwise approach to alleviate individual symptoms

Collaborate with the individual to select and institute stepwise approach to eliminating symptoms

Provide information about symptom-specific self-care measures (e.g., exercise and calcium supplementation)

Prescribe symptom-specific medication, as appropriate to practice level

Monitor changes in symptoms

Encourage individual to participate in PMS support group if available

Refer to a specialist, as appropriate

Background Readings:

Mortola, J. (2000) Premenstrual syndrome. In M. Goldman & M. Hatch (Eds.). Women and health education (114-125). San Diego: Academic Press.

Ugarriza, D., Klingner, S., & O'Brien, S. (1998) Premenstrual syndromes: Diagnosis and intervention. The Nurse Practitioner, 23, 40-58

Speroff, L., Glass, R., & Kase, N. (1999). Clinical gynecologic endocrinology and infertility (6th ed.) (557-587). Baltimore: Lippincott Williams & Wilkins.

P

Prenatal Care   6960

Definition: Monitoring and management of patient during pregnancy to prevent complications of pregnancy and promote a healthy outcome for both mother and infant

Activities:

Instruct patient on importance of regular prenatal care throughout entire pregnancy

Encourage father or significant other to participate in prenatal care

Encourage parent(s) to attend prenatal classes

Instruct patient on nutrition needed during pregnancy

Monitor nutritional status

Monitor weight gain during pregnancy

Refer patient for supplemental food programs (e.g., WIC), as appropriate

Instruct patient on appropriate exercises and rest during pregnancy

Instruct patient on desired weight gain, based on weight before pregnancy

Monitor psychosocial adjustment of patient and family during pregnancy

Monitor blood pressure

Monitor urine glucose and protein levels

Monitor hemoglobin level

Monitor ankles, hands, and face for edema

Monitor deep tendon reflexes

Instruct patient on danger signs that warrant immediate reporting

Measure fundal height and compare with gestational age

Determine the patient's feelings about an unplanned pregnancy

Determine whether an unplanned pregnancy is approved of by the family

Assist with decision to keep or relinquish infant

Counsel patient about changes in sexuality during pregnancy

Determine social support system

Assist patient to develop and use social support system

Counsel patient on ways to adapt work environment to meet physical needs of pregnancy

Give patient anticipatory guidance about physiological and psychological changes accompanying pregnancy

Assist patient in managing changes associated with pregnancy

Discuss changing body image with patient

Instruct patient on fetal growth and development

Monitor fetal heart rate

Instruct patient to monitor fetal activity

Instruct patient on self-help strategies to relieve common discomforts of pregnancy

Instruct patient on harmful effects of smoking on fetus

Refer patient to smoking cessation program, if appropriate

Instruct patient on harmful effects of alcohol and drugs, including over-the-counter drugs, on fetus

Refer patient to drug dependency treatment program, if appropriate

Instruct patient on environmental teratogens to avoid during pregnancy

Determine the image mother has of her unborn child

Guide patient in imagining her unborn child, as appropriate

Provide parent(s) the opportunity to hear fetal heart tones, as soon as possible

Provide parent(s) the opportunity to see the ultrasound image of fetus

Ascertain before birth whether parent(s) has names picked out for both genders

Refer patient to childbirth preparation class

Refer patient to child care/parenting classes, as appropriate

Background Readings:

Heamen, N. (1998), Antepartum home care for high-risk pregnant women. AACN Clinical Issues: Advanced Practice in Acute and Critical Care, 9(3), 362-376.

Olds, S.B., London, M.L., & Ladewig, P.A. (1992). Maternal-newborn nursing: A family-centered approach (4th ed.). Menlo Park, CA: Addison-Wesley.

U.S. Public Health Service. (1989). Caring for our future: The content of prenatal care: A report of the Public Health Service Panel on the Content of Prenatal Care. Washington, DC: U.S. Government Printing Office.

P

Preoperative Coordination   2880

Definition: Facilitating preadmission diagnostic testing and preparation of the surgical patient

Activities:

Review planned surgery

Obtain client history, as appropriate

Complete a physical assessment, as appropriate

Review physician's orders

Order or coordinate diagnostic testing, as appropriate

Describe and explain preadmission treatments and diagnostic tests

Interpret diagnostic test results, as appropriate

Obtain blood specimens, as appropriate

Obtain urine specimen, as needed

Notify physician of abnormal diagnostic test results

Inform patient and significant other of the date and time of surgery, time of arrival, and admission procedure

Inform the patient and significant other of the location of receiving unit, surgery, and the waiting area

Determine the patient's expectations about the surgery

Reinforce information provided by other health care providers, as appropriate

Obtain consent for treatment, as appropriate

Provide time for the patient and significant other to ask questions and voice concerns

Obtain financial clearance from third-party payers, as necessary

Discuss postoperative discharge plans

Determine ability of caretakers

Telephone the patient to verify planned surgery

Background Readings:

Burden, N. (1993). Ambulatory surgical nursing. Philadelphia: W.B. Saunders.

Muldowny, E. (1993). Establishing a preadmission clinic: A model for quality service. AORN Journal, 58(6), 1183-1191.

U.S. Department of Health and Human Services. (1993). Cataract in adults: Management of functional impairment. Rockville, MD: Agency for Health Care Policy and Research.

Preparatory Sensory Information   5580

Definition: Describing in concrete and objective terms the typical sensory experiences and events associated with an upcoming stressful health care procedure/treatment

Activities:

Identify the sequence of events and describe the environment associated with the procedure/treatment

Identify the typical sensations (what will be seen, felt, smelled, tasted, heard) the majority of patients describe as associated with each aspect of the procedure/treatment

Describe sensations in concrete, objective terms using patients' descriptive words while omitting evaluative adjectives that reflect degree of sensation or emotional response to a sensation

Present sensations and procedural/treatment events in the sequence most likely to be experienced

Link the sensations to their cause when cause may not be self-evident

Describe how long the sensations and procedural events may be expected to last, or when they may be expected to change

Personalize the information by using personal pronouns

Provide an opportunity for the patient to ask questions and clarify misunderstandings

Background Readings:

Christman, N.J., Kirchhoff, K.T., & Oakley, M.G. (1999). Preparatory sensory information. In G.M. Bulechek & J.C. McCloskey (Eds.), Nursing interventions: Effective nursing treatments (3rd ed) (pp. 398-408). Philadelphia: W.B. Saunders.

CURN Project. (1981). Preoperative sensory preparation to promote recovery. New York: Grune & Stratton.

Johnson, J.E., Fieler, V.K., Jones, L.S., Wlasowicz, G.S., & Mitchell, M.L. (1997). Self-regulation theory: Applying theory to your practice. Pittsburgh: Oncology Nursing Press.

Johnson, J.E., Fieler, V.K., Wlasowicz, G.S., Mitchell, M.L., & Jones, L.S. (1997). The effects of nursing care guided by self-regulation theory on coping with radiation therapy. Oncology Nursing Forum, 24, 1041-1050.

Sime, A.M. (1992). Sensation information. In M. Snyder (Ed.), Independent nursing interventions (2nd ed.) (pp. 165-170). Albany, NY: Delmar Publishers.

P

Presence 5340

Definition: Being with another, both physically and psychologically, during times of need

Activities:

Demonstrate accepting attitude

Verbally communicate empathy or understanding of the patient's experience

Be sensitive to the patient's traditions and beliefs

Establish trust and a positive regard

Listen to the patient's concerns

Use silence as appropriate

Touch patient to express concern as appropriate

Be physically available as a helper

Remain physically present without expecting interactional responses

Provide distance for the patient and family as needed

Offer to remain with patient during initial interactions with others in the unit

Help patient to realize that you are available, but do not reinforce dependent behaviors

Stay with patient to promote safety and reduce fear

Reassure and assist parents in their supportive role with their child

Stay with the patient and provide assurance of safety and security during periods of anxiety

Offer to contact other support persons (e.g., priest/rabbi) as appropriate

Background Readings:

Gardner, D.L. (1992). Presence. In G.M. Bulechek & J.C. McCloskey (Eds.), Nursing interventions: Essential nursing treatments (2nd ed.) (pp. 191-200). Philadelphia: W.B. Saunders.

Osterman, P., & Schwartz-Barcott, D. (1996). Presence: Four ways of being there. Nursing Forum, 31(2), 23-30.

Pederson, C. (1993). Presence as a nursing intervention with hospitalized children. Maternal-Child Nursing Journal, 21(3), 75-81.

P

Pressure Management   3500

Definition: Minimizing pressure to body parts

Activities:

Dress patient in nonrestrictive clothing

Bivalve and spread a cast to relieve pressure

Pad rough cast edges and traction connections, as appropriate

Place patient on an appropriate therapeutic mattress/bed

Place patient on a polyurethane foam pad, as appropriate

Refrain from applying pressure to the affected body part

Administer back rub/neck rub, as appropriate

Elevate injured extremity

Turn the immobilized patient at least every 2 hours, according to a specific schedule

Facilitate small shifts of body weight

Monitor skin for areas of redness and breakdown

Monitor patient's mobility and activity

Use an established risk assessment tool to monitor patient's risk factors (e.g., Braden scale)

Use appropriate devices to keep heels and bony prominences off the bed

Make bed with toe pleats

Apply heel protectors, as appropriate

Monitor the patient's nutritional status

Monitor for sources of pressure and friction

Background Readings:

Bergman-Evans, B., Cuddigan, J., & Bergstrom, N. (1994). Clinical practice guidelines: Prediction and prevention of pressure ulcers. Journal of Gerontological Nursing, 20(9), 19-26, 52.

Braden, B.J., & Bergstrom, N. (1992). Pressure reduction. In G.M. Bulechek & J.C. McCloskey (Eds.), Nursing interventions: Essential nursing treatments (2nd ed.) (pp. 94-108). Philadelphia: W.B. Saunders.

Titler, M.G., Pettit, D., Bulechek, G.M., McCloskey, J.C., Craft, M.J., Cohen, M.Z., Crossley, J.D., Denehy, J. A., Glick, O.J., Kruckeberg, T.W., Maas, M.L., Prophet, C.M., & Tripp-Reimer, T. (1991). Classification of nursing interventions for care of the integument. Nursing Diagnosis, 2(2), 45-56.

P

Pressure Ulcer Care   3520

Definition: Facilitation of healing in pressure ulcers

Activities:

Describe characteristics of the ulcer at regular intervals, including size (L×W×D), stage (I-IV), location, exudate, granulation or necrotic tissue, and epithelialization

Monitor color, temperature, edema, moisture, and appearance of surrounding skin

Keep the ulcer moist to aid in healing

Apply moist heat to ulcer to improve blood perfusion and oxygen supply to area

Cleanse the skin around the ulcer with mild soap and water

Debride ulcer, as needed

Cleanse the ulcer with the appropriate nontoxic solution, working in a circular motion from the center

Use a 19-gauge needle and 35-cc syringe to clean deep ulcers

Note characteristics of any drainage

Apply a permeable adhesive membrane to the ulcer, as appropriate

Apply saline soaks, as appropriate

Apply ointments, as appropriate

Apply dressings, as appropriate

Administer oral medications, as appropriate

Monitor for signs and symptoms of infection in the wound

Position every 1 to 2 hours to avoid prolonged pressure

Utilize specialty beds and mattresses, as appropriate

Use devices on the bed (e.g., sheepskin) that protect the individual

Ensure adequate dietary intake

Monitor nutritional status

Verify adequate caloric and high-quality protein intake

Instruct family member/caregiver about signs of skin breakdown, as appropriate

Teach individual or family member(s) wound care procedures

Initiate consultation services of the enterostomal therapy nurse, as needed

Background Readings:

Bergstrom, N., Bennett, M.A., Carlson, C.E., et al. (1994). Treatments of pressure ulcers. Clinical practice guideline. AHCPR Publication No. 95-0652. Rockville, MD: Agency for Health Care Policy and Research, Public Health Service, U.S. Department of Health and Human Services.

Frantz, R.A., & Gardner, S. (1999). Pressure ulcer care. In G.M. Bulechek & J.C. McCloskey (Eds.), Nursing interventions: Effective nursing treatments (3rd ed.) (pp. 211-223). Philadelphia: W.B. Saunders.

Frantz, R.A., Gardner, S., Specht, J.K., & McIntire, G. (2001). Integration of pressure ulcer treatment protocol into practice: Clinical outcomes and care environment attributes. Outcomes Management for Nursing Practice, 5(3), 112-120.

Hirshberg, J., Coleman, J., Marchant, B., & Rees, R.S. (2001). TGF-β3 in the treatment of pressure ulcers: A preliminary report. Advances in Skin & Wound Care, 14(2), 91-95.

Perry, A.G., & Potter, P.A. (2002). Clinical nursing skills and techniques (5th ed.) (pp. 175-191). St. Louis: Mosby.

Spungen, A.M., Koehler, K.M., Modeste-Duncan, R., Rasul, M., Cytryn, A.S., & Bauman, W.A. (2001). 9 clinical cases of non-healing pressure ulcers in patients with spinal cord injury treated with an anabolic agent: A therapeutic trial. Advances in Skin & Wound Care, 14(3), 139-144.

Whitney, J.D., Salvadalena, G., Higa, L., & Mich, M. (2001). Treatment of pressure ulcers with noncontact normothermic wound therapy: Healing and warming effects. Journal of Wound, Ostomy, and Continence Nursing, 28(5), 244-252.

Pressure Ulcer Prevention   3540

Definition: Prevention of pressure ulcers for an individual at high risk for developing them

Activities:

Use an established risk assessment tool to monitor individual's risk factors (e.g., Braden scale)

Utilize methods of measuring skin temperature to determine pressure ulcer risk, per agency protocol

Encourage individual not to smoke and to avoid alcohol use

Document any previous incidences of pressure ulcer formation

Document weight and shifts in weight

Document skin status on admission and daily

Monitor any reddened areas closely

Remove excessive moisture on the skin resulting from perspiration, wound drainage, and fecal or urinary incontinence

Apply protective barriers, such as creams or moisture-absorbing pads, to remove excess moisture, as appropriate

Turn every 1 to 2 hours, as appropriate

Turn with care (e.g., avoid shearing) to prevent injury to fragile skin

Post a turning schedule at the bedside, as appropriate

Inspect skin over bony prominences and other pressure points when repositioning at least daily

Avoid massaging over bony prominences

Position with pillows to elevate pressure points off the bed

Keep bed linens clean, dry, and wrinkle free

Make bed with toe pleats

Utilize specialty beds and mattresses, as appropriate

Use devices on the bed (e.g., sheepskin) that protect the individual

Avoid use of "donut" type devices in sacral area

Moisturize dry, unbroken skin

Avoid hot water and use mild soap when bathing

Monitor for sources of pressure and friction

Apply elbow and heel protectors, as appropriate

Facilitate small shifts of body weight frequently

Provide trapeze to assist patient in shifting weight frequently

Monitor individual's mobility and activity

Ensure adequate dietary intake, especially protein, vitamins B and C, iron, and calories, using supplements, as appropriate

Assist individual in maintaining a healthy weight

Instruct family member/caregiver on signs of skin breakdown, as appropriate

P

Background Readings:

Bergquist, S. & Frantz, R. (2001). Braden scale: Validity in community-based older adults receiving home health care. Applied Nursing Research, 14(1), 36-43.

Braden, B.J., & Bergstrom, N. (1999). Pressure ulcer reduction. In G.M. Bulechek & J.C. McCloskey (Eds.), Nursing interventions: Essential nursing treatments (3rd ed.) (pp. 193-210). Philadelphia: W.B. Saunders.

Cox, K.R., Laird, M., & Brown, J.M. (1998) Predicting and preventing pressure ulcers in adults. Nursing Management, 29(7), 41-45.

Murray, M., & Blaylock, B. (1994). Maintaining effective pressure ulcer prevention programs. MEDSURG Nursing, 3(2), 85-92.

Perry, A.G., & Potter, P.A. (2002). Clinical nursing skills and techniques (5th ed.) (pp. 165-174). St. Louis: Mosby.

Product Evaluation 7760

Definition: Determining the effectiveness of new products or equipment

Activities:

Identify need for a new product or a change in a current product

Select product(s) for evaluation

Define perspective of analysis (benefit to patient or provider)

Identify product efficacy and safety issues

Contact other agencies using the product for additional information

Define the objective of the evaluation

Write trial criteria to be used during the evaluation

Target appropriate areas in which to try a new product

Conduct staff education needed to implement trial

Complete trial evaluation forms

Solicit input from other health care providers, as needed (e.g., biomedical engineers, pharmacists, physicians, and other agencies)

Obtain patient evaluation of product, as appropriate

Determine costs for new product implementation, including training, additional supplies, and maintenance agreements

Make recommendations to the appropriate committee or individual coordinating the evaluation

Participate in ongoing monitoring of product effectiveness

Background Readings:

Bryan, B.M., & Reineke, L.A. (1989). Assessing patient care devices: An objective methodology. Nursing Management, 20(6), 57-60.

Larson, E.L., & Peters, D.A. (1986). Integrating cost analyses in quality assurance. Journal of Nursing Quality Assurance, 1(1), 1-7.

Lipetzky, P.W. (1990). Cost analysis and the clinical nurse specialist. Nursing Management, 21(8), 25-28.

Myers, S. (1990). Material management: Nurses' involvement. Nursing Management, 21(8), 30-32.

Pranger, J.K. (1990). Service-wise purchasing: A nursing contribution. Nursing Management, 21(9), 46-49.

Stahler-Wilson, J.E., & Worman, F.R. (1991). A products nurse specialist: The complete clinical shopper. Nursing Management, 22(11), 36-38.

Takiguchi, S.A., Myers, S.A., Slavish, S., & Stucke, J. (1992). Product evaluation: Air-fluidized beds in an operational setting. Nursing Management, 23(6), 42-48.

P

Program Development   8700

Definition: Planning, implementing, and evaluating a coordinated set of activities designed to enhance wellness, or to prevent, reduce, or eliminate one or more health problems for a group or community.

Activities:

Assist the group or community in identifying significant health needs or problems

Prioritize health needs of problems identified

Convene a task force, including appropriate community members, to examine the priority need or problem

Educate members of the planning group regarding the planning process as appropriate

Identify alternative approaches to address the need(s) or problem(s)

Evaluate alternative approaches detailing cost, resource needs, feasibility, and required activities

Select the most appropriate approach

Develop goals and objectives to address the need(s) or problem(s)

Describe methods, activities, and a time frame for implementation

Identify resources for and constraints on implementing the program

Plan for evaluation of the program

Gain acceptance for the program by the target group, providers, and related groups

Hire personnel to implement and manage the program

Procure equipment and supplies

Market the program to the intended participants and to supporting individuals or groups

Facilitate adoption of the program by the group or community

Monitor the progress of program implementation

Evaluate the program for relevance, efficiency, and cost-effectiveness

Modify and refine the program

Background Readings:

Clark, M. (1996). Nursing in the community (2nd ed.). Stamford CT: Appleton & Lange.
Dignan, M., & Carr. P. (1992). Program planning for health education and promotion (2nd ed.). Philadelphia: Lea & Febiger.
Spradley, B., & Allender, J. (1996). Community health nursing: Concepts and practice. Philadelphia: Lippincott.

P

Progressive Muscle Relaxation   1460

Definition: Facilitating the tensing and releasing of successive muscle groups while attending to the resulting differences in sensation

Activities:

Choose a quiet, comfortable setting

Subdue the lighting

Take precautions to prevent interruptions

Seat patient in a reclining chair, or otherwise make comfortable

Instruct patient to wear comfortable, nonrestrictive clothing

Screen for neck or back orthopedic injuries in which hyperextension of the upper spine would add discomfort and complications

Screen for increased intracranial pressure, capillary fragility, bleeding tendencies, severe acute cardiac difficulties with hypertension, or other conditions in which tensing muscles might produce greater physiological injury, and modify the technique, as appropriate

Instruct patient in jaw relaxation exercise

Have the patient tense, for 5 to 10 seconds, each of 8 to 16 major muscle groups

Tense the foot muscles for no longer than 5 seconds to avoid cramping

Instruct patient to focus on the sensations in the muscles while they are tensed

Instruct patient to focus on the sensations in the muscles while they are relaxed

Check periodically with the patient to ensure that the muscle group is relaxed

Have the patient tense the muscle group again, if relaxation is not experienced

Monitor for indicators of nonrelaxation, such as movement, uneasy breathing, talking, and coughing

Instruct the patient to breathe deeply and to slowly let the breath and tension out

Develop a personal relaxation "patter" that helps the patient to focus and feel comfortable

Terminate the relaxation session gradually

Allow time for the patient to express feelings concerning the intervention

Encourage the patient to practice between regular sessions with the nurse

Background Readings:

McCaffery, M., & Beebe, A. (1989). Pain: Clinical manual for nursing practice. St. Louis: Mosby.

Scandrett, S., & Uecker, S. (1992). Relaxation training. In G.M. Bulechek & J.C. McCloskey (Eds.), Nursing interventions: Essential nursing treatments (2nd ed.) (pp. 434-461). Philadelphia: W.B. Saunders.

Snyder, M. (1998). Progressive muscle relaxation. In M. Snyder & R. Lindquist. (Eds.), Complementary/alternative therapies in nursing (3rd ed.) (pp. 1-13). New York: Springer Publishing Company.

P

Prompted Voiding   0640

Definition: Promotion of urinary continence through the use of timed verbal toileting reminders and positive social feedback for successful toileting

Activities:

Determine ability to recognize urge to void

Keep a continence specification record for 3 days to establish voiding pattern

Use for patients not exhibiting signs and symptoms of overflow and/or reflex urinary incontinence

Establish interval of initial prompted voiding schedule, based upon voiding pattern

Establish beginning and ending time for the prompted voiding schedule, if not for 24 hours

Approach within 15 minutes of prescribed prompted voiding intervals

Allow time (5 seconds) to self-initiate a request for toileting assistance

Determine patient's awareness of continence status by asking if wet or dry

Determine accuracy of response by physically checking clothing or linens, as appropriate

Give positive feedback for accuracy of continence status response and success of maintaining continence between scheduled toileting times

Prompt (maximum of 3 times) to use toilet or substitute, regardless of continence status

Offer assistance with toileting, regardless of continence status

Provide privacy for toileting

Give positive feedback by praising desired toileting behavior

Refrain from commenting on incontinence or refusal to toilet

Inform patient of the time of next toileting session

Teach patient to consciously hold urine between toileting sessions, if not cognitively impaired

Teach patient to self-initiate requests to toilet in response to urge to void

Document outcomes of toileting session in clinical record

Discuss continence record with staff to provide reinforcement and encourage compliance with prompted voiding schedule on a weekly basis and as needed

Background Readings:

Colling, J., Ouslander, J., Hadley, B.J., Eisch, J., & Campbell, E. (1992). The effects of patterned urge response toileting (PURT) on urinary incontinence among nursing home residents. Journal of the American Geriatrics Society, 40, 135-141.

Fantl, J.A., Newman, D.K., Colling, J., et al. (1996, March). Managing acute and chronic urinary incontinence. Clinical practice guideline. Quick reference guide for clinicians, No. 2, 1996 Update. AHCPR Pub. No. 96-0686. Rockville, MD: U.S. Department of Health and Human Services, Public Health Service, Agency for Health Care and Research.

Kaltreider, D.L., Hu, T.W., Igou, J.F., Yu, L.C., & Craighead, W.E. (1990). Can reminders curb incontinence? Geriatric Nursing, 11(1), 17-19.

Lyons, S.S., & Specht, J.K.P. (1999). Research-based protocol: Prompted voiding for persons with urinary incontinence. Iowa City, IA: The University of Iowa Gerontological Nursing Interventions Research Center Research Development and Dissemination Core.

Palmer, M., Bennett, R., Marks, J., McCormick, K., & Engel, B. (1994). UI: A program that works. Journal of Long Term Care Administration, 22(2), 19-25.

P

Prosthesis Care   1780

Definition: Care of a removable appliance worn by a patient and the prevention of complications associated with its use

Activities:

Supervise initial use and care of the appliance

Inspect surrounding tissue for signs and symptoms of complications

Identify potential for alterations in body image

Identify modifications in clothing required

Cleanse the artificial appliance, as appropriate

Teach patient and family how to care for and apply the appliance

Secure the appliance in a safe manner when not in use

Remove all appliances prior to surgery, as appropriate

Background Readings:

Hanawalt, A.K., & Troutman, K. (1984). If your patient has a hearing aid. American Journal of Nursing, 84(7), 900-901.
Perry, A.G., & Potter, P.A. (1998). Clinical nursing skills and techniques. (4th ed.) St. Louis: Mosby–Year Book.

P

Pruritus Management   3550

Definition: Preventing and treating itching

Activities:

Determine the cause of the pruritus (e.g., contact dermatitis, systemic disorder, or medications)

Perform a physical examination to identify skin disruptions (e.g., lesions, blisters, ulcers, or abrasions)

Apply dressings or splints to hand or elbow during sleep to limit uncontrollable scratching, as appropriate

Apply medicated creams and lotions, as appropriate

Administer antipruritics, as indicated

Administer opiate antagonists, as indicated

Apply antihistamine cream, as appropriate

Apply cold to relieve irritation

Instruct patient to avoid perfumed bath soaps and oils

Instruct patient to run a humidifier in the home

Instruct the patient not to wear tight-fitting clothing and wool or synthetic fabrics

Instruct patient to keep fingernails trimmed short

Instruct patient to minimize sweating by avoiding warm/hot environments

Instruct patient to limit bathing to once or twice a week, as appropriate

Instruct patient to bathe in lukewarm water and pat skin dry

Instruct patient to use the palm of the hand to rub over a wide area of the skin or pinch the skin gently between thumb and index finger to relieve itching

Instruct patient with casts not to insert objects in cast opening to scratch skin

Background Readings:

Banov, C.H., Epstein, J.H., & Grayson, L.D. (1992). When an itch persists. Patient Care, March 15, 75-88.

Dewitt, S. (1990). Nursing assessment of the skin and dermatologic lesions. Nursing Clinics of North America, 25(1), 235-245.

Hagermark, O., & Wahlgren, C.F. (1995). Treatment of itch. Seminars in Dermatology, 14(4), 320-325.

Kam, P.C.A, & Tan, K.H. (1996). Pruritus—itching for a cause and relief? Anesthesia, 51, 1133-1138.

P

Quality Monitoring 7800

Definition: Systematic collection and analysis of an organization's quality indicators for the purpose of improving patient care

Activities:

Identify patient care problems or opportunities to improve care

Participate in development of quality indicators

Incorporate standards from appropriate professional groups

Use preestablished criteria when collecting data

Interview patients, families, and staff, as appropriate

Review patient care record for documentation of care, as needed

Conduct data analysis, as appropriate

Compare results of data collected with preestablished norms

Consult with nursing staff or other health professionals to develop action plans, as appropriate

Recommend changes in practice, based on findings

Report findings at staff meetings

Review and revise standards, as appropriate

Participate on quality improvement committees, as appropriate

Provide orientation about quality improvement for new employees at the unit level

Participate on intra- and interdisciplinary problem-solving teams

Background Readings:

Berwick, D.M. (1989). Continuous improvement as an ideal in health care. New England Journal of Medicine, 320(1), 53-56.

Crisler, K.S., & Richard, A.A. (2001). Using case mix and adverse event for outcome-based quality monitoring. Home Healthcare Nurse, 19(10), 613-621.

Fralic, M.F., Kowalski, P.M., & Llewellyn, F.A. (1991). The staff nurse as quality monitor. American Journal of Nursing, 91(4), 40-42.

Karon, S.L., & Zimmerman, D.R. (1998). Nursing home quality indicators and quality improvement initiatives. Topics in Health Information Management, 18(4), 46-58.

Kerfoot, K.M., & Watson, C.A. (1985). Research-based quality assurance: The key to excellence in nursing. In J.M. McCloskey & H.K. Grace (Eds.), Current issues in nursing (pp. 539-547). Boston: Blackwell Scientific.

Q

Radiation Therapy Management   6600

Definition: Assisting the patient to understand and minimize the side effects of radiation treatments

Activities:

Initiate and maintain radiation protection, according to agency protocol, for patient receiving internal radiation treatment (e.g., gold seed placement or radiopharmaceutical agents)

Explain radiation protection protocols to patient, family, and visitors

Offer diversional activities while patient is in radiation protection

Limit visitor time in the room, as appropriate

Limit staff time in the room, if patient is isolated for radiation precautions

Distance oneself from the radiation sources while giving care (e.g., stand at the head of the bed of patients with uterine implants), as appropriate

Shield oneself using a lead apron/shield while assisting with procedures involving radiation

Monitor for alterations in skin integrity and treat appropriately

Avoid use of adhesive tapes and other skin-irritating substances

Provide special skin care to tissue folds, which are prone to infection (e.g., buttocks, perineum, and groin)

Avoid application of deodorants and aftershave lotion to treated area

Discuss the need for skin care, such as maintenance of dye markings, avoidance of soap and other ointments, and protection during sunbathing or heat application

Reassure patient that hair will grow back after radiation treatment is terminated, as appropriate

Assist patient in planning for hair loss, as appropriate, by teaching about available alternatives, such as wigs, scarves, hats, and turbans.

Teach patient to gently wash and comb hair and to sleep on a silk pillowcase to prevent further hair loss, as appropriate

Monitor for indications of infection of oral mucous membranes

Encourage good oral hygiene with use of dental floss and Water Pik, as appropriate

Initiate oral health restoration activities, such as use of artificial saliva, mouth sprays, and use of sugarless mints, as appropriate

Monitor patient for anorexia, nausea, vomiting, changes in taste, esophagitis, and diarrhea, as appropriate

Promote adequate fluid and nutritional intake

Promote therapeutic diet, such as low fiber, to prevent diarrhea

Administer antiemetics, as needed, to control incidence of nausea and vomiting

Assist patient in managing fatigue by planning frequent rest periods, spacing activities, and limiting daily demands, as appropriate

Encourage rest immediately after radiation treatment

Assist patient in receiving pain management techniques that are effective and acceptable to patient

Force fluids to maintain renal and bladder hydration, as appropriate

Monitor for indications of urinary tract infection

Monitor for signs and symptoms of systemic infection, anemia, and bleeding

Facilitate patient's discussion of feelings about radiation therapy equipment, as appropriate

Facilitate expression of fears about prognosis or success of radiation treatments

R

Continued

Background Readings:

Hilderley, L.J. (1990). Radiotherapy. In S.L. Groenwald, M.H. Frogge, M. Goodman, & C.H. Yarbro (Eds.), Cancer nursing: Principles and practice. Boston: Jones & Bartlett.

Hogan, C.M. (1990). Advances in the management of nausea and vomiting. Nursing Clinics of North America, 25(2), 475-497.

Strohl, R.A. (1990). Radiation therapy: Recent advances and nursing implications. Nursing Clinics of North America, 25(2), 309-330.

Thompson, J.M., McFarland, G.K., Hirsch, J.E., & Tucker, S.M. (1998). Mosby's clinical nursing (4th ed.). St. Louis: Mosby.

R

Rape-Trauma Treatment   6300

Definition: Provision of emotional and physical support immediately following a reported rape

Activities:

Provide support person to stay with patient

Explain legal proceedings available to patient

Explain rape protocol and obtain consent to proceed through protocol

Document whether patient has showered, douched, or bathed since incident

Document mental state, physical state (clothing, dirt, and debris), history of incident, evidence of violence, and prior gynecological history

Determine presence of cuts, bruises, bleeding, lacerations, or other signs of physical injury

Implement rape protocol (e.g., label and save soiled clothing, vaginal secretions, and vaginal hair combings)

Secure samples for legal evidence

Implement crisis intervention counseling

Offer medication to prevent pregnancy, as appropriate

Offer prophylactic antibiotic medication against venereal disease

Inform patient of HIV testing, as appropriate

Give clear, written instructions about medication use, crisis support services, and legal support

Refer patient to rape advocacy program

Document according to agency policy

Background Readings:

Burgess, A.W., Fehder, W.P., & Hartman, C.R. (1995). Delayed reporting of the rape victim. Journal of Psychosocial Nursing and Mental Health Services, 33(9), 21-29.

Haber, J., McMahon, A.L., Price-Hoskins, P., & Sideleau, B.F. (1992). Comprehensive psychiatric nursing (4th ed.). St. Louis: Mosby.

Haddix-Hill, K. (1997). The violence of rape. Critical Care Nursing Clinics of North America, 9(2), 167-174.

Luckmann, J., & Sorensen, K.C. (1987). Medical-surgical nursing (3rd ed.). Philadelphia: W.B. Saunders.

May, K.A., & Mahlmeister, L.R. (1994). Maternal and neonatal nursing: Family-centered care (3rd ed.). Philadelphia: Lippincott.

R

Reality Orientation 4820

Definition: Promotion of patient's awareness of personal identity, time, and environment

Activities:

Use an approach that is consistent (e.g., kind firmness, active friendliness, passive friendliness, matter-of-fact, and no demands) when interacting with the patient and that reflects the particular needs and capabilities of that patient

Inform patient of person, place, and time, as needed

Avoid frustrating patient by quizzing with orientation questions that cannot be answered

Label items in environment to promote recognition

Provide a consistent physical environment and daily routine

Provide access to familiar objects, when possible

Dress patient in personal clothing

Avoid unfamiliar situations, when possible

Prepare patient for upcoming changes in usual routine and environment before their occurrence

Provide caregivers who are familiar to the patient

Use environmental cues (e.g., signs, pictures, clocks, calendars, and color coding of environment) to stimulate memory, reorient, and promote appropriate behavior

Provide objects that symbolize gender identity (e.g., purse or cap)

Encourage use of aids that increase sensory input (e.g., eyeglasses, hearing aids, and dentures)

Remove stimuli, when possible, that create misperception in a particular patient (e.g., pictures on the wall and television)

Provide a low-stimulation environment for patient in whom disorientation is increased by overstimulation

Provide for adequate rest/sleep/daytime naps

Limit visitors and length of visits if patient experiences overstimulation and increased disorientation from them

Provide access to current news events (e.g., television, newspapers, radio, and verbal reports), when appropriate

Approach patient slowly and from the front

Address the patient by name when initiating interaction

Use a calm and unhurried approach when interacting with the patient

Speak to patient in a slow, distinct manner with appropriate volume

Repeat verbalizations, as necessary

Use gestures/objects to increase comprehension of verbal communications

Stimulate memory by repeating patient's last expressed thought

Ask questions one at a time

Interrupt confabulation by changing the subject or responding to the feeling or theme, rather than the content of the verbalization

Avoid demands for abstract thinking, if patient can think only in concrete terms

Limit need for decision making if frustrating/confusing to patient

Give one simple direction at a time

Use picture cues to promote appropriate use of items

Provide physical prompting/posturing (e.g., moving patient's hand through necessary motions to brush teeth), as necessary for task completion

Engage patient in concrete "here and now" activities (i.e., ADLs) that focus on something outside self that is concrete and reality oriented

Involve patient in a reality orientation group setting/class, when appropriate and available

Monitor for changes in sensation and orientation

Background Readings:

Holden, U.P., & Woods, R.T. (1988). Reality orientation: Psychological approaches to the confused elderly (2nd ed.). New York: Churchill Livingstone.

Kanak, M.F. (1992). Interventions related to safety. In G.M. Bulechek & J.C. McCloskey (Eds.), Symposium on Nursing Interventions. Nursing Clinics of North America, 27(2), 371-396.

Kohout, S., Kohout, J.J., & Fleishman J.J. (1987). Reality orientation for the elderly (3rd ed.). Oradell, NJ: Medical Economics.

Parker, C., & Somers, C. (1983). Reality orientation on a geropsychiatric unit. Geriatric Nursing, 4(3), 163-165.

Spector, A., Orrell, M., Davies S., & Woods, B. (2001). Cochrane reviews. Reality orientation for dementia. Nursing Times, 97(48), 37.

R

Recreation Therapy

Definition: Purposeful use of recreation to promote relaxation and enhancement of social skills

Activities:

Assist patient/family to identify deficits in mobility

Assist to explore the personal meaning of favorite recreational activities

Monitor physical and mental capacities to participate in recreational activities

Include patient in the planning of recreational activities

Assist patient to choose recreational activities consistent with physical, psychological, and social capabilities

Assist in obtaining resources required for the recreational activity

Assist patient to identify meaningful recreational activities

Describe benefits of stimulation for a variety of sensory modalities

Provide safe recreational equipment

Observe safety precautions

Supervise recreational sessions, as appropriate

Provide new recreational activities that are age and ability appropriate, such as brewing root beer, making taffy, or visiting a horse farm

Provide recreational activities aimed at reducing anxiety (e.g., cards or puzzles)

Assist in obtaining transportation to recreational activities

Provide positive reinforcement for participation in activities

Monitor emotional, physical, and social responses to recreational activity

Background Readings:

Carlo, S., & Deichman, E.S. (1990). Enlarging the circles of interest. Nursing Homes, 39(1), 16-17.

Donaghy, P. (1991). Recreation in a nursing home: A nursing success. Australian Nurses Journal, 21(4), 14-16.

Hutchinson, S.A. (1990). The PALS program: Intergenerational remotivation. Journal of Gerontological Nursing, 16(12), 18-26, 40-42.

Lyall, J. (1993). Beyond bingo . . . activity is central to the well-being of elderly people in residential homes. Nursing Times, 89(36), 16-17.

R

Rectal Prolapse Management 0490

Definition: Prevention and/or manual reduction of rectal prolapse

Activities:

Identify patients with history of rectal prolapse

Encourage avoidance of straining at stool, lifting, and excessive standing

Instruct patient to regulate bowel function through diet, exercise, and medication, as appropriate

Assist patient to identify specific activities that have triggered rectal prolapse episodes in the past

Monitor for bowel incontinence

Monitor status of rectal prolapse

Position patient on left side with knees raised toward chest, when rectum is prolapsed

Place a water- or saline-soaked cloth over the protruding bowel to protect it from drying

Encourage patient to remain in side-lying position to facilitate return of bowel into rectum naturally

Manually reduce rectal prolapse with lubricated, gloved hand, gently applying pressure to prolapse until it returns to a normal position, as necessary

Check rectal area 10 minutes after manual reduction to ensure that prolapse is in correct position

Identify frequency of occurrence of rectal prolapse

Notify physician of change in frequency of occurrence or inability to manually reduce prolapse, as appropriate

Assist in preoperative workup, as appropriate, helping to explain the tests and reduce anxiety for the patient who will undergo surgical repair

Background Readings:

Abrams, W.B., & Berkow, R. (1990). The Merck manual of geriatrics. Rahway, NJ: Merck, Sharp & Dohme Research Laboratories.

Gillies, D.A. (1985). Nursing care for aged patients with rectal prolapse. Journal of Gerontological Nursing, 11(2), 29-33.

R

Referral   8100

Definition: Arrangement for services by another care provider or agency

Activities:

Perform ongoing monitoring to determine the need for referral

Identify preference of patient/family/significant others for referral agency

Identify health care providers' recommendation for referral, as needed

Identify nursing/health care required

Determine whether appropriate supportive care is available in the home/community

Determine whether rehabilitation services are available for use in the home

Evaluate strengths and weaknesses of family/significant others for responsibility of care

Evaluate accessibility of environmental needs for the patient in the home/community

Determine appropriate equipment for use after discharge, as necessary

Determine patient's financial resources for payment to another provider

Arrange for appropriate home care services, as needed

Encourage an assessment visit by receiving agency or other care provider, as appropriate

Contact appropriate agency/health care provider

Complete appropriate written referral

Arrange mode of transportation

Discuss patient's plan of care with next health care provider

Background Readings:

Bowles, K.H., Naylor, M.D., & Foust, J.B. (2002). Patient characteristics at hospital discharge and a comparison of home care referral decisions. Journal of the American Geriatrics Society, 50 (2), 336-342.

McClelland, E., Kelly, K., & Buckwalter, K.C. (1985). Continuity of care: Advancing the concept of discharge planning. New York: Harcourt Brace Jovanovich.

McKeehan, K.M. (1981). Continuing care. St. Louis: Mosby.

R

Religious Addiction Prevention   5422

Definition: Prevention of a self-imposed controlling religious lifestyle

Activities:

Identify individuals at risk for an excessive dependence upon religion, religious leaders, and/or religious practice

Examine religious practices in terms of balanced relationships and beliefs

Explore and encourage behaviors that contribute to growth and faith development

Explore with individuals the elements of religious addiction and freedom for religious formation

Explain how shame-based people are vulnerable to religious and ritual addiction

Examine gratitude and forgiveness as ways of defending one's self from forming religious or other addictive processes

Offer to pray for healthy, life-giving relationships with self, God/Higher Power, and others, as appropriate

Educate individuals about the process of faith development

Educate individuals about the dangers of using religion to control other persons

Promote the formation of self-help groups or support groups to explore religious balance

Identify and share resources of groups and professional counseling services within the community

Background Readings:

Booth, L. (1991). When God becomes a drug: Breaking the chains of religious addiction and abuse. Los Angeles: Jeremy P Tarcher, Inc.

Linn, M., Linn, S. F., & Linn, D. (1994). Healing spiritual abuse and religious addiction. New York: Paulist Press.

R

Religious Ritual Enhancement 5424

Definition: Facilitating participation in religious practices

Activities:

Identify patient's concerns regarding religious expression (e.g., lighting candles, fasting, circumcision ceremonies, or food practices)

Coordinate or provide healing services, communion, meditation, or prayer in place of residence or other setting

Encourage the use of and participation in usual religious rituals or practices that are not detrimental to health

Provide video or audio tapes from religious services, as available

Treat individual with dignity and respect

Provide opportunities for discussion of various belief systems and world views

Coordinate or provide transportation to worship site

Encourage ritual planning and participation, as appropriate

Encourage ritual attendance, as appropriate

Explore alternative for worship

Encourage discussion about religious concerns

Listen and develop a sense of timing for prayer or ritual

Refer patient to religious advisor of his/her choice

Assist with modifications of the ritual to meet the needs of the disabled or ill

Background Readings:

Beck, R., & Metrick, S. (1990). The art of ritual. Berkley, CA: Celestial Arts.

LeMone, P. (2001). Spiritual distress. In M.L. Maas, K.C. Buckwater, M.D. Hardy, T. Tripp-Reimer, M.G. Titler, & J.P. Specht (Eds.), Nursing care of older adults: Diagnoses, outcomes and interventions (Chapter 62). St. Louis: Mosby.

Ramshaw, E. (1987). Ritual and pastoral care. Philadelphia: Fortress Press.

Walton, D. (1995). Adapting faith rituals. Messenger, Church of the Brethren (October), p. 14.

R

Relocation Stress Reduction   5350

Definition: Assisting the individual to prepare for and cope with movement from one environment to another

Activities:

Explore if the individual has had any previous relocations

Include the individual in relocation plans, as appropriate

Explore what is most important in the individual's life (e.g., family, friends, personal belongings)

Encourage individual and family to discuss concerns regarding relocation

Explore with the individual previous coping strategies

Encourage the use of coping strategies

Appraise individual's need/desire for social support

Evaluate available support systems (e.g., extended family, community involvement, religious affiliations)

Assign a "buddy" to the individual to help acquaint him/her with the new environment

Encourage individual and/or family to seek counseling, as appropriate

Make arrangements for individual's personal items to be in place prior to relocation

Monitor for physiological and psychological signs and symptoms of relocation stress (e.g., anorexia, anxiety, depression, increased demands, and hopelessness)

Provide diversional activities (e.g., involvement in hobbies, usual activities)

Assist the individual to grieve and work through the losses of home, friends, independence

Evaluate the impact of disruption of lifestyle, loss of home, and adaptation to new a environment

Background Readings:

Castle, N. G. (2001). Relocation of the elderly. Medical Care Research and Review, 58(3), 291-333.

Jackson, B., Swanson, C., Hicks, L.E., Prokop, L., Laughlin, J. (2000). Bridge of continuity from hospital to nursing home Part II: Reducing relocation stress syndrome and interdisciplinary guide. Continuum, January-February, 9-14.

Morse, D.L. (2000). Relocation stress syndrome is real. American Journal of Nursing 100(8), 24AAAA-24DDDD.

Puskar, K.R., & Rohay, J.M. (1999). School relocation and stress in teens. Journal of School Nursing, 15(1), 16-21.

Reed, J., & Morgan, D. (1999). Discharging older people from hospital to care home: Implications for nursing. Journal of Advanced Nursing, 29(4), 819-825.

R

Reminiscence Therapy 4860

Definition: Using the recall of past events, feelings, and thoughts to facilitate pleasure, quality of life, or adaptation to present circumstances

Activities:

Choose a comfortable setting

Set aside adequate time

Identify with the patient, a theme for each session (e.g., work life)

Select an appropriately small number of participants for group reminiscence therapy

Utilize effective listening and attending skills

Determine which method of reminiscence (e.g., taped autobiography, journal, structured life review, scrapbook, open discussion and storytelling) is most effective

Introduce props that address all five senses (e.g., music for auditory, photo albums for visual, perfume for olfactory) to stimulate recall

Encourage verbal expression of both positive and negative feelings about past events

Observe body language, facial expression, and tone of voice to identify the importance of recollections to the patient

Ask open-ended questions about past events

Encourage writing about past events

Maintain focus of sessions, more on process than on an end product

Provide support, encouragement, and empathy for participant(s)

Use culturally sensitive props, themes, and techniques

Assist the person to address painful, angry, or other negative memories

Use the patient's photo albums or scrapbooks to stimulate memories

Assist the patient in creating or adding to a family tree or in recording his/her oral history

Encourage the patient to write to old friends or relatives

Use communication skills such as focusing, reflecting, and restating to develop the relationship

Comment on the affective quality accompanying the memories in an empathetic manner

Use direct questions to refocus on life events, as necessary

Inform family members about the benefits of reminiscence

Gauge the length of the session by the patient's attention span

Give immediate positive feedback to cognitively impaired patients

Acknowledge previous coping skills

Repeat sessions weekly or more often over prolonged period

Gauge the number of sessions by the patient's response and willingness to continue

Background Readings:

Brady, E.M. (1999). Stories at the hour of our death. Home Healthcare Nurse, 17(3), 176-180.

Burnside, I. (1994). Reminiscence and life review: Therapeutic interventions for older people. Nurse Practitioner, 19(4), 55-61.

Coleman, P.G. (1999). Creating a life story: The task of reconciliation. The Gerontologist, 39(2), 133-139.

Burnside, I., & Haight, B. (1992). Reminiscence and life review: Analyzing each concept. Journal of Advanced Nursing, 17, 855-862.

Haight, B.K. (2001). Life reviews: Helping Alzheimer's patients reclaim a fading past. Reflections on Nursing Leadership, 27(1), 20-22.

Hamilton, D. (1992). Reminiscence therapy. In G. Bulechek & J. McCloskey (Eds.), Nursing interventions: Treatments for nursing diagnoses (pp. 292-303). Philadelphia: W.B. Saunders.

Harrand, A.G., & Bollstetter, J.J. (2000). Developing a community-based reminiscence group for the elderly. Clinical Nurse Specialist, 14(1), 17-22.

Puentes, W.J. (2000). Using social reminiscence to teach therapeutic communication skills. Geriatric Nursing, 21(6), 315-318.

Johnson, R.A. (1999). Reminiscence therapy. In G.M. Bulechek & J. C. McCloskey (Eds.), Nursing interventions: Effective nursing treatments (3rd ed.) (pp. 371-384). Philadelphia: W.B. Saunders.

R

Reproductive Technology Management 7886

Definition: Assisting a patient through the steps of complex infertility treatment

Activities:

Provide education about various treatment modalities (e.g., intrauterine insemination, in vitro fertilization-embryo transfer (IVF-ET), gamete intrafallopian transfer (GIFT), zygote intrafallopian transfer (ZIFT), donor sperm, donor oocytes, gestational carrier, and surrogacy)

Discuss ethical dilemmas before initiating a particular treatment modality

Explore feelings about assisted reproductive technology (e.g., known vs. anonymous oocyte or sperm donors, cryopreserved embryos, selective reduction, and use of a host uterus)

Refer for preconception counseling, as needed

Teach ovulation prediction and detection techniques (e.g., basal temperature and urine testing)

Teach administration of ovulatory stimulants

Schedule tests, as needed, based on the menstrual cycle

Coordinate activities of the multidisciplinary team for treatment process

Assist out-of-town individuals in locating housing while participating in the program

Provide education to gamete donors and their partners

Collaborate with IVF team in screening and selecting gamete donors

Explore psychosocial issues involving gamete donation before administering medications for comfort

Coordinate synchronization of donor and recipient hormonal cycles

Obtain specimens for endocrine determination

Perform ultrasound exams to ascertain follicular growth

Participate in team conferences to correlate test results for evaluating oocyte maturity

Set up equipment for oocyte retrieval

Assist with freezing and preservation of embryos, as indicated

Assist with fertilization procedures

Prepare patient for embryo transfer

Provide anticipatory guidance about typical emotional reactions, including extremes of anguish and joy

Discuss risks, including the likelihood of miscarriage, ectopic pregnancy, and ovarian hyperstimulation

Teach ectopic pregnancy precautions

Teach symptoms of ovarian hyperstimulation to report

Perform pregnancy tests

Provide support for grieving when implantation fails to occur

Schedule follow-up medication, tests, and ultrasound exams

Assist with hormonal and ultrasound monitoring of early pregnancy

Refer for genetic counseling, as needed, related to maternal age at conception

Refer to infertility support groups, as needed

Follow up with patients who have stopped treatment because of pregnancy, adoption, or the decision to remain childfree

Assist patients to focus on life areas of success unrelated to fertility status

Educate in methods of securing workplace support for necessary absences during treatment

R

Provide counseling about financial and insurance issues

Participate in reporting data about treatment outcomes to national registry

Background Readings:

Berger, G.S., Goldstein, M., & Fuerst, M. (1989). The couple's guide to fertility: How new medical advances can help you have a baby. New York: Doubleday.

Bobak, I.M., & Jensen, M. (1993). Maternity & gynecologic care: The nurse and the family (5th ed.). St. Louis: Mosby.

Dunnington, R.M., & Estok, P.J. (1991). Potential psychological attachments formed by donors involved in fertility technology: Another side to infertility. Nurse Practitioner, 16(11), 41-48.

Field, P.A., & Marck, P. (1994). Uncertain motherhood: Negotiating the risks of the childbearing years. Newbury Park, CA: Sage.

Gardner, C. (Ed.). (1991). Principles of infertility nursing. Boca Raton, FL: CRC Press.

Hahn, S.J., Butkowski, C.R., & Capper, L.L. (1994). Ovarian hyperstimulation syndrome: Protocols for nursing care Journal of Gynecologic, Obstetric, and Neonatal Nursing, 23(3), 217-226.

James, C. (1992). The nursing role in assisted reproductive technologies. NAACOG's Clinical Issues in Perinatal and Women's Health Nursing, 3(2), 328-334.

Jones, S.L. (1994). Genetic-based and assisted reproductive technology of the 21st century. Journal of Obstetric, Gynecologic, and Neonatal Nursing, 23(2), 160-165.

Olshansky, E.F. (1992). Redefining the concepts of success and failure. NAACOG's Clinical Issues in Perinatal and Women's Health Nursing, 3(2), 343-346.

R

Research Data Collection 8120

Definition: Collecting research data

Activities:

Adhere to Institutional Review Board (IRB) procedures of data collection site

Inform investigator of facility rules for conducting research, as needed

Facilitate completion of consent form, as appropriate

Explain purpose of research during data collection, as appropriate

Inform patient of the obligations of being a part of the study (e.g., surveys, laboratory tests, medications)

Implement study protocol as specified and agreed upon

Monitor patient's response to research protocol

Collect data agreed upon for use in the study

Provide private space for conducting interviews and/or data collection, as needed

Assist patients to complete study questionnaires or other data collection tool, as requested

Perform activities per routine while under study observation

Discuss with investigator any patient or agency rewards for participation

Obtain summary of study results for participating staff and interested study subjects

Communicate regularly with researcher about progress of data collection, as appropriate

Record data findings clearly on provided forms

Monitor amount of participation in research studies requested of patients and staff

Background Readings:

American Nurses Association. (1985). Human rights guidelines for nurses in clinical and other research. Kansas City, MO: American Nurses Association.

Bliesmer, M., & Earle, P. (1993). Research considerations: Nursing home quality perceptions. Journal of Gerontological Nursing, 19(6), 27-34.

Burns, N., & Grove, S.K. (1997). The practice of nursing research (3rd ed.). Philadelphia: Saunders.

R

Resiliency Promotion   8340

Definition: Assisting individuals, families, and communities in development, use, and strengthening of protective factors to be used in coping with environmental and societal stressors

Activities:

Facilitate family cohesion

Encourage family support

Encourage the development of and adherence to family routines and traditions (e.g., birthdays, holidays)

Assist youth in viewing family as a resource for advice and support

Facilitate family communication

Encourage family to eat meals together on a regular basis

Link youth to interested adults in community

Provide family/community models for conventional behavior

Motivate youth to pursue academic achievement and goals

Encourage family involvement with child's school work and activities

Assist family in providing atmosphere conducive to learning

Encourage family/community to value achievement

Encourage family/community to value health

Encourage positive health seeking behaviors

Assist parents in determining age-appropriate expectations for their child

Encourage family to establish rules and consequences for child/youth behavior

Assist parents in establishing norms for parental monitoring of friends and activities

Assist youth in acquiring assertiveness skills

Assist youth in role playing decision-making skills

Assist youth in developing friendship skills

Encourage family and youth attendance at religious services and/or activities

Encourage youth involvement in school activities and/or voluntary clubs

Provide opportunities for youth involvement in community volunteer activities

Assist youth in developing social and global awareness

Promote quality, caring schools in community

Arrange to keep schools/gyms/libraries open after hours for activities

Inform and involve community in youth programs

Facilitate development and use of neighborhood resources

Assist youth/families/communities in developing optimism for the future

Background Readings:

Benson, P. (1993). The troubled journey: A portrait of 6th-12th grade youth. Minneapolis, MN: Search Institute.

Castiglia, P.T. (1993). Gangs. Journal of Pediatric Health Care, 7(1), 39-41.

Jessor, R. (1991). Risk behavior in adolescence: A psychosocial framework for understanding and action. Journal of Adolescent Health, 12(8), 597-605.

Keltner, B., Keltner, N.L., & Farren, E. (1990). Family routines and conduct disorders in adolescent girls. Western Journal of Nursing Research, 12(2), 161-1741.

McCubbin, M., & Van Riper, M. (1996). Factors influencing family functioning and the health of family members. In S.M.H. Hanson & S.T. Boyd (Eds.), Family health care nursing: Theory, practice, and research. (pp. 101-121). Philadelphia: F.A. Davis.

Respiratory Monitoring

3350

Definition: Collection and analysis of patient data to ensure airway patency and adequate gas exchange

Activities:

Monitor rate, rhythm, depth, and effort of respirations

Note chest movement, watching for symmetry, use of accessory muscles, and supraclavicular and intercostal muscle retractions

Monitor for noisy respirations, such as crowing or snoring

Monitor breathing patterns: bradypnea, tachypnea, hyperventilation, Kussmaul respirations, Cheyne-Stokes respirations, apneustic breathing, Biot's respiration, and ataxic patterns

Palpate for equal lung expansion

Percuss anterior and posterior thorax from apices to bases bilaterally

Note location of trachea

Monitor for diaphragmatic muscle fatigue (paradoxical motion)

Auscultate breath sounds, noting areas of decreased/absent ventilation and presence of adventitious sounds

Determine the need for suctioning by auscultating for crackles and rhonchi over major airways

Auscultate lung sounds after treatments to note results

Monitor PFT values, particularly vital capacity, maximal inspiratory force, forced expiratory volume in 1 second (FEV_1), and FEV_1/FVC, as available

Monitor mechanical ventilator readings, noting increases in inspiratory pressures and decreases in tidal volume, as appropriate

Monitor for increased restlessness, anxiety, and air hunger

Note changes in SaO_2, SvO_2, end-tidal CO_2, and ABG values, as appropriate

Monitor patient's ability to cough effectively

Note onset, characteristics, and duration of cough

Monitor patient's respiratory secretions

Monitor for dyspnea and events that decrease and worsen it

Monitor for hoarseness and voice changes every hour in patients with facial burns

Monitor for crepitus, as appropriate

Monitor chest x-ray reports

Open the airway, using the chin lift or jaw thrust technique, as appropriate

Place the patient on side, as indicated, to prevent aspiration; log roll if cervical aspiration is suspected

Institute resuscitation efforts, as needed

Institute respiratory therapy treatments (e.g., nebulizer), as needed

Background Readings:

Capps, J.S., & Schade, K. (1988). Work of breathing: Clinical monitoring and considerations in the critical care setting. Critical Care Nursing Quarterly, 11(3), 1-11.

Carrol, P. (1999). Evolutions/revolutions: Respiratory monitoring: Revolutions: continuous spirometry. RN, 62(5), 72-74, 77-78.

Carroll, P. (1999). Evolutions/revolutions respiratory monitoring: Evolutions: capnography. RN, 62(5), 68-71, 78.

Lane, G.H. (1990). Pulmonary therapeutic management. In L.A. Thelan, J.K. Davie, & L.D. Urden (Eds.), Textbook of critical care nursing (pp. 444-471). St. Louis: Mosby.

Nelson, D.M. (1992). Interventions related to respiratory care. In G.M. Bulechek & J.C. McCloskey (Eds.), Symposium on Nursing Interventions. Nursing Clinics of North America, 27(2), 301-324.

Respite Care   7260

Definition: Provision of short-term care to provide relief for family caregiver

Activities:

Establish a therapeutic relationship with patient/family

Monitor endurance of caregiver

Inform patient/family of available state funding for respite care

Coordinate volunteers for in-home services, as appropriate

Arrange for substitute caregiver

Follow usual routine of care

Provide care, such as exercises, ambulation, and hygiene, as appropriate

Obtain emergency telephone numbers

Determine how to contact usual caregiver

Provide emergency care, as necessary

Maintain normal home environment

Provide a report to usual caregiver on return

Background Readings:

Cowen, P.S., & Reed, D.A. (2002). Effects of respite care for children with developmental disabilities: Evaluation of an intervention for at risk families. Public Health Nursing, 19(4), 273-283.

McClelland, F., Kelly, K., & Buckwalter, K.C. (1985). Continuity of care: Advancing the concept of discharge planning. New York: Harcourt Brace Jovanovich.

McKeehan, K.M. (1981). Continuing care. St. Louis: Mosby.

Newfield, S.M., Query, B., & Drummond, J.E. (2001). Respite care users who have children with chronic conditions: Are they getting a break? Journal of Pediatric Nursing, 16(4), 234-244.

Pearson, M.A., & Theis, S.L. (1991). Program evaluation application of a comprehensive model for a community-based respite program. Journal of Community Health Nursing, 8(1), 25-31.

Perry, J., & Bontinen, K. (2001). Evaluation of a weekend respite program for persons with Alzheimer disease. Canadian Journal of Nursing Research, 33(1), 81-95.

R

Resuscitation 6320

Definition: Administering emergency measures to sustain life

Activities:

Monitor level of awareness/sensory/motor function

Use either the head tilt or jaw thrust maneuver to maintain an airway

Clear oral, nasal, and tracheal secretions, as appropriate

Administer manual ventilation, as appropriate

Perform cardiopulmonary resuscitation, as appropriate

Assist with open chest massage, as appropriate

Call "code" and obtain necessary help, as appropriate

Call for physician assistance, as needed

Connect the person to an ECG monitor

Initiate an IV line and administer IV fluids, as indicated

Provide standby equipment (and/or drugs)

Apply cardiac/apnea monitor

Check that electronic equipment is working properly

Obtain electrocardiogram

Evaluate changes in chest pain

Assist with insertion of endotracheal (ET) tube

Assess lung sounds after intubation for proper ET tube position

Assist with performing chest x-ray examination after intubation

Call for ICU bed and ventilator, as appropriate

Arrange safe transport

Background Readings:

American Heart Association (1987). Textbook of advanced cardiac life support. Dallas, TX: The Association.

Davis, A. (1987). The boundaries of intervention: Issues in the noninfliction of harm. In M. Fowler & J. Levine-Ariff (Eds.), Ethics at the bedside (pp. 50-78). Philadelphia: J.B. Lippincott.

Nelson, D.M. (1992). Interventions related to respiratory care. In G.M. Bulechek & J.C. McCloskey (Eds.), Symposium on Nursing Interventions. Nursing Clinics of North America, 27(2), 301-324.

Marco, C.A. (2001), Resuscitation research: Future directions and ethical issues. Academic Emergency Medicine, 8(8), 839-843.

R

Resuscitation: Fetus   6972

Definition: Administering emergency measures to improve placental perfusion or correct fetal acid-base status

Activities:

Monitor fetal vital signs, using auscultation and palpation or electronic fetal monitor, as appropriate

Observe for abnormal (e.g., nonreassuring) fetal heart rate signs, such as bradycardia, tachycardia, nonreactivity, variable decelerations, late decelerations, prolonged decelerations, decreased long term and/or short-term variability, and sinusoidal pattern

Include mother and support person in explanation of measures needed to enhance fetal oxygenation

Use universal precautions

Reposition mother to lateral or hands-and-knees position

Reevaluate fetal heart rate

Apply oxygen at 6 to 8 L, if positioning is ineffective in correcting abnormal or nonreassuring pattern of fetal heart rate

Initiate IV line, as appropriate

Give a bolus of IV fluid, per physician order or protocol

Monitor maternal vital signs

Perform a vaginal exam with fetal scalp stimulation

Apprise midwife or physician about outcome of resuscitation measures

Document strip interpretation, activities performed, fetal outcome, and maternal response

Apply internal monitors once the amniotic membranes are ruptured to obtain more information about the fetal heart rate response to uterine activity

Reassure and calm mother and support person(s)

Decrease uterine activity by stopping oxytocin infusion, as appropriate

Administer tocolytic medication to reduce contractions, as appropriate

Perform amnioinfusion for abnormal (e.g., nonreassuring) variable decelerations in fetal heart rate or meconium-stained amniotic fluid

Turn to left-lateral position for pushing during second-stage labor to improve placental perfusion

Coach to decrease pushing efforts for abnormal (e.g., nonreassuring) fetal heart signs to allow reestablishment of placental perfusion

Consult with obstetrician to obtain fetal blood sample, as appropriate

Anticipate requirements for mode of delivery and neonatal support, based on fetal responses to resuscitation techniques

Background Readings:

Galvan, B., Van Mullen, C., & Broekhuizen, F. (1989). Using amnioinfusion for the relief of repetitive variable decelerations during labor. Journal of Obstetric, Gynecologic, and Neonatal Nursing, 18(93), 222-229.

Knorr, L.J. (1989). Relieving fetal distress with amnioinfusion. American Journal of Maternal/Child Nursing, 14(5), 346-350.

Murray, M. (1988). Essentials of electronic fetal monitoring. Antepartal and intrapartal fetal monitoring. Washington, DC: NAACOG.

Roberts, J.E. (1989). Managing fetal bradycardia during second stage of labor. American Journal of Maternal/Child Nursing, 14(6), 394-398.

Tucker, S.M. (1992). Pocket guide to fetal monitoring (3rd ed.). St. Louis: Mosby.

R

Resuscitation: Neonate 6974

Definition: Administering emergency measures to support newborn adaptation to extrauterine life

Activities:

Set up equipment for resuscitation before birth

Test resuscitation bag, suction, and oxygen flow to ensure proper function

Place newborn under the radiant warmer

Insert laryngoscope to visualize the trachea to suction for meconium-stained fluid, as appropriate

Intubate with an endotracheal tube to remove meconium from the lower airway, as appropriate

Reintubate and suction until the return is clear of meconium

Use mechanical suction to remove meconium from lower airway

Dry with a prewarmed blanket to remove amniotic fluid, to reduce heat loss, and to provide stimulation

Position the newborn on back, with neck slightly extended to open airway

Place a rolled blanket under the shoulders to assist with correct positioning, as appropriate

Suction secretions from nose and mouth with a bulb syringe

Provide tactile stimulation by rubbing the soles of the feet or rubbing the infant's back

Monitor respirations

Monitor heart rate

Initiate positive-pressure ventilation for apnea or gasping

Use 100% oxygen at 5 to 8 L to fill resuscitation bag

Adjust bag to fill correctly

Obtain a tight seal with a mask that covers the chin, mouth, and nose

Ventilate at a rate of 40 to 60 breaths per minute using 20 to 40 cm of water for initial breaths and 15 to 20 cm of water for subsequent pressures

Auscultate to ensure adequate ventilation

Check heart rate after 15 to 30 seconds of ventilation

Give chest compressions for heart rate of <60 beats per minute or if >80 beats per minute with no increase

Compress sternum 0.5 to 0.75 inches using a 3:1 ratio for delivering 90 compressions and 30 breaths per minute

Check heart rate after 30 seconds of compressions

Continue compressions until heart rate is >80 beats per minute

Continue ventilations until adequate spontaneous respirations begin and color becomes pink

Insert endotracheal tube for prolonged ventilation or poor response to bag and mask ventilation

Auscultate bilateral breath sounds for confirmation of endotracheal tube placement

Observe for rise of chest without gastric distention to check placement

Secure airway to face with tape

Insert an orogastric catheter if ventilation is given for more than 2 minutes

Prepare medications, as needed (e.g., narcotic antagonists, epinephrine, volume expanders, and sodium bicarbonate)

Activities:—cont'd

Administer medications per order

Document time, sequence, and neonatal responses to all steps of resuscitation

Provide explanation to parents, as appropriate

Assist with neonatal transfer or transport, as appropriate

Background Readings:

American Heart Association & American Academy of Pediatrics. (1990). Textbook of neonatal resuscitation. Elk Grove Village, IL: AHA/AAP.

Keenan, W.J., Raye, J.R., & Schell, B. (April 1993). NRP instructor update. Elk Grove Village, IL: AHA/AAP.

R

Risk Identification 6610

Definition: Analysis of potential risk factors, determination of health risks, and prioritization of risk reduction strategies for an individual or group

Activities:

Institute routine risk assessment, using reliable and valid instruments

Review medical history and documents for evidence of existing or previous medical and nursing diagnoses

Maintain accurate records and statistics

Identify patient(s) with continuing care needs

Identify patient(s) with unique social circumstances that complicate a timely and efficient discharge

Determine community support systems

Determine presence and quality of family support

Determine financial resources

Determine educational status

Identify individual's and group's usual coping strategies

Determine past and current level of functioning

Determine presence/absence of basic living needs

Determine compliance with medical and nursing treatments

Prioritize areas for risk reduction, in collaboration with individual/group

Plan for risk reduction activities, in collaboration with individual/group

Identify agency resources to assist in decreasing risk factors

Determine community resources appropriate for basic living and health needs

Initiate referrals to health care personnel and/or agencies, as appropriate

Use mutual goal setting, as appropriate

Use patient contracting, as appropriate

Background Readings:

Goeppinger, J., & Labuhn, K.T. (1991). Self-health care through risk appraisal and reduction. In M. Stanhope & J. Lancaster (Eds.), Community health nursing (3rd ed.) (pp. 578-591). St. Louis: Mosby.

Titler, M.G. (1992). Interventions related to surveillance. In G.M. Bulechek & J.C. McCloskey (Eds.), Symposium on Nursing Interventions. Nursing Clinics of North America, 27(2), 495-515.

R

Risk Identification: Childbearing Family   6612

Definition: Identification of an individual or family likely to experience difficulties in parenting and prioritization of strategies to prevent parenting problems

Activities:

Determine age of mother

Determine developmental stage of parent

Determine parity of mother

Determine economic status of family

Determine educational status of mother

Determine marital status of mother

Determine literacy

Determine whether previous children born to mother are still in her care

Ascertain understanding of English or other language used in community

Determine prior involvement with social services

Determine prior history of abuse

Determine health and immunization status of siblings

Monitor behaviors that may indicate a problem with attachment

Review prenatal and intrapartal records for documented signs of prenatal attachment

Review prenatal history for factors that predispose patient to complications

Note medications that mother received during prenatal period

Review prenatal history for possible stressors affecting neonatal glucose stores (e.g., diabetes, pregnancy-induced hypertension, and cardiac or renal disorders)

Review history for abnormal prenatal growth patterns, as detected by ultrasonography or fundal changes

Review maternal history of chemical dependency, noting duration, type of drug(s) used (including alcohol), and time and strength of last dose before delivery

Determine the patient's feelings about an unplanned pregnancy

Determine whether the unplanned pregnancy is approved of by the family

Determine whether unplanned pregnancy is supported by the family

Note medications mother received during intrapartal period

Note any anesthetic or analgesic administered to mother during intrapartal period

Note presence of fetal distress

Note presence of hypoxia in infant

Review history for presence of abnormal amount of amniotic fluid, as detected by ultrasonography or fundal changes

Identify reason for separation from newborn after birth

Monitor parent-infant interactions, noting behaviors thought to indicate attachment

Refer to the appropriate community agency for follow-up, if a lag in attachment is identified

Prioritize areas for risk reduction, in collaboration with the individual or family

Plan for risk reduction activities, in collaboration with the individual or family

Continued

Background Readings:

Denehy, J.A. (1992). Interventions related to parent-infant attachment. In G.M. Bulechek & J.C. McCloskey (Eds.), Symposium on Nursing Interventions. Nursing Clinics of North America, 27(2), 425-444.

Pressler, J.L. (1990). Promoting attachment. In M.J. Craft & J.A. Denehy (Eds.), Nursing interventions for infants and children (pp. 4-17). Philadelphia: W.B. Saunders.

R

Risk Identification: Genetic   6614

Definition: Identification and analysis of potential genetic risk factors in an individual, family, or group

Activities:

Ensure privacy and confidentiality

Obtain or review a complete health history, including prenatal and obstetrical history, developmental history, and past and present health status related to the confirmed or suspected genetic condition

Obtain or review environment (e.g., potential teratogen and carcinogen exposures) and lifestyle (e.g., tobacco, alcohol, street or prescription drug exposure) history

Determine presence and quality of family support, other support systems, and previous coping skills

Obtain or review a comprehensive family history and construct at least a three-generation pedigree

Obtain documented diagnosis of affected family members

Review options for diagnostic testing that may confirm or predict the presence of a genetic disorder, such as biochemical or radiographic studies, chromosome analysis, linkage analyses, or direct DNA testing

Provide information about the diagnostic procedures

Discuss advantages, risks, and financial costs of diagnostic options

Discuss insurance and possible job discrimination issues, as relevant

Discuss issues in testing other family members, as relevant

Initiate genetic counseling intervention based upon risk identification, as appropriate

Refer to genetic health care specialists for genetic counseling as needed

Provide patient a written summary of the risk identification counseling, as indicated

Background Readings:

Andrews, L.B., Fullerton, J.E., Holtzman, N.A., & Motulsky, A.G. (1994). Assessing genetic risks: Implications for health and social policy. Institute of Medicine, Washington, DC: National Academy Press.

Cohen, F.L. (1984). Clinical genetics in nursing practice. Philadelphia: J.B. Lippincott.

R

Role Enhancement   5370

Definition: Assisting a patient, significant other, and/or family to improve relationships by clarifying and supplementing specific role behaviors

Activities:

Assist patient to identify various roles in life

Assist patient to identify usual role in family

Assist patient to identify role transition periods throughout the life span

Assist patient to identify role insufficiency

Assist patient to identify behaviors needed for new or changed roles

Assist patient to identify specific role changes required due to illness or disability

Assist adult children to accept elderly parent's dependency and the role changes involved, as appropriate

Encourage patient to identify a realistic description of change in role

Assist patient to identify positive strategies for managing role changes

Facilitate discussion of role adaptations of family to compensate for ill member's role changes

Assist patient to imagine how a particular situation might occur and how a role would evolve

Facilitate role rehearsal by having patient anticipate others' reactions to enactment

Facilitate discussion of how siblings' roles will change with newborn's arrival, as appropriate

Provide rooming-in opportunities to help clarify parents' roles, as appropriate

Facilitate discussion of role adaptations related to children's leaving home (empty nest syndrome), as appropriate

Serve as role model for learning new behaviors, as appropriate

Facilitate opportunity for patient to role play new behaviors

Facilitate discussion of expectations between patient and significant other in reciprocal role

Teach new behaviors needed by patient/parent to fulfill a role

Facilitate reference group interactions as part of learning new roles

Background Readings:

Bunten, D. (2001) Normal changes with aging. In M.L. Maas, K.C. Buckwalter, M.D. Hardy, T.T. Reimer, M.G. Titler, & J.P., Specht (Eds.), Nursing care of older adults: Diagnoses, outcomes, & interventions (pp. 615-618). St. Louis: Mosby.

Craven, R.F., & Hirnle, C.J. (2000) Fundamentals of nursing: Human health and function (3rd ed.) (p. 1237). Philadelphia: Lippincott.

Luckmann, J., & Sorensen, K.C. (1987). Medical-surgical nursing (3rd ed.). Philadelphia: W.B. Saunders.

Meleis, A. (1975). Role insufficiency and role supplementation. Nursing Research, 24(4), 254-271.

Meleis, A., & Swendson, L. (1978). Role supplementation: An empirical test of a nursing intervention. Nursing Research, 27(1), 11-18.

Moorhead, S.A. (1985). Role supplementation. In G.M. Bulechek & J.C. McCloskey (Eds.), Nursing interventions: Treatments for nursing diagnoses (pp. 152-159). Philadelphia: W.B. Saunders.

R

Seclusion   6630

Definition: Solitary containment in a fully protective environment with close surveillance by nursing staff for purposes of safety or behavior management

Activities:

Obtain a physician's order, if required by institutional policy, to use a physically restrictive intervention

Designate one nursing staff member to communicate with the patient and to direct other staff

Identify for patient and significant others those behaviors that necessitated the intervention

Explain procedure, purpose, and time period of the intervention to patient and significant others in understandable and nonpunitive terms

Explain to patient and significant others the behaviors necessary for termination of the intervention

Contract with patient (as patient is able) to maintain control of behavior

Instruct on self-control methods, as appropriate

Assist in dressing in clothing that is safe and in removing jewelry and eyeglasses

Remove all items from seclusion area that patient might use to harm self or nursing staff

Assist with needs related to nutrition, elimination, hydration, and personal hygiene

Provide food and fluids in nonbreakable containers

Provide appropriate level of supervision/surveillance to monitor patient and to allow for therapeutic actions, as needed

Acknowledge your presence to patient periodically

Administer PRN medications for anxiety or agitation

Provide for patient's psychological comfort, as needed

Monitor seclusion area for temperature, cleanliness, and safety

Arrange for routine cleaning of seclusion area

Evaluate, at regular intervals, patient's need for continued restrictive intervention

Involve patient, when appropriate, in making decisions to move to a more/less restrictive intervention

Determine patient's need for continued seclusion

Document rationale for restrictive intervention, patient's response to intervention, patient's physical condition, nursing care provided throughout intervention, and rationale for terminating the intervention

Process with the patient and staff, on termination of the restrictive intervention, the circumstances that led to the use of the intervention, as well as any patient concerns about the intervention itself

Provide the next appropriate level of restrictive intervention (e.g., physical restraint or area restriction), as needed

S

Background Readings:

Carpenito, L.J. (1989). Nursing diagnosis: Application to clinical practice (3rd ed.). New York: J.B. Lippincott.

Craig, C., Ray, F., & Hix, C. (1989). Seclusion and restraint: Decreasing the discomfort. Journal of Psychosocial Nursing and Mental Health Services, 27(7), 16-19.

Kanak, M.F. (1992). Interventions related to safety. In G.M. Bulechek & J.C. McCloskey (Eds.), Symposium on Nursing Interventions. Nursing Clinics of North America, 27(2), 371-395.

Kirkpatrick, H. (1989). A descriptive study of seclusion: The unit environment, patient behavior, and nursing interventions. Archives of Psychiatric Nursing, 3(1), 3-9.

Munns, D., & Nolan, L. (1990). Potential for violence: Self-directed or directed at others. In M. Maas, K.C. Buckwalter, & M. Hardy (Eds.), Nursing diagnoses and interventions for the elderly (pp. 551-560). Menlo Park, CA: Addison-Wesley.

Thackrey, M. (1987). Therapeutics for aggression: Psychological/physical crisis intervention. New York: Human Sciences Press.

Security Enhancement   5380

Definition: Intensifying a patient's sense of physical and psychological safety

Activities:

Provide a nonthreatening environment

Demonstrate calmness

Spend time with patient

Offer to remain with patient in a new environment during initial interactions with others

Stay with the patient and provide assurance of safety and security during periods of anxiety

Present change gradually

Discuss upcoming changes (e.g., an interward transfer) before event

Avoid causing intense emotional situations

Give pacifier to infant, as appropriate

Hold a young child or infant, as appropriate

Facilitate a parent's staying overnight with a hospitalized child

Facilitate maintenance of patient's usual bedtime rituals

Encourage family to provide personal items for patient's use or enjoyment

Listen to patient's/family's fears

Encourage exploration of the dark, as appropriate

Leave light on at night, as needed

Discuss specific situations or individuals that seem threatening to the patient or family

Explain all tests and procedures to patient/family

Answer questions about health status in an honest manner

Help the patient/family identify what factors increase sense of security

Assist patient to identify usual coping responses

Assist patient to use coping responses that have been successful in the past

Background Readings:

Luckmann, J., & Sorensen, K.C. (1987). Medical-surgical nursing (3rd ed.). Philadelphia: W.B. Saunders.

Reynolds, E.A., & Ramenofsky, M.L. (1988). The emotional impact of trauma on toddlers. MCN: American Journal of Maternal Child Nursing, 13(2), 106-109.

Schepp, K.G. (1990). Factors influencing the coping effort of mothers of hospitalized children. Nursing Research, 40(1), 42-46.

Wong, D.L. (1993). Whaley & Wong's essentials of pediatric nursing (4th ed.). Unit 8: Impact of hospitalization on the child and family (pp. 582-707). St. Louis: Mosby.

S

Sedation Management   2260

Definition: Administration of sedatives, monitoring of the patient's response, and provision of necessary physiological support during a diagnostic or therapeutic procedure

Activities:

Review patient's health history and results of diagnostic tests to determine if patient meets agency criteria for conscious sedation by a registered nurse

Ask patient or family about any previous experiences with conscious sedation

Check for drug allergies

Determine last food and fluid intake

Review other medications patient is taking and verify absence of contraindications for sedation

Instruct the patient and/or family about effects of sedation

Obtain informed written consent

Evaluate the patient's level of consciousness and protective reflexes before administering sedation

Obtain baseline vital signs, oxygen saturation, EKG, height, and weight

Ensure that emergency resuscitation equipment is readily available, specifically source to deliver 100% O_2, emergency medications, and a defibrillator

Initiate an IV line

Administer medication per physician's order or protocol, titrating carefully according to patient's response

Monitor the patient's level of consciousness and vital signs, oxygen saturation, and EKG per agency protocol

Monitor the patient for adverse effects of medication, including agitation, respiratory depression, hypotension, undue somnolence, hypoxemia, arrhythmias, apnea, or exacerbation of a preexisting condition

Ensure availability of and administer antagonists, as appropriate per physician's order or protocol

Determine if the patient meets discharge or transfer criteria (i.e., Aldrete scale), per agency protocol

Document actions and patient response, per agency policy

Discharge or transfer patient, per agency protocol

Provide written discharge instructions, per agency protocol

Background Readings:

American Academy of Pediatrics. (1992). Guidelines for monitoring and management of pediatric patients during and after sedation for diagnostic and therapeutic procedures. Pediatrics, 89(6), 1110-1114.

Holzman, R.S., Cullen, D.J., Eichron, J.H., Philip, J.J. (1994). Guidelines for sedation by nonanesthesiologists during diagnostic and therapeutic procedures. Clinical Anesthesia, 6(4), 265-276.

Somerson, S.J., Husted, C.W. & Siclia, M.R. (1995). Insights into conscious sedation. American Journal of Nursing, 95, 25-32.

Somerson, S.J., Somerson, S.W., & Sicilia, M.R. (1999) Conscious sedation. In G.M. Bulechek & J.C. McCloskey (Eds.), Nursing interventions: Effective nursing treatments (3rd ed.) (pp. 297-310). Philadelphia: W.B. Saunders Company.

Watson, D. (1990). Monitoring the patient receiving local anesthesia. Denver, CO: AORN.

S

Seizure Management   2680

Definition: Care of a patient during a seizure and the postictal state

Activities:

Guide movements to prevent injury

Monitor direction of head and eyes during seizure

Loosen clothing

Remain with patient during seizure

Maintain airway

Establish IV access, as appropriate

Apply oxygen, as appropriate

Monitor neurological status

Monitor vital signs

Reorient after seizure

Record length of seizure

Record seizure characteristics: body parts involved, motor activity, and seizure progression

Document information about seizure

Administer medication, as appropriate

Administer anticonvulsants, as appropriate

Monitor antiepileptic drug levels, as appropriate

Monitor postictal period duration and characteristics

Background Readings:

Ackerman, L.L. (1992). Interventions related to neurological care. In G.M. Bulechek & J.C. McCloskey (Eds.), Symposium on Nursing Interventions. Nursing Clinics of North America, 27(2), 325-346.

Brewer, K., & Sperling, M.R. (1988). Neurosurgical treatment of intractible epilepsy. Journal of Neuroscience Nursing, 20(6), 366-372.

Cammermeyer, M., & Appledorn, C. (Eds.). (1990). Core curriculum for neuroscience nursing (3rd ed.) (pp. Ig1-Ig3). Chicago: American Association of Neuroscience Nurses.

Graham, O., Naveau, I., & Cummings, C. (1989). A model for ambulatory care of patients with epilepsy and other neurological disorders. Journal of Neuroscience Nursing, 21(2), 108-112.

Johanson, B.C., Wells, S.J., Hoffmeister, D., & Dungca, C.U. (1988). Standards for critical care (3rd ed.). St. Louis: Mosby.

LeMone, P., & Burke, K.M. (2000). Medical-surgical nursing: Critical thinking in client care, (2nd ed.) (pp. 1719-1727). Upper Saddle River, NJ: Prentice Hall Health

Santilli, N., & Sierzant, T.L. (1987). Advances in the treatment of epilepsy. Journal of Neuroscience Nursing, 19(3), 141-155.

S

Seizure Precautions   2690

Definition: Prevention or minimization of potential injuries sustained by a patient with a known seizure disorder

Activities:

Provide low-height bed, as appropriate

Escort patient during off-ward activities, as appropriate

Monitor drug regimen

Monitor compliance in taking antiepileptic medications

Have patient/significant other keep record of medications taken and occurrence of seizure activity

Instruct patient not to drive

Instruct patient about medications and side effects

Instruct family/significant other about seizure first aid

Monitor antiepileptic drug levels, as appropriate

Instruct patient to carry medication alert card

Remove potentially harmful objects from the environment

Keep suction at bedside

Keep ambu bag at bedside

Keep oral or nasopharyngeal airway at bedside

Use padded side rails

Keep side rails up

Instruct patient on potential precipitating factors

Instruct patient to call if aura occurs

Background Readings:

Ackerman, L.L. (1992). Interventions related to neurological care. In G.M. Bulechek & J.C. McCloskey (Eds.), Symposium on Nursing Interventions. Nursing Clinics of North America, 27(2), 325-346.

Brewer, K., & Sperling, M.R. (1988). Neurosurgical treatment of intractible epilepsy. Journal of Neuroscience Nursing, 20(6), 366-372.

Cammermeyer, M., & Appledorn, C. (Eds.). (1990). Core curriculum for neuroscience nursing (3rd ed.) (pp. Ig1-Ig3). Chicago: American Association of Neuroscience Nurses.

Graham, O., Naveau, I., & Cummings, C. (1989). A model for ambulatory care of patients with epilepsy and other neurological disorders. Journal of Neuroscience Nursing, 21(2), 108-112.

Johanson, B.C., Wells, S.J., Hoffmeister, D., & Dungca, C.U. (1988). Standards for critical care (3rd ed.). St. Louis: Mosby.

LeMone, P., & Burke, K.M. (2000). Medical-surgical nursing: Critical thinking in client care, (2nd ed.) (pp. 1719-1727). Upper Saddle River, NJ: Prentice Hall Health.

Santilli, N., & Sierzant, T.L. (1987). Advances in the treatment of epilepsy. Journal of Neuroscience Nursing, 19(3), 141-155.

S

Self-Awareness Enhancement   5390

Definition: Assisting a patient to explore and understand his/her thoughts, feelings, motivations, and behaviors

Activities:

Encourage patient to recognize and discuss thoughts and feelings

Assist patient to realize that everyone is unique

Assist patient to identify the values that contribute to self-concept

Assist patient to identify usual feelings about self

Share observation or thoughts about patient's behavior or response

Facilitate patient's identification of usual response patterns to various situations

Assist patient to identify life priorities

Assist patient to identify the impact of illness on self-concept

Verbalize patient's denial of reality, as appropriate

Confront patient's ambivalent (angry or depressed) feelings

Make observation about patient's current emotional state

Assist patient to accept dependency on others, as appropriate

Assist patient to change view of self as victim by defining own rights, as appropriate

Assist patient to be aware of negative self-statements

Assist patient to identify guilty feelings

Help patient identify situations that precipitate anxiety

Explore with patient the need to control

Assist patient to identify positive attributes of self

Assist patient/family to identify reasons for improvement

Assist patient to identify abilities, learning styles

Assist patient to reexamine negative perceptions of self

Assist patient to identify source of motivation

Assist patient to identify behaviors that are self-destructive

Facilitate self-expression with peer group

Assist patient to recognize contradictory statements

Background Readings:

Luckmann, J., & Sorensen, K.C. (1987). Medical-surgical nursing (3rd ed.). Philadelphia: W.B. Saunders.
Potter, P.A., & Perry, A.G. (1998). Fundamentals of nursing: Concepts, process, and practice (4th ed.). St. Louis: Mosby.
Sorensen, K., & Luckmann, J. (1986). Basic nursing: A psychophysiologic approach (2nd ed.). Philadelphia: W.B. Saunders.

Self-Care Assistance   1800

Definition: Assisting another to perform activities of daily living

Activities:

Monitor patient's ability for independent self-care

Monitor patient's need for adaptive devices for personal hygiene, dressing, grooming, toileting, and eating

Provide desired personal articles (e.g., deodorant, toothbrush, and bath soap)

Provide assistance until patient is fully able to assume self-care

Assist patient in accepting dependency needs

Use consistent repetition of health routines as a means of establishing them

Encourage patient to perform normal activities of daily living to level of ability

Encourage independence, but intervene when patient is unable to perform

Teach parents/family to encourage independence, to intervene only when the patient is unable to perform

Establish a routine for self-care activities

Consider age of patient when promoting self-care activities

Background Readings:

Lantz, J., Penn, C., Stamper, J., & Natividad, P. (1991). Self-care deficit. In M. Maas, K. Buckwalter, & M. Hardy (Eds.), Nursing diagnoses and interventions for the elderly (pp. 285-312). Redwood City, CA: Addison-Wesley.

Potter, P.A., & Perry, A.G. (1998). Fundamentals of nursing: Concepts, process, and practice (4th ed.). St. Louis: Mosby.

Sorensen, K., & Luckmann, J. (1986). Basic nursing: A psychophysiologic approach (2nd ed.). Philadelphia: W.B. Saunders.

Styker, R. (1977). Rehabilitative aspects of acute and chronic nursing care. Philadelphia: W.B. Saunders.

Taylor, C.M. (1987). Nursing diagnosis cards. Springhouse, PA: Springhouse.

S

Self-Care Assistance: Bathing/Hygiene   1801

Definition: Assisting patient to perform personal hygiene

Activities:

Place towels, soap, deodorant, shaving equipment, and other needed accessories at bedside in bathroom

Provide desired personal articles (e.g., deodorant, toothbrush, and bath soap)

Facilitate patient's brushing teeth, as appropriate

Facilitate patient's bathing self, as appropriate

Monitor cleaning of nails, according to patient's self-care ability

Facilitate maintenance of patient's usual bedtime routines, presleep cues/props, and familiar objects (e.g., for children, a favorite blanket/toy, rocking, pacifier, or story; for adults, a book to read or a pillow from home), as appropriate

Encourage parent/family participation in usual bedtime rituals, as appropriate

Provide assistance until patient is fully able to assume self-care

Background Readings:

Craven, R.F., & Hirnle, C.J. (2000) Fundamentals of nursing: Human health and function (3rd ed.) (pp. 696-701). Philadelphia: Lippincott.

Sorensen, K., & Luckmann, J. (1986). Basic nursing: A psychophysiologic approach (2nd ed.). Philadelphia: W.B. Saunders.

Taylor, C.M. (1987). Nursing diagnosis cards. Springhouse, PA: Springhouse.

Tracy, C.A. (1992). Hygiene assistance. In G.M. Bulechek & J.C. McCloskey (Eds.), Nursing interventions: Essential nursing treatments (2nd ed.) (pp. 24-33). Philadelphia: W.B. Saunders.

S

Self-Care Assistance: Dressing/Grooming   1802

Definition: Assisting patient with clothes and makeup

Activities:

Inform patient of available clothing for selection

Provide patient's clothes in accessible area (e.g., at bedside)

Provide personal clothing, as appropriate

Be available for assistance in dressing, as necessary

Facilitate patient's combing hair, as appropriate

Facilitate patient's shaving self, as appropriate

Maintain privacy while the patient is dressing

Help with laces, buttons, and zippers, as needed

Use extension equipment for pulling on clothing, if appropriate

Offer to launder clothing, as necessary

Place removed clothing in laundry

Offer to hang up clothing or place in dresser

Offer to rinse special garments, such as nylons

Provide fingernail polish, if requested

Provide makeup, if requested

Reinforce efforts to dress self

Facilitate assistance of a barber or beautician, as necessary

Background Readings:

Craven, R.F., & Hirnle, C.J. (2000) Fundamentals of nursing: Human health and function (3rd ed.) (pp. 708-712). Philadelphia: Lippincott.

Potter, P.A., & Perry, A.G. (1998). Fundamentals of nursing: Concepts, process, and practice (4th ed.). St. Louis: Mosby.

Sorensen, K., & Luckmann, J. (1986). Basic nursing: A psychophysiologic approach (2nd ed.). Philadelphia: W.B. Saunders.

Taylor, C.M. (1987). Nursing diagnosis cards. Springhouse, PA: Springhouse.

S

Self-Care Assistance: Feeding 1803

Definition: Assisting a person to eat

Activities:

Identify prescribed diet

Set food tray and table attractively

Create a pleasant environment during mealtime (e.g., put bedpans, urinals, and suctioning equipment out of sight)

Provide for adequate pain relief before meals, as appropriate

Provide for oral hygiene before meals

Fix food on tray, as necessary, such as cutting meat or peeling an egg

Open packaged foods

Avoid placing food on a person's blind side

Describe location of food on tray for person with vision impairment

Place patient in comfortable eating position

Protect patient's clothing with a bib, as appropriate

Provide a drinking straw, as needed or desired

Provide foods at most appetizing temperatures

Note intake, as appropriate

Encourage patient to eat in dining room, if available

Provide adaptive devices to facilitate patient's feeding self (e.g., long handles, handle with large circumference, or small strap on utensils), as needed

Use a cup with a large handle, if necessary

Use unbreakable and weighted dishes and glasses, as necessary

Provide frequent cuing and close supervision, as appropriate

Background Readings:

Evans, N.J. (1992). Feeding. In G.M. Bulechek & J.C. McCloskey (Eds.), Nursing interventions: Essential nursing treatments (2nd ed.) (pp. 48-60). Philadelphia: W.B. Saunders.

Potter, P.A., & Perry, A.G. (1998). Fundamentals of nursing: Concepts, process and practice (4th ed.). St. Louis: Mosby.

Sorensen, K., & Luckmann, J. (1986). Basic nursing: A psychophysiologic approach (2nd ed.). Philadelphia: W.B. Saunders.

Taylor, C.M. (1987). Nursing diagnosis cards. Springhouse, PA: Springhouse.

S

Self-Care Assistance: IADL   1805

Definition: Assisting and instructing a person to perform instrumental activities of daily living (IADL) needed to function in the home or community

Activities:

Determine individual's need for assistance with instrumental activities of daily living (e.g., shopping, cooking, housekeeping, laundry, use of transportation, managing money, managing medications, use of communication, and use of time)

Determine needs for safety-related changes in the home (e.g., wider door frames to allow for wheelchair access to bathroom, removal of scatter rugs)

Determine needs for home enhancements to offset disabilities (e.g., large numbers on telephones, increased volume of telephone ringer, laundry and other facilities located on main floor; side rails in hallways, grab-bars in bathrooms)

Provide for methods of contacting support and assistance people (e.g., lifeline; list of telephone numbers for police, fire, poison control, and assistance people)

Instruct individual on alternative methods of transportation (e.g., buses and bus schedules, taxis, city or county transportation for disabled people)

Provide cognitive enhancing techniques (e.g., up-to-date calendars, clearly legible and understandable lists such as medication times, easy-to-see clocks)

Obtain transportation enhancements to offset disabilities (e.g., hand controls on cars, wide rearview mirror), as appropriate

Obtain tools to assist in daily activities (e.g., ability to reach items in cupboards, closets, on countertops, on stovetops, in refrigerator, and ability to operate household equipment such as stoves and microwaves)

Determine financial resources and personal preferences regarding modifications to home or car

Instruct individual to wear clothing with short or tight-fitting sleeves when cooking

Verify adequacy of lighting throughout house, especially in working areas (e.g., kitchen, bathroom), and at night (e.g., appropriately placed nightlights)

Instruct individual not to smoke in bed or while reclining, or after taking mind-altering medication

Verify presence of safety equipment in home (e.g., smoke detectors, carbon monoxide detectors, fire extinguishers, hot water heater set to 120 degrees Fahrenheit)

Determine whether individual's monthly income is sufficient to cover ongoing expenses

Obtain visual safety devices or techniques (e.g., painting edges of steps bright yellow, rearrange furniture for safety when walking, reduced clutter throughout walkways of house, nonskid surfaces installed in showers and bathtubs)

Assist individual in establishing methods and routines for cooking, cleaning, and shopping

Instruct individual and caregiver on what to do in the event the individual suffers from a fall or other injury (e.g., how to gain access to emergency services, how to prevent further injury)

Determine if physical or cognitive ability is stable or declining and respond to changes in either accordingly

Consult with occupational and/or physical therapist to deal with physical disability

Instruct assisting person in completing appropriate setting-up tasks so that individual can complete task (e.g., chop up vegetables so individual can cook with them, place clothing to wear for the day in an easy-to-reach place, unpack groceries on countertop for eventual storage)

Provide appropriate container for used sharps, as appropriate

Instruct individual on appropriate and safe storage for medications

Continued

S

Activities:—cont'd

Instruct individual on appropriate use of monitoring equipment (e.g., glucose-monitoring device, lancets)

Instruct individual on appropriate methods of dressing wounds and appropriate disposal of soiled dressings

Verify that individual is able to open medication containers

Refer to family and community services, as needed

Background Readings:

Eliopoulos, C. (1999). Manual of gerontologic nursing (2nd ed.). St. Louis: Mosby.

Lawton, H.P., & Brody, E.M. (1969). Assessment of older people: Self maintaining and instrumental activities of daily living. Gerontologist, 9, 179-186

Lueckenotte, A. (2000). Gerontologic nursing, (2nd ed.). St. Louis: Mosby.

Perry, A.G., & Potter, P.A. (2002). Clinical nursing skills and techniques (5th ed.) (pp. 1093-1113). St. Louis: Mosby.

S

Self-Care Assistance: Toileting

1804

Definition: Assisting another with elimination

Activities:

Remove essential clothing to allow for elimination

Assist patient to toilet/commode/bedpan/fracture pan/urinal at specified intervals

Consider patient's response to lack of privacy

Provide privacy during elimination

Facilitate toilet hygiene after completion of elimination

Replace patient's clothing after elimination

Flush toilet/cleanse elimination utensil

Institute a toileting schedule, as appropriate

Instruct patient/appropriate others in toileting routine

Institute bathroom rounds, as appropriate and needed

Provide assistive devices (e.g., external catheter or urinal), as appropriate

Background Readings:

Potter, P.A., & Perry, A.G. (1998). Fundamentals of nursing: Concepts, process, and practice (4th ed.). St. Louis: Mosby.

Sorensen, K., & Luckmann, J. (1986). Basic nursing: A psychophysiologic approach (2nd ed.). Philadelphia: W.B. Saunders.

Taylor, C.M. (1987). Nursing diagnosis cards. Springhouse, PA: Springhouse.

S

Self-Care Assistance: Transfer   1806

Definition: Assisting a person to change body location

Activities:

Determine current ability of individual to transfer self (e.g., muscle strength, level of ability, endurance)

Determine current ability of individual to comprehend instructions, and to stand and bear weight

Determine presence of medical or orthopedic instability that may impede transfer

Determine presence of orthostatic hypotension

Select transfer technique that is appropriate for the individual

Identify ways to prevent injury during transfer

Instruct individual on appropriate techniques for transfer from one area to another (e.g., from bed to chair, from chair to bed, from wheelchair to vehicle, from vehicle to wheelchair)

Demonstrate the technique, as appropriate

Provide support for body and extremities during transfer, as appropriate

Instruct individual on transfer with the goal of reaching the highest level of independence

Provide assistive devices (e.g., bars attached to walls, ropes attached to headboard or footboard for help in moving to center or edge of bed) to help individual transfer independently, as appropriate

Instruct individual in appropriate use of ambulatory aids (e.g., crutches, wheelchairs, walkers, trapeze bar, cane)

Utilize transfer belt, as appropriate

Provide encouragement to individual as he/she learns to transfer independently

Document progress, as appropriate

Background Readings:

Harkness, G.A. & Dincher, J.R. (1999). Medical-surgical nursing: Total patient care (10th ed.) (pp. 420-423). St. Louis: Mosby.

Perry, A.G., & Potter, P.A. (2002). Clinical nursing skills & techniques (5th ed.) (pp. 806-815). St. Louis: Mosby.

Smeltzer, S.C., & Bare, B.G. (1996). Brunner and Suddarth's textbook of medical-surgical nursing (8th ed.) (pp. 335-341). Philadelphia: Lippincott.

S

Self-Esteem Enhancement

5400

Definition: Assisting a patient to increase his/her personal judgment of self-worth

Activities:

Monitor patient's statements of self-worth

Determine patient's locus of control

Determine patient's confidence in own judgment

Encourage patient to identify strengths

Encourage eye contact in communicating with others

Reinforce the personal strengths that patient identifies

Provide experiences that increase patient's autonomy, as appropriate

Assist patient to identify positive responses from others

Refrain from negatively criticizing

Refrain from teasing

Convey confidence in patient's ability to handle situation

Assist in setting realistic goals to achieve higher self-esteem

Assist patient to accept dependence on others, as appropriate

Assist patient to reexamine negative perceptions of self

Encourage increased responsibility for self, as appropriate

Assist patient to identify the impact of peer group on feelings of self-worth

Explore previous achievements

Explore reasons for self-criticism or guilt

Encourage the patient to evaluate own behavior

Encourage patient to accept new challenges

Reward or praise patient's progress toward reaching goals

Facilitate an environment and activities that will increase self-esteem

Assist patient to identify significant effects of culture, religion, race, gender, and age on self-esteem

Instruct parents on the importance of their interest and support in their children's development of a positive self-concept

Instruct parents to set clear expectations and to define limits with their children

Teach parents to recognize children's accomplishments

Monitor frequency of self-negating verbalizations

Monitor lack of follow-through in goal attainment

Monitor levels of self-esteem over time, as appropriate

Make positive statements about patient

Background Readings:

Bunten, D. Normal changes with aging. (2001). In M.L. Maas, K.C. Buckwalter, M.D. Hardy, T.T. Reimer, M.G. Titler, & J.P. Specht (Eds.), Nursing care of older adults: Diagnoses, outcomes, & interventions (p. 519). St. Louis: Mosby.

Byers, P.H. (1990). Enhancing the self-esteem of inpatient alcoholics. Issues in Mental Health Nursing, 11(4), 337-346.

Luckmann, J., & Sorensen, K.C. (1987). Medical-surgical nursing (3rd ed.). Philadelphia: W.B. Saunders.

Norris, J., & Kunes-Connell, M. (1985). Self-esteem disturbance. Nursing Clinics of North America, 20(4), 745-761.

Reasoner, R.W. (1983). Enhancement of self-esteem in children and adolescents. Family and Community Health, 6(2), 51-63.

Whall, A.L., & Parent, C.J. (1991). Self-esteem disturbance. In M. Maas, K. Buckwalter, & M. Hardy (Eds.), Nursing diagnosis and interventions for the elderly (pp. 480-488). Redwood City, CA: Addison-Wesley.

S

Self-Hypnosis Facilitation   5922

Definition: Teaching and monitoring the use of a self-initiated hypnotic state for therapeutic benefit

Activities:

Determine whether the patient is an appropriate candidate for self-hypnosis (e.g., see literature-based recommendations in the background readings)

Utilize self-hypnosis as an adjunct to other treatment modalities (e.g., individual hypnotherapy by a therapist, individual psychotherapy, group therapy, family therapy, etc.), as deemed appropriate

Introduce the patient to the concept of self-hypnosis as a therapeutic modality

Identify with the patient those problems/issues that are amenable to treatment with self-hypnosis

Assist the patient to identify treatment goals

Provide the patient with an individualized procedure for the process of self-hypnosis that reflects his/her specific needs and goals

Assist the patient to identify appropriate induction techniques (e.g., arm gravitational techniques, eye fixation techniques, simple muscle relaxation, visualization exercises, attention to breathing, and repetition of key words/phrases)

Assist the patient to identify appropriate deepening techniques (e.g., movement of a hand to the face, imagery escalation technique, and others)

Encourage the patient to become proficient at self-hypnosis by practicing the technique

Contract for a practice schedule with the patient, if needed

Monitor the patient's response to self-hypnosis on an ongoing basis

Solicit the patient's feedback regarding his/her comfort with the procedure and experience of self-hypnosis

Assist the patient to process and interpret what occurs as a result of the self-hypnosis sessions

Recommend modifications in the patient's practice of self-hypnosis (frequency, intensity, specific techniques) based on his/her response and level of comfort

Assist the patient to evaluate progress made towards therapy goals

Background Readings:

Fromm, E., & Kahn, S. (1990). Self-hypnosis. The Chicago paradigm. New York: The Guilford Press.

Haber, J. (1997). Mood disorders. In J. Haber, B. Krainovich-Miller, A. Leach McMahon, P. Price-Hoskins (Eds.), Comprehensive psychiatric nursing (5th ed.) (pp. 603-651). St. Louis: Mosby.

Meyer, R.G. (1992). Practical clinical hypnosis. New York: Lexington Books, Macmillan, Inc.

Sanders, S. (1991). Clinical self-hypnosis. New York: The Guilford Press.

Shames, K.H., & Hover-Kramer, D. (2001). Self-care modalities. In N.C. Frisch & L.E. Frisch (Eds.), Psychiatric mental health nursing (2nd ed.) (pp. 761-777). Albany, NY: Delmar.

Zarren, J.I., & Eimer, B.N. (2002). Brief cognitive hypnosis. Facilitating the change of dysfunctional behavior. New York: Springer.

S

Self-Modification Assistance 4470

Definition: Reinforcement of self-directed change initiated by the patient to achieve personally important goals

Activities:

Encourage the patient to examine personal values and beliefs and satisfaction with them

Appraise the patient's reasons for wanting to change

Assist the patient in identifying a specific goal for change

Assist the patient in identifying target behaviors that need to change to achieve the desired goal

Appraise the patient's present knowledge and skill level in relationship to the desired change

Appraise the patient's social and physical environment for extent of support of desired behaviors

Explore with the patient potential barriers to change behavior

Identify with the patient the most effective strategies for behavior change

Explain to the patient the importance of self-monitoring in attempting behavior change

Assist the patient in identifying the frequency with which specific behaviors occur

Assist the patient in developing a portable, easy-to-use coding sheet to aid in recording behaviors (may be a graph or chart)

Instruct the patient to record the incidence of behaviors for at least 3 days, up to 2 to 3 weeks

Encourage the patient to identify appropriate, meaningful reinforcers/rewards

Encourage the patient to choose a reinforcer/reward that is significant enough to sustain the behavior

Assist the patient in developing a list of valued extrinsic and intrinsic rewards

Encourage the patient to begin with extrinsic rewards and progress to intrinsic rewards

Instruct the patient that reward list may include manners in which the nurse, family, or friends can assist the patient in behavior change

Assist the patient in formulating a systematic plan for behavior change

Encourage the patient to identify steps that are manageable in size and able to be accomplished in a set amount of time

Foster moving toward primary reliance on self-reinforcement vs. family or nurse for rewards

Instruct the patient on how to move from continuous reinforcement to intermittent reinforcement

Assist the patient in evaluating progress by comparing records of previous behavior with present behavior

Encourage the patient to develop a visual measure of changes in behavior (e.g., a graph)

Foster flexibility during the shaping plan, promoting complete mastery of one step before advancing to the next

Encourage the patient to adjust the shaping plan to enhance behavior change, if needed (e.g., size of steps or reward)

Assist the patient in identifying the circumstances or situations in which the behavior occurs (e.g., cues/triggers)

Assist the patient in identifying even small successes

Explain to the patient the function of cues/triggers in producing behavior

Assist the patient in appraising the physical, social, and interpersonal settings for the existence of cues/triggers

Encourage the patient to develop a "cue analysis sheet" that illustrates links between cues and behaviors

Continued

Activities:—cont'd

Instruct the patient on the use of "cue expansion": increasing the number of cues that prompt a desired behavior

Instruct the patient on the use of "cue restriction or limitation": decreasing the frequency of cues that elicit an undesirable behavior

Assist the patient in identifying methods of controlling behavioral cues

Assist the patient in identifying existent behaviors that are habitual or automatic (e.g., brushing teeth and tying shoes)

Assist the patient in identifying existing paired stimuli and habitual behavior (e.g., eating a meal and brushing teeth afterward)

Encourage the patient to pair a desired behavior with an existing stimulus or cue (e.g., exercising after work every day)

Encourage the patient to continue pairing desired behavior with existing stimuli until it becomes automatic or habitual

Explore with the patient the potential use of meditation or progressive relaxation in attempting behavior change

Explore with the patient the possibility of using role playing to clarify behaviors

Background Readings:

Hill, L., & Smith, N. (1985). Self-care nursing. Englewood Cliffs, NJ: Prentice-Hall.

Pender, N.J. (1982). Health promotion in nursing practice. Norwalk, CT: Appleton-Century-Crofts.

Pender, N.J. (1985). Self modification. In G.M. Bulechek & J.C. McCloskey (Eds.), Nursing interventions: Treatments for nursing diagnoses (pp. 80-91). Philadelphia: W.B. Saunders.

Simons, M.R. (1992). Interventions related to compliance. In G.M. Bulechek & J.C. McCloskey (Eds.), Symposium on Nursing Interventions. Nursing Clinics of North America, 27(2), 477-494.

Stuart, R.B. (1977). Behavioral self-management. New York: Brunner/Mazel.

Watson, D.L., & Tharp, R.G. (1993). Self-directing behavior: Self-modification for personal adjustment (2nd ed.). Monterey, CA: Brooks/Cole Publishing.

S

Self-Responsibility Facilitation   4480

Definition: Encouraging a patient to assume more responsibility for own behavior

Activities:

Hold patient responsible for own behavior

Discuss with patient the extent of responsibility for present health status

Determine whether patient has adequate knowledge about health care condition

Encourage verbalizations of feelings, perceptions, and fears about assuming responsibility

Monitor level of responsibility that patient assumes

Encourage independence, but assist patient when unable to perform

Discuss consequences of not dealing with own responsibilities

Encourage admission of wrongdoing, as appropriate

Set limits on manipulative behaviors

Refrain from arguing or bargaining about the established limits with the patient

Encourage patient to take as much responsibility for own self-care, as possible

Assist parents in identifying age-appropriate tasks for which child could be responsible, as appropriate

Encourage parents to clearly communicate expectations for responsible behavior in child, as appropriate

Encourage parents to follow through on expectations for responsible behavior in child, as appropriate

Assist patients to identify areas in which they could readily assume more responsibility

Facilitate family support for new level of responsibility sought or attained by patient

Assist with creating a timetable to guide increased responsibility in the future

Provide positive feedback for accepting additional responsibility and/or behavior change

Background Readings:

Arnold, L.J. (1990). Codependency. Part I: Origins, characteristics. AORN Journal, 51(5), 1341-1348.

Arnold, L.J. (1990). Codependency. Part II: The hospital as a dysfunctional family. AORN Journal, 51(6), 1581-1584.

Arnold, L.J. (1990). Codependency. Part III: Strategies for healing. AORN Journal, 52(1), 85-89.

Barnsteiner, J.H., & Gillis-Donovan, J. (1990). Being related and separate: A standard for therapeutic relationships. MCN: American Journal of Maternal Child Nursing, 15(4), 223-228.

Hall, S.F., & Wray, L.M. (1989). Codependency. Nurses who give too much. American Journal of Nursing, 89(11), 1456-1460.

Johnson, P.A., & Gaines, S.K. (1988). Helping families to help themselves. MCN: American Journal of Maternal Child Nursing, 13(5), 336-339.

Luckmann, J., & Sorensen, K.C. (1987). Medical-surgical nursing (3rd ed.). Philadelphia: W.B. Saunders.

S

Sexual Counseling 5248

Definition: Use of an interactive helping process focusing on the need to make adjustments in sexual practice or to enhance coping with a sexual event/disorder

Activities:

Establish a therapeutic relationship, based on trust and respect

Establish the length of the counseling relationship

Provide privacy and ensure confidentiality

Inform patient early in the relationship that sexuality is an important part of life and that illness, medications, and stress (or other problems/events patient is experiencing) often alter sexual functioning

Tell the patient that you are prepared to answer any questions about sexual functioning

Provide information about sexual functioning, as appropriate

Preface questions about sexuality with a statement that tells the patient that many people experience sexual difficulties

Begin with the least sensitive topics and proceed to the more sensitive

Discuss the effect of the illness/health situation on sexuality

Discuss the effect of medication on sexuality, as appropriate

Discuss the effect of changes in sexuality on significant others

Discuss the patient's knowledge about sexuality in general

Encourage patient to verbalize fears and to ask questions

Identify learning objectives necessary to reach goals

Discuss necessary modifications in sexual activity, as appropriate

Help patient to express grief and anger about alterations in body functioning/appearance, as appropriate

Avoid displaying aversion to an altered body part

Introduce patient to positive role models who have successfully conquered a similar problem, as appropriate

Provide factual information about sexual myths and misinformation that patient may verbalize

Discuss alternative forms of sexual expression that are acceptable to patient, as appropriate

Instruct the patient only on techniques compatible with values/beliefs

Instruct the patient on use of medication(s) (e.g., bronchodilators) to enhance ability to perform sexually, as appropriate

Determine amount of sexual guilt associated with the patient's perception of the causative factors of illness

Avoid prematurely terminating discussion of guilt feelings, even when these seem unreasonable

Include the spouse/sexual partner in the counseling as much as possible, as appropriate

Use humor and encourage patient to use humor to relieve anxiety or embarrassment

Provide reassurance that current and new sexual practices are healthy, as appropriate

Provide reassurance and permission to experiment with alternative forms of sexual expression, as appropriate

Provide referral/consultation with other members of the health care team, as appropriate

Refer the patient to a sex therapist, as appropriate

Background Readings:

Hines, J., & Daines, M.A. (1987). Sexuality and the renal patient. Nursing Times, 83(20), 35-36.

Kerfoot, K.M., & Buckwalter, K.C. (1985). Sexual counseling. In G.M. Bulechek & J.C. McCloskey (Eds.), Nursing interventions: Treatments for nursing diagnoses (pp. 127-138). Philadelphia: W.B. Saunders.

Muir, A. (2000). Counselling patients who have sexual difficulties. Professional Nurse, 15(11), 723-726.

Steinke, E.E. (2000). Sexual counseling after myocardial infraction. American Journal of Nursing, 100(12), 38-44.

S

Shift Report   8140

Definition: Exchanging essential patient care information with other nursing staff at change of shift

Activities:

Review pertinent demographic data, including name, age, and room number

Identify chief complaint and reason for admission, as appropriate

Summarize significant health history, as necessary

Identify key medical and nursing diagnoses, as appropriate

Identify resolved medical and nursing diagnoses, as appropriate

Present information succinctly, focusing on recent and significant data needed by nursing staff assuming responsibility for care

Describe treatment regimen, including diet, fluid therapy, medications, and exercise

Identify laboratory and diagnostic tests to be completed during the next 24 hours

Review recent pertinent laboratory and diagnostic test results, as appropriate

Describe health status data, including vital signs and signs and symptoms present during the shift

Describe nursing interventions being implemented

Describe patient and family response to nursing interventions

Summarize progress toward goals

Summarize discharge plans, as appropriate

Background Readings:

Donaghue, A.M., & Reiley, P.J. (1981). Some do's and don'ts for giving reports. Nursing, 11(11), 117.

Kron, T., & Gray, A. (1987). The management of patient care. Putting leadership skills to work (6th ed.). Philadelphia: W.B. Saunders.

Lamond, D. (2000). The information content of the nurse change of shift report: A comparative study. Journal of Advanced Nursing, 31(4), 794-804.

Priest, C.S., & Holmberg, S.K. (2000). A new model for the mental health nursing change of shift report. Journal of Psychosocial Nursing and Mental Health Service, 38(8), 36-45.

Richard, J.A. (1988). Congruence between intershift reports and patients' actual conditions. Image, 20(1), 4-6.

S

Shock Management   4250

Definition: Facilitation of the delivery of oxygen and nutrients to systemic tissue with removal of cellular waste products in a patient with severely altered tissue perfusion

Activities:

Monitor vital signs, orthostatic blood pressure, mental status, and urinary output

Monitor laboratory evidence of inadequate tissue perfusion (e.g., increased lactic acid levels, decreased arterial pH levels), as available

Administer crystalloid IV fluids, as appropriate

Administer vasoactive medications, as appropriate

Provide oxygen therapy and/or mechanical ventilation, if necessary

Monitor trends in hemodynamic parameters (e.g., central venous pressure, pulmonary capillary/artery wedge pressure)

Monitor fetal heart rate for bradycardia (<110 beats/min) or tachycardia (>160 beats/min) lasting longer than 10 minutes, if appropriate

Draw blood for measurement of ABGs and monitor tissue oxygenation

Maintain patent IV access

Administer fluids to maintain blood pressure and cardiac output, as appropriate

Monitor determinants of tissue oxygen delivery (e.g., PaO_2, SaO_2, hemoglobin levels, and cardiac output), if available

Note tachycardia or bradycardia, decreased blood pressure, or abnormally low systemic arterial pressure, as well as pallor, cyanosis, and diaphoresis

Monitor for symptoms of respiratory failure (e.g., low PaO_2, elevated $PaCO_2$ levels, respiratory muscle fatigue)

Monitor lab values for changes in oxygenation or acid-base balance, as appropriate

Monitor serum glucose and treat abnormal levels, as appropriate

Monitor coagulation studies and complete blood count (CBC) with WBC differential

Utilize arterial line monitoring to improve accuracy of blood pressure readings, as appropriate

Monitor fluid status, including intake and output, as appropriate

Monitor renal function (e.g., BUN, Cr levels), if appropriate

Insert urinary catheter, as appropriate

Insert NG tube to suction and monitor secretions, as appropriate

Position the patient for optimal perfusion

Offer emotional support to the patient and family

Encourage realistic expectations for the patient and family

S

Background Readings:

Gulanick, M., & Ruback, C. (1999). Shock management. In G.M. Bulechek & J.C. McCloskey (Eds.), Nursing interventions: Effective nursing treatments (3rd ed.) (pp. 311-324). Philadelphia: W.B. Saunders.

Khalaf, S., & DeBlieux, P.M.C. (2001). Managing shock: The role of vasoactive agents, part 1. The Journal of Critical Illness, 16(6), 281-287.

Khalaf, S., & DeBlieux, P.M.C. (2001). Managing shock: The role of vasoactive agents, part 2. The Journal of Critical Illness, 16(7), 334-338.

McCance, K.L., & Huether, S.E. (2002). Pathophysiology: The biologic basis for disease in adults & children (4th ed.) (pp.1483-1492). St. Louis: Mosby.

Porth, C.M. (2002). Pathophysiology: Concepts of altered health states (6th ed.) (pp. 558-569). Philadelphia: Lippincott.

Shock Management: Cardiac   4254

Definition: Promotion of adequate tissue perfusion for a patient with severely compromised pumping function of the heart

Activities:

Auscultate lung sounds for crackles or other adventitious sounds

Note signs and symptoms of decreased cardiac output

Monitor for symptoms of inadequate coronary artery perfusion (e.g., ST changes on EKG or angina), as appropriate

Monitor coagulation studies, including prothrombin time (PT), partial thromboplastin time (PTT), fibrinogen, fibrin degradation/split products, and platelet counts, as appropriate

Maintain fluid balance by administering IV fluids or diuretics, as appropriate

Administer positive inotropic/contractility medications

Promote optimal preload to improve contractility while minimizing heart failure (e.g., administer nitroglycerine and maintain pulmonary capillary/artery wedge pressure within prescribed range), as appropriate

Promote afterload reduction (e.g., with vasodilators or intraaortic balloon pumping), as appropriate

Promote coronary artery perfusion (e.g., maintain mean arterial pressure >60 mm Hg and control tachycardia), as appropriate

Background Readings:

Cullen, L.M. (1992). Interventions related to circulatory care. In G.M. Bulechek & J.C. McCloskey (Eds.), Symposium on Nursing Interventions. Nursing Clinics of North America, 27(2), 445-476.

Johanson, B.C., Wells, S.J., Hoffmeister, D., & Dungca, C.U. (1988). Standards for critical care (3rd ed.). St. Louis: Mosby.

Olson, J., & Larsen, E. (1985). Cardiogenic shock. Emergency Care Quarterly, 1(2), 19-27.

Rice, V. (1991). Shock, a clinical syndrome: An update: 3. Therapeutic management. Critical Care Nurse, 11(6), 34-39.

Whitman, G. (1993). Shock. In M.R. Kinney, D.R. Packa, & S.B. Dunbar (Eds.), AACN's clinical reference for critical-care nursing (pp. 133-172). St. Louis: Mosby.

S

Shock Management: Vasogenic   4256

Definition: Promotion of adequate tissue perfusion for a patient with severe loss of vascular tone

Activities:

Perform dressing changes to prevent infection and/or promote healing, as appropriate

Limit invasive monitoring, to extent possible, to decrease the chance of infection

Administer antibiotics on schedule, if appropriate

Administer antihistamine medications, as appropriate

Administer epinephrine SQ emergently for anaphylaxis, if appropriate

Administer antiinflammatory medications, if appropriate

Remove stimuli precipitating neurogenic reaction, if appropriate

Treat hyperthermia with antipyretic drugs, a cooling mattress, or a sponge bath

Prevent or control shivering with medication or by wrapping the extremities

Monitor coagulation studies, including prothrombin time (PT), partial thromboplastin time (PTT), fibrinogen, fibrin degradation/split products, and platelet counts, as appropriate

Background Readings:

Cullen, L.M. (1992). Interventions related to circulatory care. In G.M. Bulechek & J.C. McCloskey (Eds.), Symposium on Nursing Interventions. Nursing Clinics of North America, 27(2), 445-476.

Hardaway, R. (1988). Vasodilative shock. In R. Hardaway (Ed.), Shock: The reversible stage of dying (pp. 311-314). Littleton, MA: PSG Publishing.

Hughes, M. (1990). Critical care nursing for the patient with a spinal cord injury. Critical Care Nursing Clinics of North America, 2(1), 33-40.

Johanson, B.C., Wells, S.J., Hoffmeister, D., & Dungca, C.U. (1988). Standards for critical care (3rd ed.). St. Louis: Mosby.

Rice, V. (1991). Shock, a clinical syndrome: An update: 3. Therapeutic management. Critical Care Nurse, 11(6), 34-39.

Schwenker, D. (1990). Cardiovascular considerations in the critical phase: Spinal cord injury. Critical Care Nursing Clinics of North America, 2(3), 363-367.

Tribett, D. (1993). Immulogic data acquisitions. In M. Kinney, D. Packa, & S. Dunbar (Eds.), AACN's clinical reference for critical-care nursing (3rd ed.) (pp. 1030-1031). St. Louis: Mosby.

S

Shock Management: Volume   4258

Definition: Promotion of adequate tissue perfusion for a patient with severely compromised intravascular volume

Activities:

Monitor for signs and symptoms of persistent bleeding (e.g., check all secretions for frank or occult blood)

Monitor the patient closely for hemorrhage

Prevent blood volume loss (e.g., apply pressure to site of bleeding)

Administer IV fluids, as appropriate

Note hemoglobin/hematocrit level before and after blood loss, as indicated

Administer blood products (e.g., platelets or fresh frozen plasma), as appropriate

Monitor coagulation studies, including prothrombin time (PT), partial thromboplastin time (PTT), fibrinogen, fibrin degradation/split products, and platelet counts, as appropriate

Apply MAST trousers, if appropriate

Background Readings:

Cullen, L.M. (1992). Interventions related to circulatory care. In G.M. Bulechek & J.C. McCloskey (Eds.), Symposium on Nursing Interventions. Nursing Clinics of North America, 27(2), 445-476.

Harvey, C. (1991). Critical care obstetrics. Rockville, MD: Aspen Publishing.

Johanson, B.C., Wells, S.J., Hoffmeister, D., & Dungca, C.U. (1988). Standards for critical care (3rd ed.). St. Louis: Mosby.

Kaldor, P. (1988). Medical and surgical therapies for gastrointestinal problems. In M. Kinney, D. Packa, & S. Dunbar (Eds.), AACN's clinical reference for critical-care nursing (pp. 1363-1366). St. Louis: Mosby.

Kitt, S., & Karser, J. (1990). Emergency nursing: A physiological and clinical perspective. Philadelphia: W.B. Saunders.

Rice, V. (1991). Shock, a clinical syndrome: An update: 3. Therapeutic management. Critical Care Nurse, 11(6), 34-39.

Whitman, G. (1993). Shock. In M.R. Kinney, D.R. Packa, & S.B. Dunbar (Eds.), AACN's clinical reference for critical-care nursing (pp. 133-172). St. Louis: Mosby.

S

Shock Prevention   4260

Definition: Detecting and treating a patient at risk for impending shock

Activities:

Monitor circulatory status: BP, skin color, skin temperature, heart sounds, heart rate and rhythm, presence and quality of peripheral pulses, and capillary refill

Monitor for signs of inadequate tissue oxygenation

Monitor for apprehension, increased anxiety, and changes in mental status

Monitor temperature and respiratory status

Monitor intake and output

Monitor laboratory values, especially hemoglobin and hematocrit levels, clotting profile, ABG and electrolyte levels, cultures, and chemistry profile

Monitor invasive hemodynamic parameters, as appropriate

Note bruising, petechiae, and condition of mucous membranes

Note color, amount, and frequency of stools, vomitus, and nasogastric drainage

Test urine for blood, glucose, and protein, as appropriate

Monitor abdominal pain and girth

Monitor for signs/symptoms of ascites

Monitor for early compensatory responses to fluid loss: increased heart rate, decreased BP, orthostatic hypotension, decreased urinary output, narrowed pulse pressure, decreased capillary refill, apprehension, pale and cool skin, and diaphoresis

Monitor for early signs of cardiogenic shock: declining cardiac output and urinary output, increasing SVR and PCWP, crackles in the lungs, S_3 and S_4 heart sounds, and tachycardia

Monitor for early signs of septic shock: warm, flushed, dry, skin; increasing cardiac output and temperature; and declining SVR and PAP

Monitor for early signs of allergic reactions: wheezing, hoarseness, chest tightness, dyspnea, itching, hives and wheals, angioedema, GI upset, anxiety, and restlessness

Monitor possible sources of fluid loss: chest tube, wound, and nasogastric drainage; diarrhea; vomiting; and increasing abdominal and extremity girth

Place patient in supine position with legs elevated to increase preload, as appropriate

Institute and maintain airway patency, as appropriate

Administer antiarrhythmic agents, as appropriate

Administer IV fluid challenge while monitoring cardiac loading pressures, cardiac output, and urinary output, as appropriate

Administer IV and/or oral fluids, as appropriate

Administer packed red blood cells and/or fresh frozen plasma, as appropriate

Administer diuretics, as appropriate

Administer vasodilators, as appropriate

Initiate early administration of antimicrobial agents and closely monitor their effectiveness, as appropriate

Insert and maintain large bore IV access

Administer oxygen and/or mechanical ventilation, as appropriate

Administer antiinflammatory agents and/or bronchodilators, as appropriate

Continued

Activities:—cont'd

Administer subcutaneous, IV, or endotracheal epinephrine, as appropriate

Teach patient to avoid known allergens and how to use an anaphylaxis kit, as appropriate

Perform skin testing to determine agents causing anaphylaxis and/or allergic reactions, as appropriate

Advise patients at risk for severe allergic reactions to undergo desensitization therapy

Instruct patient and/or family on precipitating factors of shock

Instruct patient and family about signs/symptoms of impending shock

Instruct patient and family about steps to take with onset of shock symptoms

Background Readings:

Price, S.A., & Wilson, L.M. (1986). Pathophysiology: Clinical concepts of disease processes (3rd ed.). New York: McGraw-Hill.

Thelan, L.A., & Urden, L.D. (1998). Critical care nursing: Diagnosis and management (3rd ed.). St. Louis: Mosby.

Thompson, J.M., McFarland, G.K., Hirsch, J.E., & Tucker, S.M. (1993). Mosby's clinical nursing (3rd ed.). St. Louis: Mosby.

Titler, M.G. (1992). Interventions related to surveillance. In G.M. Bulechek & J.C. McCloskey (Eds.), Symposium on Nursing Interventions. Nursing Clinics of North America, 27(2), 495-516.

S

Sibling Support   7280

Definition: Assisting a sibling to cope with a brother or sister's illness/chronic condition/ disability

Activities:

Explore what sibling knows about brother or sister

Appraise stress in sibling related to condition of affected brother or sister

Appraise sibling's coping with illness/disability of brother or sister

Facilitate family members' awareness of sibling's feelings

Provide information about common sibling responses and what other family members can do to help

Perform sibling advocacy role (e.g., in case of life-threatening situations when anxiety is high and parents or other family members are unable to perform that role)

Recognize that each sibling responds differently

Encourage parents or other family members to provide honest information to sibling

Encourage parents to arrange for care of young sibling in their own home, if possible

Assist sibling to maintain and/or modify usual routines and activities of daily living, as necessary

Promote communication between well sibling and affected brother or sister

Value each child individually, avoiding comparisons

Help child to see differences/similarities between self and sibling with special needs

Encourage sibling to visit affected brother or sister

Explain to visiting sibling what is being done in care of affected brother or sister

Encourage well sibling to participate in care of the affected brother or sister, as appropriate

Teach well sibling ways to interact with affected sister/brother

Permit siblings to settle own difficulties

Recognize and respect sibling who may not be emotionally ready to visit an affected brother or sister

Respect well sibling's reluctance to be with or to include child with special needs in activities

Encourage maintenance of parental or family interactional patterns

Assist parents to be fair in terms of discipline, resources, attention

Assist sibling to clarify and explore concerns

Use drawings, puppetry, and dramatic play to see how younger sibling perceives events

Clarify sibling concern about contracting the illness of the affected child, and develop strategies for coping with concern

Teach pathology of disease to sibling, according to developmental stage and learning style

Use concrete substitutes for sibling who is unable to visit affected brother or sister (e.g., pictures and videos)

Explain to young siblings that they are not the cause of illness

Teach well sibling strategies for meeting own emotional and developmental needs

Praise siblings when they have been patient, have sacrificed, or have been particularly helpful

Acknowledge the personal strengths siblings have and their abilities to cope with stress successfully

Provide referral to peer sibling group, as appropriate

Continued

Activities:—cont'd

Provide community resource referrals to sibling, as necessary

Communicate situation to the school nurse to promote support for well sibling, in accord with parental wishes

Background Readings:

Craft, M.J., & Craft, J. (1989). Perceived changes in siblings of hospitalized children: A comparison of parent and sibling report. Children's Health Care, 18(1), 42-49.

Craft, M.J., & Denehy, J.A. (Eds.). (1990). Nursing interventions for infants and children. Philadelphia: W.B. Saunders.

Craft, M.J., & Willadsen, J.A. (1992). Interventions related to family. In G.M. Bulechek & J.C. McCloskey (Eds.), Symposium on Nursing Interventions. Nursing Clinics of North America, 27(2), 517-540.

Ross-Alaolmolki, K. (1990). Coping with family loss: The death of a sibling. In M.J. Craft & J.A. Denehy (Eds.), Nursing interventions for infants and children (pp. 213-277). Philadelphia: W.B. Saunders.

Wong, D.L. (1997). Whaley and Wong's nursing care of infants and children (5th ed.). St. Louis: Mosby.

S

Simple Guided Imagery   6000

Definition: Purposeful use of imagination to achieve relaxation and/or direct attention away from undesirable sensations

Activities:

Screen for severe emotional problems, history of psychiatric illness, hallucinations, decreased energy, or inability to concentrate

Describe the rationale for and the benefits, limitations, and types of guided imagery techniques available

Elicit information on past coping experiences to determine whether guided imagery might be helpful

Determine capability for doing non–nurse-guided imagery (e.g., alone or with tape)

Encourage the individual to choose from a variety of guided imagery techniques (e.g., nurse-guided, taped)

Instruct the individual to assume a comfortable position, with nonrestrictive clothing and eyes closed

Provide comfortable environment without interruptions, as possible (e.g., supply headphones)

Discuss an image the patient has experienced that is pleasurable and relaxing, such as lying on a beach, watching a new snow fall, floating on a raft, or watching the sun set

Individualize the images chosen, considering religious or spiritual beliefs, artistic interest, or other individual preferences

Choose a scene that involves as many of the five senses as possible

Make suggestions to induce relaxation (e.g., peaceful images, pleasant sensations, or rhythmic breathing)

Use modulated voice when guiding the imagery experience

Have the patient travel mentally to the scene and assist in describing the setting in detail

Use permissive directions and suggestions when leading the imagery, such as "perhaps," "if you wish," or "you might like"

Have the patient slowly experience the scene; how does it look? smell? sound? feel? taste?

Use words or phrases that convey pleasurable images, such as floating, melting, releasing, and so on

Develop a cleansing or clearing portion of imagery (e.g., all pain appears as red dust and washes downstream in a creek as you enter)

Assist the patient to develop a method of ending the imagery technique, such as counting slowly while breathing deeply; slow movements; and thoughts of being relaxed, refreshed, and alert

Encourage patient to express thoughts and feelings regarding the experience

Prepare patient for unexpected (but often therapeutic) experiences, such as crying

Instruct patient to practice the imagery, if possible

Tape-record the imaged experience, if useful

Plan with patient an appropriate time to do guided imagery

Use the imagery techniques preventively

Plan follow-up to assess effects of imagery and any resultant changes in sensation and perception

Use guided imagery alone or in conjunction with other measures, as appropriate

Evaluate and document response to guided imagery

S

Continued

Background Readings:

Dossey, B. (1995). Using imagery to help heal your patient. American Journal of Nursing 95 (6), 41-46.

Herr, K.A., & Mobily, P.R. (1992). Interventions related to pain. In G.M. Bulechek & J.C. McCloskey (Eds.), Symposium on Nursing Interventions. Nursing Clinics of North America, 27(2), 347-370.

McCaffery, M., & Beebe, A. (1989). Pain: Clinical manual for nursing practice. St. Louis: Mosby–Year Book.

Scandrett-Hibdon, S., & Uecker, S. (1992). Relaxation training. In G.M. Bulechek & J.C. McCloskey (Eds.), Nursing interventions: Essential nursing treatments (2nd ed.) (pp. 434-461). Philadelphia: W.B. Saunders.

Sodergren, K.M (1992). Guided imagery. In M. Snyder (Ed.), Independent nursing interventions (2nd ed.) (pp. 95-109). Albany, NY: Delmar Publishers, Inc.

Teirnan, P.J. (1994). Independent nursing interventions: Relaxation and guided imagery in critical care. Critical Care Nurse, 14(5), 47-51.

S

Simple Massage   1480

Definition: Stimulation of the skin and underlying tissues with varying degrees of hand pressure to decrease pain, produce relaxation, and/or improve circulation

Activities:

Screen for contraindications, such as decreased platelets, decreased skin integrity, deep vein thrombosis, and hypersensitivity to touch

Determine the patient's degree of psychological comfort with touch

Select the area or areas of the body to be massaged

Prepare a warm, comfortable environment without distractions

Place in a position that facilitates massage

Apply moist heat before massage or during massage to other areas of the body, as indicated

Drape to expose only area to be massaged, as needed

Use warm lotion, oil, or dry powder to reduce friction (no lotion or oils on head or scalp), assessing for any sensitivity or contraindications

Massage, using continuous, even, and rhythmical movements

Massage the hands or feet, if other areas are inconvenient, or if more comfortable for the patient

Establish a period of time for massage that achieves the desired response

Adapt massage area, technique, and pressure to patient's perception of comfort and purpose of massage

Encourage patient to deep breathe and relax during massage

Encourage patient to concentrate on the good feelings of the massage

Avoid lengthy conversation during the massage, unless it is used as a distraction technique

Avoid massaging over areas of open lesion or tender skin

Instruct patient at completion of massage to rest until ready and then to move slowly

Use massage alone or in conjunction with other measures, as appropriate

Evaluate and document response to massage

Background Readings:

Herr, K.A., & Mobily, P.R. (1992). Interventions related to pain. In G.M. Bulechek & J.C. McCloskey (Eds.), Symposium on Nursing Interventions. Nursing Clinics of North America, 27(2), 347-370.

McCaffery, M., & Beebe, A. (1989). Pain. Clinical manual for nursing practice. St. Louis: Mosby.

Perry, A.G., & Potter, P.A. (1998). Clinical nursing skills and techniques, (4th ed.). St. Louis: Mosby.

Smith, M.C., Kemp, J., Hemphill, L. & Vojir, C.P. (2002). Outcomes of therapeutic massage for hospitalized cancer patients. Journal of Nursing Scholarship, 34(3), 257-267.

Snyder, M. (1992). Massage. In M. Snyder (Ed.), Independent nursing interventions (2nd ed.) (pp. 199-205). Albany, NY: Delmar Publishers.

S

Simple Relaxation Therapy   6040

Definition: Use of techniques to encourage and elicit relaxation for the purpose of decreasing undesirable signs and symptoms such as pain, muscle tension, or anxiety

Activities:

Describe the rationale for relaxation and the benefits, limits, and types of relaxation available (e.g., music therapy, meditation, and progressive muscle relaxation)

Determine whether any relaxation intervention in the past has been useful

Consider the individual's willingness to participate, ability to participate, preference, past experiences, and contraindications, before selecting a specific relaxation strategy

Provide detailed description of chosen relaxation intervention

Create a quiet, nondisrupting environment with dim lights and comfortable temperature, when possible

Instruct the individual to assume a comfortable position, with nonrestrictive clothing and eyes closed

Individualize the content of the relaxation intervention (e.g., by asking for suggestions of changes)

Elicit behaviors that are conditioned to produce relaxation, such as deep breathing, yawning, abdominal breathing, or peaceful imaging

Instruct patient to relax and let the sensations happen

Use low tone of voice with a slow, rhythmical pace of words

Demonstrate and practice the relaxation technique with the patient

Encourage return demonstrations of techniques, if possible

Anticipate the need for the use of relaxation

Provide written information about preparing and engaging in relaxation techniques

Encourage frequent repetition or practice of technique(s) selected

Provide undisturbed time, because patient may fall asleep

Encourage control of when the relaxation technique is performed

Regularly evaluate individual's report of relaxation achieved; and periodically monitor muscle tension, heart rate, blood pressure, and skin temperature, as appropriate

Plan to provide regular reinforcement for the use of relaxation, such as praising efforts and acknowledging positive outcomes

Develop a tape of the relaxation technique for the individual to use, as appropriate

Use relaxation therapy alone or in conjunction with other measures, as appropriate

Evaluate and document the response to relaxation therapy

Background Readings:

Herr, K.A., & Mobily, P.R. (1992). Interventions related to pain. In G.M. Bulechek & J.C. McCloskey (Eds.), Symposium on Nursing Interventions. Nursing Clinics of North America, 27(2), 347-370.

McCaffery, M., & Beebe, A. (1989). Pain. Clinical manual for nursing practice. St. Louis: Mosby.

Scandrett-Hibdon, S., & Uecker, S. (1992). Relaxation training. In G.M. Bulechek & J.C. McCloskey (Eds.), Nursing interventions: Essential nursing treatments (2nd ed.) (pp. 434-461). Philadelphia: W.B. Saunders.

S

Skin Care: Donor Site 3582

Definition: Prevention of wound complications and promotion of healing at the donor site.

Activities:

Verify that a complete history has been obtained and a physical exam has been performed prior to skin graft surgery

Provide adequate pain control (e.g., medication, music therapy, distraction, massage)

Incorporate moist wound healing techniques for skin autografts

Cover donor site for skin autografts postoperatively with an alginate and a transparent, semi-occlusive dressing, per agency protocol

Inspect the dressing daily, per agency protocol

Monitor for signs of infection (e.g., fever, pain) and other postoperative complications

Keep skin donor site clean, dry, and free from pressure

Instruct individual to keep healed skin donor site soft and pliable with cream (e.g., lanolin, olive oil)

Instruct individual to avoid exposing skin donor site to extremes in temperature, external trauma, and sunlight

Background Readings:

Mendez-Eastman, S.K. (2001). Skin grafting: Preoperative, intraoperative, and postoperative care. Plastic Surgical Nursing, 21(1), 49-51.

Smeltzer, S.C., & Bare, B.G. (1996). Brunner and Suddarth's textbook of medical-surgical nursing (8th ed.) (pp. 805, 1535-1536, 1567). Philadelphia: Lippincott.

S

Skin Care: Graft Site   3583

Definition: Prevention of wound complications and promotion of graft site healing

Activities:

Verify that a complete history has been obtained and a physical exam has been performed prior to skin graft surgery

Apply dressings made of cotton or gauze to maintain adequate tension on the graft site, per agency protocol

Provide adequate pain control (e.g., medication, music therapy, distraction, massage)

Elevate graft site until graft-host circulation develops (approximately one week), then allow the graft site to be in a dependent position for progressively longer periods of time, per agency protocol

Utilize needle aspiration to evacuate fluids from beneath the graft to maintain close contact between the recipient bed and the graft during the postoperative revascularization period

Avoid "rolling" the blebs of fluid to the edge of the graft during the postoperative revascularization period

Avoid friction and shearing forces at new graft site

Limit patient activity to bed rest until graft adheres

Instruct the patient to keep the affected part immobilized as much as possible during healing

Inspect the dressing daily, per agency protocol

Monitor color, warmth, capillary refill, and turgor of graft, if site is not dressed

Monitor for signs of infection (e.g., fever, pain) and other postoperative complications

Incorporate aggressive efforts to prevent development of pneumonia, pulmonary emboli, and pressure ulcers during period of immobility

Provide emotional support, understanding, and consideration to patient and family members in times when graft does not take

Support patient to appropriately ventilate anger, hostility, and frustration if graft does not take

Instruct patient on methods to protect the graft area from mechanical and thermal assaults (e.g., exposure to sun, use of heating pads)

Instruct patient to utilize compression stockings, pads, or straps to protect the graft site

Instruct patients to regularly apply artificial lubrication to graft site, as necessary

Instruct patient that protection of graft site may be necessary for years following the graft

Instruct patient that smoking decreases blood supply to the graft-recipient bed interface and increases chances of graft failure, and thus should be avoided

S

Background Readings:

Donato, M.C., Novicki, D.C., & Blume, P.A. (2000). Skin grafting: Historic and practical approaches. Clinics in Podiatric Medicine and Surgery, 17(4), 561-598.

Lewis, S.M., Heitkemper, M.M., & Dirksen, S.R. (2000). Medical-surgical nursing: Assessment and management of clinical problems (5th ed.) (pp. 515-516, 543-544). St. Louis: Mosby.

Mendez-Eastman, S.K. (2001). Skin grafting: Preoperative, intraoperative, and postoperative care. Plastic Surgical Nursing, 21(1), 49-51.

Smeltzer, S.C., & Bare, B.G. (1996). Brunner and Suddarth's textbook of medical-surgical nursing (8th ed.) (pp. 1534-1536, 1567). Philadelphia: Lippincott.

Waymack, P., Duff, R.G., & Sabolinski, M. (2000). The effect of a tissue engineered bilayered living skin analog, over meshed split-thickness autografts on the healing of excised burn wounds. Burns, 26, 609-619.

White, L., & Duncan, G. (2002). Medical-surgical nursing: An integrated approach (2nd ed.) (p. 522). Ft. Wayne, IN: Delmar/Thomson Learning.

Skin Care: Topical Treatments   3584

Definition: Application of topical substances or manipulation of devices to promote skin integrity and minimize skin breakdown

Activities:

Avoid using rough-textured bed linens

Clean with antibacterial soap, as appropriate

Dress patient in nonrestrictive clothing

Dust the skin with medicated powder, as appropriate

Remove adhesive tape and debris

Provide support to edematous areas (e.g., pillow under arms and scrotal support), as appropriate

Apply lubricant to moisten lips and oral mucosa, as needed

Administer back rub/neck rub, as appropriate

Change condom catheter, as appropriate

Apply diapers loosely, as appropriate

Place on incontinence pads, as appropriate

Massage around the affected area

Apply appropriately fitting ostomy appliance, as needed

Cover the hands with mittens, as appropriate

Provide toilet hygiene, as needed

Refrain from giving local heat applications

Refrain from using an alkaline soap on the skin

Soak in a colloidal bath, as appropriate

Keep bed linen clean, dry, and wrinkle free

Turn the immobilized patient at least every 2 hours, according to a specific schedule

Use devices on the bed (e.g., sheepskin) that protect the patient

Apply heel protectors, as appropriate

Apply drying powders to deep skinfolds

Initiate consultation services of the enterostomal therapy nurse, as needed

Apply clear occlusive dressing (e.g., Tegaderm or Duoderm), as needed

Apply topical antibiotic to the affected area, as appropriate

Apply topical antiinflammatory agent to the affected area, as appropriate

Apply emollients to the affected area

Apply topical antifungal agent to the affected area, as appropriate

Apply topical debriding agent to the affected area, as appropriate

Paint or spray skin warts with liquid nitrogen, as appropriate

Inspect skin of patients at risk of breakdown daily

Document degree of skin breakdown

Add moisture to environment with a humidifier, as needed

Continued

Background Readings:

Frantz, R.A., & Gardner, S. (1994). Management of dry skin. Journal of Gerontological Nursing, 20(9), 15-18.

Hardy, M.A. (1992). Dry skin care. In G.M. Bulechek & J.C. McCloskey (Eds.), Nursing interventions: Essential nursing treatments (2nd ed.) (pp. 34-47). Philadelphia: W.B. Saunders.

Kemp, M.G. (1994). Protecting the skin from moisture and associated irritants. Journal of Gerontological Nursing, 20(9), 8-14.

Titler, M.G., Pettit, D., Bulechek, G.M., McCloskey, J.C., Craft, M.J., Cohen, M.Z., Crossley, J.D., Denehy, J.A., Glick, O.J., Kruckeberg, T.W., Maas, M.L., Prophet, C.M., & Tripp-Reimer, T. (1991). Classification of nursing interventions for care of the integument. Nursing Diagnosis, 2(2), 45-56.

S

Skin Surveillance   3590

Definition: Collection and analysis of patient data to maintain skin and mucous membrane integrity

Activities:

Inspect condition of surgical incision, as appropriate

Observe extremities for color, warmth, swelling, pulses, texture, edema, and ulcerations

Inspect skin and mucous membranes for redness, extreme warmth, or drainage

Monitor skin for areas of redness and breakdown

Monitor for sources of pressure and friction

Monitor for infection, especially of edematous areas

Monitor skin and mucous membranes for areas of discoloration and bruising

Monitor skin for rashes and abrasions

Monitor skin for excessive dryness and moistness

Inspect clothing for tightness

Monitor skin color

Monitor skin temperature

Note skin or mucous membrane changes

Institute measures to prevent further deterioration, as needed

Instruct family member/caregiver about signs of skin breakdown, as appropriate

Background Readings:

Deters, G.R. (1991). Management of patients with dermatologic problems. In S.C. Smeltzer, & B.G. Bare (Eds.), Brunner and Suddarth's textbook of medical-surgical nursing (5th ed.) (pp. 809-837). Philadelphia: J.B. Lippincott.

Sundberg, M.C. (1989). Promoting personal hygiene and skin integrity. In M.C. Sundberg, Fundamentals of nursing with clinical procedures (2nd ed.) (pp. 570-600). Boston: Jones & Bartlett.

Titler, M.G., Pettit, D., Bulechek, G.M., McCloskey, J.C., Craft, M.J., Cohen, M.Z., Crossley, J.D., Denehy, J.A., Glick, O.J., Kruckeberg, T.W., Maas, M.L., Prophet, C.M., & Tripp-Reimer, T. (1991). Classification of nursing interventions for care of the integument. Nursing Diagnosis, 2(2), 45-56.

S

Sleep Enhancement 1850

Definition: Facilitation of regular sleep/wake cycles

Activities:

Determine patient's sleep/activity pattern

Approximate patient's regular sleep/wake cycle in planning care

Explain the importance of adequate sleep during pregnancy, illness, psychosocial stresses, etc.

Determine the effects of the patient's medications on sleep pattern

Monitor/record patient's sleep pattern and number of sleep hours

Monitor patient's sleep pattern, and note physical (e.g., sleep apnea, obstructed airway, pain/discomfort, and urinary frequency) and/or psychological (e.g., fear or anxiety) circumstances that interrupt sleep

Instruct patient to monitor sleep patterns

Monitor participation in fatigue-producing activities during wakefulness to prevent overtiredness

Adjust environment (e.g., light, noise, temperature, mattress, and bed) to promote sleep

Encourage patient to establish a bedtime routine to facilitate transition from wakefulness to sleep

Facilitate maintenance of patient's usual bedtime routines, presleep cues/props, and familiar objects (e.g., for children, a favorite blanket/toy, rocking, pacifier, or story; for adults, a book to read, etc.), as appropriate

Assist to eliminate stressful situations before bedtime

Monitor bedtime food and beverage intake for items that facilitate or interfere with sleep

Instruct patient to avoid bedtime foods and beverages that interfere with sleep

Assist patient to limit daytime sleep by providing activity that promotes wakefulness, as appropriate

Instruct patient how to perform autogenic muscle relaxation or other nonpharmacological forms of sleep inducement

Initiate/implement comfort measures of massage, positioning, and affective touch

Promote an increase in number of hours of sleep, if needed

Provide for naps during the day, if indicated, to meet sleep requirements

Group care activities to minimize number of awakenings; allow for sleep cycles of at least 90 minutes

Adjust medication administration schedule to support patient's sleep/wake cycle

Instruct the patient and significant others about factors (e.g., physiological, psychological, lifestyle, frequent work shift changes, rapid time zone changes, excessively long work hours, and other environmental factors) that contribute to sleep pattern disturbances

Identify what sleep medications patient is taking

Encourage use of sleep medications that do not contain REM sleep suppressor(s)

Regulate environmental stimuli to maintain normal day-night cycles

Discuss with patient and family sleep-enhancing techniques

Provide pamphlet with information about sleep enhancement techniques

S

Background Readings:

Glick, O.J. (1992). Interventions related to activity and movement. In G.M. Bulechek & J.C. McCloskey (Eds.), Symposium on Nursing Interventions. Nursing Clinics of North America, 27(2), 541-554.

Guyton, A. (1991). Textbook of medical physiology (8th ed.). Philadelphia: W.B. Saunders.

McFarland, G.K., & McFarlane, E.A. (1997). Nursing diagnosis and intervention (3rd ed.). St. Louis: Mosby.

Prinz, P., Vitiello, M., Raskind, M., et al. (1990). Geriatrics: Sleep disorders and aging. New England Journal of Medicine, 322(8), 520.

Schibler, K.D., & Fay, S.A. (1990). Sleep promotion. In M.J. Craft & J.A. Denehy (Eds.), Nursing interventions for infants and children (pp. 285-303). Philadelphia: W.B. Saunders.

Treatment of sleep disorders of older people. (1990). National Institutes of Health Consensus Development Conference, 8(3), 1-22.

Smoking Cessation Assistance   4490

Definition: Helping another to stop smoking

Activities:

Record current smoking status and smoking history

Determine patient's readiness to learn about smoking cessation

Monitor patient's readiness to attempt to quit smoking

Give smoker clear, consistent advice to quit smoking

Help patient identify reasons to quit and barriers to quitting

Instruct patient on the physical symptoms of nicotine withdrawal (e.g., headache, dizziness, nausea, irritability, and insomnia)

Reassure patient that physical withdrawal symptoms from nicotine are temporary

Inform patient about nicotine replacement products (e.g., patch, gum, nasal spray, inhaler) to help reduce physical withdrawal symptoms

Assist patient to identify psychosocial aspects (e.g., positive and negative feelings associated with smoking) that influence smoking behavior

Assist patient in developing a smoking cessation plan that addresses psychosocial aspects that influence smoking behavior

Assist patient to recognize cues that prompt him/her to smoke (e.g., being around others who smoke, frequenting places where smoking is allowed)

Assist patient to develop practical methods to resist cravings (e.g., spend time with nonsmoking friends, frequent places where smoking is not allowed, relaxation exercises)

Help choose best method for giving up cigarettes, when patient is ready to quit

Help motivated smokers to set a quit date

Provide encouragement to maintain a smoke-free lifestyle (e.g., make the quit day a celebration day; encourage self-rewards at specific intervals of smoke-free living, such as at 1 week, 1 month, 6 months; encourage saving money used previously on smoking materials to buy a special reward)

Encourage patient to join a smoking cessation support group that meets weekly

Refer to group programs or individual therapists, as appropriate

Assist patient with any self-help methods

Help patient plan specific coping strategies and resolve problems that result from quitting

Advise to avoid dieting while trying to give up smoking because it can undermine chances of quitting

Advise to work out a plan to cope with others who smoke and to avoid being around them

Inform patient that dry mouth, cough, scratchy throat, and feeling on edge are symptoms that may occur after quitting; the patch or gum may help with cravings

Advise patient to keep a list of "slips" or near slips, what causes them, and what he/she learned from them

Advise patient to avoid smokeless tobacco, dipping, and chewing as these can lead to addiction and/or health problems including oral cancer, gum problems, loss of teeth, and heart disease

Manage nicotine replacement therapy

Contact national and local resource organizations for resource materials

Follow patient for 2 years after quitting if possible, to provide encouragement

Arrange to maintain frequent telephone contact with patient (e.g., to acknowledge that withdrawal is difficult, to reinforce the importance of remaining abstinent, to offer congratulations on progress)

S

Continued

Activities:—cont'd

Help patient deal with any lapses (e.g., reassure patient that he/she is not a "failure," reassure that much can be learned from this temporary regression, assist patient in identifying reasons for the relapse)

Support patient who begins smoking again by helping to identify what has been learned

Encourage the relapsed patient to try again

Promote policies that establish and enforce smoke-free environment

Serve as a nonsmoking role model

Background Readings:

Lenaghan, N.A. (2000). The nurse's role in smoking cessation. MEDSURG Nursing, 9(6), 298-312.

O'Connell, K.A. (1990). Smoking cessation: Research on relapse crises. In J.J. Fitzpatrick, R.L. Taunton, & J.Z. Benoliel (Eds.), Annual Review of Nursing Research, 8, 83-100. New York: Springer Publishing.

O'Connell, K.A., & Koerin, C.A. (1999). Smoking cessation assistance. In G.M. Bulechek & J.C. McCloskey (Eds.), Nursing interventions: Effective nursing treatments (3rd ed.) (pp. 438-450). Philadelphia: W.B. Saunders.

U.S. Department of Health and Human Services. (1997). Smoking cessation: Clinical practice guideline No. 18. Rockville, MD: Agency for Health Care Policy & Research.

Wewers, M.E., & Ahijeoych, K.L. (1996). Smoking cessation interventions in chronic illness. In J.J. Fitzpatrick & J. Norbeck. (Eds.), Annual Review of Nursing Research, 14, 75-93.

S

Socialization Enhancement   5100

Definition: Facilitation of another person's ability to interact with others

Activities:

Encourage enhanced involvement in already established relationships

Encourage patience in developing relationships

Encourage relationships with persons who have common interests and goals

Encourage social and community activities

Encourage sharing of common problems with others

Encourage honesty in presenting oneself to others

Encourage involvement in totally new interests

Encourage respect for the rights of others

Refer patient to interpersonal skills group or program in which understanding of transactions can be increased, as appropriate

Allow testing of interpersonal limits

Give feedback about improvement in care of personal appearance or other activities

Help patient increase awareness of strengths and limitations in communicating with others

Use role playing to practice improved communication skills and techniques

Provide role models who express anger appropriately

Confront patient about impaired judgment, when appropriate

Request and expect verbal communication

Give positive feedback when patient reaches out to others

Encourage patient to change environment, such as going outside for walks or to movies

Facilitate patient input and planning of future activities

Encourage small group planning for special activities

Explore strengths and weaknesses of current network of relationships

Background Readings:

Drury, J., & Akins, J. (1991). Sensory/perceptual alterations. In M. Maas, K. Buckwalter, & M. Hardy (Eds.), Nursing diagnoses and interventions for the elderly (pp. 369-389). Redwood City, CA: Addison-Wesley.

Elsen, J., & Blegen, M. (1991). Social isolation. In M. Maas, K. Buckwalter, & M. Hardy (Eds.). Nursing diagnoses and interventions for the elderly (pp. 519-529). Redwood City, CA: Addison-Wesley.

Pender, N.J. (1982). Health promotion in nursing practice (pp. 367-382). Norwalk, CT: Appleton-Century-Crofts.

S

Specimen Management 7820

Definition: Obtaining, preparing, and preserving a specimen for a laboratory test

Activities:

Obtain required sample, according to protocol

Instruct patient how to collect and preserve specimen, as appropriate

Provide specimen container required

Apply special specimen collection devices, as needed, for infants, toddlers, or impaired adults

Assist with the biopsy of a tissue or organ, as appropriate

Assist with aspiration of fluid from a body cavity, as appropriate

Store specimen collected over time, according to protocol

Seal all specimen containers to prevent leakage or contamination

Label specimen with appropriate data

Place specimen in appropriate container for transport

Arrange transport of the specimen to the laboratory

Order specimen-related routine laboratory tests, as appropriate

Background Readings:

Perry, A.G., & Potter, P.A. (1998). Clinical nursing skills and techniques (4th ed.). St. Louis: Mosby.

Smith, S., & Duell, D. (1992). Clinical nursing skills (3rd ed.). Los Altos, CA: National Nursing Review.

S

Spiritual Growth Facilitation 5426

Definition: Facilitation of growth in patient's capacity to identify, connect with, and call upon the source of meaning, purpose, comfort, strength, and hope in his/her life

Activities:

Demonstrate caring presence and comfort by spending time with patient, patient's family, and significant others

Encourage conversation that assists the patient in sorting out spiritual concerns

Model healthy relating and reasoning skills

Assist patient with identifying barriers and attitudes that hinder growth or self-discovery

Offer individual and group prayer support, as appropriate

Encourage participation in devotional services, retreats, and special prayer/study programs

Promote relationships with others for fellowship and service

Encourage use of spiritual celebration and rituals

Encourage patient's examination of his/her spiritual commitment based on beliefs and values

Provide an environment that fosters a meditative/contemplative attitude for self-reflection

Assist the patient to explore beliefs as related to healing of body, mind, and spirit

Refer to support groups, mutual self-help or other spiritually based programs, as appropriate

Refer for pastoral care or to primary spiritual caregiver as issues warrant

Refer for additional guidance and support in the body, mind, and spirit connection, as needed

Background Readings:

Carson, V.B. (1993). Spirituality: Generic or Christian. Journal of Christian Nursing, 4, 24-27.

Hawks, S., Hull, M., Thalman, R., & Ridhins, P.M. (1995). Review of spiritual health: Definition, role, & intervention strategies in health promotion. American Journal of Health Promotion, 9(5), 371-377.

Oldnall, A. (1996). A critical analysis of nursing: Meeting the spiritual needs of patients. Journal of Advanced Nursing, 23, 138-144.

Reed, P.G. (1991). Preferences for spiritually related nursing interventions among terminally ill and nonterminally ill hospitalized adults and well adults. Applied Nursing Research, 4(3), 122-128.

Reed, P.G. (1992). An emerging paradigm for the investigation of spirituality in nursing. Research in Nursing & Health, 15, 349-357.

Schnorr, M.A. (1990). Spiritual caregiving: A key component of parish nursing. In P.A. Solari-Twadell, A.M. Djupe, & M.A. McDermott (Eds.), Parish nursing: The developing practice. Park Ridge, IL: National Parish Nurse Resource Center.

S

Spiritual Support   5420

Definition: Assisting the patient to feel balance and connection with a greater power

Activities:

Use therapeutic communications to establish trust and demonstrate empathy

Utilize tools to monitor and evaluate spiritual well-being, as appropriate

Encourage individual to review past life and focus on events and relationships that provided spiritual strength and support

Treat individual with dignity and respect

Encourage life review through reminiscence

Encourage participation in interactions with family members, friends, and others

Provide privacy and quiet times for spiritual activities

Encourage participation in support groups

Teach methods of relaxation, meditation, and guided imagery

Share own beliefs about meaning and purpose, as appropriate

Share own spiritual perspective, as appropriate

Provide opportunities for discussion of various belief systems and world views

Be open to individual's expressions of concern

Pray with the individual

Provide spiritual music, literature, or radio or TV programs to the individual

Be open to individual's expressions of loneliness and powerlessness

Encourage chapel service attendance, if desired

Encourage the use of spiritual resources, if desired

Provide desired spiritual articles, according to individual preferences

Refer to spiritual advisor of individual's choice

Use values clarification techniques to help individual clarify beliefs and values, as appropriate

Be available to listen to individual's feelings

Express empathy with individual's feelings

Facilitate individual's use of meditation, prayer, and other religious traditions and rituals

Listen carefully to individual's communication, and develop a sense of timing for prayer or spiritual rituals

Assure individual that nurse will be available to support individual in times of suffering

Be open to individual's feelings about illness and death

Assist individual to properly express and relieve anger in appropriate ways

Background Readings:

Dossey, B.M. (1998). Attending to holistic care. American Journal of Nursing, 98(8), 35-38.

Harris Sumner, C. (1998). Recognizing and responding. American Journal of Nursing, 98(1), 26-30.

Harvey, S.A. (2001). S.C.A.L.E.—Spiritual care at life's end: A multi-disciplinary approach to end-of-life issues in a hospital setting. Medical Reference Services Quarterly, 20(4), 63-71.

LeMone, P. (2001). Spiritual distress. In M.L. Maas, K.C. Buckwater, M.D. Hardy, T. Tripp-Reimer, M.G. Titler, & J.P. Specht (Eds.), Nursing care of older adults: Diagnoses, outcomes and interventions (Chapter 62). St. Louis: Mosby.

Maddox, M. (2002). Spiritual assessments in primary care. The Nurse Practitioner, 27(2), 12, 14.

S

Meraviglia, M.G. (1999). Critical analysis of spirituality and its empirical indicators: Prayer and meaning in life. Journal of Holistic Nursing, 17(1), 18-33.

Penrod Hermann, C. (2001). Spiritual needs of dying patients: A qualitative study. Oncology Nursing Forum, 28(1), 67-72.

Vandenbrink, R.A. (2001). Spiritual assessment: Comparing the tools. Journal of Christian Nursing, 18(3), 24-27.

Van Dover, L.J., & Bacon, J.M. (2001). Spiritual care in nursing practice: A close-up view. Nursing Forum, 36(3), 18-30.

S

Splinting 0910

Definition: Stabilization, immobilization, and/or protection of an injured body part with a supportive appliance

Activities:

Position body part with sandbags or other device, as appropriate

Support the affected body part

Apply an air splint, as appropriate

Apply a sling to rest an injured body part

Pad injured area to prevent friction from the appliance, as appropriate

Splint an injured leg in an extended position, as appropriate

Splint an injured arm in a flexed or extended position, as appropriate

Move the injured extremity as little as possible

Stabilize proximal and distal joints in the splint, when possible

Monitor circulation in affected body part

Monitor for bleeding at injury site

Monitor skin integrity under supportive appliance

Support feet using a footboard, as appropriate

Support paralyzed hands in a functional position

Encourage isometric exercises, as appropriate

Teach patient how to observe and care for the splint

Background Readings:

Perry, A.G., & Potter, P.A. (1998). Clinical nursing skills and techniques (4th ed.). St. Louis: Mosby.

Ruda, S.C. (1991). Common ankle injuries of the athlete. Nursing Clinics of North America, 26(1), 167-180.

Smith, S., & Duell, D. (1992). Clinical nursing skills (3rd ed). Los Altos, CA: National Nursing Review.

S

Sports-Injury Prevention: Youth   6648

Definition: Reduce the risk of sports-related injury in young athletes

Activities:

Encourage general fitness as prerequisite to participation in sports

Encourage modification of game rules according to age and ability of participants

Inform parents of the differences between recreational and organized competitive sports

Assist athlete in finding a sport that is a good fit with interests and abilities and that will promote the development of life-long fitness behaviors

Assist parents and athletes to set realistic goals for participation

Provide resources for parents, athletes, and coaches concerning the psychosocial aspects of sports involvement

Encourage appropriate matching of competitors by age, weight, and stage of physical maturation

Monitor adherence to recommended training guidelines and correct biomechanics

Monitor compliance with safety rules

Monitor field of play for safe playing conditions

Monitor proper use and condition of safety equipment

Encourage appropriate supervision for training, recreation, and competitive events

Monitor sports physicals to ensure they are complete before participation

Encourage use of warm-up and cool-down activities to prevent injuries

Use certified athletic trainers for competitive sports at the junior and senior high school levels

Ensure medical coverage at competitive sporting events, as appropriate

Develop an emergency plan in case of serious injury

Coordinate preseason seminars for athletes, families, and coaches, to increase awareness of injury prevention

Collaborate with other professionals in planning programs related to injury prevention

Inform parents and athletes of steps they can take to prevent injuries

Inform parents and athletes of signs and symptoms of overuse injuries, dehydration, heat exhaustion, use of performance-enhancing drugs, eating disorders, menstrual dysfunction, and stress

Collect data on injury type, rate, treatment, and referrals

Monitor the long-term health of athletes

Monitor return of injured athletes to participation to prevent reinjury

Provide emotional support for athletes experiencing injury

Arrange for coaches to get annual CPR and first aid training

Communicate with coaches the importance of emphasizing "fun" in sports

Ensure that coaches are well informed of normal childhood development and the physical, emotional, and social needs of children

Communicate information about special health care concerns of individual athletes, as appropriate

Develop oversight groups to ensure education of school and volunteer coaches

Inform parents of qualifications and behavior expected of coaches

Encourage parents to become involved in their children's sports programs

Continued

S

Monitor athletes for sports-related stress and provide referrals for athletes with emotional/psychosocial concerns

Teach relaxation techniques and coping strategies to athletes, coaches, and parents

Advocate for the health of young athletes

Background Readings:

American College of Sports Medicine. (1994). The prevention of sport injuries of children and adolescents. Journal of American Academy of Physician's Assistants, 7(6), 437-442.

Dyment, P. (1991). Sports medicine: Health care for young athletes. Elk Grove Village, IL.: The American Academy of Pediatrics.

Hutchinson, M.R. (1997). Cheerleading injuries, patterns, prevention, case reports. The Physician and Sports Medicine, 15(9), 83-86, 89-91, 96.

Overbaugh, K., & Allen, J. (1994). The adolescent athlete. Part I: Pre-season preparation and examination. Journal of Pediatric Health Care, 8(4), 146-151.

Overbaugh, K., & Allen, J. (1994). The adolescent athlete. Part II: Injury patterns and prevention. Journal of Pediatric Health Care, 8(5), 203-211.

Petlichkoff, L.M. (1992). Youth sport participation and withdrawal: Is it simply a matter of FUN? Pediatric Exercise Science, 4, 105-110.

S

Staff Development   7850

Definition: Developing, maintaining, and monitoring competence of staff

Activities:

Identify learning needs of staff (e.g., new or change in policy and procedures, new hire to organization, transfer within organization, new job requirements, cross-training, equipment upgrades, emerging trends, skills training)

Identify learner characteristics (e.g., literacy, language, educational background, previous experience, age, motivation, attitude)

Identify performance problem(s) (e.g., knowledge deficit, skill deficit, motivational deficit), as needed

Identify instructional goal(s) (e.g., inform staff of changes, provide knowledge and skills, improve proficiency, improve competence)

Identify standard(s) of learning achievement (e.g., psychomotor, interpersonal, critical thinking)

Determine instructional learning objectives

Identify instructional content

Identify instructional constraints (e.g., time, cost, equipment availability)

Identify resources that support instruction (e.g., expert consultation, learning materials, time, fiscal resources)

Identify appropriate individual(s) to provide instruction

Organize and develop instructional content

Design teaching and learning activities

Design methods of pre and post assessment/evaluation

Provide instructional program (e.g., self-directed learning packets, classroom presentation, small group presentation, on-the-job training)

Evaluate effectiveness of the instruction

Provide feedback on results of staff development instruction to appropriate individuals

Monitor competence of staff skills

Conduct periodic review of competencies

Determine needed frequency of staff development instruction in order to maintain competency

Provide financial assistance and time off to attend educational programs as required by job

Encourage participation in peer review

Encourage reading of professional journals

Encourage participation in professional organizations

Background Readings:

Alspach, J.G. (1995). The educational process in nursing staff development. St. Louis: Mosby.

Kelly, K.J. (1992). Nursing staff development: Current competence, future focus. Philadelphia: J.B. Lippincott.

Rodriguez, L., Patton, C., Stiesmeyer, J.K., & Teikmanis, M.L. (Eds.). (1996). Manual of staff development. St. Louis: Mosby.

S

Staff Supervision 7830

Definition: Facilitating the delivery of high-quality patient care by others

Activities:

Create a work environment that validates the importance of each employee to the organization

Acknowledge an employee's area of expertise

Select a management style appropriate to the work situation and employee characteristics

Encourage open communication

Identify opportunities for participation in decision making

Provide a job description for all new employees

Provide clear expectations for job performance

Share evaluation methods used with employee

Foster teamwork and a sense of purpose for the work group

Set goals for staff, as appropriate

Consider employee growth in work assignments

Share information about the organization and future plans

Listen to employee concerns and suggestions

Provide feedback on work performance at regular intervals

Provide coaching and encouragement

Reinforce good/excellent performance verbally

Provide recognition for behavior that supports organizational goals

Maintain an attitude of trust of others

Seek advice from employees, as appropriate

Use informal networks to accomplish goals

Provide challenges and opportunities for employee growth

Monitor quality of work performance

Monitor quality of employee's relationships with other health care providers

Document strengths and weaknesses of employee

Counsel, when appropriate

Facilitate employee opportunities to be "winners"

Seek information on employee concerns for patient care and the work environment

Seek feedback from patients concerning care provided

Encourage staff to solve own problems

Initiate disciplinary action, as appropriate, following policies and procedures

Counsel employee on how to improve performance, as appropriate

Set time frames for needed behavior changes, as appropriate

Provide reeducation, as needed, to improve performance

Complete evaluation forms at appropriate time intervals

Discuss evaluation results privately

Background Readings:

Buccheri, R.C. (1986). Nursing supervision: A new look at an old role. Nursing Administration Quarterly, 11(1), 11-25.

Christen, J.W. (1987). The changing nature of first-line supervision. The Health Care Supervisor, 5(2), 65-70.

Hersey, P. (1989). Situational leadership in nursing. Norwalk, CT: Appleton & Lange.

Hersey, P., & Blanchard, K. (1996). Management of organizational behavior: Utilizing human resources (7th ed.). Englewood Cliffs, NJ: Prentice-Hall.

Swansburg, R.C. (1990). Management and leadership for nurse managers. Boston: Jones & Bartlett Publishers.

S

Subarachnoid Hemorrhage Precautions 2720

Definition: Reduction of internal and external stimuli or stressors to minimize risk of rebleeding prior to aneurysm surgery

Activities:

Manipulate lighting for therapeutic benefit

Place patient in a private room

Restrict visitors

Decrease stimuli in patient's environment

Maintain hemodynamic parameters within prescribed limits

Monitor neurological status

Give sedation, as needed

Restrict TV, radio, and other stimulants

Avoid taking rectal temperatures

Administer stool softeners

Administer anticonvulsants, as appropriate

Monitor ICP and CPP

Monitor pulse and BP

Monitor intake and output

Administer pain medications PRN

Restrict physical activity

Implement seizure precautions

Monitor serum electrolyte levels

Monitor hemoglobin/hematocrit levels

Background Readings:

Ackerman, L.L. (1992). Interventions related to neurological care. In G.M. Bulechek & J.C. McCloskey (Eds.), Symposium on Nursing Interventions. Nursing Clinics of North America, 27(2), 325-346.

Cammermeyer, M., & Appeldorn, C. (Eds.). (1990). Core curriculum for neuroscience nursing (3rd ed.) (pp. Ia1-Ia4). Chicago: American Association of Neuroscience Nurses.

Hummel, S.K. (1989). Cerebral vasospasm: Current concepts of pathogenesis and treatment. Journal of Neuroscience Nursing, 21(4), 216-224.

Johanson, B.C., Wells, S.J., Hoffmeister, D., & Dungca, C.U. (1988). Standards for critical care (3rd ed.). St. Louis: Mosby.

MacDonald, E. (1989). Aneurysmal subarachnoid hemorrhage. Journal of Neuroscience Nursing, 21(5), 313-321.

Marshall, S.B., Marshall, L.F., Vos, H.R., et al. (1990). Neuroscience critical care: Pathophysiology and patient management. Philadelphia: W.B. Saunders.

S

Substance Use Prevention   4500

Definition: Prevention of an alcoholic or drug use lifestyle

Activities:

Assist individual to tolerate increased levels of stress, as appropriate

Prepare individual for difficult or painful events

Reduce irritating or frustrating environmental stress

Reduce social isolation, as appropriate

Support measures to regulate the sale and distribution of alcohol to minors

Lobby for increased drinking age

Recommend responsible changes in the alcohol and drug curricula for primary grades

Conduct programs in schools on the avoidance of drugs and alcohol as recreational activities

Encourage responsible decision making about lifestyle choices

Recommend media campaigns on substance use issues in the community

Instruct parents in the importance of example regarding substance use

Instruct parents and teachers in the identification of signs and symptoms of addiction

Assist individual to identify substitute tension-reducing strategies

Support or organize community groups to reduce injuries associated with alcohol, such as SADD and MADD

Survey students in grades 1 to 12 on the use of alcohol and drugs and alcohol-related behaviors

Instruct parents to support school policy that prohibits drug and alcohol consumption at extracurricular activities

Assist in the organization of substance-free activities for teenagers for such functions as prom and homecoming

Facilitate coordination of efforts between various community groups concerned with substance use

Encourage parents to participate in children's activities beginning in preschool through adolescence

Background Readings:

Finley, B. (1989). The role of the psychiatric nurse in the community substance abuse prevention program. Nursing Clinics of North America, 24(1), 121-136.

Hagemaster, J. (1999). Substance use prevention. In G.M. Bulechek & J.C. McCloskey (Eds.), Nursing interventions: Effective nursing treatments (3rd ed.) (pp. 482-490). Philadelphia: W.B. Saunders Company.

Hahn, E.J (1995). Predicting Head Start parent involvement in an alcohol and other drug prevention program. Nursing Research, 44(1), 45-51.

Solari-Twadell, P.A. (1990). Recreational drugs: Societal and professional issues. Nursing Clinics of North America, 26(2), 499-509

S

Substance Use Treatment   4510

Definition: Supportive care of patient/family members with physical and psychosocial problems associated with the use of alcohol or drugs

Activities:

Establish a therapeutic relationship with patient

Identify with patient those factors (e.g., genetic, psychological distress, and stress) that contribute to chemical dependency

Encourage patient to take control over own behavior

Assist patient/family to identify use of denial as a substitute for confronting the problem

Help family members recognize that chemical dependency is a family disease

Determine substance(s) used

Discuss with patient the impact of substance use on medical condition or general health

Discuss with patient the effect of associations with other users during leisure or work time

Determine history of drug/alcohol use

Assist patient to identify the negative effects of chemical dependency on health, family, and daily functioning

Instruct patient/family that the volume/frequency of substance use leading to dependency varies greatly among patients

Discuss effect of substance use on relationships with family, co-workers, and friends

Identify constructive goals with patient to provide alternatives to the use of substances to reduce stress

Assist the patient to determine whether moderation is an acceptable goal, considering health status

Facilitate support by significant others

Provide support to family or significant others, as appropriate

Set limits that benefit the patient and show caring

Screen patient at frequent intervals for continued substance use, using urine screens or breath analysis, as appropriate

Encourage patient to keep a detailed chart of substance use to evaluate progress

Assist the patient to evaluate the amount of time spent using the substance and the usual patterns within the day

Assist patient to select an alternative activity that is incompatible with the substance abused

Assist patient to learn alternate methods of coping with stress or emotional distress

Determine whether codependent relationships exist in the family

Identify support groups in the community for long-term substance abuse treatment

Instruct patient and family about drugs used to treat specific substance used

Background Readings:

Adams, F.A. (1988). Drug dependency in hospital patients. American Journal of Nursing, 88(4), 477-482.

Captain, C. (1989). Family recovery from alcoholism. Nursing Clinics of North America, 24(1), 55-67.

Chychula, N.M., & Okore, C. (1990). The cocaine epidemic: Treatment options for cocaine dependence. Nurse Practitioner, 15(8), 33-40.

Hough, G.S. (1976). A behavioral approach to alcoholism. Nursing Clinics of North America, 11(3), 507-515.

Kinney, J. (1996). Clinical manual of substance abuse (2nd ed.). St. Louis: Mosby.

Mittleman, J.S., Mittleman, R.E., & Elser, B. (1984). Cocaine. American Journal of Nursing, 84(9), 1092-1095.

Potter, P.A., & Perry, A.G. (1998). Fundamentals of nursing: Concepts, process and practice (4th ed.). St. Louis: Mosby.

Starling, B.P., & Martin, A.C. (1990). Adult survivors of parental alcoholism: Implications for primary care. Nurse Practitioner, 15(7), 16-24.

Substance Use Treatment: Alcohol Withdrawal   4512

Definition: Care of the patient experiencing sudden cessation of alcohol consumption

Activities:

Create a low-stimulation environment for detoxification

Monitor vital signs during withdrawal

Monitor for delirium tremens (DTs)

Administer anticonvulsants or sedatives, as appropriate

Medicate to relieve physical discomfort, as needed

Approach abusive patient behavior in a neutral manner

Address hallucinations in a therapeutic manner

Maintain adequate nutrition and fluid intake

Administer vitamin therapy as appropriate

Monitor for covert alcohol consumption during detoxification

Listen to patient's concerns about alcohol withdrawal

Provide emotional support to patient/family, as appropriate

Provide verbal reassurance, as appropriate

Provide reality orientation, as appropriate

Reassure patient that depression and fatigue commonly occur during withdrawal

Background Readings:

Haber, J., McMahon, A.L., Price-Hoskins, P., & Sideleau, B.F. (1997). Comprehensive psychiatric nursing (5th ed.). St. Louis: Mosby–Year Book.

Joyce, C. (1989). The woman alcoholic. American Journal of Nursing, 89(10), 1314-1316.

Powell, A.F., & Minick, M.P. (1988). Alcohol withdrawal syndrome. American Journal of Nursing, 88(3), 312-315.

Wilson, H.S., & Kneisl, C.R. (1992). Psychiatric nursing (4th ed.). Menlo Park, CA: Addison-Wesley.

S

Substance Use Treatment: Drug Withdrawal   4514

Definition: Care of a patient experiencing drug detoxification

Activities:

Provide symptom management during the detoxification period

Determine history of substance use

Discuss with patient the role that drugs play in his/her life

Assist the patient to recognize that drugs provide a sense of assertiveness, heightened self-esteem, and frustration tolerance

Assist the patient to identify other means of relieving frustrations and increasing self-esteem

Monitor for paranoia and hesitancy to trust others during the detoxification period

Encourage self-disclosure

Monitor for body image distortions and anorexia

Provide adequate nutrition

Monitor for hypertension and tachycardia

Monitor for depression and/or suicidal tendencies

Medicate to relieve symptoms during withdrawal, as appropriate

Encourage exercise to stimulate the release of endorphins

Encourage involvement in a support group, such as Narcotics Anonymous

Facilitate family support

Background Readings:

Acee, A.M., & Smith, D. (1987). Crack. American Journal of Nursing, 87(5), 614-617.

Nuckols, C.C., & Greeson, J. (1989). Cocaine addiction: Assessment and intervention. Nursing Clinics of North America, 24(1), 33-43.

Varcarolis, E.M. (2000). Psychiatric nursing clinical guide (pp. 255-288). Philadelphia: W.B. Saunders Company.

S

Substance Use Treatment: Overdose   4516

Definition: Monitoring, treatment, and emotional support of a patient who has ingested prescription or over-the-counter drugs beyond the therapeutic range

Activities:

Facilitate collection of toxicology screens of blood, urine, and gastric contents

Identify amount and type of drug or combination of drugs ingested and time of ingestion, when possible

Determine whether alcohol was also ingested

Monitor respiratory, cardiac, and neurological status

Induce emesis in the conscious patient only after a strong acid or base substance has been ruled out

Lavage with normal saline using a large-bore gastric tube, as appropriate

Administer ipecac, as appropriate

Administer activated charcoal when substance used is unknown, as appropriate

Administer drug-specific antidotes when the drug that was used is known

Monitor fluid and electrolyte levels, liver function tests, blood counts, and arterial blood gas levels

Monitor for urinary retention and/or renal failure

Monitor for convulsions, seizures, and CNS depression or stimulation

Provide emotional support to patient and family

Provide nonjudgmental support for the conscious patient

Facilitate verbalization about the incident

Identify whether a traumatic life event is associated with the overdose

Monitor for lingering suicidal tendencies

Encourage family support of patient

Monitor patient's ability to verbalize feelings

Monitor ability to deal with strong emotions, such as anger and remorse

Explore constructive release mechanisms

Explore patient's feelings about psychiatric consultation

Facilitate follow-up counseling, when the diagnosis of overdose is confirmed

Facilitate admission to a chemical dependency treatment center, as appropriate

S

Background Readings:

Cooper, K.L. (1989). Drug overdose. American Journal of Nursing, 89(9), 1146-1148.

Johanson, B.C., Wells, S.J., Hoffmeister, D., & Dungca, C.U. (1988). Standards for critical care (3rd ed.). St. Louis: Mosby.

Varcarolis, E.M. (2000). Psychiatric nursing clinical guide (pp. 255-288). Philadelphia: W.B. Saunders Company.

Suicide Prevention 6340

Definition: Reducing the risk for self-inflicted harm with intent to end life

Activities:

Determine presence and degree of suicidal risk

Determine if patient has available means to follow through with suicide plan

Consider hospitalization of patient who is at serious risk for suicidal behavior

Treat and manage any psychiatric illness or symptoms that may be placing patient at risk for suicide (e.g., mood disorder, hallucinations, delusions, panic, substance abuse, grief, personality disorder, organic impairment, crisis)

Administer medications to decrease anxiety, agitation, or psychosis and to stabilize mood, as appropriate

Advocate for quality-of-life and pain control issues

Conduct mouth checks following medication administration to ensure that patient is not "cheeking" the medications for later overdose attempt

Provide small amounts of prescribed medications that may be lethal to those at risk to decrease the opportunity for suicide, as appropriate

Monitor for medication side effects and desired outcomes

Involve patient in planning his/her own treatment, as appropriate

Instruct patient in coping strategies (e.g., assertiveness training, impulse control, and progressive muscle relaxation), as appropriate

Contract (verbally or in writing) with patient for "no self-harm" for a specified period of time, recontracting at specified time intervals, as appropriate

Implement necessary actions to reduce an individual's immediate distress when negotiating a no-self-harm or safety contract

Identify immediate safety needs when negotiating a no–self-harm or safety contract

Assist the individual in discussing his/her feelings about the contract

Observe individual for signs of incongruence that may indicate lack of commitment to fulfilling the contract

Take action to prevent individual from harming or killing self, when contract is a no–self-harm or safety contract (e.g., increased observation, removal of objects that may be used to harm self)

Interact with the patient at regular intervals to convey caring and openness and to provide an opportunity for patient to talk about feelings

Use direct, nonjudgmental approach in discussing suicide

Encourage patient to seek out care providers to talk as urge to harm self occurs

Avoid repeated discussion of suicide history by keeping discussions present- and future-oriented

Discuss plans for dealing with suicidal ideation in the future (e.g., precipitating factors, whom to contact, where to go for help, ways to alleviate impulses to harm self)

Assist patient to identify network of supportive persons and resources (e.g., clergy, family care providers)

Initiate suicide precautions (e.g., ongoing observation and monitoring of the patient, provision of a protective environment) for the patient who is at serious risk of suicide

Place patient in least restrictive environment that allows for necessary level of observation

Continue regular assessment of suicidal risk (at least daily) in order to adjust suicide precautions appropriately

Consult with treatment team before modifying suicide precautions

Search the newly hospitalized patient and personal belongings for weapons/potential weapons during inpatient admission procedure, as appropriate

Search environment routinely and remove dangerous items to maintain it as hazard free

Limit access to windows, unless locked and shatterproof, as appropriate

Limit patient use of potential weapons (e.g., sharps and ropelike objects)

Monitor patient during use of potential weapons (e.g., razor)

Utilize protective interventions (e.g., area restrictions, seclusion, physical restraints) if patient lacks the restraint to refrain from harming self, as needed

Communicate risk and relevant safety issues to other care providers

Assign hospitalized patient to a room located near nursing station for ease in observation, as appropriate

Increase surveillance of hospitalized patients at times when staffing is predictably low (e.g., staff meetings, change of shift report, staff mealtimes, nights, weekends, times of chaos on nursing unit)

Consider strategies to decrease isolation and opportunity to act on harmful thoughts (e.g., use of a sitter)

Observe, record, and report any change in mood or behavior that may signify increasing suicidal risk and document results of regular surveillance checks

Explain suicide precautions and relevant safety, issues to the patient/family/significant others (e.g., purpose, duration, behavioral expectations, and behavioral consequences)

Facilitate support of patient by family and friends

Involve family in discharge planning (e.g., illness/medication teaching, recognition of increasing suicidal risk, patient's plan for dealing with thoughts of harming self, community resources)

Refer patient to mental health care provider (e.g., psychiatrist or psychiatric/mental health advanced practice nurse) for evaluation and treatment of suicidal ideation and behavior, as needed

Provide information about what community resources and outreach programs are available

Improve access to mental health services

Increase the public's awareness that suicide is a preventable health problem

Background Readings:
Conwell, Y. (1997). Management of suicidal behavior in the elderly. Psychiatric Clinics of North America, 20(3), 667-683.
Drew, B.L. (2001). Self-harm behavior and no-suicide contracting in psychiatric inpatient settings. Archives of Psychiatric Nursing, 15(3), 99-106.
Hirschfeld, R.M.A., & Russel, J.M. (1997). Assessment and treatment of suicidal patients. New England Journal of Medicine, 337(13), 910-915.
Potter, M.L., & Dawson, A.M. (2001). From safety contract to safety agreement. Journal of Psychosocial Nursing, 39(8), 38-45.
Schultz, J.M., & Videbeck, S.D. (1998). Lippincott's manual of psychiatric nursing care plans. Philadelphia: Lippincott.
Suicide Prevention and Advocacy Network (1998). Working draft 2—National strategy for suicide prevention. Available on-line: http://www.spanusa.org/draft.htm
Valente, S.M., & Trainor, D. (1998). Rational suicide among patients who are terminally ill. Official Journal of the Association of Operating Room Nurses, 68(2), 252-255, 257-258, 260-264.

S

Supply Management 7840

Definition: Ensuring acquisition and maintenance of appropriate items for providing patient care

Activities:

Identify items commonly used for patient care

Determine stock level needed for each item

Add new items to inventory list, as appropriate

Check items for expiration dates at specific intervals

Inspect integrity of sterile packages

Ensure that supply area is cleaned regularly

Avoid stockpiling expensive items

Order new or replacement equipment, as necessary

Ensure that maintenance requirements on special equipment are completed

Order patient education materials, as appropriate

Order specialty items for patient, as appropriate

Charge patient for supplies, as appropriate

Mark unit/agency equipment for identification, as appropriate

Review supply budget, as appropriate

Background Readings:

Keller, R.A. (1992). Buying smart . . . purchasing equipment and supplies. Emergency, 24(1), 78-80.
Rowland H.S., & Rowland, B.L. (1992). Nursing administration handbook (3rd ed.). Gaithersburg; MD: Aspen.
Stasen, L. (1982). Key business skills for nurse managers. Philadelphia: J.B. Lippincott.

S

Support Group 5430

Definition: Use of a group environment to provide emotional support and health-related information for members

Activities:

Determine level and appropriateness of patient's present support system

Use a support group during transitional stages to help patient adjust to a new lifestyle

Determine purpose of the group and nature of the group process

Create a relaxed, accepting atmosphere

Clarify early on the goals of the group and the members' and leader's responsibilities

Use a written contract, if deemed appropriate

Choose members who can contribute to and benefit from group interaction

Form a group of optimal size: 5 to 12 members

Address the issue of mandatory attendance

Address the issue of whether new members can join at any time

Establish a time and place for the group meeting

Meet in 1- to 2-hour sessions, as appropriate

Begin and end on time, and expect participants to remain until the conclusion

Arrange chairs in a circle in close proximity

Schedule a limited number of sessions (usually 6 to 12), in which the work of the group will be accomplished

Publicize membership policies to avoid problems that may arise as the group progresses

Monitor and direct active involvement of group members

Encourage expression and sharing of experiential knowledge

Encourage expression of mutual aid

Encourage appropriate referrals to professionals for information

Emphasize personal responsibility and control

Maintain positive pressure for behavior change

Emphasize the importance of active coping

Identify topic themes that occur in the group discussion

Do not allow group to become a nonproductive social gathering

Assist the group to progress through the stages of group development: from orientation through cohesiveness to termination

Attend to the needs of the group as a whole, as well as the needs of individual members

Use a co-leader, as appropriate

Background Readings:

Cole, S., O'Connor, S., & Bennett, L. (1979). Self-help groups for clinic patients with chronic illness. Primary Care, 6(2), 325-340.

Kinney, C.K.D., Mannetter, R., & Carpenter, M. (1992). Support groups. In G.M. Bulechek & J.C. McCloskey (Eds.), Nursing interventions: Essential nursing treatments (2nd ed.) (pp. 326-339). Philadelphia: W.B. Saunders.

Snyder, M. (1992). Groups. In M. Snyder (Ed.), Independent nursing interventions (2nd ed.) (pp. 244-255). Albany, NY: Delmar Publishers.

S

Support System Enhancement   5440

Definition: Facilitation of support to patient by family, friends, and community

Activities:

Assess psychological response to situation and availability of support system

Determine adequacy of existing social networks

Identify degree of family support

Identify degree of family financial support

Determine support systems currently used

Determine barriers to using support systems

Monitor current family situation

Encourage the patient to participate in social and community activities

Encourage relationships with persons who have common interests and goals

Refer to a self-help group, as appropriate

Assess community resource adequacy to identify strengths and weaknesses

Refer to a community-based promotion/prevention/treatment/rehabilitation program, as appropriate

Provide services in a caring and supportive manner

Involve family/significant others/friends in care and planning

Explain to concerned others how they can help

Background Readings:

Pflederer, S. (1990). Using friends as a social support system for children. In M.J. Craft & J.A. Denehy (Eds.), Nursing interventions for infants and children (pp. 201-212). Philadelphia: W.B. Saunders.

Tse, A.M., & Perez-Woods, R.C. (1990). Providing support. In M.J. Craft & J.A. Denehy (Eds.), Nursing interventions for infants and children (pp. 181-200). Philadelphia: W.B. Saunders.

S

Surgical Assistance   2900

Definition: Assisting the surgeon/dentist with operative procedures and care of the surgical patient

Activities:

Determine the equipment, instruments, and supplies needed for care of the patient in surgery, and make arrangements for availability

Assemble equipment, instruments, and supplies for the surgery

Prepare supplies, drugs, and solutions for use, as indicated

Check instruments and arrange in order of use

Turn on and position lights

Position instrument and supply tables near the operative field

Anticipate and provide needed supplies and instruments throughout the procedure

Grasp tissue, as appropriate

Dissect tissue, as appropriate

Irrigate and suction surgical wound, as appropriate

Protect tissue, as appropriate

Provide surgical exposure

Provide hemostasis, as appropriate

Clean instruments periodically to remove blood and fat

Assist in estimating blood loss

Prepare and care for specimens, as appropriate

Communicate information to the surgical team, as appropriate

Communicate patient status and progress to family, as appropriate

Arrange for equipment needed immediately after surgery

Assist in transferring patient to the cart or bed and transport to appropriate postanesthesia or postoperative care area

Report to the postanesthesia or postoperative nurse pertinent information about the patient and procedure performed

Document information, per agency policy

Assist with removal of equipment, supplies, and instruments after surgery

Background Readings:

Association of Operating Room Nurses. (1993). Standards and recommended practices. Denver: AORN.

Fairchild, S. (1993). Perioperative nursing: Principles and practice. Boston: Jones & Bartlett.

Kneedler, J., & Dodge, G. (1994). Perioperative patient care: The nursing perspective. Boston: Jones & Bartlett.

Rockroth, J. (1993). RN first assistant (2nd ed.). Philadelphia: J.B. Lippincott.

S

Surgical Precautions   2920

Definition: Minimizing the potential for iatrogenic injury to the patient related to a surgical procedure

Activities:

Check ground isolation monitor

Verify the correct functioning of equipment

Check suction for adequate pressure and complete assembly of canisters, tubing, and catheters

Remove any unsafe equipment

Verify consent for surgery and other treatments, as appropriate

Verify with the patient or appropriate others the procedure and surgical site

Verify that patient's identification band and blood band are correct

Ask patient or appropriate other to state patient's name

Ensure documentation and communication of any allergies

Count sponges, sharps, and instruments before, during, and after surgery, per agency policy

Record results of counts, per agency policy

Remove and store prostheses appropriately

Provide an electrosurgical unit, grounding pad, and active electrode, as appropriate

Verify integrity of electrical cords

Verify proper functioning of electrosurgical unit

Verify absence of cardiac pacemaker, other electrical implant, or metal prostheses contraindicating use of electrosurgical cautery

Verify that the patient is not touching metal

Inspect the patient's skin at the site of grounding pad

Apply grounding pad to dry, intact skin with minimal hair, over large muscle mass, and as close to the operative site as possible

Verify that prep solutions are nonflammable

Protect grounding pad from prep and irrigation solutions and damage

Apply and use holster to store active electrode during surgery

Adjust coagulation and cutting currents, as instructed by physician or per agency policy

Inspect the patient's skin for injury after use of electrosurgery

Document appropriate information on the operative record

Background Readings:

Association of Operating Room Nurses. (1993). Standards and recommended practices. Denver: AORN.

Emergency Care Research Institute. (1990). Electrosurgery. In Operating room risk management. Plymouth Meeting, PA: Emergency Care Research Institute.

Fairchild, S. (1993). Perioperative nursing: Principles and practice. Boston: Jones & Bartlett.

Kneedler, J., & Dodge, G. (1994). Perioperative patient care: The nursing perspective. Boston: Jones & Bartlett.

S

Surgical Preparation   2930

Definition: Providing care to a patient immediately prior to surgery and verifying required procedures/tests and documentation in the clinical record

Activities:

Identify patient's level of anxiety/fear concerning the surgical procedure

Reinforce preoperative teaching information

Complete preoperative checklist

Ensure that patient is NPO, as appropriate

Ensure that a completed history and physical exam findings are recorded in the chart

Verify that the surgical consent form is properly signed

Verify that the required lab and diagnostic test results are in the chart

Verify that blood transfusions are available, as appropriate

Verify that an EKG has been completed, as appropriate

List allergies on the front of the chart

Communicate special care considerations such as blindness, hearing loss, or handicap to OR staff, as appropriate

Determine whether patient's wishes about health care are known (e.g., advance directives, organ donor cards)

Verify that patient identification band, allergy band, and blood bands are readable and in place

Remove jewelry and/or tape rings in place, as appropriate

Remove nail polish, makeup, and hairpins, as appropriate

Remove dentures, glasses, contacts, or other prosthesis, as appropriate

Ensure that money or valuables are in a safe place, as appropriate

Administer bowel preparation medications, as appropriate

Explain preoperative medications that will be used, as appropriate

Administer and document preoperative medications, as appropriate

Start IV therapy, as directed

Send required medications or equipment with patient to the OR, as appropriate

Insert NG tube or Foley catheter, as appropriate

Explain tubing and equipment associated with preparation activities

Administer surgical shave, scrub, shower, enema, and/or douche, as appropriate

Apply antiembolism stockings, as appropriate

Apply sequential compression device sleeves, as appropriate

Instruct patient to void immediately prior to administration of preoperative medications, as appropriate

Check that patient is in proper attire according to institutional policy

Support patient with high anxiety/fear level

Assist patient onto gurney for transport, as appropriate

Provide time for family members to speak with patient prior to transport

Encourage parents to accompany child to the OR, as appropriate

S

Continued

Activities:—cont'd

Provide information to family concerning waiting areas and visiting times for surgical patients

Support family members, as appropriate

Prepare room for patient's return after surgery

Background Readings:

Perry, A.G., & Potter, P.A. (1998). Clinical nursing skills and techniques (4th ed.). St. Louis: Mosby–Year Book.

Smith, S., & Duell, D. (1992). Clinical nursing skills (3rd ed.). Los Altos, CA: National Nursing Review.

Sorensen, K., & Luckmann, J. (1986). Basic nursing: A psychophysiologic approach (2nd ed.). Philadelphia: W.B. Saunders.

S

Surveillance   6650

Definition: Purposeful and ongoing acquisition, interpretation, and synthesis of patient data for clinical decision making

Activities:

Determine patient's health risk(s), as appropriate

Obtain information about normal behavior and routines

Ask patient for her/his perception of health status

Select appropriate patient indices for ongoing monitoring, based on patient's condition

Ask patient about recent signs, symptoms, or problems

Establish the frequency of data collection and interpretation, as indicated by status of the patient

Facilitate acquisition of diagnostic tests, as appropriate

Interpret results of diagnostic tests, as appropriate

Retrieve and interpret laboratory data; contact physician, as appropriate

Explain diagnostic test results to patient and family

Monitor patient's ability to do self-care activities

Monitor neurological status

Monitor behavior patterns

Monitor emotional state

Monitor vital signs, as appropriate

Collaborate with physician to institute invasive hemodynamic monitoring, as appropriate

Collaborate with physician to institute ICP monitoring, as appropriate

Monitor comfort level, and take appropriate action

Monitor coping strategies used by patient and family

Monitor changes in sleep patterns

Monitor oxygenation and initiate measures to promote adequate oxygenation of vital organs

Initiate routine skin surveillance in high-risk patient

Monitor for signs and symptoms of fluid and electrolyte imbalance

Monitor tissue perfusion, as appropriate

Monitor for infection, as appropriate

Monitor nutritional status, as appropriate

Monitor gastrointestinal function, as appropriate

Monitor elimination patterns, as appropriate

Monitor for bleeding tendencies in high-risk patient

Note type and amount of drainage from tubes and orifices and notify the physician of significant changes

Troubleshoot equipment and systems to enhance acquisition of reliable patient data

Compare current status with previous status to detect improvements and deterioration in patient's condition

Initiate and/or change medical treatment to maintain patient parameters within the limits specified by the physician, using established protocols

S

Continued

Activities:—cont'd

Facilitate acquisition of interdisciplinary services (e.g., pastoral services or audiology), as appropriate

Obtain a physician consult when patient data indicate a needed change in medical therapy

Institute appropriate treatment, using standing orders

Prioritize actions, based on patient status

Analyze physician orders in conjunction with patient status to ensure safety of the patient

Obtain consultation from the appropriate health care worker to initiate new treatment or change existing treatments

Background Readings:

Dougherty, C.M. (1992). Surveillance. In G.M. Bulechek & J.C. McCloskey (Eds.), Nursing interventions: Essential nursing treatments (2nd ed.) (pp. 500-511). Philadelphia: W.B. Saunders.

Titler, M.G. (1992). Interventions related to surveillance. In G.M. Bulechek & J.C. McCloskey (Eds.), Symposium on Nursing Interventions. Nursing Clinics of North America, 27(2), 495-517.

S

Surveillance: Community   6652

Definition: Purposeful and ongoing acquisition, interpretation, and synthesis of data for decision making in the community

Activities:

Identify the purpose, procedure, and reporting mechanisms for required and voluntary health data reporting systems

Collect data related to health events such as diseases and injuries to be reported

Establish frequency of data collection and analysis

Report data using standard reporting mechanisms

Collaborate with other agencies in the collection, analysis, and reporting of data

Follow up on reports to appropriate agencies to ensure accuracy and usefulness of information

Instruct patients, families, and agencies regarding the importance of follow-up of contagious disease treatment

Participate in program development (e.g., teaching, policy making, lobbying) as associated with community data collection and reporting

Use reports to recognize need for additional data collection, analysis, and interpretation

Background Readings:

Block, A.B., Onorato, I.M., Ihle, W.W., Hadler, J.L., Hayden, C.H., & Snider, D.E. (1996). The need for epidemic intelligence. Public Health Reports, 111(1), 26-33.

Clemen-Stone, S., McGuire, S., & Eigisti, D. (1997). Comprehensive community health nursing: Family, aggregate, and community practice. St. Louis: Mosby.

Harkness, G. (1995). Epidemiology in nursing practice. St. Louis: Mosby.

U.S. Department of Health & Human Services. (1991). Healthy People 2000: National health promotion and disease prevention objectives. Washington, DC: U.S. Government Printing Office.

U.S. Department of Health & Human Services. (1995). Healthy People 2000: Midcourse review and 1995 revisions. Washington, DC: U.S. Government Printing Office.

Valanais, B. (1992). Epidemiology in nursing and health care (2nd ed.). Norwalk, CT: Appleton & Lange.

S

Surveillance: Late Pregnancy 6656

Definition: Purposeful and ongoing acquisition, interpretation, and synthesis of maternal-fetal data for treatment, observation, or admission

Activities:

Review obstetrical history, if available

Determine maternal-fetal health risk(s) through client interview

Establish gestational age by reviewing history or calculating expected date of confinement (EDC) from last menstrual period

Monitor maternal vital signs

Monitor behavior of woman and support person

Implement electronic fetal monitoring

Inquire about presence and quality of fetal movement

Monitor for signs of premature labor (e.g., >4 contractions per hour, backache, cramping, show, and pelvic pressure from 20 to 37 weeks of gestation), as appropriate

Monitor for signs of pregnancy-induced hypertension (e.g., hypertension, headache, blurred vision, nausea, vomiting, visual alterations, hyperreflexia, edema, and proteinuria), as appropriate

Monitor elimination patterns, as appropriate

Monitor for signs of urinary tract infection, as appropriate

Facilitate acquisition of diagnostic tests, as appropriate

Interpret results of diagnostic tests, as appropriate

Retrieve and interpret laboratory data; contact physician, as appropriate

Explain diagnostic test results to patient and family

Initiate interventions for IV therapy, fluid resuscitation, and medication administration, as ordered

Monitor comfort level, and take appropriate action

Monitor nutritional status, as appropriate

Monitor changes in sleep patterns, as appropriate

Obtain history of sexually transmitted diseases and frequency of intercourse, as appropriate

Monitor uterine activity (e.g., frequency, duration, and intensity of contractions)

Perform Leopold maneuver to determine fetal position

Note type, amount, and onset of vaginal drainage

Perform speculum exam for diagnosis of spontaneous rupture of amniotic membranes, unless there is evidence of frank bleeding

Test amniotic fluid (e.g., nitrazine, ferning, and pooling), as appropriate

Obtain cervical cultures, as appropriate (e.g., history of beta-streptococcal infection, herpes, or prolonged rupture of membranes)

Examine cervix for dilatation, effacement, softening, position, and station

Perform ultrasonography to determine fetal presentation or placental position, as appropriate

Institute appropriate treatment, using standing orders

Prioritize actions, based on patient status (e.g., treat, continue to observe, admit, or discharge)

Background Readings:

Angelini, D.J., Zannieri, C.L., Silva, V.B., et al. (1990). Toward a concept of triage for labor and delivery: Staff perceptions and role utilization. Journal of Perinatal & Neonatal Nursing, 4(3), 1-11.

Eganhouse, D.J. (1991). A comparative study of variables differentiating false labor from early labor. Journal of Perinatology, 11(3), 249-257.

S

Surveillance: Remote Electronic   6658

Definition: Purposeful and ongoing acquisition of patient data via electronic modalities (telephone, video conference, e-mail) from distant locations, as well as interpretation and synthesis of patient data for clinical decision making with individuals or populations

Activities:

Determine that you are interacting with the patient or, if with someone else, that you have the patient's permission to interact with him/her

Identify self with name, credentials, organization; let caller know if call is being recorded (e.g., for quality monitoring)

Inform patient about interaction process and obtain consent

Determine patient's health risk(s), as appropriate

Obtain information about usual patient behavior and routines

Establish the frequency of data collection and interpretation, as indicated by status of the patient

Monitor incoming data for validity and reliability

Interpret results of diagnostic indicators such as vital signs, glucose readings, EKGs

Collaborate/consult with physician resources, as necessary

Explain test results and interventions to patient and family

Monitor comfort level, and take appropriate action

Monitor coping strategies and actions used by patient and family

Initiate skin surveillance in high-risk patient when high-resolution video monitoring in use

Monitor for potential problems based on current status (i.e., infection, fluid and electrolyte balance, tissue perfusion, nutrition, and elimination)

Troubleshoot all equipment and systems to enhance acquisition of reliable patient data

Coordinate placement/replacement/setup of equipment/supplies

Compare current status with previous status to detect improvements and or deterioration in patient's condition

Initiate and/or change medical treatment to maintain patient parameters within the limits specified by the physician, using established guidelines

Facilitate acquisition of interdisciplinary services (e.g., pastoral services), as appropriate

Prioritize actions based on patient status

Analyze physician orders in conjunction with patient status to ensure safety of the patient

Obtain consultation from appropriate health care worker to initiate new treatment or change existing treatments

Advocate for patient's welfare, as necessary

Maintain confidentiality, keeping in mind the specific threats to confidentiality implicit in the electronic modality in use

Determine need, and establish time intervals, for further intermittent assessment

Document assessments, advice, instructions, or other information given to patient according to specified guidelines

Determine how patient or family member can be reached for future surveillance, as appropriate

Document permission for return call and identify person(s) able to receive call

Identify or aggregate data that has programmatic or population implications

S

Background Readings:

AAACN/ANA Task Force. (1997). Nursing in ambulatory care: The future is here. Washington, DC: American Nurses Publishing.

American Academy of Ambulatory Nursing. (1997). Telephone nursing practice administration and practice standards. Pitman, NJ: Anthony J. Jannetti, Inc.

Wheeler, S.Q., & Windt, J.H. (Eds.) (1993). Telephone triage: Theory, practice, and protocol development. Albany, NY: Delmar.

S

Surveillance: Safety   6654

Definition: Purposeful and ongoing collection and analysis of information about the patient and the environment for use in promoting and maintaining patient safety

Activities:

Monitor patient for alterations in physical or cognitive function that might lead to unsafe behavior

Monitor environment for potential safety hazards

Determine degree of surveillance required by patient, based on level of functioning and the hazards present in environment

Provide appropriate level of supervision/surveillance to monitor patient and to allow for therapeutic actions, as needed

Place patient in least restrictive environment that allows for necessary level of observation

Initiate and maintain precaution status for patient at high risk for dangers specific to the care setting

Communicate information about patient's risk to other nursing staff

Background Readings:

Dougherty, C.M. (1992). Surveillance. In G.M. Bulechek & J.C. McCloskey (Eds.), Nursing interventions: Essential nursing treatments (2nd ed.) (pp. 500-511). Philadelphia: W.B. Saunders.

Kanak, M.F. (1992). Interventions related to safety. In G.M. Bulechek & J.C. McCloskey (Eds.), Symposium on Nursing Interventions. Nursing Clinics of North America, 27(2), 371-396.

Kozier, B., & Erb, G. (1987). Fundamentals of nursing: Concepts and procedures (3rd ed.). Menlo Park, CA: Addison-Wesley.

Nightingale, F. (1969). Notes on nursing: What it is and what it is not. New York: Dover Publications.

S

Sustenance Support   7500

Definition: Helping a needy individual/family to locate food, clothing, or shelter

Activities:

Determine adequacy of patient's financial situation

Determine adequacy of food supplies in home

Inform individual/families about how to access local food pantries and free lunch programs, as appropriate

Inform individual/families about how to access low-rent housing and subsidy programs, as appropriate

Inform individual/families about rental laws and protections

Inform individual/families of available emergency housing shelter programs, as appropriate

Arrange transportation to emergency housing shelter, as appropriate

Discuss with the individual/families available job service agencies, as appropriate

Arrange for transportation to job services, if necessary

Inform individual/families of agency providing clothing assistance, as appropriate

Arrange transportation to agency providing clothing assistance, as necessary

Inform individual/families of agency programs for support, such as Red Cross and Salvation Army, as appropriate

Discuss with the individual/families financial aid support available

Assist individual/families to complete forms for assistance, such as housing and financial aid

Inform individual/families of available free health clinics

Assist individual/families to reach free health clinics

Inform individual/families of eligibility requirements for food stamps

Inform individual/families of available schools and/or day care centers, as appropriate

Background Readings:

Boyer, D.E., & Heppner, I. (1992). Community mental health: Problem identification and treatment. In M. Stanhope & J. Lancaster (Eds.), Community health nursing (3rd ed.) (pp. 351-363). St. Louis: Mosby.

Hymovich, D.P., & Barnard, M.U. (1979). Family health care (2nd ed.) (pp. 165-182). New York: McGraw-Hill.

S

Suturing   3620

Definition: Approximating edges of a wound using sterile suture material and a needle

Activities:

Identify patient allergies to anesthetics, tape, and/or povidone-iodine or other topical solutions

Identify history of keloid formation, as appropriate

Refer deep, facial, joint, or potentially infected wounds to a physician

Immobilize a frightened child or confused adult, as appropriate

Shave hair from the immediate wound site

Cleanse the surrounding skin with soap and water or other mild antiseptic solution

Use sterile technique

Administer a topical or injectable anesthetic to the area, as appropriate

Allow sufficient time for the anesthetic to numb the area

Select an appropriate gauge suture material

Determine method of suturing (continuous or interrupted) most appropriate for the wound

Position the needle so that it enters and exits perpendicular to the skin surface

Pull the needle through, following the line or curve of the needle itself

Pull the suture tight enough to not buckle the skin

Secure the suture line with square knots

Cleanse the area before applying an antiseptic or dressing

Apply a dressing, as appropriate

Instruct patient on how to care for the suture line, including signs and symptoms of infection

Instruct patient when sutures should be removed

Remove sutures, as indicated

Schedule return visit, as appropriate

Background Readings:

Hamilton, H.K. (Ed.) (1983). Procedures: Bedside care, life support, equipment, precautions. Springhouse, PA: Intermed Communications.

Meeker, M.H., & Rothrock, J.C. (1998). Alexander's care of the patient in surgery. (11th ed.) St. Louis: Mosby.

Sorensen, K., & Luckmann, J. (1986). Basic nursing: A psychophysiologic approach (2nd ed.). Philadelphia: W.B. Saunders.

S

Swallowing Therapy   1860

Definition: Facilitating swallowing and preventing complications of impaired swallowing

Activities:

Collaborate with other members of health care team (i.e., occupational therapist, speech pathologist, and dietician) to provide continuity in patient's rehabilitative plan

Determine patient's ability to focus attention on learning/performing eating and swallowing tasks

Remove distractions from environment prior to working with patient on swallowing

Provide privacy for patient, as desired or indicated

Position self so that patient can see and hear you speak

Explain rationale of swallowing regimen to patient/family

Collaborate with speech therapist to instruct patient's family about swallowing exercise regimen

Provide/use assistive devices, as appropriate

Avoid use of drinking straws

Assist patient to sit in an erect position (as close to 90 degrees as possible) for feeding/exercise

Assist patient to position head in forward flexion in preparation for swallowing ("chin tuck")

Assist patient to maintain sitting position for 30 minutes after completing meal

Instruct patient to open and close mouth in preparation for food manipulation

Instruct patient not to talk during eating, if appropriate

Guide patient in phonating staccato "ahs" to promote soft palate elevation, if appropriate

Provide a lollipop for patient to suck on to enhance tongue strength, if appropriate

Assist hemiplegic patient to sit with affected arm forward on table

Assist patient to place food at back of mouth and on unaffected side

Monitor for signs and symptoms of aspiration

Monitor patient's tongue movements while eating

Monitor for sealing of lips during eating, drinking, and swallowing

Monitor for signs of fatigue during eating, drinking, swallowing

Provide rest period before eating/exercise to prevent excessive fatigue

Check mouth for pocketing of food after eating

Instruct patient to reach for particles of food on lips or chin with tongue

Assist patient to remove food particles from lips and chin if unable to extend tongue

Instruct family/caregiver how to position, feed, and monitor patient

Instruct patient/caregiver on nutritional requirements and dietary modifications, in collaboration with dietician

Instruct patient/caregiver on emergency measures for choking

Instruct patient/caregiver how to check for pocketed food after eating

Provide written instructions, as appropriate

Provide scheduled practice sessions for family/caregiver, as needed

Provide/monitor consistency of food/liquid based on findings of swallowing study

Consult with therapist and/or physician to gradually advance consistency of patient's food

Continued

Activities:—cont'd

Assist to maintain adequate caloric and fluid intake

Monitor body weight

Monitor body hydration (e.g., intake, output, skin turgor, mucous membranes)

Provide mouth care as needed

Background Readings:

Baker, D.M. (1993). Assessment and management of impairments in swallowing. Nursing Clinics of North America, 28(4), 793-806.

Davies, P. (1993). Steps to follow: A guide to the treatment of adult hemiplegia based on the concept of K & B Bobath. New York: Springer-Verlag.

Emick-Herring, B., & Wood, P. (1990). A team approach to neurologically based swallowing disorders. Rehabilitation Nursing, 15(3) 126-132.

Glick, O.J. (1992). Interventions related to activity and movement. In G.M. Bulechek & J.C. McCloskey (Eds.), Symposium on Nursing Interventions. Nursing Clinics of North America, 27(2), 541-568.

Killen, J.M. (1996). Understanding dysphagia: Interventions for care. MEDSURG Nursing, 5,(2), 99-105.

Maat, M.T., & Tandy, L. (1991). Impaired swallowing. In M. Maas, K. Buckwalter, & M. Hardy (Eds.), Nursing diagnoses and interventions for the elderly (pp. 106-116). Redwood City, CA: Addison-Wesley.

McHale, J.M., Phipps, M.A., Horvath, K., & Schmelz, J. (1998). Expert nursing knowledge in the care of patients at risk for impaired swallowing. Image: Journal of Nursing Scholarship, 30(2), 137-141.

S

Teaching: Disease Process 5602

Definition: Assisting the patient to understand information related to a specific disease process

Activities:

Appraise the patient's current level of knowledge related to specific disease process

Explain the pathophysiology of the disease and how it relates to anatomy and physiology, as appropriate

Review patient's knowledge about condition

Acknowledge patient's knowledge about condition

Describe common signs and symptoms of the disease, as appropriate

Explore with patient what she/he has already done to manage the symptoms

Describe the disease process, as appropriate

Identify possible etiologies, as appropriate

Provide information to the patient about condition, as appropriate

Identify changes in physical condition for patient

Avoid empty reassurances

Provide reassurance about patient's condition, as appropriate

Provide the family/significant other(s) with information about the patient's progress, as appropriate

Provide information about available diagnostic measures, as appropriate

Discuss lifestyle changes that may be required to prevent future complications and/or control the disease process

Discuss therapy/treatment options

Describe rationale behind management/therapy/treatment recommendations

Encourage the patient to explore options/get a second opinion, as appropriate or indicated

Describe possible chronic complications, as appropriate

Instruct the patient on measures to prevent/minimize side effects of treatment for the disease, as appropriate

Instruct the patient on measures to control/minimize symptoms, as appropriate

Explore possible resources/support, as appropriate

Refer the patient to local community agencies/support groups, as appropriate

Instruct the patient on which signs and symptoms to report to health care provider, as appropriate

Provide the phone number(s) to call if complications occur

Reinforce information provided by other health care team members, as appropriate

Background Readings:

Rakel, B.A. (1992). Interventions related to patient teaching. In G.M. Bulechek & J.C. McCloskey (Eds.), Symposium on Nursing Interventions. Nursing Clinics of North America, 27(2), 397-424.

Springhouse Corporation. (1987). Core teaching topics. In Patient teaching (Nurse's Reference Library): Learning needs, discharge preparation, tips and checklists (pp. 83-89). Springhouse, PA: Springhouse Corporation.

Teaching: Foot Care 5603

Definition: Preparing a patient at risk and/or significant other to provide preventive foot care

Activities:

Determine current level of knowledge and skills related to foot care

Determine current foot care practices

Provide information related to the level of risk for injury

Recommend toenail and callus trimming by a specialist, as appropriate

Provide written foot care guidelines

Assist in developing a plan for daily foot assessment and care at home

Determine capacity to carry out foot care (i.e., visual acuity, physical mobility, and judgment)

Recommend assistance of a significant other with foot care if vision is impaired or if there are problems with mobility

Recommend daily foot inspection over all surfaces and between the toes, looking for redness, swelling, warmth, dryness, maceration, tenderness, or open areas

Instruct individual to use a mirror or the assistance of another to carry out foot inspection, as needed

Recommend daily washing of feet with warm water and mild soap

Recommend thoroughly drying feet after washing them, especially between the toes

Instruct individual to hydrate the skin daily by brief soaking or bathing in room temperature water, followed by application of an emollient

Provide information regarding the relationship between neuropathy, injury, and vascular disease and the risk for ulceration and lower extremity amputation in persons with diabetes

Advise individual when it is appropriate to contact a health professional (e.g., the presence of a nonhealing or infected lesion)

Advise regarding appropriate self-care measures for minor foot problems

Caution about potential sources of injury to the feet, (e.g., heat, cold, cutting corns or calluses, chemicals, use of strong antiseptics or astringents, use of adhesive tape, and going barefoot or wearing thongs or open-toe shoes)

Instruct on proper technique for toenail trimming (i.e., cutting relatively straight across, following the contour of the toe, and filing sharp edges with an emery board)

Instruct on care of soft calluses including gentle buffing with a towel or pumice stone after a bath

Recommend specialist care for fungal infection, thick or ingrown toenails, corns, or calluses, as indicated

Describe appropriate shoes (i.e., low-heeled with a shape that matches foot shape; adequate depth of toe box; soles made of material that will absorb shock; adjustable fit by lace or straps; uppers made of breathable, soft, and flexible materials; changes made for gait and limb length disorders; and potential for modification if necessary)

Describe appropriate socks (i.e., absorbent material and nonconstricting)

Recommend guidelines to be followed when purchasing new shoes including having feet properly measured and fitted at the time of purchase

Recommend wearing new shoes only for a few hours at a time for the first two weeks

Instruct individual to inspect inside shoes daily for foreign objects, nail points, torn linings, and rough areas

Instruct individual to change shoes two times, (e.g., 12 noon and 5 PM) each day to avoid local repetitive pressure

Explain the necessity for prescriptive footwear or orthotics, as appropriate

Caution about clothing and activities that cause pressure on nerves and blood vessels, including elastic bands on socks and crossing legs

Advise individual to stop smoking, as appropriate

Include the family/significant others in instruction, as appropriate

Reinforce information provided by other health professionals, as appropriate

Background Readings:

American Diabetes Association. (1998). Preventive foot care in people with diabetes. Diabetes, 21(12), 2178-2179.

Collier, J.H., Kinion, E.S., & Brodbeck, C.A. (1996). Evolving role of CNSs in developing risk-anchored preventive interventions. Clinical Nurse Specialist, 10(3), 131-136, 143.

Culleton, J.L. (1999). Preventing diabetic foot complications. Postgraduate Medicine, 106(1), 78-84.

Kruger, S., & Guthrie, D. (1992). Foot care: Knowledge retention and self-care practices. The Diabetes Educator, 18(6), 487-490.

Litzelman, D.K., Slemenda, C.W., Langefeld, C.D., Hays, L.M., Welch, M.A., Bild, D.E., Ford, E.S., Vinicor, F. (1993). Reduction of lower extremity clinical abnormalities in patients with non-insulin-dependent diabetes. A randomized controlled trial. Annals of Internal Medicine, 119(1), 36-41.

Mayfield, J.A., Reiber, G.E., Sanders, L.J., Janise, D., & Pogach, L.M. (1998). Preventive foot care in people with diabetes. Diabetes Care, 21(12), 2161-2177.

Plummer E.S., & Albert, S.G. (1995). Foot care assessment in patients with diabetes: A screening algorithm for patient education and referral. The Diabetic Educator, 21(1), 47-51.

Reiber, G.E., Pecoraro, R.E., & Koepsell, T.D. (1992). Risk factors for amputation in patients with diabetes mellitus. A case control study. Annals of Internal Medicine, 117(2), 97-105.

T

Teaching: Group 5604

Definition: Development, implementation, and evaluation of a patient teaching program for a group of individuals experiencing the same health condition

Activities:

Provide an environment conducive to learning

Include the family/significant others, as appropriate

Establish the need for a program

Determine administrative support

Determine budget

Coordinate resources within the facility to form a planning/advisory committee that can contribute to positive outcomes for the program and provide a forum for ensuring commitment to the program

Utilize community resources, as appropriate

Define potential target population(s)

Write program goals

Outline major content area(s)

Write learning objectives

Write a job description for a coordinator responsible for patient education

Select a coordinator

Preview available educational materials

Develop new educational materials, as appropriate

List possible teaching strategies, educational materials, and learning activities

Train the teaching personnel, as appropriate

Educate the staff about the patient teaching program, as appropriate

Provide a written schedule, including dates, times, and places of the teaching sessions/classes to the staff and/or patient(s), as appropriate

Determine appropriate days/times to reach maximum number of patients

Prepare announcements/memos to publicize outcomes, as appropriate

Control the size and competencies of the group, as appropriate

Orient patient(s)/significant others to educational program and the objectives it is designed to accomplish

Provide for special needs of learners (e.g., handicap access, portable oxygen), as appropriate

Adapt the educational methods/materials to the group's learning needs/characteristics, as appropriate

Provide group instruction

Evaluate the patient's progress in the program and mastery of content

Document the patient's progress on the permanent medical record

Revise teaching strategies/learning activities, if necessary, to increase learning

Provide forms for the patient to evaluate the program

Provide for further individual instruction, as appropriate

Evaluate the extent to which program goals were attained

Communicate the program's goal attainment evaluation to the planning/advisory committee

Hold summative evaluation sessions for the planning/advisory committee to revamp the program as appropriate

Document the number of patients who have attained the learning objectives

Refer the patient to other specialists/agencies to meet the learning objectives, as appropriate

Background Readings:

Bastable, S.B. (1997). Nurse as educator: Principles of teaching and learning (pp. 264-266). Boston: Jones & Bartlett Publishers.

Rakel, B.A. (1992). Interventions related to patient teaching. In G.M. Bulechek & J.C. McCloskey (Eds.), Symposium on Nursing Interventions. Nursing Clinics of North America, 27(2), 397-424.

Redman, B.K. (1997). Teaching: Theory, and interpersonal techniques. In B.K. Redman (Ed.), The process of patient education (8th ed.). St. Louis: Mosby–Year Book.

T

Teaching: Individual   5606

Definition: Planning, implementation, and evaluation of a teaching program designed to address a patient's particular needs

Activities:

Establish rapport

Establish teacher credibility, as appropriate

Determine the patient's learning needs

Appraise the patient's current level of knowledge and understanding of content

Appraise the patient's educational level

Appraise the patient's cognitive, psychomotor, and affective abilities/disabilities

Determine the patient's ability to learn specific information (i.e., developmental level, physiological status, orientation, pain, fatigue, unfulfilled basic needs, emotional state, and adaptation to illness)

Determine the patient's motivation to learn specific information (i.e., health beliefs, past noncompliance, bad experiences with health care/learning, and conflicting goals)

Enhance the patient's readiness to learn, as appropriate

Set mutual, realistic learning goals with the patient

Identify learning objectives necessary to reach goals

Determine the sequence for presenting the information

Appraise the patient's learning style

Select appropriate teaching methods/strategies

Select appropriate educational materials

Tailor the content to the patient's cognitive, psychomotor, and/or affective abilities/disabilities

Adjust instruction to facilitate learning, as appropriate

Provide an environment conducive to learning

Instruct the patient, when appropriate

Evaluate the patient's achievement of the stated objectives

Reinforce behavior, as appropriate

Correct information misinterpretations, as appropriate

Provide time for the patient to ask questions and discuss concerns

Select new teaching methods/strategies, if previous ones were ineffective

Refer the patient to other specialists/agencies to meet the learning objectives, as appropriate

Document the content presented, the written materials provided, and the patient's understanding of the information or patient behaviors that indicate learning on the permanent medical record

Include the family/significant others, as appropriate

Background Readings:

Kemp, J.E. (1990). The instructional design process. New York: Harper & Row.

Rakel, B.A. (1992). Interventions related to patient teaching. In G.M. Bulechek & J.C. McCloskey (Eds.), Symposium on Nursing Interventions. Nursing Clinics of North America, 27(2), 397-424.

Redman, B.K. (1993). The process of patient education (7th ed.). St. Louis: Mosby.

Springhouse. (1987). How to teach patients. In Patient teaching (Nurse's Reference Library): Learning needs, discharge preparation, tips and checklists (pp. 83-89). Springhouse, PA: Springhouse.

Springhouse (1987). Principles of patient teaching. In Patient teaching manual (Vols. 1 & 2) (pp. 1-26). Springhouse, PA: Springhouse.

Teaching: Infant Nutrition   5626

Definition: Instruction on nutrition and feeding practices during the first year of life

Activities:

Provide parents with written materials appropriate to identified knowledge needs

Instruct parent/caregiver of infant 0-3 months to:

  feed only breast milk or formula for first year (no solids before 4 months)
  always hold infant when giving bottle
  never prop bottle or give bottle in bed
  avoid putting cereal in bottle (only formula or breast milk)
  limit water intake to ½ oz to 1 oz at a time, 4 oz daily
  avoid use of honey or corn syrup
  allow nonnutritive sucking
  discard leftover formula and clean bottle after every feeding

Instruct parent/caregiver of infant 4-6 months to:

  introduce solids (pureed) without added salt or sugar
  introduce iron-fortified infant cereal
  introduce one new food at a time
  avoid giving juice or sweetened drinks
  feed from a spoon only

Instruct parent/caregiver of infant 7-9 months to:

  introduce finger foods when infant can sit up
  introduce cup when infant can sit up
  have infant join family at mealtimes
  let infant begin self-feedings and observe to avoid choking
  offer fluids after solids
  avoid sugary desserts and soda
  offer a variety of foods according to the food pyramid
  introduce limited amounts of diluted juice in a cup

Instruct parent/caregiver of infant 10-12 months to:

  offer three meals and healthy snacks
  begin to wean from bottle
  avoid fruit drinks and flavored milk
  begin table foods
  allow infant to feed self with a spoon

Continued

T

Background Readings:

Barnes, L. A. (Ed.). (1993). Pediatric nutrition handbook (3rd ed.). Elk Grove Village, IL: American Academy of Pediatrics.

California Department of Health Services WIC Supplemental Nutrition Branch. (1998a). Feeding your baby 6-12 months [Brochure]. Sacramento, CA: California Department of Health Services WIC Supplemental Nutrition Branch.

California Department of Health Services WIC Supplemental Nutrition Branch. (1998b). Feeding your baby birth to 8 months [Brochure]. Sacramento, CA: California Department of Health Services, WIC Supplemental Nutrition Branch.

California Department of Health Services WIC Supplemental Nutrition Branch. (1997). Feeding your 1-3 year old [Brochure]. Sacramento, CA: California Department of Health Services WIC Supplemental Nutrition Branch.

Formon, S.J. (1993). Nutrition of normal infants. St. Louis: Mosby.

Satter, E., & Sharkey, P.B. (1997). Ellyn Satter's nutrition and feeding for infants and children: Handout masters. Madison, WI: E. Satter & P.B. Sharkey.

T

Teaching: Infant Safety 5628

Definition: Instruction on safety during first year of life

Activities:
Provide parents with written materials appropriate to identified knowledge needs

Instruct parent/caregiver of infant 0-3 months to:
>   install and use car seat according to manufacturer's recommendations
>   place infant on back to sleep and keep loose bedding, pillows, and toys out of crib
>   use only cribs that are safe
>   avoid use of jewelry or cords/chains on infant
>   use and maintain all equipment properly (e.g. swings, strollers, playpens, port-a-cribs)
>   avoid holding infant while smoking or drinking hot liquids
>   hold infant when feeding, avoid propping of bottle, and test formula temperature
>   monitor experienced/trained child care providers
>   prevent falls
>   test water temperature of bath
>   keep pets at a safe distance from infant
>   never shake, toss, or swing infant in the air

Instruct parent/caregiver of infant 4-6 months to:
>   avoid use of walkers or jumpers due to danger of injury and detrimental effects on muscle development
>   never leave infant unattended in the bath, grocery cart, high chair, on sofa, etc.
>   evaluate hanging crib toys
>   use a safe high chair when infant is able to sit
>   feed only soft or mashed foods
>   remove small objects from infant's reach

Instruct parent/caregiver of infant 7-9 months to:
>   avoid sources of lead poisoning
>   keep dangerous items out of infant's reach
>   provide barriers to dangerous areas
>   supervise infant's activity at all times

Instruct parent/caregiver of infant 10-12 months to:
>   provide protection from glass furniture, sharp edges, unstable furniture, and appliances
>   store all cleaning supplies, medications, and personal care products out of infant's reach
>   use childproof latches on cupboards
>   prevent infant's access to upper story windows, balconies, and stairs
>   keep infant away from ponds, pools, toilets, and all containers with liquid to prevent drowning
>   select toys according to manufacturer's age recommendations
>   ensure multiple barriers to pool/hot tub area

Continued

T

Background Readings:

American Academy of Pediatrics. (1994a). 1 to 2 years: Safety for your child [Brochure]. Elk Grove Village, IL: American Academy of Pediatrics.

American Academy of Pediatrics. (1994b). 2 to 4 years: Safety for your child [Brochure]. Elk Grove Village, IL: American Academy of Pediatrics.

American Academy of Pediatrics. (1994c). 6 to 12 months: Safety for your child [Brochure]. Elk Grove Village, IL: American Academy of Pediatrics.

American Academy of Pediatrics. (1994d). Birth to 6 months: Safety for your child [Brochure]. Elk Grove Village, IL: American Academy of Pediatrics.

California Center for Childhood Injury Prevention. (1997). Safe home assessment program. San Diego, CA: California Center for Childhood Injury Prevention.

California Department of Health Services Childhood Lead Poisoning Prevention Branch. (1994). Lead: Simple things that you can do to prevent childhood lead poisoning [Brochure]. Sacramento, CA: California Department of Health Services Childhood Lead Poisoning Prevention Branch.

T

Teaching: Infant Stimulation 5605

Definition: Teaching parents and caregivers to provide developmentally appropriate sensory activities to promote development and movement during the first year of life

Activities:

Teach normal infant development

Assist parents to identify infant readiness cues and responses to stimulation

Protect infant from overstimulation

Assist parents to set up routine for infant stimulation

Teach parents/caregivers to perform activities that encourage movement and/or provide sensory stimulation

Have parents demonstrate techniques learned during teaching

Instruct parents of infants 0-4 months to:
  promote face-to-face interaction with infant
  talk, sing, and smile at infant while giving care, describing care to infant
  praise infant for all efforts to respond to stimulation
  tell infant his/her name frequently
  whisper to infant
  touch and hug infant frequently
  respond to crying by holding, rocking, singing, talking, walking, repositioning, rubbing/massaging
    back, wrapping, as appropriate
  rock infant in either an upright or cradle position
  sponge or tub bathe using various massaging strokes with a soft washcloth or sponge and pat dry with
    soft towel
  massage infant by rubbing lotion in gentle but firm strokes
  rub soft toys on infant's body
  encourage infant to feel different textures and identify them for infant
  blow air in circles on alert infant's arms, legs, and tummy
  encourage infant to grasp soft toys or caregiver's fingers
  promote shaking of rattles, encouraging auditory following
  provide opportunities for infant to reach for objects
  encourage visual following of objects
  reposition infant every hour unless sleeping, placing in infant seat, swing, stroller, as appropriate
  place infant on tummy while awake to encourage head lifting
  position infant on back under cradle gym
  play peek-a-boo with infant
  encourage infant to look in mirror

Instruct parents of infants 5-8 months to:
  place infant on tummy, putting caregiver's palms on soles of infant's feet, and push gently forward
  stand infant on caregiver's lap, swaying side to side
  encourage infant to lay on back and kick with feet
  lay infant on back or tummy and help to roll over
  provide opportunity for infant to explore cloth or soft plastic books
  introduce infant to body parts
  encourage infant to use toys for teething
  play pat-a-cake with infant
  hide objects and let infant look for them
  encourage infant to bang toys together
  encourage hand transfer of toys
  place infant in high chair, encouraging infant to feel food and feed self
  dance with infant while holding infant upright

T

Continued

Activities:—cont'd

Instruct parents of infants 9-12 months to:

    pull infant to standing, holding onto hands for stabilization

    guide infant to walk, holding infant by hands/wrists with arms above head

    encourage ball play (e.g., rolling, grasping, stopping, retrieving)

    introduce use of cup at meal times, assisting infant to grasp and put to mouth

    wave bye-bye to infant, encouraging infant to imitate

    take infant on a house tour, identifying objects and rooms

    play follow the leader, practicing imitation of infant noises, animals, or songs

    say words to infant, encouraging infant to say them back

    demonstrate how to remove objects from and replace them in a container

    demonstrate stacking objects

Background Readings:

Broussard, A.B., Kidman, S. (1990). Incorporating infant stimulation concepts into prenatal classes. JOGNN, 19(5), 381-387.

Harrison, L.L. (1985). Effects of early supplemental stimulation programs for premature infants: Review of the literature. Maternal Child Nursing, 14(2), 125.

Health First, Infant Stimulation. Retrieved February 14, 2002, from http://www.health-first.org/health_info/your_health_first/kids/infant_stim.cfm

Korner, A.F. (1990). Infant stimulation: Issues of theory and research. Clinics in Perinatology, 17(1), 173-184.

Ludington-Hoe, S.M. (1988). Case study in infant stimulation: Lessons for newborn and parent. Early Child Development and Care, 36, 1-24.

Mayes, L.C. Early childhood stimulation, Yale University Expert's Opinions. Retrived February 14, 2002, from http://www.health-first.org/health_info/your_health_first/kids/infant_stim.cfm

T

Teaching: Preoperative   5610

Definition: Assisting a patient to understand and mentally prepare for surgery and the postoperative recovery period

Activities:

Inform the patient and significant other(s) of the scheduled date, time, and location of surgery

Inform the patient/significant other(s) how long the surgery is expected to last

Determine the patient's previous surgical experiences and level of knowledge related to surgery

Appraise the patient's/significant other(s) anxiety related to surgery

Provide time for the patient to ask questions and discuss concerns

Describe the preoperative routines (e.g., anesthesia, diet, bowel preparation, tests/labs, voiding, skin preparation, IV therapy, clothing, family waiting area, transportation to operating room), as appropriate

Describe any preoperative medications, the effects these will have on the patient, and the rationale for using them

Inform the significant other(s) of the place to wait for the results of the surgery, as appropriate

Conduct a tour of the postsurgical unit(s) and waiting area(s), as appropriate

Introduce the patient to the staff who will be involved in the surgery/postoperative care, as appropriate

Reinforce the patient's confidence in the staff involved, as appropriate

Provide information on what will be heard, smelled, seen, tasted, or felt during the event

Discuss possible pain control measures

Explain the purpose of frequent postoperative assessments

Describe the postoperative routines/equipment (e.g., medications, respiratory treatments, tubes, machines, support hose, surgical dressings, ambulation, diet, family visitation) and explain their purpose

Instruct the patient on the technique of getting out of bed, as appropriate

Evaluate the patient's ability to return demonstrate getting out of bed, as appropriate

Instruct the patient on the technique of splinting his/her incision, coughing, and deep breathing

Evaluate the patient's ability to return demonstrate splinting incision, coughing, and deep breathing

Instruct the patient on how to use the incentive spirometer

Evaluate the patient's ability to return demonstrate proper use of the incentive spirometer

Instruct the patient on the technique of leg exercises

Evaluate the patient's ability to return demonstrate leg exercises

Stress the importance of early ambulation and pulmonary care

Inform the patient how he/she can aid in recuperation

Reinforce information provided by other health care team members, as appropriate

Determine the patient's expectations of the surgery

Correct unrealistic expectations of the surgery, as appropriate

Provide time for the patient to rehearse events that will happen, as appropriate

Instruct the patient to use coping techniques directed at controlling specific aspects of the experience (e.g., relaxation, imagery), as appropriate

Include the family/significant others, as appropriate

Continued

Background Readings:

Butcher, L. (1999). Teaching: Preoperative. In G.M. Bulechek & J.C. McCloskey (Eds.), Nursing interventions: Effective nursing treatments (3rd ed.) (pp. 224-233). Philadelphia: W.B. Saunders Company.

Cipperley, J.A., Butcher, L.A., Hayes, J.E. (1995). Research utilization: The development of a preoperative teaching protocol. MEDSURG Nursing, 4(3), 199-306.

Horsley, J.A. (1981). Structured preoperative teaching. CURN Project. New York: Grune & Stratton.

Rakel, B.A. (1992). Interventions related to patient teaching. In G.M. Bulechek & J.C. McCloskey (Eds.), Symposium on Nursing Interventions. Nursing Clinics of North America, 27(2), 397-424.

Springhouse. (1987). Core teaching topics. In Patient teaching (Nurse's Reference Library): Learning needs, discharge preparation, tips and checklists (pp. 83-99). Springhouse, PA: Springhouse.

T

Teaching: Prescribed Activity/Exercise   5612

Definition: Preparing a patient to achieve and/or maintain a prescribed level of activity

Activities:

Appraise the patient's current level of exercise and knowledge of prescribed activity/exercise

Inform the patient of the purpose for, and the benefits of, the prescribed activity/exercise

Instruct the patient how to perform the prescribed activity/exercise

Instruct the patient how to monitor tolerance of the activity/exercise

Instruct the patient how to keep an exercise diary, as appropriate

Inform the patient what activities are appropriate based on physical condition

Instruct the patient how to safely progress activity/exercise

Caution the patient on the dangers of overestimating capabilities, as appropriate

Warn the patient of the effects of extreme heat and cold, as appropriate

Instruct the patient on methods to conserve energy, as appropriate

Instruct the patient about how to properly stretch before and after activity/exercise and the rationale for doing so, as appropriate

Instruct the patient how to warm up and cool down before and after activity/exercise and the importance of doing so, as appropriate

Instruct the patient on good posture and body mechanics, as appropriate

Observe the patient perform the prescribed activity/exercise

Provide information on available assistive devices that may be used to facilitate performance of the required skill, as appropriate

Instruct the patient on the assembly, use, and maintenance of assistive devices, as appropriate

Assist the patient to incorporate activity/exercise regimen into daily routine/lifestyle

Assist the patient to properly alternate periods of rest and activity

Refer the patient to physical therapist/occupational therapist/exercise physiologist, as appropriate

Reinforce information provided by other health care team members, as appropriate

Include the family/significant others, as appropriate

Provide information on available community resources/support groups to increase the patient's compliance with activity/exercise, as appropriate

Refer the patient to a rehabilitation center, as appropriate

Background Readings:

Rakel, B.A. (1992). Interventions related to patient teaching. In G.M. Bulechek & J.C. McCloskey (Eds.), Symposium on Nursing Interventions. Nursing Clinics of North America, 27(2), 397-424.

Springhouse. (1987). Core teaching topics. In Patient teaching (Nurse's Reference Library): Learning needs, discharge preparation, tips and checklists (pp. 83-89). Springhouse, PA: Springhouse.

T

Teaching: Prescribed Diet   5614

Definition: Preparing a patient to correctly follow a prescribed diet

Activities:

Appraise the patient's current level of knowledge about prescribed diet

Determine the patient's/significant other's feelings/attitude toward prescribed diet and expected degree of dietary compliance

Instruct the patient on the proper name of the prescribed diet

Explain the purpose of the diet

Inform the patient about how long the diet should be followed

Instruct the patient about how to keep a food diary, as appropriate

Instruct the patient on allowed and prohibited foods

Inform the patient of possible drug-food interactions, as appropriate

Assist the patient to accommodate food preferences into the prescribed diet

Assist the patient in substituting ingredients to conform favorite recipes to the prescribed diet

Instruct the patient about how to read labels and select appropriate foods

Observe the patient's selection of foods appropriate to prescribed diet

Instruct the patient about how to plan appropriate meals

Provide written meal plans, as appropriate

Recommend a cookbook that includes recipes consistent with the diet, as appropriate

Reinforce information provided by other health care team members, as appropriate

Refer patient to dietitian/nutritionist, as appropriate

Include the family/significant others, as appropriate

Background Readings:

Rakel, B.A. (1992). Interventions related to patient teaching. In G.M. Bulechek & J.C. McCloskey (Eds.), Symposium on Nursing Interventions. Nursing Clinics of North America, 27(2), 397-424.

Snetselaar, L. (1987). Teaching patients, families and communities about nutrition. In C.E. Smith (Ed.), Patient education: Nurses in partnership with other health professionals (pp. 297-330). Philadelphia: W.B. Saunders.

Springhouse. (1987). Core teaching topics. In Patient teaching (Nurse's Reference Library): Learning needs, discharge preparation, tips and checklists (pp. 83-89). Springhouse, PA: Springhouse.

T

Teaching: Prescribed Medication   5616

Definition: Preparing a patient to safely take prescribed medications and monitor for their effects

Activities:

Instruct the patient to recognize distinctive characteristics of the medication(s), as appropriate

Inform the patient of both the generic and brand names of each medication

Instruct the patient on the purpose and action of each medication

Explain how health care providers choose the most appropriate medication

Instruct the patient on the dosage, route, and duration of each medication

Instruct the patient on the proper administration/application of each medication

Review patient's knowledge of medications

Acknowledge patient's knowledge of medications

Evaluate the patient's ability to self-administer medications

Instruct the patient to perform needed procedures before taking a medication (e.g., check pulse, glucose), as appropriate

Inform the patient what to do if a dose of medication is missed

Instruct the patient on which criteria to use when deciding to alter the medication dosage/schedule, as appropriate

Inform the patient of consequences of not taking or abruptly discontinuing medication(s), as appropriate

Instruct the patient on specific precautions to observe when taking medication(s) (e.g., no driving/using power tools), as appropriate

Instruct the patient on possible adverse effects of each medication

Instruct the patient how to relieve and/or prevent certain side effects, as appropriate

Instruct the patient on appropriate actions to take if side effects occur

Instruct the patient on the signs and symptoms of overdosage/underdosage

Inform the patient of possible drug-food interactions, as appropriate

Instruct the patient how to properly store the medication(s)

Instruct the patient on the proper care of devices used for administration

Instruct the patient on proper disposal of needles and syringes at home, as appropriate, and where to dispose of the sharps container in his/her community

Provide the patient with written information about the action, purpose, side effects, and so on, of medications

Assist the patient to develop a written medication schedule

Instruct the patient to carry documentation of his/her prescribed medication regimen

Instruct the patient how to fill his/her prescription(s), as appropriate

Inform the patient of possible changes in appearance and/or dosage when filling generic medication prescription(s)

Warn the patient of the risks associated with taking expired medication

Caution the patient against giving prescribed medication to others

Determine the patient's ability to obtain required medications

Provide information on medication reimbursement, as appropriate

T

Continued

Activities:—cont'd

Provide information on cost savings programs/organizations to obtain medications and devices, as appropriate

Provide information on medication alert devices and how to obtain them

Reinforce information provided by other health care team members, as appropriate

Include the family/significant others, as appropriate

Background Readings:

Devine, E.C., & Reifschneider, E. (1995). A meta-analysis of the effects of psychoeducational care in adults with hypertension. Nursing Research, 44(4), 237-245.

Doak, C.C. (1996). Teaching patients with low literacy skills. (2nd ed.). Philadelphia: J.B. Lippincott.

Hayes, K.S. (1998). Randomized trial of geragogy-based medication instruction in the emergency department. Nursing Research, 47(4), 211-218.

Kleoppel, J.W., & Henry, D.W. (1987). Teaching patients, families, and communities about their medications. In C.E. Smith (Ed.), Patient education: Nurses in partnership with other health professionals (pp. 271-296). Philadelphia: W.B. Saunders.

Proos, M., Reiley, P., Eagan, J., Stengrevics, S., Castile, J., & Arian, D. (1992). A study of the effects of self-medication on patients' knowledge of and compliance with their medication regimen. Journal of Nursing Care Quality, (Special Report), 18-26.

Rakel, B.A. (1992). Interventions related to patient teaching. In G.M. Bulechek & J.C. McCloskey (Eds.), Symposium on Nursing Interventions. Nursing Clinics of North America, 27(2), 397-424.

Springhouse Corporation. (1987). Core teaching topics. In Patient teaching: Learning needs, discharge preparation, tips and checklists (pp. 83-99). Springhouse, PA: Springhouse Corporation.

Springhouse Corporation. (1987). Drug therapy. In Patient teaching manual (Vol. 1) (pp. 401-503). Springhouse, PA: Springhouse Corporation.

T

Teaching: Procedure/Treatment 　　5618

Definition: Preparing a patient to understand and mentally prepare for a prescribed procedure or treatment

Activities:

Inform the patient/significant other(s) about when and where the procedure/treatment will take place, as appropriate

Inform the patient/significant other(s) about how long the procedure/treatment is expected to last

Tell the patient/significant other(s) who will be performing the procedure/treatment

Reinforce the patient's confidence in the staff involved, as appropriate

Determine the patient's previous experience(s) and level of knowledge related to procedure/treatment

Explain the purpose of the procedure/treatment

Describe the preprocedure/pretreatment activities

Explain the procedure/treatment

Obtain/witness patient's informed consent for the procedure/treatment according to agency policy, as appropriate

Instruct the patient on how to cooperate/participate during the procedure/treatment, as appropriate

Involve child in procedure (e.g., allow child to hold bandage) but don't give a choice about completing procedure

Conduct a tour of the procedure/treatment room and waiting area, as appropriate

Introduce the patient to the staff who will be involved in the procedure/treatment, as appropriate

Explain the need for and function of certain equipment (e.g., monitoring devices)

Discuss the need for special measures during the procedure/treatment, as appropriate

Provide information on what will be heard, smelled, seen, tasted, or felt during the procedure/treatment

Describe the postprocedure/posttreatment assessments and activities and the rationale for them

Inform the patient how he/she can aid in recuperation

Reinforce information provided by other health care team members, as appropriate

Provide time for the patient to rehearse events that will happen, as appropriate

Instruct the patient to use coping techniques directed at controlling specific aspects of the experience (e.g., relaxation and imagery), as appropriate

Provide distraction that will divert child's attention away from procedure

Provide information on when and where results will be available and indicate who will explain them

Determine the patient's expectations of the procedure/treatment

Correct unrealistic expectations of the procedure/treatment, as appropriate

Discuss alternative treatments, as appropriate

Provide time for the patient to ask questions and discuss concerns

Include the family/significant others, as appropriate

Background Readings:

Monroe, D. (1989). Patient teaching for x-ray and other diagnostics. RN, 52(12), 36-40.

Rakel, B.A. (1992). Interventions related to patient teaching. In G.M. Bulechek & J.C. McCloskey (Eds.), Symposium on Nursing Interventions. Nursing Clinics of North America, 27(2), 397-424.

Springhouse. (1987). Core teaching topics. In Patient teaching (Nurse's Reference Library): Learning needs, discharge preparation, tips and checklists (pp. 83-89). Springhouse, PA: Springhouse.

Wong, D.L. (1998). Whaley and Wong's nursing care of infants and children (6th ed.). St. Louis: Mosby.

T

Teaching: Psychomotor Skill   5620

Definition: Preparing a patient to perform a psychomotor skill

Activities:

Demonstrate the skill for the patient

Give clear, step-by-step directions

Instruct the patient to perform the skill one step at a time

Inform the patient of the rationale for performing the skill in the specified manner

Guide the patients' body so that he/she can experience the physical sensations that accompany the correct motions, as appropriate

Provide written information/diagrams, as appropriate

Provide practice sessions (spaced to avoid fatigue, but often enough to prevent excessive forgetting), as appropriate

Provide adequate time for task mastery

Observe patient return demonstrate the skill

Provide frequent feedback to patient on what he/she is doing correctly and incorrectly, so that bad habits are not formed

Provide information on available assistive devices that may be used to facilitate performance of the required skill, as appropriate

Instruct the patient on the assembly, use, and maintenance of assistive devices, as appropriate

Include the family/significant others, as appropriate

Background Readings:

Rakel, B.A. (1992). Interventions related to patient teaching. In G.M. Bulechek & J.C. McCloskey (Eds.), Symposium on Nursing Interventions. Nursing Clinics of North America, 27(2), 397-424.

Springhouse. (1987). Patient teaching (Nurse's Reference Library): Learning needs, discharge preparation, tips and checklists. Springhouse, PA: Springhouse.

T

Teaching: Safe Sex   5622

Definition: Providing instruction concerning sexual protection during sexual activity

Activities:

Discuss patient's attitudes about various birth control methods

Instruct patient on the use of effective birth control methods, as appropriate

Incorporate religious beliefs into discussions of birth control, as appropriate

Discuss abstinence as a means of birth control, as appropriate

Encourage patient to be selective when choosing sexual partners, as appropriate

Stress the importance of knowing the partner's sexual history, as appropriate

Instruct patient on low-risk sexual practices, such as those that avoid bodily penetration or the exchange of body fluids, as appropriate

Instruct patient on the importance of good hygiene, lubrication, and voiding after intercourse, to decrease susceptibility to infections

Endorse use of condoms, as appropriate

Instruct patient on how to choose condoms and keep them intact, as appropriate

Instruct patient on proper application and removal of condoms, as appropriate

Discuss with patient ways to convince partners to use condoms

Instruct patient on spermicidal products that can enhance protection from sexually transmitted diseases, as appropriate

Provide patient with condoms/spermicidal products, as appropriate

Encourage patient at high risk for sexually transmitted diseases to seek regular examinations

Refer patient with sexual problem or questions to appropriate health care provider, as appropriate

Plan sex education classes for group of patients, as appropriate

Background Readings:

Andrist, L.C. (1988). Taking a sexual history and educating clients about safe sex. Nursing Clinics of North America, 23(4), 959-973.

Dirubbo, N.E. (1987). The condom barrier. American Journal of Nursing, 98(10), 1306-1309.

Hajagos, K., Geiser, P., Parker, B. & Tesfa, A. (1998). Safer-sex education for persons with mental illness. Journal of Psychosocial Nursing and Mental Health Services, 36(8), 33-39.

Lewis, H.R., & Lewis, M.E. (1987). What you and your patients need to know about safer sex. RN, 50(9), 53-55, 56, 59.

T

Teaching: Sexuality   5624

Definition: Assisting individuals to understand physical and psychosocial dimensions of sexual growth and development

Activities:

Create an accepting, nonjudgmental atmosphere

Explain human anatomy and physiology of the male and female body

Explain the anatomy and physiology of human reproduction

Discuss signs of fertility (related to ovulation and menstrual cycle)

Explain emotional development during childhood and adolescence

Facilitate communication between children or adolescents, and parents

Support parents' role as the primary sexuality educators of their children

Educate parents on sexual growth and development through the life span

Provide parents with a bibliography of sexuality education materials

Discuss what values are, how we obtain them, and their effect on our choices in life

Facilitate the children's and adolescents' awareness of family, peer, societal, and media influence on values

Use appropriate questions to assist children and adolescents to reflect on what is important personally

Discuss peer and social pressure in relation to sexual activity

Explore the meaning of sexual roles

Discuss sexual behavior and appropriate ways to express one's feelings and needs

Inform children and adolescents of the benefits of postponing sexual activity

Educate children and adolescents on the negative consequences of early childbearing (e.g., poverty and loss of education and career opportunities)

Teach children and adolescents about AIDs and other sexually transmitted diseases

Promote responsibility for sexual behavior

Discuss benefits of abstinence

Inform children and adolescents about effective contraceptives

Inform adolescents about accessibility of contraceptives and how to obtain them

Assist adolescents in choosing an appropriate contraceptive, as appropriate

Facilitate role playing where decision making and assertive communication skills may be practiced to resist peer and social pressures of sexual activity

Enhance self-esteem through peer role modeling and role playing

Background Readings:

Howard, M., & McCabe, J. (1990). Helping teenagers postpone sexual involvement. Family Planning Perspectives, 22(1), 21-26.

Kirby, D., Barth, R., Leland, N., & Fetro, J. (1991). Reducing the risk: Impact of a new curriculum on sexual risk-taking. Family Planning Perspectives, 23(6), 253-263.

Roth, B. (1993). Fertility awareness as a component of sexuality education. Nurse Practitioner, 18(3), 40-53.

Smith, M. (1993). Pediatric sexuality: Promoting normal sexual development in children. Nurse Practitioner, 18(8), 37-44.

Stevens-Simon, C. (1993). Clinical applications of adolescent female sexual development. Nurse Practitioner, 18(12), 18-29.

Vincent, M.L., Clearie, A.F., & Schluchter, M.D. (1987). Reducing adolescent pregnancy through school and community-based education. Journal of American Medical Association, 257(24), 3382-3385.

Teaching: Toddler Nutrition   5630

Definition: Instruction on nutrition and feeding practices during the second and third years of life

Activities:
Provide parents with written materials appropriate to identified knowledge needs

Instruct parent/caregiver of toddler 13-18 months to:
   discontinue bottle feeding
   offer textured solids
   continue use of spoon and self-feeding
   introduce dairy products
   provide healthy snacks
   offer small portions and frequent feedings
   avoid "diet" food/drinks (e.g., nonfat milk, diet soda)
   avoid force feeding as there is decreased appetite

Instruct parent/caregiver of toddler 19-24 months to:
   encourage drinking water for thirst
   limit fluids before meals
   offer foods high in iron and protein
   have regular mealtimes and eat as a family
   increase or decrease foods, as appropriate
   avoid fruit drinks and flavored milk
   read the labels for nutritive content
   discontinue bottle feeding

Instruct parent/caregiver of toddler 25-36 months to:
   give child healthy food choices
   encourage child to eat raw/cooked vegetables
   provide healthy snacks between meals
   be creative in food preparation for picky eater
   offer small portions of food
   limit fat content in foods
   have child participate in food preparation
   offer iron-fortified cereals, avoiding high-sugar cereals
   increase protein foods
   include all food groups
   avoid use of food as a reward

Background Readings:

Barnes, L.A. (Ed.). (1993). Pediatric nutrition handbook (3rd ed.). Elk Grove Village, IL: American Academy of Pediatrics Committee on Nutrition.
California Department of Health Services WIC Supplemental Nutrition Branch. (1998a). Feeding your baby 6-12 months [Brochure]. Sacramento, CA: California Department of Health Services WIC Supplemental Nutrition Branch.
California Department of Health Services WIC Supplemental Nutrition Branch. (1998b). Feeding your baby birth to 8 months [Brochure]. Sacramento, CA: California Department of Health Services, WIC Supplemental Nutrition Branch.
California Department of Health Services WIC Supplemental Nutrition Branch. (1997). Feeding your 1-3 year old [Brochure]. Sacramento, CA: California Department of Health Services WIC Supplemental Nutrition Branch.
Formon, S.J. (1993). Nutrition of normal infants. St. Louis: Mosby.
Satter, E. & Sharkey, P.B. (1997). Ellyn Satter's nutrition and feeding for infants and children: Handout masters. Madison, WI: E. Satter & P.B. Sharkey.

T

Teaching: Toddler Safety   5632

Definition: Instruction on safety during the second and third years of life

Activities:
Provide parents with written materials appropriate to identified knowledge needs

Instruct parent/caregiver of toddler 13-18 months to:
    supervise child outdoors
    install car seat and use it according to manufacturer's recommendations
    educate child about dangers of throwing and hitting
    prevent access to electrical outlets, cords, and electrical equipment/appliances/tools
    store weapons and weapon-like items under lock and key
    educate child about safe ways of interacting with pets
    secure doors/gates to prevent child's access to dangerous areas (e.g. street, driveway, pool)
    dispose of and/or remove the doors to unused refrigerators, ice chests, and other air-tight containers
    use back burners of the stove, install knob covers, and/or restrict child's access to kitchen
    set home water heater temperature to between 120° and 130° Fahrenheit

Instruct parent/caregiver of toddler 19-24 months to:
    store sharp objects, appliances, and kitchen items out of child's reach
    instruct child on dangers of the street
    store all cleaning supplies, medications, and personal care products out of child's reach
    ensure multiple barriers to pool/hot tub area

Instruct parent/caregiver of toddler 25-36 months to:
    instruct child on dangers of weapons
    select toys according to manufacturer's age recommendations
    provide supervision and instruct about safe use of large climbing and riding toys
    store matches/lighters out of child's reach and instruct child on the dangers of fire and fire starters
    always supervise child around swimming pools, ponds, hot tubs
    instruct child about stranger danger and good touch/bad touch
    provide an approved helmet for bike riding and instruct child to always wear it
    prevent child's access to upper story windows, balconies, and stairs
    closely supervise child when out in public settings
    instruct child how to get adult help when he/she feels scared or in danger

Background Readings:

American Academy of Pediatrics. (1994a). Birth to 6 months: Safety for your child [Brochure]. Elk Grove Village, IL: American Academy of Pediatrics.

American Academy of Pediatrics. (1994b). 6 to 12 months: Safety for your child [Brochure]. Elk Grove Village, IL: American Academy of Pediatrics.

American Academy of Pediatrics. (1994c). 1 to 2 years: Safety for your child [Brochure]. Elk Grove Village, IL: American Academy of Pediatrics.

American Academy of Pediatrics. (1994d). 2 to 4 years: Safety for your child [Brochure]. Elk Grove Village, IL: American Academy of Pediatrics.

California Center for Childhood Injury Prevention. (1997). Safe home assessment program. San Diego, CA: California Center for Childhood Injury Prevention.

California Department of Health Services Childhood Lead Poisoning Prevention Branch. (1994). Lead: Simple things that you can do to prevent childhood lead poisoning [Brochure]. Sacramento, CA: California Department of Health Services Childhood Lead Poisoning Prevention Branch.

T

Teaching: Toilet Training   5634

Definition: Instruction on determining the child's readiness and strategies to assist the child to learn independent toileting skills.

Activities:

Instruct parent about how to determine the child's physical readiness for toilet training:

child is at least 18-24 months of age; children from 24-36 months are more mature and likely to succeed

child shows evidence of being able to hold urine before voiding

child recognizes urge to go or that he/she has just voided or defecated

child shows some regularity in elimination patterns

child has the ability to navigate to the toilet/potty, sit on it, and get off when elimination has been completed

child has the ability to remove and replace clothing before and after elimination

child has the ability to wipe self and wash hands after elimination

Instruct parent about how to determine the child's psychosocial readiness for toilet training:

child expresses interest in and desire to participate/cooperate in toileting

child has vocabulary to communicate need to eliminate

child is anxious to please parents

child readily imitates the behaviors of others

Instruct parent about how to determine parental/family readiness for toilet training:

parent has knowledge and time to devote to training process

parent/family is experiencing no major transitions during or shortly after the process (e.g., change of job or residence, divorce, birth of another child)

parent has realistic expectations about child development and the time and energy needed to successfully complete the process

parents understand child may regress during times of stress or illness

Provide information on strategies to promote toilet training:

dress the child in loose, easy-to-remove clothing

agree on vocabulary to be used during training process

provide opportunities for child to observe others during the toileting process

take the child to the potty to introduce him/her to the equipment and process

take the child to the potty on a regular basis and encourage him/her to sit

reinforce the child's success with any part of the process

consider the child's temperament or behavior style when planning strategies

expect and ignore accidents

communicate strategies, expectations, and progress to other care providers

Support parents throughout this process

Encourage parents to be flexible and creative in developing and implementing training strategies

Provide additional information, as requested or needed

Background Readings:

Brazelton, T.B., Christophersen, E.R., Frauman, A.C., Gorski, P.A., Poole, J.M., Stradtler, A.C., & Wright, C.D. (1999). Instruction, timelines, and medical influences affecting toilet training. Pediatrics, 103(6), 1353-1358.

Doran, J., & Lister, A. (1998). Toilet training: Meeting the needs of children and parents. Community Practitioner, 71(5), 179-180.

Kinservik, M.A., & Friedhoff, M.M. (2000). Control issues in toilet training. Pediatric Nursing, 26(3), 267-274.

Stadtler, A.C., Gorski, P.A., & Brazelton, T.B. (1999). Toilet training methods, clinical interventions, and recommendations. Pediatrics, 103(6), 1359-1361.

T

Technology Management   7880

Definition: Use of technical equipment and devices to monitor patient condition or sustain life

Activities:

Change or replace patient care equipment, per protocol

Provide standby equipment, as appropriate

Maintain equipment in good working order

Correct malfunctioning equipment

Zero and calibrate equipment, as appropriate

Keep emergency equipment in an appropriate and readily accessible place

Ensure proper grounding of electronic equipment

Plug equipment into electrical outlets connected to an emergency power source

Have equipment periodically checked by bioengineering, as appropriate

Recharge batteries in portable patient care equipment

Set alarm limits on equipment, as appropriate

Respond to equipment alarms appropriately

Consult with other health care team members, and recommend equipment/devices for patient use

Use alterations in machine-derived data as an impetus for reassessing the patient

Compare machine-derived data with nurse's perception of patient's condition

Explain potential risks and benefits of using this technology

Facilitate obtaining informed consent, as appropriate

Place bedside equipment strategically to maximize patient access and prevent tripping over tubes and cords

Become knowledgeable about the equipment and proficient in using it

Teach patient and family how to operate equipment, as appropriate

Teach patient and family the expected outcomes and side effects associated with using the equipment

Facilitate ethical decision making related to use of life-sustaining and life-support technologies, as appropriate

Demonstrate to family members how to communicate with patient connected to life-support equipment

Facilitate interaction between family members and patient who is receiving life-support therapy

Monitor the effect of equipment use on the physiological, psychological, and social functioning of the patient and family

Monitor effectiveness of the technology on patient outcomes

T

Background Readings:

Alexander, J.W., & Mark, B. (1990). Technology and structure of nursing organizations. Nursing and Health Care, 11(4), 195-199.

Jacox, A. (1990). Nursing and technology. Nursing Economics, 8(2), 116-119.

Jacox, A., Pillar, B., & Redman, B.K. (1990). A classification of nursing technology. Nursing Outlook, 38(2), 81-85.

McCauley, M.D., & Von Reuden, K.T. (1988). Noninvasive monitoring of the mechanically ventilated patient. Critical Care Nursing Quarterly, 11(3), 36-49.

McConnell, E. (1990). The impact of machines on the work of critical care nurses. Critical Care Nursing Quarterly, March, 45-52.

Pillar, B., Jacox, A.K., & Redman, B.K. (1990). Technology, its assessment and nursing. Nursing Outlook, 38(1), 16-19.

T

Telephone Consultation   8180

Definition: Eliciting patient's concerns; listening; and providing support, information, or teaching in response to patient's stated concerns, over the telephone

Activities:

Identify self with name and credentials, organization; let caller know if call is being recorded (e.g., for quality monitoring), using voice to create therapeutic relationship

Inform patient about call process and obtain consent

Consider cultural, socioeconomic barriers to patient's response

Obtain information about purpose of the call (e.g., medical diagnoses if any, health history, and current treatment regimen)

Identify concerns about health status

Establish level of caller's knowledge and source of that knowledge

Determine patient's ability to understand telephone teaching/instructions (e.g., hearing deficits, confusion, language barriers)

Provide means of overcoming any identified barrier to learning or use of support system(s)

Identify degree of family support and involvement in care

Inquire about related complaints/symptoms/ (according to standard protocol, if available)

Obtain data related to effectiveness of current treatment(s) if any, by consulting and citing approved references as sources (e.g., "American Red Cross suggests . . .")

Determine psychological response to situation and availability of support system(s)

Determine safety risk to caller and/others

Determine whether concerns require further evaluation (use standard protocol)

Provide clear instructions on how to access needed care, if concerns are immediate

Provide information about treatment regimen and resultant self-care responsibilities, as necessary, according to scope of practice and established guidelines

Provide information about prescribed therapies and medications, as appropriate

Provide information about health promotion/health education, as appropriate,

Identify actual/potential problems related to implementation self-care regimen

Make recommendations about regimen changes as appropriate (using established guidelines if available)

Consult with physician/primary care provider about changes in the treatment regimen, as necessary

Provide information about community resources, educational programs, support groups, and self-help groups, as indicated

Provide services in a caring and supportive manner

Involve family/significant others in the care and planning

Answer questions

Determine caller's understanding of information provided

Maintain confidentiality, as indicated

Document any assessments, advice, instructions, or other information given to patient according to specified guidelines

Follow guidelines for investigating or reporting suspected child, elder, or spousal abuse situations

Follow up to determine disposition; document disposition and patient's intended action(s)

Activities:—cont'd

Determine need, and establish time intervals for, further intermittent assessment, as appropriate

Determine how patient or family member can be reached for a return telephone call, as appropriate

Document permission for return call and identify persons able to receive call information

Discuss and resolve problem calls with supervisory/collegial help

Background Readings:

American Academy of Ambulatory Nursing. (1997). Telephone nursing practice administration and practice standards. Pitman, NJ: Anthony J. Jannetti, Inc.

Anderson, K., Qiu, Y., Whittaker, A.R., & Lucas, M. (2001). Breath sounds, asthma, and the mobile phone. Lancet, 358(9290), 1343-1344.

Haas, S.A., & Androwich, I.A. (1999). Telephone consultation. In G.M. Bulechek & J.C. McCloskey (Eds.), Nursing interventions: Effective nursing treatments (3rd ed.) (pp. 670-685). Philadelphia: W.B. Saunders.

Hagan, L., Morin, D., & Lepine, R. (2000). Evaluation of telenursing outcomes: Satisfaction, self-care practices, and cost savings. Public Health Nursing, 17(4), 305-313.

Larson-Dahn, M. L. (2001). Tel-eNurse practice: Quality of care and patient outcomes. Journal of Nursing Administration, 31(3), 145-152.

Poole, S. G., Schmitt, B.D., Carruth, T., Peterson-Smith, A.A., & Slusarski, M. (1993). After-hours telephone coverage: The application of an area-wide telephone triage and advice system for pediatric practices. Pediatrics, 92(5), 670-679.

Wheeler, S., & Siebelt, B. (1997). Calling all nurses: How to perform telephone triage. Nursing, 97(7), 37-41.

T

Telephone Follow-Up 8190

Definition: Providing results of testing or evaluating patient's response and determining potential for problems as a result of previous treatment, examination, or testing, over the telephone

Activities:

Determine that you are actually speaking to the patient or, if someone else, that you have the patient's permission to give information to the person

Identify self with name and credentials, organization; let caller know if call is being recorded (e.g., for quality monitoring)

Inform patient about call process and obtain consent

Notify patient of test results, as indicated (positive results with significant health implications, such as biopsy results, should not be given over the phone by the nurse)

Use intermediary services such as language relay services, TTY/TDD (text telephone for hearing- and speech-impaired persons), or emerging telecommunication technologies such as computer networks or visual displays, as appropriate

Assist with prescription refills, according to established guidelines

Solicit and answer questions

Provide information about community resources, educational programs, support groups, and self-help groups, as indicated

Establish a date and time for follow-up care or referral appointment

Provide information about treatment regimen and resultant self-care responsibilities, as necessary, according to scope of practice and established guidelines

Maintain confidentiality

Do not leave follow-up messages on answering machines or voice mail, to ensure confidentiality

Document any assessments, advice, instructions, or other information given to patient according to specified guidelines

Determine how patient or family member can be reached for a return telephone call, as appropriate

Document permission for return call and identify persons able to receive call information

Background Readings:

AAACN/ANA Task Force. (1997). Nursing in ambulatory care: The future is here. Washington, DC: American Nurses Publishing.

American Academy of Ambulatory Nursing. (1997). Telephone nursing practice administration and practice standards. Pitman, NJ: Anthony J. Jannetti, Inc.

Anderson, K, Oiu, Y., Wittaker, A.R., & Lucas, M. (2001). Breath sounds, asthma, and the mobile phone. Lancet, 358, 1343-1344.

Hagan, L. Morin, D., & Lepine, R. (2000). Evaluation of telenursing outcomes: Satisfaction, self-care practices, and cost savings. Public Health Nursing, 17(4), 305-313.

Larson-Dahn, M.L. (2001). Tel-eNurse practice: Quality of care and patient outcomes. Journal of Nursing Administration, 31(3), 145-152.

Pidd, H., McGrory, K.J., & Payne, S.R. (2000). Telephone follow-up after urological surgery. Professional Nurse, 15(7), 449-451.

Weaver, L.A., & Doran, K.A. (2001). Telephone follow-up after cardiac surgery. American Journal of Nursing, 101(5), 24OO, 24QQ, 24SS, passim.

T

Temperature Regulation   3900

Definition: Attaining and/or maintaining body temperature within a normal range

Activities:

Monitor temperature at least every 2 hours, as appropriate

Monitor newborn's temperature until stabilized

Institute use of a continuous core temperature monitoring device, as appropriate

Monitor blood pressure, pulse, and respiration, as appropriate

Monitor skin color and temperature

Monitor for and report signs and symptoms of hypothermia and hyperthermia

Promote adequate fluid and nutritional intake

Wrap infant immediately after birth to prevent heat loss

Maintain warm body temperature of newborn

Apply stockinette cap to prevent heat loss of newborn

Teach patients how to prevent heat exhaustion and heat stroke

Place newborn in isolette or under warmer, as needed

Discuss importance of thermoregulation and possible negative effects of excess chilling, as appropriate

Teach patients, particularly elderly patients, actions to prevent hypothermia from cold exposure

Teach indications of heat exhaustion and appropriate emergency treatment, as appropriate

Teach indications of hypothermia and appropriate emergency treatment, as appropriate

Use heat mattress and warm blankets to adjust altered body temperature, as appropriate

Adjust environmental temperature to patient's needs

Give appropriate medication to prevent or control shivering

Administer antipyretic medication, as appropriate

Use cooling mattress and tepid baths to adjust altered body temperature, as appropriate

Background Readings:

Beutler, B., & Beutler, S. (1992). Pathogenesis of fever. In J.B. Wyngaarden, L.H. Smith, Jr., & J.C. Bennett, Jr. (Eds.), Cecil textbook of medicine (19th ed.) (pp. 1568-1571). Philadelphia: W.B. Saunders.

Thomas, K.A. (1991). The emergence of body temperature biorhythm in preterm infants. Nursing Research, 40(2), 98-102.

Thompson, J.M., McFarland, G.K., Hirsch, J.E., & Tucker, S.M. (1998). Mosby's clinical nursing (4th ed.). St. Louis: Mosby.

T

Temperature Regulation: Intraoperative   3902

Definition: Attaining and/or maintaining desired intraoperative body temperature

Activities:

Adjust operating room temperature for therapeutic effect

Set up and regulate appropriate warming/cooling devices

Apply head covering

Cover patient with reflective blanket

Provide or set up humidifier for anesthetic gases

Transport neonates and infants in heated isolette

Cover exposed body parts

Warm or cool all irrigating, IV, and skin preparation solutions, as appropriate

Provide and regulate blood warmer, as appropriate

Warm surgical sponges

Continuously monitor patient temperature

Monitor room temperature

Monitor and maintain temperature of warming/cooling devices

Monitor and maintain temperature of irrigating solutions

Cover patient with heated blanket for transport to postanesthesia care unit

Document information, per agency policy

Background Readings:

Association of Operating Room Nurses. (1989). Intraoperative phase. In B. Bailes (Ed.), Perioperative nursing research: A ten year review. Denver: AORN.

Biddle, C., & Biddle, W. (1985). A plastic head cover to reduce surgical heat loss. Geriatric Nursing–American Journal of Care for the Aging, 6(1), 39-41.

Closs, J., MacDonald, J., & Hawthorn, P. (1986). Factors affecting perioperative body temperature. Journal of Advanced Nursing, 11(6), 739-744.

Craven, R.F., & Hirnle, C.J. (2000) Fundamentals of nursing: Human health and function (3rd ed.) (p. 595). Philadelphia: Lippincott.

Roizen, M., Sohn, Y.J., L'Hommedieu, C.S., et al. (1980). Operating room temperature prior to surgical draping: Effect on patient temperature in recovery room. Anesthesia and Analgesia, 59(11), 852-855.

Wehmer, M., & Baldwin, B. (1986). Inadvertent hypothermia: Clinical nursing research. AORN Journal, 44(5), 788-793.

White, H.E., Thurston, N.E., Blackmore, K.A., et al. (1987). Body temperature in elderly surgical patients. Research in Nursing and Health, 10(5), 317-321.

T

Temporary Pacemaker Management   4092

Definition: Temporary support of cardiac pumping though the insertion and use of temporary pacemakers

Activities:

Perform a comprehensive appraisal of peripheral circulation (e.g., check peripheral pulses, edema, capillary refill), skin temperature, and diaphoresis

Ensure ongoing monitoring of bedside EKG by qualified individuals

Note frequency and duration of dysrhythmias

Monitor hemodynamic response to dysrhythmias

Facilitate acquisition of a 12-lead EKG, as appropriate

Monitor sensorium and cognitive abilities

Monitor blood pressure at specified intervals and with changes in patient's condition

Monitor heart rate and rhythm at specified intervals and with changes in patient's condition

Obtain informed consent for insertion of transvenous or epicardial transthoracic temporary pacemaker

Prepare skin on chest and back by washing with soap and water and trim body hair with scissors, not razor, as necessary

Assist with insertion of device (e.g., transvenous or epicardial transthoracic temporary pacemaker), as appropriate

Apply external transcutaneous pacemaker electrodes to the left anterior chest and to the posterior chest, as appropriate

Provide sedation and analgesia for patients receiving external transcutaneous pacemakers

Inspect skin frequently to prevent potential burns for patients receiving external transcutaneous pacemakers

Set rate (usually 60 to 80 beat/min) as directed by physician

Set output at intermediate output (approximately 5 mA) and decrease until capture is lost (usually at less than 2 mA), then set output at 2 to 3 times the output required for capture, or as directed by physician, for transvenous or epicardial transthoracic temporary pacemakers

Initiate pacing by slowly increasing the energy level (milliamperes or Joules), until consistent capture occurs (capture threshold) for external transcutaneous pacemaker

Assist with chest x-ray examination after insertion of tranvenous temporary pacemaker, if pacemaker is transvenous or epicardial transthoracic

Monitor for presence of paced rhythm or resolution of initiating dysrhythmia

Ensure that all equipment is grounded and in good working order

Wear gloves when adjusting electrodes

Insulate electrode wires when not in use

Monitor for signs of improved cardiac output at specified intervals after initiation of pacing (e.g. improved urine output, warm and dry skin, freedom from chest pain, stable vital signs, absence of JVD and crackles, improved level of consciousness), per facility protocol

Palpate peripheral pulses at specified intervals, per facility protocol, to ensure adequate perfusion with paced beats

Monitor for potential complications associated with pacemaker insertion (e.g., pneumothorax, hemothorax, myocardial perforation, cardiac tamponade, hematoma, PVCs, infections, hiccups, muscle twitches)

Monitor for failure to pace and determine cause (e.g., battery failure, lead dislodgment, wire fracture, disconnected wire or cable), as appropriate

T

Continued

Activities:—cont'd

Monitor for failure to capture and determine cause (e.g., lead dislodgment or malposition, battery failure, pacing at voltage below capture threshold, faulty connections, lead fracture, ventricular perforation), as appropriate

Monitor for failure to sense and determine cause (e.g., sensitivity set too high, battery failure, malposition of catheter lead, lead fracture, pulse generator failure, lead insulation break), as appropriate

Instruct patient and family member(s) regarding symptoms to report (e.g., dizziness, fainting, prolonged weakness, nausea, palpitations, chest pain, difficulty breathing, discomfort at insertion or external electrode site, electrical shocks)

Teach patient and family member(s) precautions and restrictions required while temporary pacemaker is in place (e.g., limitation of movement, avoid handling the pacemaker)

Background Readings:

Alspach, J. G. (1998). Core curriculum for critical care nursing. (5th ed.). Philadelphia: W. B. Saunders.
Lynn-McHale, D. J., & Carlson, K. K. (2001). AACN procedure manual for critical care (4th ed.). Philadelphia: W. B. Saunders.

T

Therapeutic Play 4430

Definition: Purposeful and directive use of toys or other materials to assist children in communicating their perception and knowledge of their world and to help in gaining mastery of their environment

Activities:

Provide a quiet environment that is free from interruptions

Provide sufficient time to allow for effective play

Structure play session to facilitate desired outcome

Communicate the purpose of play session to child and parent

Discuss play activities with family

Set limits for therapeutic play session

Provide safe play equipment

Provide developmentally appropriate play equipment

Provide play equipment that stimulates creative, expressive play

Provide play equipment that stimulates role playing

Provide real or simulated hospital or medical equipment to encourage expression of knowledge and feelings about hospitalization, treatments, or illness

Supervise therapeutic play sessions

Encourage child to manipulate play equipment

Encourage child to share feelings, knowledge, and perceptions

Validate child's feelings expressed during the play session

Communicate acceptance of feelings, both positive and negative, expressed through play

Observe the child's use of play equipment

Monitor child's reactions and anxiety level throughout play session

Identify child's misconceptions or fears through comments made during (hospital role) play session

Continue play sessions on a regular basis to establish trust and reduce fear of unfamiliar equipment or treatments, as appropriate

Record observations made during play session

Background Readings:

Hart, R., Powell, M.A., Mather, P.L., & Slack, J.L. (1992). Therapeutic play activities for hospitalized children. St. Louis: Mosby–Year Book.

Snyder, M. (1992). Play. In M. Snyder (Ed.), Independent nursing interventions (2nd ed.) (pp. 287-293). Albany, NY: Delmar Publishers, Inc.

Tiedeman, M.E., Simon, K.A., & Clatworthy, S. (1990). Communication through therapeutic play. In M.J. Craft & J.A. Denehy (Eds.), Nursing interventions for infants and children (pp. 93-110). Philadelphia: W.B. Saunders.

Vessey, J.A., & Mahon, M.M. (1990). Therapeutic play and the hospitalized child. Journal of Pediatric Nursing, 5(5), 328-333.

T

Therapeutic Touch   5465

Definition: Attuning to the universal healing field, seeking to act as an instrument for healing influence, and using the natural sensitivity of the hands to gently focus and direct the intervention process

Activities:

Focus awareness on the inner self

Focus on the intention to facilitate wholeness and healing at all levels of consciousness

Place the hands 1 to 2 inches from the patient's body

Begin the assessment by moving the hands slowly and steadily over as much of the patient as possible, from head to toe and front to back

Note the overall pattern of the energy flow, especially any areas of disturbance such as congestion or unevenness, which may be perceived through very subtle cues in the hands, for example, temperature change, tingling, or other subtle feelings of movement

Focus intention on facilitating symmetry and healing in disturbed areas

Begin by moving the hands in very gentle downward movements through the patient's energy field, thinking of the patient as a unitary whole and facilitating an open and balanced energy flow

Continue the treatment by very gently facilitating the flow of healing energy into areas of disturbance

Finish when it is judged that the appropriate amount of change has taken place (i.e., for an infant, 1 to 2 minutes; for an adult, 5 to 7 minutes), keeping in mind the importance of gentleness

Note whether the patient has experienced a relaxation response and any related outcomes

Background Readings:

Engle, V.F., & Graney, M.J. (2000). Biobehavioral effects of theraputic touch. Journal of Nursing Scholarship, 32(3), 287-293.

Krieger, D. (1979). The therapeutic touch. Englewood Cliffs, NJ: Prentice-Hall.

Meehan, T.C. (1999). Therapeutic touch. In G.M. Bulechek & J.C. McCloskey (Eds.), Nursing interventions: Essential nursing treatments (3rd ed.) (pp. 173-188). Philadelphia: W.B. Saunders.

O'Mathuna, D.P. (2000). Evidence-based practice and reviews of therapeutic touch. Journal of Nursing Scholarship, 32(3), 279-285.

Quinn, J. (1984). Therapeutic touch as energy exchange: Testing the theory. Advances in Nursing Science, 6(2), 42-49.

T

Therapy Group   5450

Definition: Application of psychotherapeutic techniques to a group, including the utilization of interactions between members of the group

Activities:

Determine the purpose of the group (e.g., maintenance of reality testing, facilitation of communication, examination of interpersonal skills, and/or support) and the nature of the group process

Form a group of optimal size: 5 to 12 members

Choose group members who are willing to participate actively and take responsibility for own problems

Determine whether level of motivation is high enough to benefit from group therapy

Use a coleader, as appropriate

Address the issue of mandatory attendance

Address the issue of whether new members can join at any time

Establish a time and place for the group meeting

Meet in 1- to 2-hour sessions, as appropriate

Begin and end on time and expect participants to remain until the conclusion

Arrange chairs close together in a circle

Move the group to the working stage as quickly as possible

Assist the group in forming therapeutic norms

Help the group to work through resistance to change

Give group members a sense of direction that enables them to identify and resolve each step of development

Use the technique of "process illumination" to encourage exploration of the significance of the message

Encourage self-disclosure and discussion of the past only as they relate to the function and goals of the group

Use the technique of "here and now activation" to move the focus from the generic to the personal, from the abstract to the specific

Encourage members to share things they have in common with each other

Encourage members to share their anger, sadness, humor, mistrust, and other feelings with each other

Assist members in the process of exploration and acceptance of any anger felt toward the group leader and others

Confront behaviors that threaten group cohesion (e.g., tardiness, absences, disruptive extragroup socialization, subgrouping, and scapegoating)

Provide social reinforcement (verbal and nonverbal) for desired behaviors/responses

Provide structured group exercises, as appropriate, to promote group function and insight

Use role playing and problem solving, as appropriate

Help members provide feedback to each other, so that they develop insights into their own behavior

Incorporate leaderless sessions, when appropriate to the goals and function of the group

Conclude session with a summary of the proceedings

Meet individually with the member who desires premature termination to examine rationale for this

Assist member to terminate from the group, if appropriate

Assist group to review the history and a member's relationship with the group when someone leaves

Continued

Activities:—cont'd

Recruit new members, as appropriate, to maintain the integrity of the group

Provide an individualized orientation session for each new member of the group before first group session

Background Readings:

Lassiter, P.G. (1992). Working with groups in the community. In M. Stanhope & J. Lancaster (Eds.), Community health nursing (3rd ed.) (pp. 277-291). St. Louis: Mosby.

Snyder, M. (1992). Groups. In M. Snyder (Ed.), Independent nursing interventions (2nd ed.) (pp. 244-255). Albany, NY: Delmar Publishers.

Wieland, V., & Cummings, S. (1992). Group psychotherapy. In G.M. Bulechek & J.C. McCloskey (Eds.), Nursing interventions: Essential nursing treatments (2nd ed.) (pp. 340-351). Philadelphia: W.B. Saunders.

Yalom, I.D. (1985). The theory and practice of group psychotherapy (3rd ed.). New York: Basic Books.

T

Total Parenteral Nutrition (TPN) Administration   1200

Definition: Preparation and delivery of nutrients intravenously and monitoring of patient responsiveness

Activities:

Assist with insertion of central line

Insert peripheral IV central catheter, per agency protocol

Ascertain correct placement of IV central catheter by x-ray examination

Maintain central line patency and dressing, per agency protocol

Monitor for infiltration and infection

Check the TPN solution to ensure that correct nutrients are included, as ordered

Maintain sterile technique when preparing and hanging TPN solutions

Use an infusion pump for delivery of TPN solutions

Maintain a constant flow rate of TPN solution

Avoid rapidly replacing lagging TPN solution

Monitor patient's weight daily

Monitor intake and output

Monitor serum albumin, total protein, electrolyte, and glucose levels and chemistry profile

Monitor vital signs

Monitor urine glucose for glycosuria, acetone, and protein

Administer insulin, as ordered, to maintain serum glucose level in the designated range, as appropriate

Report abnormal signs and symptoms associated with TPN to the physician, and modify care accordingly

Maintain universal precautions

Background Readings:

Thelan, L.A., & Urden, L.D. (1998). Critical care nursing: Diagnosis and management (4th ed.). St. Louis: Mosby.

Travenol Laboratories. (1982). Fundamentals of nutritional support. Deerfield, IL: Travenol Laboratories, Hospital Division.

T

Touch 5460

Definition: Providing comfort and communication through purposeful tactile contact

Activities:

Observe cultural taboos about touch

Give a reassuring hug, as appropriate

Put arm around patient's shoulders, as appropriate

Hold patient's hand to provide emotional support

Apply gentle pressure at wrist, hand, or shoulder of seriously ill patient

Rub back in synchrony with patient's breathing, as appropriate

Stroke body part in slow, rhythmical fashion, as appropriate

Massage around painful area, as appropriate

Elicit from parents common actions used to soothe and calm their child

Hold infant or child firmly and snugly

Encourage parents to touch newborn or ill child

Surround premature infant with blanket rolls (nesting)

Swaddle infant snugly in a blanket to keep arms and legs close to the body

Place infant on mother's body immediately after birth

Encourage mother to hold, touch, and examine the infant while umbilical cord is being severed

Encourage parents to hold infant

Encourage parents to massage infant

Demonstrate quieting techniques for infants

Provide appropriate pacifier for nonnutritive sucking for newborns

Provide oral stimulation exercises before tube feedings for premature infants

Background Readings:

Molsberry, D., & Shogan, M.G. (1990). Communicating through touch. In M.J. Craft & J.A. Denehy (Eds.), Nursing interventions for infants and children (pp. 127-150). Philadelphia: W.B. Saunders.

Snyder, M., & Nojima, Y. Purposeful touch. In M. Snyder & R. Lindquist. (Eds.), Complementary/alternative therapies in nursing (3rd ed.) (pp. 149-158). New York: Springer Publishing Company.

Sorensen, K.C., & Luckmann, J. (1986). Basic nursing: A psychophysiologic approach. Philadelphia: W.B. Saunders.

Weiss, S.J. (1988). Touch. In J. Fitzpatrick, R. Taunton, & J. Benoliel (Eds.), Annual review of nursing research, 6, (pp. 3-27). New York: Springer.

Weiss, S.J. (1992). The tactile environment of caregiving: Implications for health science and health care. The Science of Caring, 3(2), 33-40.

T

Traction/Immobilization Care   0940

Definition: Management of a patient who has traction and/or a stabilizing device to immobilize and stabilize a body part

Activities:

Position in proper body alignment

Maintain proper position in bed to enhance traction

Ensure that proper weights are being applied

Ensure that the ropes and pulleys hang freely

Ensure that the pull of ropes and weights remains along the axis of the fractured bone

Brace traction weights while moving patient

Maintain traction at all times

Monitor self-care ability while in traction

Monitor external fixation device

Monitor pin insertion sites

Monitor skin and bony prominences for signs of skin breakdown

Monitor circulation, movement, and sensation of affected extremity

Monitor for complications of immobility

Perform pin insertion site care

Administer appropriate skin care at friction points

Provide trapeze for movement in bed, as appropriate

Instruct on bracing device care, as needed

Instruct on external fixation device care, as needed

Instruct on pin site care, as needed

Instruct in importance of adequate nutrition for bone healing

Background Readings:

Davis, F.A. (1989). Taber's cyclopedic medical dictionary (16th ed.). Philadelphia: F.A. Davis.

Mourad, L.A. (1991). Orthopedic disorders: Mosby's clinical nursing series. St. Louis: Mosby.

Phipps, W.J., Long, B.C., & Woods, N.F. (1998). Medical-surgical nursing: Concepts and clinical practice (6th ed.). St. Louis: Mosby.

T

Transcutaneous Electrical Nerve Stimulation (TENS)   1540

Definition: Stimulation of skin and underlying tissues with controlled, low-voltage electrical vibration via electrodes

Activities:

Discuss the rationale for and limits and potential problems of TENS with the patient, family, and/or significant others

Determine whether a recommendation for TENS is appropriate

Discuss therapy with physician and obtain prescription for TENS, if appropriate

Select stimulation site, considering alternate sites when direct application is not possible (e.g., adjacent to, distal to, between affected areas and the brain, and contralateral)

Determine therapeutic amplitude, rate, and pulse width

Give thorough verbal and written instructions on the use of TENS

Apply electrodes to the site of stimulation

Adjust the amplitude, rate, and/or pulse width to predetermined settings indicated

Maintain stimulation for predetermined interval (continuous or intermittent)

Instruct the patient to adjust the site and settings to achieve the desired response based on individual tolerance, if appropriate

Observe patient application of TENS and inspection of skin surfaces

Inspect or instruct patient to inspect sites of electrodes for possible skin irritation at every application or at least every 12 hours, as appropriate

Use TENS alone or in conjunction with other measures, as appropriate

Evaluate and document the effectiveness of TENS in altering pain sensation periodically

Background Readings:

Herr, K.A., & Mobily, P.R. (1992). Interventions related to pain. In G.M. Bulechek & J.C. McCloskey (Eds.), Symposium on Nursing Interventions. Nursing Clinics of North America, 27(2), 347-370.

McCaffery, M., & Beebe, A. (1989). Pain. Clinical manual for nursing practice (pp. 158-171). St. Louis: Mosby.

T

Transport   0960

Definition: Moving a patient from one location to another

Activities:

Determine amount and type of assistance needed

Discuss need for relocation

Assist patient in receiving all necessary care (e.g., personal hygiene, gathering belongings) before performing the transfer, as appropriate

Make sure the new location for the patient is ready

Raise and move patient with a hydraulic lift, as necessary

Move patient using a transfer board, as necessary

Transfer patient from a bed to stretcher, or vice versa, using a turning sheet, as appropriate

Use a belt to assist a patient who can stand with assistance, as appropriate

Use an incubator, stretcher, or bed to move a weak, injured, or surgical patient from one area to another

Use a wheelchair to move a patient unable to walk

Cradle and carry an infant or small child

Assist patient to ambulate using your body as a human crutch, as appropriate

Evacuate patient, using an appropriate method, in emergencies such as fire, hurricane, or tornado

Maintain traction devices during move, as appropriate

Provide escort during transport, as needed

Use an ambulance for a seriously injured patient

Provide a clinical report about patient to the receiving location, as appropriate

Arrange for community transportation, as needed

Background Readings:

Kozier, B., & Erb, G. (1989). Techniques in clinical nursing (3rd ed.). Menlo Park, CA: Addison-Wesley.

Perry, A.G., & Potter, P.A. (1998). Clinical nursing skills and techniques. (4th ed.) St. Louis: Mosby–Year Book.

Sorensen, K., & Luckmann, J. (1986). Basic nursing: A psychophysiologic approach (2nd ed.). Philadelphia: W.B. Saunders.

Stabl, L. (1996). How to transfer patients to other units. American Journal of Nursing, 96(8), 57-58

T

Trauma Therapy: Child   5410

Definition: Use of an interactive helping process to resolve a trauma experienced by a child

Activities:

Teach specific stress management techniques before trauma exploration to restore a sense of control over thoughts and feelings

Explore the trauma and its meaning to the child

Use developmentally appropriate language to ask about the trauma

Use relaxation and desensitization procedures to assist the child to describe the event

Establish trust, safety, and the right to gain access to carefully guarded trauma material by monitoring reactions to the disclosure

Proceed with therapy at the child's own pace

Establish a signal the child can give if the trauma-focused work becomes overwhelming

Focus therapy on self-regulation and rebuilding a sense of security

Use art and play to promote expression

Involve the parents or appropriate caretakers in therapy, as appropriate

Educate the parents about their child's response to the trauma and about the process of therapy

Assist parents in resolving their own emotional distress about the trauma

Assist appropriate others to provide support

Avoid involving parents or caretakers if they are the cause of the trauma

Assist the child to reconsider assumptions made about the traumatic event with step-by-step analysis of any perceptive and cognitive distortions

Explore and correct inaccurate attributions regarding the trauma, including omen formation and survivor's guilt

Help identify and cope with feelings

Explain the grief process to the child and parent(s), as appropriate

Assist the child to examine any distorted assumptions and conclusions

Assist child in reestablishing a sense of security and predictability in his/her life

Assist child to integrate the restructured trauma events into history and life experience

Address posttrauma role functioning in family life, peer relationships, and school performance

Background Readings:

Clark, C.C. (1997). Posttraumatic stress disorder: How to support healing. American Journal of Nursing, 97(8), 27-33.

DiPalma, L.M. (1997). Integrating trauma theory into nursing practice and education. Clinical Nurse Specialist, 11(3), 102-107.

Pifferbaum, B. (1997). Posttraumatic stress disorder in children: A review of the last 10 years. Journal of the American Academy of Child and Adolescent Psychiatry, 36(11), 1503-1511.

T

Triage: Disaster 6362

Definition: Establishing priorities of patient care for urgent treatment while allocating scarce resources

Activities:

Ready an area and equipment for triage

Acquire information about the nature of the problem, emergency, accident, or disaster

Consider the resources that are available

Contact appropriate personnel

Evaluate critical patients from the field first

Evacuate injured, as appropriate

Participate in prioritization of patients for treatment

Monitor for and treat life-threatening injuries or immediate needs

Identify the patient's chief complaint

Obtain information about the patient's medical history

Check for medical alert tags, as appropriate

Conduct a primary survey of all body systems, as appropriate

Initiate appropriate emergency measures, as indicated

Perform a secondary body system survey, as appropriate

Attach appropriate identification as indicated by patient's status

Assist with performance of diagnostic tests as indicated by the patient's condition

Background Readings:

Kenner, C.V., Guzetta, C.E., & Dossey, B.M. (1985). Critical care nursing: Body, mind, and spirit (2nd ed.). Boston: Little, Brown, & Co.

Mezza, I. (1992). Triage: Setting priorities for health care. Nursing Forum, 27(2), 15-19.

Pepe, P.E. (1988). Whom to resuscitate. In J.M. Civetta, R.W. Taylor, & R.K. Kirby (Eds.), Critical care. Philadelphia: Lippincott.

T

Triage: Emergency Center   6364

Definition: Establishing priorities and initiating treatment for patients in an emergency center

Activities:

Monitor breathing and circulation

Perform crisis intervention, as appropriate

Diffuse escalating violence, as appropriate

Take patients requiring urgent care to treatment area immediately

Evaluate and transfer mothers in labor

Explain the triage process to those presenting for service

Monitor vital signs

Perform a physical examination relevant to chief complaint

Obtain a pertinent medical history

Identify current medications

Classify according to acuity of condition

Refer patients with nonurgent care needs to clinics, other primary care providers, or health department

Contact poison control resource and initiate treatment, as appropriate

Splint possibly fractured extremities, as appropriate

Perform initial burn care, as appropriate

Control bleeding

Dress wounds

Preserve amputated parts

Initiate treatment protocols

Order diagnostic tests, as appropriate

Assign patients to physicians and/or treatment teams

Provide information to receiving caregiver

Monitor patients waiting to be seen

Serve as liaison between health care team and persons in waiting area

Answer questions from patients and families

Reassure patients and families

Perform grief counseling

Take phone calls from persons requesting information

Control traffic flow of visitors and patients

Background Readings:

Donatelli, N.S., Flaherty, L., Greenberg, L., Larson, L., & Newberry, L. (Eds.). (1995). Standards of emergency nursing practice (3rd ed.). New York: Mosby.

Emergency Nurses Association. (1996). Standards of emergency nursing practice. Chicago: Emergency Nurses Association.

Triage: Telephone   6366

Definition: Determining the nature and urgency of a problem(s) and providing directions for the level of care required, over the telephone

Activities:

Identify self with name and credentials, organization; let caller know if call is being recorded (e.g., for quality monitoring)

Display willingness to help (e.g., ask "How may I help?")

Obtain information about purpose of the call (e.g., nature of crisis, symptoms, medical diagnosis, health history, and current treatment regimen)

Consider cultural, socioeconomic barriers to patient's response

Identify patient's concerns about health status

Speak directly to the patient whenever possible

Direct, assist, and calm caller by giving simple instructions for action, as needed

Inquire about related complaint/symptoms (according to standard guidelines, if available)

Use standardized symptom-based guidelines to identify and evaluate significant data and classify urgency of symptoms, as available

Prioritize reported symptoms, addressing those with highest possible risk first

Obtain data related to effectiveness of current treatment(s), if any

Determine whether concerns require further evaluation (use standard guidelines, if available)

Provide first aid instructions or emergency directions for crises (e.g., CPR instructions or birthing) using standard guidelines

Stay on the line while contacting emergency services, according to organization's protocol

Provide clear directions for transport to the hospital, as needed

Advise patient on options for referral and/or intervention

Provide information about treatment regimen and resultant self-care responsibilities, as necessary, according to scope of practice and established guidelines

Confirm patient's understanding of advice or directions through verbalization

Determine need, and establish time intervals for, further intermittent assessment

Document any assessments, advice, instructions, or other information given to patient according to specified guidelines

Determine how patient or family member can be reached for return telephone calls, as appropriate

Document permission for return call and identify persons able to receive call information

Follow up, as necessary, to determine disposition; document disposition and patient's intended action

Maintain confidentiality, as indicated

Discuss and resolve problem calls with supervisory/collegial help

Background Readings:

American Academy of Ambulatory Nursing. (1997). Telephone nursing practice administration and practice standards. Pitman, NJ: Anthony J. Jannetti, Inc.

Janowski, M. (1995). Is telephone triage calling you? American Journal of Nursing, 95(1), 59-62.

Katz, H.P. (1990). Telephone medicine, triage and training: A handbook for primary care health professionals. Philadelphia: F.A. Davis Company.

Stock, C.M. (1995). Standardization of telephone triage: Is it time? Journal of Nursing Law, 2(2), 19-25.

Wheeler, S., & Siebelt, B. (1997). Calling all nurses: How to perform telephone triage. Nursing, 97(7), 37-41.

T

Truth Telling   5470

Definition: Use of whole truth, partial truth, or decision delay to promote the patient's self-determination and well-being

Activities:

Clarify own values about the particular situation

Clarify the values of the patient, family, health care team, and institution about the particular situation

Clarify own knowledge base and communication skills about the situation

Determine patient's desire for truth in the situation

Point out discrepancies between the patient's expressed beliefs and behaviors, as appropriate

Collaborate with other health care providers about the choice of options (i.e., whole truth, partial truth, or decision delay) and their needed participation in the options

Determine risks to patient and self associated with each option

Choose one of the options, based on the ethics of the situation and leaning more favorably toward the use of truth or partial truth

Establish a trusting relationship

Deliver the truth with sensitivity, warmth, and directness

Make the time to deal with the consequences of the truth

Refer to another if that person has better rapport, better knowledge and skills to deliver the truth, or more time and ability to deal with the consequences of telling the truth

Remain with the patient to whom you have told the truth and be prepared to clarify, give support to, and receive disapproval from that patient

Be physically present to communicate caring and support, if decision to withhold information has been made

Choose decision delay when there is missing information, lack of knowledge, and lack of rapport

Attend to verbal and nonverbal cues during the communication process

Monitor the patient's responses to the interaction, including alterations in pain, restlessness, anxiety, mood change, involvement in care, ability to synthesize new information, ability to verbalize feelings, and reported satisfaction with care, as appropriate

Document the patient's responses at various stages of the intervention

Background Readings:

Erde, E.L., Nadal, E.C., & Scholl, T.O. (1988). On truth telling and the diagnosis of Alzheimer's disease. Journal of Family Practice, 26(4), 401-406.

Gadow, S. (1981). Truth: Treatment of choice, scarce resource, or patient's right? Journal of Family Practice, 13(6), 857-860.

High, D.M. (1989). Truth telling, confidentiality, and the dying patient: New dilemmas for the nurse. Nursing Forum, 24(1), 5-10.

Williamson, C.B., & Livingston, D.J. (1992). Truth telling. In G.M. Bulechek & J.C. McCloskey (Eds.), Nursing interventions: Essential nursing treatments (2nd ed.) (pp. 151-167). Philadelphia: W.B. Saunders.

T

Tube Care   1870

Definition: Management of a patient with an external drainage device exiting the body

Activities:

Maintain patency of tube, as appropriate

Keep the drainage container at the proper level

Provide sufficiently long tubing to allow freedom of movement, as appropriate

Secure tubing, as appropriate, to prevent pressure and accidental removal

Monitor patency of catheter, noting any difficulty in drainage

Monitor amount, color, and consistency of drainage from tube

Empty the collection appliance, as appropriate

Ensure proper placement of the tube

Ensure functioning of tube and associated equipment

Connect tube to suction, as appropriate

Irrigate tube, as appropriate

Change tube routinely, as indicated by agency protocol

Inspect the area around the tube insertion site for redness and skin breakdown, as appropriate

Administer skin care at the tube insertion site, as appropriate

Assist the patient in securing tube(s) and/or drainage devices while walking, sitting, and standing, as appropriate

Encourage periods of increased activity, as appropriate

Monitor patient's and family members' responses to presence of external drainage devices

Clamp tubing, if appropriate, to facilitate ambulation

Teach patient and family the purpose of the tube and how to care for it, as appropriate

Provide emotional support to deal with long-term use of tubes and/or external drainage devices, as appropriate

Background Readings:

Ahrens, T.S. (1993). Pulmonary data aquisition. In M.R. Kinney, D.R. Packa, & S.B. Dunbar (Eds.), AACN's clinical reference for critical-care nursing (pp. 689-700). St. Louis: Mosby.

Johanson, B.C., Wells, S.J., Hoffmeister, D., & Dungca, C.U. (1988). Standards for critical care (pp. 67-73). St. Louis: Mosby.

Nelson, D.M. (1992). Interventions related to respiratory care. In G.M. Bulechek & J.C. McCloskey (Eds.), Symposium on Nursing Interventions. Nursing Clinics of North America, 27(2), 301-324.

Suddarth, D. (1991). The Lippincott manual of nursing practice (5th ed.) (pp. 196-198). Philadelphia: J.B. Lippincott.

T

Tube Care: Chest 1872

Definition: Management of a patient with an external water-seal drainage device exiting the chest cavity

Activities:

Monitor for signs and symptoms of pneumothorax

Ensure that all tubing connections are securely attached and taped

Keep the drainage container below chest level

Provide sufficiently long tubing to allow freedom of movement, as appropriate

Anchor the tubing securely

Monitor x-ray reports for tube position

Monitor chest tube tidaling/output and air leaks

Monitor for bubbling of the suction chamber of the chest tube drainage system and tidaling in water-seal chamber

Monitor patency of chest tube by stripping and milking tube

Monitor for crepitus around chest tube site

Observe for signs of intrapleural fluid accumulation

Observe volume, shade, color, and consistency of drainage from lung, and record appropriately

Observe for signs of infection

Assist patient to cough, deep breathe, and turn every 2 hours

Clean around the tube insertion site

Change dressing around chest tube every 48 to 72 hours and as needed

Use petroleum jelly gauze for dressing change

Ensure that chest tube bottle/pleurovac is maintained in an upright position

Change bottle/pleurovac, as needed

Background Readings:

Ahrens, T.S. (1993). Pulmonary data acquisition. In M.R. Kinney, D.R. Packa, & S.B. Dunbar (Eds.), AACN's clinical reference for critical-care nursing (pp. 689-700). St. Louis: Mosby.

Johanson, B.C., Wells, S.J., Hoffmeister, D., & Dungca, C.U. (1988). Standards for critical care (3rd ed.). St. Louis: Mosby.

Nelson, D.M. (1992). Interventions related to respiratory care. In G.M. Bulechek & J.C. McCloskey (Eds.), Symposium on Nursing Interventions. Nursing Clinics of North America, 27(2), 301-324.

Suddarth, D. (1991). The Lippincott manual of nursing practice (5th ed.) (pp. 196-198). Philadelphia: J.B. Lippincott.

Thelan, L.A., & Urden, L.D. (1998). Critical care nursing: Diagnosis and management. (3rd ed.) St. Louis: Mosby.

T

Tube Care: Gastrointestinal   1874

Definition: Management of a patient with a gastrointestinal tube

Activities:

Monitor for correct placement of the tube, per agency protocol

Verify placement with x-ray exam, per agency protocol

Connect tube to suction, if indicated

Secure tube to appropriate body part, with consideration for patient comfort and skin integrity

Irrigate tube, per agency protocol

Monitor for sensations of fullness, nausea, and vomiting

Monitor bowel sounds

Monitor for diarrhea

Monitor fluid and electrolyte status

Monitor amount, color, and consistency of nasogastric output

Replace the amount of gastrointestinal output with the appropriate IV solution, as ordered

Provide nose and mouth care 3 to 4 times daily or as needed

Provide hard candy or chewing gum to moisten mouth, as appropriate

Initiate and monitor delivery of enteral tube feedings, per agency protocol, as appropriate

Teach patient and family how to care for tube, when indicated

Provide skin care around tube insertion site

Remove tube when indicated

Background Readings:

Bowers, S. (1996). Tubes: A nurses' guide to enteral feeding devices. MEDSURG Nursing, 5(5) 313-326.

Perry, A.G., & Potter, P.A. (1998). Clinical nursing skills and techniques. St. Louis: Mosby.

Thompson, J.M., McFarland, G.K., Hirsch, J.E., & Tucker, S.M. (1998). Mosby's clinical nursing (4th ed.). St. Louis: Mosby–Year Book.

T

Tube Care: Umbilical Line   1875

Definition: Management of a newborn with an umbilical catheter

Activities:

Assist with or insert umbilical catheter in appropriate neonates (e.g., birthweight of <1500 grams or shock)

Check position of catheter with x-ray examination

Infuse medication and nutrients, as ordered or per protocol

Obtain venous or arterial pressures, as appropriate

Apply antiseptic medication to umbilical stump, per protocol

Flush catheter with heparinized solution, as appropriate

Change stopcock daily and as needed

Secure connections with tape, as needed, to keep line intact

Cleanse outer surface with alcohol, as needed

Stabilize catheter with tape

Restrain ankles and wrists

Document infant's response to restraints, per protocol

Provide frequent range of motion to restrained limbs

Cleanse umbilical stump with alcohol, as needed

Position infant on back

Document appearance of umbilical site and nurse's actions

Observe for signs requiring catheter removal (e.g., pulseless leg, darkening of toes, hypertension, redness around umbilicus, and visible clots in catheter)

Remove catheter, as appropriate per order or protocol, by withdrawing catheter slowly over 5 minutes

Apply pressure to umbilicus or clamp vessel with hemostat

Leave umbilicus uncovered

Observe for hemorrhage

Background Readings:

Merenstein, G.B., & Gardner, S.L. (1993). Handbook of neonatal intensive care. St. Louis: Mosby.

Pernoll, M.L., Benda, G.I., & Babson, S.G. (1986). Diagnosis and management of the fetus and neonate at risk: A guide for team care. St. Louis: Mosby.

T

Tube Care: Urinary   1876

Definition: Management of a patient with urinary drainage equipment

Activities:

Maintain a closed urinary drainage system

Maintain patency of urinary catheter system

Irrigate urinary catheter system using sterile technique, as appropriate

Cleanse surrounding skin area at regular intervals

Change the urinary catheter at regular intervals

Change the urinary drainage apparatus at regular intervals

Clean the urinary catheter externally at the meatus

Note urinary drainage characteristics

Clamp suprapubic or retention catheter, as ordered

Position patient and urinary drainage system to promote urinary drainage

Empty urinary drainage apparatus at specified intervals

Disconnect leg bag at night and connect to bedside drainage bag

Check leg bag straps for constriction at regular intervals

Maintain meticulous skin care for patients with a leg bag

Cleanse urinary drainage equipment per agency protocol

Obtain urine specimen through closed urinary drainage system's port

Monitor for bladder distention

Remove catheter as soon as possible

Background Readings:

Matthews, S.D., & Courts, N.F. (2001). Orthotopic neobladder surgery: Nursing care promotes independence in patient with bladder cancer. American Journal of Nursing, 101 (Critical Care Extra), 24AA, 24CC, 24EE.

O'Connell-Smeltzer, S.C., (1988). Management of a patient with a renal and urinary dysfunction. In L. Brunner, & D. Suddarth (Eds.), Textbook of medical-surgical nursing (6th ed.) (pp. 1009-1032). Philadelphia: J.B. Lippincott.

Sundberg, M.C. (1989). Aspirating a small-volume fresh urine specimen from an indwelling catheter. In Fundamentals of nursing with clinical procedures (2nd ed.) (pp. 264-265). Boston: Jones & Bartlett.

Sundberg, M.C. (1989). Care and maintenance of an indwelling catheter. In Fundamentals of Nursing with clinical procedures (2nd ed.) (pp. 261-263). Boston: Jones & Bartlett.

T

Tube Care: Ventriculostomy/Lumbar Drain   1878

Definition: Management of a patient with an external cerebrospinal fluid drainage system

Activities:

Monitor drainage trends

Monitor amount/rate of cerebrospinal fluid (CSF) drainage

Monitor CSF drainage characteristics: color, clarity, and consistency

Record CSF drainage

Change or empty drainage bag, as needed

Administer antibiotics

Monitor insertion site for infection

Reinforce an insertion site dressing, as needed

Restrain patient, as needed

Explain and reinforce mobility restrictions to patient

Monitor for CSF rhinorrhea/otorrhea

Background Readings:

Ackerman, L.L. (1992). Interventions related to neurological care. In G.M. Bulechek & J.C. McCloskey (Eds.), Symposium on Nursing Interventions. Nursing Clinics of North America, 27(2), 325-346.

Hichman, K.M., & Muwaswes, M. (1990). Intracranial pressure monitoring: Review of risk factors associated with infection. Heart & Lung, 19(1), 84-90.

Hickey, J.V. (1992). The clinical practice of neurological and neurosurgical nursing (3rd ed.). Philadelphia: J.B. Lippincott.

Mayhall, G., Archer, N., Lamb, V.A., et al. (1984). Ventriculostomy related infection: A prospective epidemiologic study. New England Journal of Medicine, 310(9), 553-559.

Robinet, K. (1985). Increased intracranial pressure: Management with an intraventricular catheter. Journal of Neurosurgical Nursing, 17(2), 95-104.

T

Ultrasonography: Limited Obstetric   6982

Definition: Performance of ultrasound exams to determine ovarian, uterine, or fetal status

Activities:

Determine indication for ultrasound (U/S) imaging

Set up equipment

Instruct patient and family about exam indication(s) and procedure

Prepare patient physically and emotionally for procedure

Place transducer on abdomen or in vagina, as appropriate

Obtain clear picture of anatomical structures on the monitor

Determine position and size of uterus, and endometrial thickness, as appropriate

Determine location and size of ovaries, as appropriate

Monitor follicular growth throughout ovulation, as appropriate

Monitor gestational sac growth and location

Monitor fetal parameters, including number, size, cardiac activity, presentation, and position

Locate placenta

Observe for placental abnormalities, as appropriate

Measure amniotic fluid indexes

Monitor fetal breathing movements, gross movements, and tone

Identify fetal structures to parents, as appropriate

Provide picture of fetus(es), as appropriate

Discuss test results with primary practitioner, consultants, and patient, as appropriate

Schedule additional tests or procedures, as necessary

Clean equipment

Document findings

Background Readings:

Association of Women's Health, Obstetric, and Neonatal Nurses. (1993). Nursing practice competencies and educational guidelines for limited ultrasound examinations in obstetric and gynecologic/infertility settings. Washington, DC: AWHONN.

Kohn, C.L., Nelson, A., & Weiner, S. (1980). Gravidas' responses to realtime ultrasound fetal images. Journal of Obstetric, Gynecologic & Neonatal Nursing, 9(2), 77-80.

Lumley, J. (1990). Through a glass darkly: Ultrasound and prenatal bonding. Birth, 17(4), 214-217.

Milne, L.S., & Rich, O.J. (1981). Cognitive and affective aspects of the response of pregnant women to sonography. Maternal-Child Nursing Journal, 10(1), 15-39.

NAACOG. (1991). NAACOG committee opinion: The nurse's role in ultrasound. Washington, DC: NAACOG.

U

Unilateral Neglect Management 2760

Definition: Protecting and safely reintegrating the affected part of the body while helping the patient adapt to disturbed perceptual abilities

Activities:

Monitor for abnormal responses to three primary types of stimuli: sensory, visual, and auditory

Evaluate baseline mental status, comprehension, motor function, sensory function, attention span, and affective responses

Provide realistic feedback about patient's perceptual deficit

Perform personal care in a consistent manner with thorough explanation

Ensure that affected extremities are properly and safely positioned

Adapt the environment to the deficit by focusing on the unaffected side during the acute period

Supervise and/or assist in transferring and ambulating

Touch unaffected shoulder when initiating conversation

Place food and beverages within field of vision and turn plate, as necessary

Rearrange the environment to use the right or left visual field; position personal items, television, or reading materials within view on unaffected side

Give frequent reminders to redirect the patient's attention, cuing the patient to the environment

Avoid rapid movement in the room

Avoid moving objects in the environment

Position bed in room so that individuals approach and care for patient on unaffected side

Keep side rail up on affected side, as appropriate

Instruct patient to scan from left to right

Provide range of motion and massage to affected side

Encourage patient to touch and use affected body part

Consult with occupational and physical therapists concerning timing and strategies to facilitate reintegration of neglected body parts and function

Gradually focus patient's attention to the affected side, as patient demonstrates an ability to compensate for neglect

Gradually move personal items and activity to affected side, as patient demonstrates an ability to compensate for neglect

Stand on affected side when ambulating with patient, as patient demonstrates an ability to compensate for neglect

Assist patient with activities of daily living from affected side, as patient demonstrates an ability to compensate for neglect

Assist patient to bathe and groom affected side first, as patient demonstrates an ability to compensate for neglect

Focus tactile and verbal stimuli on affected side, as patient demonstrates an ability to compensate for neglect

Instruct caregivers on the cause, mechanisms, and treatment of unilateral neglect

Include family in rehabilitation process to support the patient's efforts and assist with care, as appropriate

Background Readings:

Kalbach, L.R. (1991). Unilateral neglect: Mechanisms and nursing care. Journal of Neuroscience Nursing, 23(2), 125-129.

Martin, N., Holt, N.B., & Hicks, D. (1981). Comprehensive rehabilitation nursing. New York: McGraw-Hill.

Matteson, M.A., & McConnell, E.S. (1988). Gerontological nursing: Concepts and practice. Philadelphia: W.B. Saunders.

Urinary Bladder Training   0570

Definition: Improving bladder function for those with urge incontinence by increasing the bladder's ability to hold urine and the patient's ability to suppress urination

Activities:

Determine ability to recognize urge to void

Encourage patient to keep a voiding diary

Keep a continence specification record for 3 days to establish voiding pattern

Assist patient to identify patterns of incontinence

Review voiding diary with patient

Establish interval of initial toileting schedule, based on voiding pattern

Establish beginning and ending time for toileting schedule, if not for 24 hours

Establish interval for toileting of not less than 1 hour and preferably not less than 2 hours

Toilet patient or remind patient to void at prescribed intervals

Provide privacy for toileting

Use power of suggestion (e.g., running water or flushing toilet) to assist patient to void

Avoid leaving patient on toilet for more than 5 minutes

Reduce toileting interval by one half hour if there are more than three incontinence episodes in 24 hours

Maintain toileting interval if there are three or fewer incontinence episodes in 24 hours

Increase toileting interval by one half hour if patient is unable to void at two or more scheduled toileting times

Increase the toileting interval by 1 hour if patient has no incontinence episodes for 3 days until optimal 4-hour interval is achieved

Express confidence that continence can be improved

Teach the patient to consciously hold urine until the scheduled toileting time

Discuss daily record of continence with patient to provide reinforcement

Background Readings:

Smith, D.A., & Newman, D.K. (1990). Urinary incontinence: A problem not often assessed or treated. Focus on Geriatric Care and Rehabilitation, 3(10), 1-9.

Specht, J., Tunink, P., Maas, M., & Bulechek, G. (1991). Urinary incontinence. In M. Maas, K.C. Buckwalter, & M.A. Hardy (Eds.), Nursing diagnoses and interventions for the elderly (pp. 181-204). Redwood City, CA: Addison-Wesley.

U

Urinary Catheterization 0580

Definition: Insertion of a catheter into the bladder for temporary or permanent drainage of urine

Activities:

Explain procedure and rationale for the intervention

Assemble appropriate catheterization equipment

Maintain strict aseptic technique

Insert straight or retention catheter into the bladder, as appropriate

Use smallest size catheter, as appropriate

Connect retention catheter to a bedside drainage bag or leg bag

Secure catheter to skin, as appropriate

Maintain a closed urinary drainage system

Monitor intake and output

Perform or teach patient to perform clean intermittent catheterization, when appropriate

Perform post-void residual catheterization, as needed

Background Readings:

Norton, B.A., & Miller, A.M. (1986). Skills for professional nursing practice (pp. 641-648). Norwalk, CT: Appleton-Century-Crofts.

Potter, P.A., & Perry, A.G. (1993). Fundamentals of nursing (3rd ed.) (pp. 1097-1114). St. Louis: Mosby.

U

Urinary Catheterization: Intermittent   0582

Definition: Regular periodic use of a catheter to empty the bladder

Activities:

Perform a comprehensive urinary assessment focusing on causes of incontinence (e.g., urinary output, urinary voiding pattern, cognitive function, preexisting urinary problems)

Teach patient/family purpose, supplies, method, and rationale of intermittent catheterization

Teach patient/family clean intermittent catheterization technique

Monitor technique of staff who perform intermittent catheterization in day-care/school settings and document as required by state regulations

Determine child's readiness and willingness to perform intermittent self-catheterization

Instruct designated staff how to monitor and support child performing self-catheterization at school

Provide quiet private room for procedure

Provide child a private place at school to store catheterization supplies in a school bag or other carrying case that is acceptable to child

Monitor child performing self-catheterization on a regular basis and provide continued instruction and support, as needed

Demonstrate procedure and have a return demonstration, as appropriate

Assemble appropriate catheterization equipment

Use clean or sterile technique for catheterization

Determine catheterization schedule based on a comprehensive urinary assessment

Adjust frequency of catheterization to maintain output of 300 cc or less for adults

Maintain patient on prophylactic antibacterial therapy for 2 to 3 weeks at initiation of intermittent catheterization, as appropriate

Complete a urinalysis about every 2 weeks to 1 month

Establish a catheterization schedule based on individual needs

Maintain a detailed record of catheterization schedule, fluid intake, and output

Teach patient/family signs and symptoms of urinary tract infection

Monitor color, odor, and clarity of urine

Background Readings:

Smigielski, P.A., & Mapel, J.R. (1990). Bowel and bladder maintenance. In M.J. Craft, & J.A. Denehy (Eds.), Nursing interventions for infants and children. (pp. 355-377). Philadelphia: W.B. Saunders.

Specht, J.P., Maas, M.L., Willett, S., & Myers, N. (1992). Intermittent catheterization. In G.M. Bulechek, & J.C. McCluskey (Eds.), Nursing interventions: Essential nursing treatments (2nd ed.) (pp. 61-72). Philadelphia: W.B. Saunders.

U

Urinary Elimination Management 0590

Definition: Maintenance of an optimum urinary elimination pattern

Activities:

Monitor urinary elimination including frequency, consistency, odor, volume, and color as appropriate

Monitor for signs and symptoms of urinary retention

Identify factors that contribute to incontinence episodes

Teach patient signs and symptoms of urinary tract infection

Note time of last urinary elimination, as appropriate

Instruct patient/family to record urinary output, as appropriate

Insert urethral suppository, as appropriate

Obtain midstream voided specimen for urinalysis, as appropriate

Refer to physician if signs and symptoms of urinary tract infection occur

Teach patient to obtain midstream urine specimens at first sign of return of infection

Instruct patient to respond immediately to urge to void, as appropriate

Teach patient to drink eight ounces of liquid with meals, between meals, and in early evening

Assist patient with development of toileting routine, as appropriate

Instruct patient to empty bladder prior to relevant procedures

Record time of first voiding following procedure, as appropriate

Restrict fluids, as needed

Instruct patient to monitor for signs and symptoms of urinary tract infection

Background Readings:

Smigielski, P.A., & Mapel, J.R. (1990). Bowel and bladder maintenance. In M.J. Craft & J.A. Denehy (Eds.), Nursing interventions for infants and children. (pp. 355-377). Philadelphia: W.B. Saunders.

Specht, J., Tunink, P., Maas, M., & Bulechek, G. (1991). Urinary incontinence. In M. Maas, K.C. Buckwalter, & M.A. Hardy (Eds.), Nursing diagnoses and interventions for the elderly (pp. 181-204). Redwood City, CA: Addison-Wesley.

U

Urinary Habit Training   0600

Definition: Establishing a predictable pattern of bladder emptying to prevent incontinence for persons with limited cognitive ability who have urge, stress, or functional incontinence

Activities:

Keep a continence specification record for 3 days to establish voiding pattern

Establish interval of initial toileting schedule, based on voiding pattern and usual routine (e.g., eating, rising, and retiring)

Establish beginning and ending time for the toileting schedule, if not for 24 hours

Establish interval for toileting of preferably not less than 2 hours

Assist patient to toilet and prompt to void at prescribed intervals

Provide privacy for toileting

Use power of suggestion (e.g., running water or flushing toilet) to assist patient to void

Avoid leaving patient on toilet for more than 5 minutes

Reduce toileting interval by one half hour if there are more than two incontinence episodes in 24 hours

Maintain toileting interval if there are two or fewer incontinence episodes in 24 hours

Increase the toileting interval by one half hour if patient has no incontinence episodes in 48 hours until optimal 4-hour interval is achieved

Discuss daily record of continence with staff to provide reinforcement and encourage compliance with toileting schedule

Maintain scheduled toileting to assist in establishing and maintaining voiding habit

Give positive feedback or positive reinforcement (e.g., 5 minutes of social conversation) to patient when he/she voids at scheduled toileting times, and make no comment when patient is incontinent

Background Readings:

Ouslander, J., & Uman, G. (1985). Urinary incontinence: Opportunities for research, education, and improvements in medical care in the nursing home setting. In E.L. Schneider (Ed.), The teaching nursing home. New York: Raven Press.

Specht, J., Tunink, P., Maas, M., & Bulechek, G. (1991). Urinary incontinence. In M. Maas, K.C. Buckwalter, & M.A. Hardy (Eds.), Nursing diagnoses and interventions for the elderly (pp. 181-204). Redwood City, CA: Addison-Wesley.

U

Urinary Incontinence Care 0610

Definition: Assistance in promoting continence and maintaining perineal skin integrity

Activities:

Identify multifactorial causes of incontinence (e.g., urinary output, voiding pattern, cognitive function, preexisting urinary problems, post-void residual, and medications)

Provide privacy for elimination

Explain etiology of problem and rationale for actions

Monitor urinary elimination, including frequency, consistency, odor, volume, and color

Discuss procedures and expected outcomes with patient

Assist to develop/maintain a sense of hope

Modify clothing and environment to provide easy access to toilet

Assist to select appropriate incontinence garment/pad for short-term management while more definitive treatment is designed

Provide protective garments, as needed

Cleanse genital skin area at regular intervals

Provide positive feedback for any decrease in episodes of incontinence

Limit fluids for 2 to 3 hours before bedtime, as appropriate

Schedule diuretic administration to have least impact on lifestyle

Instruct patient/family to record urinary output and pattern, as appropriate

Instruct patient to drink a minimum of 1500 cc fluids a day

Instruct in ways to avoid constipation or stool impaction

Limit ingestion of bladder irritants (e.g., colas, coffee, tea, and chocolate)

Obtain urine for culture and sensitivity testing, as needed

Monitor effectiveness of surgical, medical, pharmacological, and self-prescribed treatments

Monitor bowel habits

Refer to urinary continence specialist, as appropriate

Background Readings:

McCormick, K.A., & Palmer, M.N. (1992). Urinary incontinence in older adults. In J.J. Firtzpatrick, R.L. Taunton, & A.K. Jacox (Eds.), Annual review of nursing research, 10, (pp. 25-53). New York: Springer.

McCormick, K.A., Scheve, A.A.S., & Leahy, E. (1988). Nursing management of urinary incontinence in geriatric inpatients. Nursing Clinics of North America, 23(1), 231-264.

National Institutes of Health. (1988). Urinary incontinence in adults. Consensus Department Conference Statement. 7(5). Bethesda, MD: Office of Medical Application of Research, NIH.

Specht, J., Tunink, P., Maas, M., & Bulechek, G.M. (1991). Urinary incontinence. In M. Maas, K.C. Buckwalter, & M. Hardy (Eds.), Nursing diagnoses and interventions for the elderly (pp. 181-204). Redwood City, CA: Addison-Wesley.

Urinary Incontinence Guideline Panel. (1992). Urinary incontinence in adults. Clinical practice guideline. AHCPR Pub. No. 92-0038. Rockville, MD: Agency for Health Care Policy and Research, Public Health Service, U.S. Department of Health and Human Services.

U

Urinary Incontinence Care: Enuresis 0612

Definition: Promotion of urinary continence in children

Activities:

Assist with diagnostic evaluation (e.g., physical exam, cystogram, cystoscopy, and lab tests) to rule out physical causes

Interview parent to obtain data about toilet-training history, voiding pattern, urinary tract infections, and food sensitivities

Determine frequency, duration, and circumstances of enuresis

Discuss effective and ineffective methods of prior treatment

Monitor family's and child's level of frustration and stress

Perform physical exam

Discuss techniques to use in reducing enuresis (e.g., nightlight, restricted fluid intake, scheduling nocturnal bathroom trips, and use of alarm system)

Encourage child to verbalize feelings

Emphasize child's strengths

Encourage parents to demonstrate love and acceptance at home to counteract peer ridicule

Discuss psychosocial dynamics of enuresis with parents (e.g., familial patterns, family disruption, self esteem issues, and self-limiting characteristic)

Administer medications as appropriate for short-term control

Background Readings:

Mott, S.R., James, S.R., & Sperhac, A.M. (1990). Nursing care of children and families (2nd ed.). Redwood City, CA: Addison-Wesley.

Wong, D.L. (1997). Whaley & Wong's essentials of pediatric nursing. (5th ed.). St. Louis: Mosby.

U

Urinary Retention Care   0620

Definition: Assistance in relieving bladder distention

Activities:

Perform a comprehensive urinary assessment focusing on incontinence (e.g., urinary output, urinary voiding pattern, cognitive function, and preexisting urinary problems)

Monitor use of nonprescription agents with anticholinergic or alpha-agonist properties

Monitor effects of prescribed pharmaceuticals, such as calcium channel blockers and anticholinergics

Provide privacy for elimination

Use the power of suggestion by running water or flushing the toilet

Stimulate the reflex bladder by applying cold to the abdomen, stroking the inner thigh, or running water

Provide enough time for bladder emptying (10 minutes)

Use spirits of wintergreen in bedpan or urinal

Provide Crede maneuver, as necessary

Use double-voiding technique

Insert urinary catheter, as appropriate

Instruct patient/family to record urinary output, as appropriate

Instruct in ways to avoid constipation or stool impaction

Monitor intake and output

Monitor degree of bladder distention by palpation and percussion

Assist with toileting at regular intervals, as appropriate

Catheterize for residual, as appropriate

Implement intermittent catheterization, as appropriate

Refer to urinary continence specialist, as appropriate

Background Readings:

Norton, B.A., & Miller, A.M. (1986). Skills for professional nursing practice (pp. 629-656). Norwalk, CT: Appleton-Century-Crofts.

Potter, P.A., & Perry, A.G. (1998). Fundamentals of nursing (4th ed.). St. Louis: Mosby.

U

Values Clarification   5480

Definition: Assisting another to clarify her/his own values in order to facilitate effective decision making

Activities:

Think through the ethical and legal aspects of free choice, given the particular situation, before beginning the intervention

Create an accepting, nonjudgmental atmosphere

Use appropriate questions to assist the patient in reflecting on the situation and what is important personally

Use a value sheet clarifying technique (written situation and questions), as appropriate

Pose reflective, clarifying questions that give the patient something to think about

Encourage patient to make a list of what is important and not important in life and the time spent on each

Encourage patient to list values that guide behavior in various settings and types of situations

Help patient define alternatives and their advantages and disadvantages

Encourage consideration of the issues and consequences of behavior

Help patient to evaluate how values are in agreement with or in conflict with those of family members/significant others

Support patient's decision, as appropriate

Use multiple sessions, as directed by the specific situation

Avoid use of this intervention with persons with serious emotional problems

Avoid use of cross-examining questions

Background Readings:

Seroka, A.M. (1994). Values clarification and ethical decision making. Seminars for Nurse Managers, 2(1), 8-15.

Wilberding, J.Z. (1992). Values clarification. In G.M. Bulechek & J.C. McCloskey (Eds.), Nursing interventions: Essential nursing treatments (2nd ed.) (pp. 315-325). Philadelphia: W.B. Saunders.

V

Vehicle Safety Promotion   9050

Definition: Assisting individuals, families, and communities to increase awareness of measures to reduce unintentional injuries in motorized and nonmotorized vehicle

Activities:

Determine current awareness of vehicular safety, as appropriate

Identify the safety needs of target audience

Identify individuals and groups at high risk for vehicular injury

Identify safety hazards in environment

Eliminate safety hazards in the environment when possible

Give information about risks associated with motorized or nonmotorized vehicle use, as indicated

Teach high-risk populations about vehicular hazards and risks (e.g., drinking, risk-taking behaviors, noncompliance with laws)

Collaborate with community agencies in educational efforts to promote vehicle safety (e.g., schools, police, local health department, child safety coalitions)

Provide literature about importance of vehicle safety and methods to increase it

Educate about rules of the road for drivers of motorized and nonmotorized vehicles

Educate about the importance of proper and regular use of protective devices to decrease risk of injury (e.g., car seats, seat belts, helmets)

Emphasize importance of always wearing seat belts

Encourage drivers not to start automobile until all passengers are restrained

Encourage adults to role-model the use of seat belts and safe driving practices

Provide information about proper adjustment so seat belts are comfortable and safe

Monitor parents' use of approved child safety seats and seat belts

Educate about proper installation of child safety seats

Instruct parents to secure infants in child safety seats and children under 13 years of age in the back seat of automobile

Encourage parents to take child safety seats when traveling (e.g., airplane, train, bus)

Demonstrate strategies parents can use to keep children occupied while restrained in seat belts or child safety seats

Praise children and families for proper and regular use of safe practices in vehicles

Make child safety seats available to all families through community service agencies

Inform parents of the importance of selecting a bicycle that fits child properly and adjusting it periodically as the child grows

Encourage use of adaptive devices to increase vehicle safety (e.g., mirrors, horns, reflective devices, lights)

Stress importance of always wearing helmets and bright or reflective clothing on bicycles, motorcycles, and other motorized vehicles (e.g., all-terrain vehicles, snow mobiles)

Emphasize importance of wearing shoes and protective clothing while on motorized and nonmotorized vehicles

Monitor community injury rates to determine further educational need

Support legislative initiatives that promote and enforce vehicular safety

Background Readings:

Arneson, S.W., & Triplett, J.L. (1990). Riding with Bucklebear: An automobile safety program for preschoolers. Journal of Pediatric Nursing, 5(2), 115-122.

Foss, R.D. (1989). Evaluation of a community-wide incentive program to promote safety restraint use. American Journal of Public Health, 79(3), 304-306.

National Child Safety Council. (1989). Official bike safety manual. Jackson, MS: NCSC.

Otis, J., Lesage, D., Godin, G., Brown, B., Farley, C., & Lambert, J. (1992). Predicting and reinforcing children's intentions to wear protective helmets while bicycling. Public Health Reports, 107(3), 283-289.

Solis, G.R. (1991). Evaluation of a children's safety fair. Pediatric Nursing, 17(3), 255-258.

Watts, D., O'Shea, N., Ile, A., Flynn, E., Trask, A., & Kelleher, D. (1997). Effect of a bicycle safety program and free bicycle safety program and free bicycle helmet distribution on the use of bicycle helmets by elementary school children. Journal of Emergency Nursing, 23(5), 417-419.

V

Venous Access Device (VAD) Maintenance 2440

Definition: Management of the patient with prolonged venous access via tunneled and nontunneled (percutaneous) catheters and implanted ports

Activities:

Determine the type of VAD in place

Maintain aseptic technique whenever VAD is manipulated

Maintain universal precautions

Verify infusate orders, as applicable

Determine flow rate, reservoir capacity, and placement for implanted pumps

Determine if the VAD is to be utilized for blood sampling

Change tubing, dressings, and caps according to agency policy

Maintain occlusive dressing

Monitor for signs of catheter occlusion

Use fibrinolytic agents to open occluded VAD, as appropriate and according to agency policy

Maintain saline lock, as indicated

Maintain accurate record of infusate

Monitor fluid status, as appropriate

Monitor for signs and symptoms associated with local and systemic infection (e.g., redness, swelling, tenderness, fever, malaise)

Determine patient's and/or family's understanding of the purpose, care, and maintenance of the VAD

Instruct patient and/or family on maintenance of device

Background Readings:

Dool, J. (1993). Central venous access devices—issues for staff education and clinical competence. Nursing Clinics of North America, 28(4), 973-984.

Evans Orr, M. (1993). Issues in the management of percutaneous central venous catheters. Nursing Clinics of North America, 28(4), 911-919.

Freedman, S.E., & Bosserman, G. (1993). Tunneled catheters: Technologic advances and nursing care issues. Nursing Clinics of North America, 28(4), 851-858.

Gullo, S.M. (1993). Implanted ports: Technologic advances and nursing care issues. Nursing Clinics of North America, 28(4), 859-871.

Intravenous Nursing Society. (1990). Intravenous nursing standards of practice. Belmont, MA: Intravenous Nursing Society.

Perry, A. G., & Potter, P. A. (1998). Caring for venous access devices in clinical nursing: Skills and techniques (pp. 696-708). St. Louis: Mosby.

Ventilation Assistance   3390

Definition: Promotion of an optimal spontaneous breathing pattern that maximizes oxygen and carbon dioxide exchange in the lungs

Activities:

Maintain a patent airway

Position to alleviate dyspnea

Position to facilitate ventilation/perfusion matching ("good lung down"), as appropriate

Assist with frequent position changes, as appropriate

Position to minimize respiratory efforts (e.g., elevate the head of the bed and provide overbed table for patient to lean on)

Monitor the effects of position change on oxygenation: ABG, SaO_2, SvO_2, end-tidal CO_2, Q_{sp}/Q_t, $A\text{-}aDO_2$ levels

Encourage slow deep breathing, turning, and coughing

Use fun techniques to encourage deep breathing for children (e.g., blow bubbles with bubble blower; blow on pinwheel, whistle, harmonica, balloons, party blowers; have blowing contest using ping-pong balls, feathers, etc.)

Assist with incentive spirometer, as appropriate

Auscultate breath sounds, noting areas of decreased or absent ventilation and presence of adventitious sounds

Monitor for respiratory muscle fatigue

Initiate and maintain supplemental oxygen, as prescribed

Administer appropriate pain medication to prevent hypoventilation

Ambulate patient three to four times per day, as appropriate

Monitor respiratory and oxygenation status

Administer medications (e.g., bronchodilators and inhalers) that promote airway patency and gas exchange

Teach pursed-lip breathing techniques, as appropriate

Teach breathing techniques, as appropriate

Initiate a program of respiratory muscle strength and/or endurance training, as appropriate

Initiate resuscitation efforts, as appropriate

Background Readings:

Carrol, P. (1986). Caring for ventilator patients. Nursing 86, 16(2), 34-39.

Glennon, S. (1993). Mechanical support of ventilation. In M.R. Kinney, D.R. Backa, & S.B. Dunbar (Eds.), AACN's clinical reference for critical-care nursing (pp. 828-840). St. Louis: Mosby.

Lane, G.H. (1990). Pulmonary therapeutic management. In L.A. Thelan, J.K. Davie, & L.D. Urden (Eds.), Textbook of critical care nursing (pp. 444-471). St. Louis: Mosby.

Nelson, D.M. (1992). Interventions related to respiratory care. In G.M. Bulechek & J.C. McCloskey (Eds.), Symposium on Nursing Interventions. Nursing Clinics of North America, 27(2), 301-324.

Wong, D.L. (1998). Whaley and Wong's nursing care of infants and children (6th ed.). St. Louis: Mosby.

V

Visitation Facilitation   7560

Definition: Promoting beneficial visits by family and friends

Activities:

Determine patient's preferences for visitation and release of information

Consider legal/ethical implications regarding patient and family visitation and information rights

Determine need for limited visitation, such as too many visitors, patient's being impatient or tired, or physical status

Determine need for more visits from family and friends

Identify specific problems with visits, if any

Establish flexible, patient-centered visiting policies, as appropriate

Prepare the environment for visitation

Discuss visiting policy with family members/significant others

Discuss policy for overnight stay of family members/significant others

Discuss family's understanding of patient's condition

Negotiate family's/significant others' responsibilities and activities to assist patient, such as feeding

Establish optimal times for family/significant others to visit patient

Provide rationale for limited visiting time

Evaluate periodically with both the family and the patient whether visitation practices are meeting the needs of the patient/family, and revise accordingly

Inform visitors, including children, what they may expect to see and hear before their first hospital visitation, as appropriate

Explain procedure being done

Encourage the family member to use touch, as well as verbal communication, as appropriate

Provide a chair at the bedside

Be flexible with visitation while facilitating periods of rest

Monitor patient's response to family visitation

Note patient's verbal and nonverbal cues regarding visitation

Facilitate visitation of children, as appropriate

Encourage use of the telephone to maintain contact with significant others, as appropriate

Screen visitors, especially children, for communicable diseases before visitation

Clarify the meaning of what the family member perceived during the visit

Provide support and care for family members after visitation, as needed

Provide family with unit telephone number to call when they go home

Inform family that a nurse will call at home if significant change in patient status occurs

Provide sleeping arrangements for relatives close to the unit, as appropriate

Assist family members to find adequate lodging and meals

Inform family that they may have the right to 12 weeks of unpaid leave of absence from work

Answer questions and give explanations of care in terms that visitors can understand

Convey feelings of acceptance to visitors

V

Facilitate meeting/consultation with physician and other care providers

Debrief visitors, including children, after the visit

Assist parents to plan for ongoing support of children after the visit

Arrange animal visitation, as appropriate

Background Readings:

Daly, J. M. (1999). Visitation facilitation. In G.M. Bulecheck & J.C. McCloskey (Eds.), Nursing interventions: Effective nursing treatments. Philadelphia: W.B. Saunders Company.

Halm, M. (1990). The effect of support groups on anxiety of family members during critical illness. Heart & Lung, 19(1), 62-71.

Kleiber, C., Montgomery, L.A., Craft-Rosenberg, M. (1995). Information needs of the siblings of critically ill children. Children's Health Care, 24, 47-60.

Krapohl, G.L. (1995). Visiting hours in the adult intensive care unit: Using research to develop a system that works. Dimensions of Critical Care Nursing, 14(5), 245-258.

Lazure, L. L. A. (1997). Strategies to increase patient control of visiting. Dimensions of Critical Care Nursing, 16(1), 11-19.

Montgomergy, L.A., Kleiber, C., Nicholson, A., & Craft-Rosenberg, M. (1997). A research-based sibling visitation program for the neonatal I.C.U. Critical Care Nurse, 17, 29-40.

Titler, M.G., Cohen, M.Z., & Craft, M.J. (1991). Impact of critical hospitalization: Perceptions of patients, spouses, children, and nurses. Heart & Lung, 20(2), 174-181.

V

Vital Signs Monitoring 6680

Definition: Collection and analysis of cardiovascular, respiratory, and body temperature data to determine and prevent complications

Activities:

Monitor blood pressure, pulse, temperature, and respiratory status, as appropriate

Note trends and wide fluctuations in blood pressure

Monitor blood pressure while patient is lying, sitting, and standing before and after position change, as appropriate

Monitor blood pressure after patient has taken medications, if possible

Auscultate blood pressures in both arms and compare, as appropriate

Monitor blood pressure, pulse, and respirations before, during, and after activity, as appropriate

Initiate and maintain a continuous temperature monitoring device, as appropriate

Monitor for and report signs and symptoms of hypothermia and hyperthermia

Monitor presence and quality of pulses

Take apical and radial pulses simultaneously and note the difference, as appropriate

Monitor for pulsus paradoxus

Monitor for pulsus alternans

Monitor for a widening or narrowing pulse pressure

Monitor cardiac rhythm and rate

Monitor heart tones

Monitor respiratory rate and rhythm (e.g., depth and symmetry)

Monitor lung sounds

Monitor pulse oximetry

Monitor for abnormal respiratory patterns (e.g., Cheyne-Stokes, Kussmaul, Biot, apneustic, ataxic, respiration and excessive sighing)

Monitor skin color, temperature, and moistness

Monitor for central and peripheral cyanosis

Monitor for clubbing of nailbeds

Monitor for presence of Cushing triad (e.g., wide pulse pressure, bradycardia, and increase in systolic BP)

Identify possible causes of changes in vital signs

Check periodically the accuracy of instruments used for acquisition of patient data

Background Readings:

Erickson, R.S., & Yount, S.J. (1991). Comparison of tympanic and oral temperatures in surgical patients. Nursing Research, 40(2), 90-93.

Thelan, L.A., & Urden, L.D. (1998). Critical care nursing: Diagnosis and management (3rd ed.). St. Louis: Mosby.

Titler, M.G. (1992). Interventions related to surveillance. In G.M. Bulechek & J.C. McCloskey (Eds.), Symposium on Nursing Interventions. Nursing Clinics of North America, 27(2), 495-516.

V

Vomiting Management   1570

Definition: Prevention and alleviation of vomiting

Activities:

Assess emesis for color, consistency, blood, timing, and extent to which it is forceful

Measure or estimate emesis volume

Suggest carrying plastic bag for emesis containment

Determine vomiting frequency and duration, using such scales as Duke Descriptive Scales and Rhodes Index of Nausea and Vomiting (INV) Form 2

Obtain a complete pretreatment history

Obtain dietary history containing the person's likes, dislikes, and cultural food preferences

Identify factors (e.g., medication and procedures) that may cause or contribute to vomiting

Ensure that effective antiemetic drugs are given to prevent vomiting when possible

Control environmental factors that may evoke vomiting (e.g., aversive smells, sound, and unpleasant visual stimulation)

Reduce or eliminate personal factors that precipitate or increase the vomiting (anxiety, fear, and lack of knowledge)

Position to prevent aspiration

Maintain oral airway

Provide physical support during vomiting (such as assisting person to bend over or supporting the person's head)

Provide comfort (such as cool cloths to forehead, sponging face, or clean dry clothes) during/after the vomiting episode

Demonstrate acceptance of vomiting and collaborate with the person when selecting a vomiting control strategy

Use oral hygiene to clean mouth and nose

Clean up after the vomiting episode with special attention to removal of odors

Wait at least 30 minutes after vomiting episode before offering more fluids to patient (assuming normal gastrointestinal tract and normal peristalsis)

Begin by offering fluids that are clear and free of carbonation

Gradually increase fluids if no vomiting occurs over a 30-minute period

Monitor for damage to esophagus and posterior pharynx if vomiting and retching are prolonged

Monitor fluid and electrolyte balance

Encourage rest

Utilize nutritional supplements if necessary to maintain body weight

Weigh patient regularly

Teach the use of nonpharmacological techniques (e.g., biofeedback, hypnosis, relaxation, guided imagery, music therapy, distraction, acupressure) to manage vomiting

Encourage the use of nonpharmacological techniques along with other vomiting control measure

Inform other health care professionals and family members of any nonpharmacological strategies being used by the patient

Assist patient and family to seek and provide support for themselves

Monitor effects of vomiting management throughout

Continued

Background Readings:

Fessele, K.S. (1996). Managing the multiple causes of nausea and vomiting in the patient with cancer. Oncology Nursing Forum, 23(9), 1409-1417.

Grant, M. (1987). Nausea, vomiting, and anorexia. Seminars in Oncology Nursing, 3(4), 227-286.

Hogan, C.M. (1990). Advances in the management of nausea and vomiting. Nursing Clinics of North America, 25(2), 475-497.

Larson, P., Halliburton, P., & DiJulio, J. (1993). Nausea, vomiting, and retching. In V. Carrier-Kohlman, A.M. Lindsey, & C.M. West (Eds.), Pathophysiological phenomena in nursing human responses to illness. Philadelphia, W.B. Saunders Company.

Rhodes, V.A. (1990). Nausea, vomiting, and retching. Nursing Clinics of North America, 25(4), 885-900.

V

Weight Gain Assistance   1240

Definition: Facilitating gain of body weight

Activities:

Refer for diagnostic workup to determine cause of being underweight, as appropriate

Weigh patient at specified intervals, as appropriate

Discuss possible causes of low body weight

Monitor for nausea and vomiting

Determine cause of nausea and/or vomiting, and treat appropriately

Administer medications to reduce nausea and pain before eating, as appropriate

Monitor daily calories consumed

Monitor serum albumin, lymphocyte, and electrolyte levels

Encourage increased calorie intake

Instruct on how to increase calorie intake

Provide a variety of high-calorie nutritious foods from which to select

Consider patient's food preferences, as governed by personal choices and cultural and religious preferences

Provide oral care before meals, as needed

Provide rest periods, as needed

Ensure that patient is in a sitting position before eating or feeding

Assist with eating, or feed patient, as appropriate

Provide foods appropriate for patient: general diet, mechanical soft diet, blenderized or commercial formula via nasogastric or gastrostomy tube, or total parental nutrition, as ordered by physician

Create a pleasant, relaxing environment at mealtime

Serve food in a pleasant, attractive manner

Discuss with patient and family socioeconomic factors contributing to inadequate nutrition

Discuss with patient and family perceptions or factors interfering with ability or desire to eat

Refer to community agencies that can assist in acquiring food, as appropriate

Teach patient and family meal planning, as appropriate

Recognize that weight loss may be part of the natural progression of a terminal illness (e.g., cancer)

Instruct patient and family members on realistic expected outcomes regarding illness and the potential for weight gain

Determine patient's preferences regarding favorite foods, seasonings, and temperature

Provide dietary supplements, as appropriate

Create a social setting for food consumption, as appropriate

Teach patient and family how to buy low-cost, nutritious foods, as appropriate

Reward patient for weight gain

Chart weight gain progress and post in a strategic location

Encourage attendance at support groups, as appropriate

W

Continued

Background Readings:

Cluskey, M., & Dunton, N. (1999). Serving meals of reduced portion size did not improve appetite among elderly in a personal-care section of a long-term-care community. Journal of the American Dietetic Association, 99(6), 733-735.

Ferguson, M., Cook, A., Bender, S., Rimmasch, H., & Voss, A. (2001). Diagnosing and treating involuntary weight loss. MED-SURG Nursing, 10(4), 165-175.

Seligman, P.A., Fink, R., & Massey-Seligman, E.J. (1998). Approach to the seriously ill or terminal cancer patient who has a poor appetite. Seminars in Oncology, 25(2, Suppl 6), 33-34.

Thelan, L.A., & Urden, L.D. (1998). Critical care nursing: Diagnosis and management (3rd ed.). St. Louis: Mosby.

Wakefield, B. (2001). Altered nutrition: Less than body requirements. In M.L. Maas, K.C. Buckwater, M.D. Hardy, T. Tripp-Reimer, M.G. Titler, & J.P. Specht (Eds.), Nursing care of older adults: Diagnoses, outcomes and interventions (Chapter 13). St. Louis: Mosby.

W

Weight Management   1260

Definition: Facilitating maintenance of optimal body weight and percent body fat

Activities:

Discuss with individual the relationships among food intake, exercise, weight gain, and weight loss

Discuss with individual the medical conditions that may affect weight

Discuss with individual the habits and customs and cultural and heredity factors that influence weight

Discuss risks associated with being over- and underweight

Determine individual motivation for changing eating habits

Determine individual's ideal body weight

Determine individual's ideal percent body fat

Develop with the individual a method to keep a daily record of intake, exercise sessions, and/or changes in body weight

Encourage individual to write down realistic weekly goals for food intake and exercise and to display them in a location where they can be reviewed daily

Encourage individual to chart weekly weights, as appropriate

Encourage individual to consume adequate amounts of water daily

Plan rewards with the individual to celebrate reaching short-term and long-term goals

Inform individual about whether support groups are available for assistance

Assist in developing well-balanced meal plans consistent with level of energy expenditure

Background Readings:

National Institutes of Health. (2000). The practical guide: Identification, evaluation, and treatment of overweight and obesity in adults. NIH Publication Number 00-4084. Washington, DC: US Department of Health and Human Services.

Thelan, L.A., & Urden, L.D. (1998). Critical care nursing: Diagnosis and management (3rd ed.). St. Louis: Mosby.

Whitney, E.N., & Cataldo, C.B. (1991). Understanding normal and clinical nutrition (3rd ed.). St. Paul, MN: West Publishing.

W

Weight Reduction Assistance 1280

Definition: Facilitating loss of weight and/or body fat

Activities:

Determine patient's desire and motivation to reduce weight or body fat

Determine with the patient the amount of weight loss desired

Set a weekly goal for weight loss

Post the weekly goal in a strategic location

Weigh patient weekly

Chart progress toward reaching final goal, and post in a strategic location

Reward patient when goals are attained

Encourage use of internal reward systems when goals are accomplished

Set a realistic plan with the patient to include reduced food intake and increased energy expenditure

Determine current eating patterns by having patient keep a diary of what, when, and where he/she eats

Assist patient to identify motivation for eating and internal and external cues associated with eating

Encourage substitution of undesirable habits with desirable habits

Post reminder and encouragement signs to do health-promotion behaviors, rather than eating

Assist with adjusting diet to lifestyle and activity level

Facilitate patient participation in at least one energy-expending activity three times a week

Provide information about amount of energy expended with specific physical activities

Assist in selection of activities according to amount of desired energy expenditure

Plan an exercise program, taking into consideration the patient's limitations

Develop a daily meal plan with a well-balanced diet, reduced calories, and reduced fat, as appropriate

Encourage use of sugar substitute, as appropriate

Recommend adoption of diets that will lead to achievement of long-range goals for weight loss

Encourage attendance at support groups for weight loss (e.g., TOPS or Weight Watchers)

Refer to a community weight control program, as appropriate

Instruct on how to read labels when purchasing food, to control amount of fat and calorie density of food to be consumed

Instruct on how to calculate percentage of fat in food products

Teach food selection, in restaurants and social gatherings, that is consistent with planned calorie and nutrient intake

Discuss with patient and family the influence of alcohol consumption on food ingestion

Background Readings:

Thelan, L.A., & Urden, L.D. (1998). Critical care nursing: Diagnosis and management (3rd ed.). St. Louis: Mosby.

Whitney, E.N., & Cataldo, C.B. (1991). Understanding normal and clinical nutrition. St. Paul, MN: West Publishing.

National Institutes of Health. (2000) The practical guide: Identification, evaluation, and treatment of overweight and obesity in adults. NIH Publication Number 00-4084. Washington, DC: U.S. Department of Health and Human Services.

W

Wound Care 3660

Definition: Prevention of wound complications and promotion of wound healing

Activities:

Remove dressing and adhesive tape

Shave the hair surrounding the affected area, as needed

Monitor characteristics of the wound, including drainage, color, size, and odor

Measure the wound bed, as appropriate

Remove embedded material (e.g., splinter, tick, glass, gravel, metal), as needed

Cleanse with normal saline or a nontoxic cleanser, as appropriate

Place affected area in a whirlpool bath, as appropriate

Provide incision site care, as needed

Administer skin ulcer care, as needed

Apply an appropriate ointment to the skin/lesion, as appropriate

Apply a dressing, appropriate for wound type

Reinforce the dressing, as needed

Maintain sterile dressing technique when doing wound care, as appropriate

Change dressing according to amount of exudate and drainage

Inspect the wound with each dressing change

Compare and record regularly any changes in the wound

Position to avoid placing tension on the wound, as appropriate

Reposition patient at least every 2 hours, as appropriate

Encourage intake of fluids, as appropriate

Refer to wound ostomy clinician, as appropriate

Refer to dietitian, as appropriate

Apply TENS (transcutaneous electrical nerve stimulation) unit for wound healing enhancement, as appropriate

Place pressure-relieving devices (e.g., low-air-loss, foam, or gel mattresses; heel or elbow pads; chair cushion), as appropriate

Assist patient and family to obtain supplies

Instruct patient and family on storage and disposal of dressings and supplies

Instruct patient or family member(s) in wound care procedures

Instruct patient and family on signs and symptoms of infection

Document wound location, size, and appearance

Background Readings:

Bryant, R.A. (2000). Acute and chronic wounds: Nursing management. St. Louis: Mosby.

Dwyer, F.M., & Keeler, D. (1997). Protocols for wound management. Nursing Management, 28(7), 45-49.

Hall, P., & Schumann, L. (2001). Wound care: Meeting the challenge. Journal of the American Academy of Nurse Practitioners, 13(6), 258-266.

Thompson, J. (2000). A practical guide to wound care. RN, 63(1), 48-52.

W

Wound Care: Closed Drainage   3662

Definition: Maintenance of a pressure drainage system at the wound site

Activities:

Empty the closed wound drainage system, according to procedure

Record the volume and characteristics of the drainage at appropriate intervals

Obtain specimens, as needed

Cleanse the collection device, as needed

Check the patency of the unit

Prevent kinking of the tubing

Inspect the sutures, holding the collection device in place

Number the collection devices, if more than one exist

Secure the closed drainage appliance to the patient's clothing or bedding, as appropriate

Discard soiled dressings, supplies, and drainage in an appropriate manner

Background Readings:

Perry, A.G., & Potter, P.A. (1998). Clinical nursing skills and techniques. (4th ed.) St. Louis: Mosby.

Sorensen, K., & Luckmann, J. (1986). Basic nursing: A psychophysiologic approach (2nd ed.). Philadelphia: W.B. Saunders.

W

Wound Irrigation   3680

Definition: Flushing of an open wound to cleanse and remove debris and excessive drainage

Activities:

Identify any allergies, especially to iodine-like products

Explain the procedure to the patient, using sensory preparation

Medicate the patient before the irrigation, as needed for pain control

Protect patient's clothing from soiling by the irrigation, solution or wound drainage

Monitor the amount and type of wound drainage present with each dressing change

Position the patient so that irrigating solution can be collected by a basin, depending on the wound's location

Maintain a sterile field during the irrigation procedure, as appropriate

Irrigate wound with appropriate solution, using a large irrigating syringe

Avoid aspirating the solution back into the syringe

Attach a catheter to the syringe for irrigation of small openings

Avoid forcing the catheter into an abdominal wound, to prevent perforation of the intestine

Instill the irrigation solution slowly, reaching all areas

Cleanse from cleanest to dirtiest areas of the wound

Continue irrigating the wound until the prescribed volume is used or the solution returns clear

Position the patient after the irrigation to facilitate drainage

Cleanse and dry the area around the wound after the procedure

Protect surrounding tissue from skin breakdown

Pack the wound with the appropriate type of sterile dressing

Apply a sterile dressing, as appropriate

Monitor progress of granulating tissue

Report any sign of infection and/or necrosis to the physician

Dispose of soiled dressing and supplies appropriately

Background Readings:

Kozier, B., & Erb, G. (1989). Techniques in clinical nursing (3rd ed.). Menlo Park, CA: Addison-Wesley.

Perry, A.G., & Potter, P.A. (1998). Clinical nursing skills and techniques (4th ed.). St. Louis: Mosby.

Smith, S., & Duell, D. (1992). Clinical nursing skills (3rd ed.). Los Altos, CA: National Nursing Review.

Sorensen, K., & Luckmann, J. (1986). Basic nursing: A psychophysiologic approach (2nd ed.). Philadelphia: W.B. Saunders.

W

PART FOUR

NIC Interventions Linked to NANDA Diagnoses

Introduction to Linkages with NANDA

This section of the book provides linkages between the North American Nursing Diagnosis Association's (NANDA) diagnoses and the Nursing Interventions Classification (NIC) interventions. The 514 NIC interventions included in this edition are linked to NANDA's 156 diagnoses from the 2001 edition.* A *linkage* is defined as a relationship or association between a nursing diagnosis and a nursing intervention that causes them to occur together in order to obtain an outcome or the resolution of a patient's problem. Linkages facilitate the diagnostic reasoning and clinical decision making of the nurse by identifying nursing interventions that are treatment options for resolution of a nursing diagnosis. They can also assist those who are designing clinical nursing information systems to structure their databases.

The included lists of nursing interventions for each nursing diagnosis are comprehensive, including multiple interventions. The following three levels of interventions are provided for each diagnosis:

1st level: Priority Interventions: These are the most likely/most obvious intervention(s) to resolve the diagnosis. They were selected because of a good match with the diagnosis' etiology and/or the defining characteristics, have more activities that will resolve the problem, can be used in more settings, and are better known from research and clinical use to address the diagnosis.

2nd level: Suggested Interventions: These are interventions that are likely to address the diagnosis but not as likely as the priority interventions for the majority of patients with the diagnosis. These are sometimes mentioned in the literature as addressing the diagnosis but not mentioned as often, and they may address only selected etiologies or characteristics.

3rd level: Additional Optional: These are interventions that apply only to some patients with the diagnosis, allowing a nurse to further tailor the plan of care to the individual.

The listing of three levels of interventions provides a comprehensive list of interventions for each diagnosis. The list assists the nurse in the selection of interventions, but is not prescriptive. The nurse uses clinical reasoning and judgment with each individual patient, family, or group to determine the appropriate choice of interventions.

The following steps are suggested when using the linkage list:

1. Review the priority nursing interventions for first consideration as the treatment of choice for resolution of a nursing diagnosis.
2. Review other interventions in the suggested list because these are considered most essential for resolution of the diagnosis.
3. Review the additional suggestions for interventions that may also be used for resolution of the nursing diagnosis.

The second edition of NIC described in detail the methods that were initially used to develop this linkage list. For subsequent editions, the previous linkages were updated by the editors, who added the new diagnoses and interventions and their appropriate linkages. We also included some feedback from users who indicated some additions and deletions.

---

*NANDA's diagnoses of Altered Tissue Perfusion and Sensory Perceptual Alterations are listed individually by type.

In addition to these linkages of NIC with NANDA diagnoses, we have completed linkages for the interventions in the second edition of NIC with Omaha system problems[4] and with NOC (first edition) outcomes.[3] The third edition of NIC has also been linked with resident assessment protocols (RAPs) used in nursing homes[2] and OASIS (Outcome and Assessment Information Set) currently mandated for collection for Medicare/Medicaid–covered patients receiving skilled home care.[1] These are available in monograph form from the Center for Nursing Classification and Clinical Effectiveness (http://www.nursing.uiowa.edu/cnc). In 2001, work was completed to link NANDA, NIC, and NOC by the Iowa group. This work has been published by Mosby in a book[5] with an electronic link, which provides a format to build customized care plans. A software program providing users with the three standardized languages and the linkages is also available from Mosby. The provision of links among the three classifications will facilitate the use of standardized language in clinical practice and documentation systems, as well as in education.

References

1. Center for Nursing Classification. (2001). NIC interventions and NOC outcomes linked to the OASIS Information Set. Iowa City: Center for Nursing Classification.
2. Cox, R.A. (2000). Standardized nursing language in long term care. Iowa City: Center for Nursing Classification.
3. Iowa Intervention Project. (1998). NIC interventions linked to NOC outcomes. Iowa City, IA: Center for Nursing Classification, College of Nursing, The University of Iowa.
4. Iowa Intervention Project. (1996). NIC interventions linked to Omaha system problems. Iowa City, IA: Center for Nursing Classification, College of Nursing, The University of Iowa.
5. Johnson, M., Bulechek, G., Dochterman, J.M., Maas, M., & Moorhead, S. (2001). Nursing diagnoses, Outcomes, and interventions: NANDA, NOC, and NIC Linkages. St. Louis: Mosby.
6. North American Nursing Diagnosis Association. (2001). NANDA nursing diagnoses: Definitions and classification 2001-2002. Philadelphia: North American Nursing Diagnosis Association.

Activity Intolerance

DEFINITION: Insufficient physiological or psychological energy to endure or complete required or desired daily activities.

SUGGESTED NURSING INTERVENTIONS FOR PROBLEM RESOLUTION:

Activity Therapy
Art Therapy
Animal-Assisted Therapy
Body Mechanics Promotion
Energy Management
Exercise Promotion: Strength Training

Music Therapy
Self-Care Assistance
Self-Care Assistance: IADL
Self-Care Assistance: Transfer
Therapeutic Play
Teaching: Prescribed Activity/Exercise

ADDITIONAL OPTIONAL INTERVENTIONS:

Autogenic Training
Biofeedback
Cardiac Care: Rehabilitative
Dysrhythmia Management
Environmental Management
Environmental Management: Comfort
Exercise Promotion
Exercise Promotion: Stretching
Exercise Therapy: Ambulation
Exercise Therapy: Balance
Exercise Therapy: Joint Mobility
Exercise Therapy: Muscle Control
Hypnosis
Labor Suppression

Medication Management
Meditation Facilitation
Mutual Goal Setting
Nutrition Management
Oxygen Therapy
Pain Management
Progressive Muscle Relaxation
Sleep Enhancement
Smoking Cessation Assistance
Spiritual Support
Therapeutic Touch
Visitation Facilitation
Weight Management

Note: Highlighted interventions are priority interventions, those most likely to resolve the nursing diagnosis.

Activity Intolerance, Risk for

DEFINITION: At risk for experiencing insufficient physiological or psychological energy to endure or complete required or desired daily activities.

SUGGESTED NURSING INTERVENTIONS FOR PROBLEM RESOLUTION:

Counseling
Dementia Management
Emotional Support
Energy Management
Exercise Promotion
Exercise Promotion: Strength Training
Exercise Promotion: Stretching
Exercise Therapy: Ambulation
Exercise Therapy: Balance
Exercise Therapy: Joint Mobility

Exercise Therapy: Muscle Control
Hope Instillation
Nutrition Management
Oxygen Therapy
Pain Management
Security Enhancement
Self-Care Assistance: IADL
Self-Esteem Enhancement
Sleep Enhancement
Teaching: Prescribed Activity/Exercise

ADDITIONAL OPTIONAL INTERVENTIONS:

Medication Management
Mutual Goal Setting
Positioning
Smoking Cessation Assistance

Surveillance
Vital Signs Monitoring
Weight Management

Adjustment, Impaired

DEFINITION: Inability to modify lifestyle/behavior in a manner consistent with a change in health status.

SUGGESTED NURSING INTERVENTIONS FOR PROBLEM RESOLUTION:

Behavior Modification
Complex Relationship Building
Coping Enhancement
Counseling
Crisis Intervention
Decision-Making Support
Health System Guidance

Mutual Goal Setting
Pass Facilitation
Relocation Stress Support
Role Enhancement
Surveillance
Teaching: Disease Process

ADDITIONAL OPTIONAL INTERVENTIONS:

Anticipatory Guidance
Anxiety Reduction
Caregiver Support
Sibling Support
Support Group

Therapy Group
Truth Telling
Values Clarification
Vital Signs Monitoring

Airway Clearance, Ineffective

DEFINITION: Inability to clear secretions or obstructions from the respiratory tract to maintain a clear airway

SUGGESTED NURSING INTERVENTIONS FOR PROBLEM RESOLUTION:

Airway Insertion and Stabilization
Airway Management
Airway Suctioning
Anxiety Reduction
Artificial Airway Management
Aspiration Precautions
Asthma Management
Chest Physiotherapy
Cough Enhancement
Mechanical Ventilation

Mechanical Ventilatory Weaning
Medication Administration:
   Inhalation
Oxygen Therapy
Positioning
Respiratory Monitoring
Resuscitation: Neonate
Surveillance
Ventilation Assistance
Vital Signs Monitoring

ADDITIONAL OPTIONAL INTERVENTIONS:

Acid-Base Management
Acid-Base Management: Respiratory Acidosis
Acid-Base Management: Respiratory Alkalosis
Allergy Management
Anaphylaxis Management
Dysrhythmia Management
Emergency Care
Emotional Support
Endotracheal Extubation
Energy Management

Fluid Management
Fluid Monitoring
Infection Control
Infection Protection
Intravenous (IV) Insertion
Intravenous (IV) Therapy
Phlebotomy: Arterial Blood Sample
Smoking Cessation Assistance
Tube Care: Chest

Anxiety

DEFINITION: Vague uneasy feeling of discomfort or dread accompanied by an autonomic response (the source often nonspecific or unknown to the individual); a feeling of apprehension caused by anticipation of danger. It is an alerting signal that warns of impending danger and enables the individual to take measures to deal with threat.

SUGGESTED NURSING INTERVENTIONS FOR PROBLEM RESOLUTION:

Anxiety Reduction
Calming Technique
Coping Enhancement
Dementia Management

Dementia Management: Bathing
Examination Assistance
Presence
Telephone Consultation

ADDITIONAL OPTIONAL INTERVENTIONS:

Allergy Management
Anger Control Assistance
Animal-Assisted Therapy
Anticipatory Guidance
Art Therapy
Asthma Management
Autogenic Training
Behavior Management: Self-Harm
Biofeedback
Childbirth Preparation
Counseling
Crisis Intervention
Distraction
Elopement Precautions
Energy Management
Environmental Management
Exercise Promotion: Stretching
Genetic Counseling
Grief Work Facilitation: Perinatal Death
High-Risk Pregnancy Care
Humor
Hypnosis
Labor Induction

Labor Suppression
Medication Prescribing
Meditation Facilitation
Music Therapy
Premenstrual Syndrome Management
Progressive Muscle Relaxation
Relocation Stress Reduction
Reminiscence Therapy
Reproductive Technology Management
Security Enhancement
Self-Hypnosis Facilitation
Simple Guided Imagery
Simple Relaxation Therapy
Support Group
Teaching: Individual
Teaching: Preoperative
Teaching: Prescribed Medication
Teaching: Procedure/Treatment
Trauma Therapy: Child
Urinary Incontinence Care: Enuresis
Visitation Facilitation
Vital Signs Monitoring

Aspiration, Risk for

DEFINITION: At risk for entry of gastrointestinal secretions, oropharyngeal secretions, solids, or fluids into tracheobronchial passages.

SUGGESTED NURSING INTERVENTIONS FOR PROBLEM RESOLUTION:

Airway Suctioning
Amnioinfusion
Artificial Airway Management
Aspiration Precautions
Cough Enhancement
Neurologic Monitoring
Positioning
Postanesthesia Care

Respiratory Monitoring
Resuscitation: Neonate
Sedation Management
Surveillance
Swallowing Therapy
Teaching: Infant Safety
Teaching: Toddler Safety
Vomiting Management

ADDITIONAL OPTIONAL INTERVENTIONS:

Asthma Management
Enteral Tube Feeding
Feeding
Gastrointestinal Intubation

Mechanical Ventilation
Mechanical Ventilatory Weaning
Medication Administration: Enteral
Vital Signs Monitoring

Autonomic Dysreflexia

DEFINITION: Life-threatening, uninhibited sympathetic response of the nervous system to a noxious stimulus after a spinal cord injury at T7 or above.

SUGGESTED NURSING INTERVENTIONS FOR PROBLEM RESOLUTION:

Airway Management
Anxiety Reduction
Bowel Management
Dysreflexia Management
Fluid Management

Fluid Monitoring
Positioning
Temperature Regulation
Urinary Elimination Management
Vital Signs Monitoring

ADDITIONAL OPTIONAL INTERVENTIONS:

Cough Enhancement
Exercise Promotion
Exercise Therapy: Joint Mobility
Exercise Therapy: Muscle Control
Infection Control
Infection Protection
Intravenous (IV) Insertion
Intravenous (IV) Therapy
Medication Administration

Medication Management
Neurologic Monitoring
Nutrition Management
Skin Surveillance
Surveillance
Surveillance: Safety
Urinary Catheterization
Urinary Catheterization: Intermittent

Autonomic Dysreflexia, Risk for

DEFINITION: At risk for life-threatening, uninhibited response of the sympathetic nervous system post spinal shock, in an individual with spinal cord injury or lesion at T6 or above (has been demonstrated in patients with injuries at T7 and T8).

SUGGESTED NURSING INTERVENTIONS FOR PROBLEM RESOLUTION:

Airway Management	Fluid Monitoring
Anxiety Reduction	Positioning
Bowel Management	Temperature Regulation
Dysreflexia Management	Urinary Elimination Management
Fluid Management	Vital Signs Monitoring

ADDITIONAL OPTIONAL INTERVENTIONS:

Cough Enhancement	Medication Management
Exercise Promotion	Neurologic Monitoring
Exercise Therapy: Joint Mobility	Nutrition Management
Exercise Therapy: Muscle Control	Skin Surveillance
Infection Control	Surveillance
Infection Protection	Surveillance: Safety
Intravenous (IV) Insertion	Urinary Catheterization
Intravenous (IV) Therapy	Urinary Catheterization: Intermittent
Medication Administration	

Body Image, Disturbed

DEFINITION: Confusion in mental picture of one's physical self.

SUGGESTED NURSING INTERVENTIONS FOR PROBLEM RESOLUTION:

Active Listening
Amputation Care
Anxiety Reduction
Body Image Enhancement
Coping Enhancement
Counseling
Developmental Enhancement: Adolescent
Emotional Support
Grief Work Facilitation
Ostomy Care
Pain Management
Presence

Self-Awareness Enhancement
Self-Care Assistance
Self-Esteem Enhancement
Socialization Enhancement
Suicide Prevention
Support Group
Support System Enhancement
Surveillance: Safety
Therapy Group
Values Clarification
Weight Management
Wound Care

ADDITIONAL OPTIONAL INTERVENTIONS:

Anticipatory Guidance
Bowel Incontinence Care: Encopresis
Calming Technique
Childbirth Preparation
Cognitive Restructuring
Decision-Making Support
Lactation Counseling

Mutual Goal Setting
Patient Contracting
Prenatal Care
Teaching: Sexuality
Truth Telling
Urinary Incontinence Care: Enuresis

Body Temperature, Risk for Imbalanced

DEFINITION: At risk for failure to maintain body temperature.

SUGGESTED NURSING INTERVENTIONS FOR PROBLEM RESOLUTION:

Cerebral Edema Management
Environmental Management
Environmental Management: Comfort
Fever Treatment
Fluid Management
Fluid Monitoring

Malignant Hyperthermia Precautions
Postanesthesia Care
Temperature Regulation
Temperature Regulation: Intraoperative
Vital Signs Monitoring

ADDITIONAL OPTIONAL INTERVENTIONS:

Bathing
Energy Management
Heat/Cold Application
Hemodynamic Regulation
Kangaroo Care

Medication Management
Nutrition Management
Resuscitation: Neonate
Skin Surveillance
Surveillance

Bowel Incontinence

DEFINITION: Change in normal bowel habits characterized by involuntary passage of stool.

SUGGESTED NURSING INTERVENTIONS FOR PROBLEM RESOLUTION:

Bowel Incontinence Care
Bowel Incontinence Care: Encopresis
Bowel Irrigation
Bowel Management
Bowel Training
Dementia Management

Diarrhea Management
Perineal Care
Rectal Prolapse Management
Self-Care Assistance: Toileting
Teaching: Toilet Training

ADDITIONAL OPTIONAL INTERVENTIONS:

Bathing
Emotional Support
Environmental Management
Exercise Promotion

Exercise Therapy: Ambulation
Nutrition Management
Skin Surveillance

Breastfeeding, Effective

DEFINITION: Mother-infant dyad/family exhibits adequate proficiency and satisfaction with breastfeeding process.

SUGGESTED NURSING INTERVENTIONS FOR PROBLEM RESOLUTION:

Anticipatory Guidance
Attachment Promotion
Lactation Counseling

Parent Education: Infant
Teaching: Individual

ADDITIONAL OPTIONAL INTERVENTIONS:

Infant Care
Nutrition Therapy
Support Group
Teaching: Infant Nutrition

Teaching: Infant Safety
Teaching: Infant Stimulation
Weight Management

Breastfeeding, Ineffective

DEFINITION: Dissatisfaction or difficulty a mother, infant, or child experiences with the breastfeeding process.

SUGGESTED NURSING INTERVENTIONS FOR PROBLEM RESOLUTION:

Breastfeeding Assistance
Emotional Support
Kangaroo Care
Lactation Counseling
Lactation Suppression
Nutrition Management

Parent Education: Infant
Teaching: Individual
Teaching: Infant Nutrition
Telephone Consultation
Weight Management

ADDITIONAL OPTIONAL INTERVENTIONS:

Bottle Feeding
Pain Management
Patient Rights Protection
Sleep Enhancement

Support Group
Teaching: Infant Safety
Teaching: Infant Stimulation

Breastfeeding, Interrupted

DEFINITION: Break in the continuity of the breastfeeding process as a result of inability or inadvisability to put baby to breast for feeding.

SUGGESTED NURSING INTERVENTIONS FOR PROBLEM RESOLUTION:

Bottle Feeding
Coping Enhancement
Emotional Support
Health System Guidance
Lactation Counseling
Lactation Suppression

Nonnutritive Sucking
Parent Education: Infant
Teaching: Individual
Teaching: Infant Nutrition
Wound Care

ADDITIONAL OPTIONAL INTERVENTIONS:

Active Listening
Anticipatory Guidance
Anxiety Reduction
Behavior Modification
Body Image Enhancement
Discharge Planning

Nutritional Counseling
Referral
Simple Relaxation Therapy
Support Group
Teaching: Infant Stimulation

Breathing Pattern, Ineffective

DEFINITION: Inspiration and/or expiration that does not provide adequate ventilation.

SUGGESTED NURSING INTERVENTIONS FOR PROBLEM RESOLUTION:

Airway Management
Asthma Management
Anxiety Reduction
Cough Enhancement
Mechanical Ventilation
Mechanical Ventilatory Weaning
Medication Administration

Medication Administration: Nasal
Oxygen Therapy
Progressive Muscle Relaxation
Respiratory Monitoring
Surveillance
Ventilation Assistance
Vital Signs Monitoring

ADDITIONAL OPTIONAL INTERVENTIONS:

Acid-Base Monitoring
Airway Insertion and Stabilization
Airway Suctioning
Allergy Management
Analgesic Administration
Artificial Airway Management
Aspiration Precautions
Chest Physiotherapy
Endotracheal Extubation
Emergency Care
Emotional Support
Energy Management
Exercise Promotion
Fluid Management

Fluid Monitoring
Intravenous (IV) Insertion
Intravenous (IV) Therapy
Neurologic Monitoring
Nutrition Management
Medication Management
Pain Management
Phlebotomy: Arterial Blood Sample
Phlebotomy: Venous Blood Sample
Positioning
Presence
Resuscitation
Smoking Cessation Assistance
Tube Care: Chest

Cardiac Output, Decreased

DEFINITION: Inadequate blood pumped by the heart to meet metabolic demands of the body.

SUGGESTED NURSING INTERVENTIONS FOR PROBLEM RESOLUTION:

Acid-Base Management
Acid-Base Management: Metabolic Acidosis
Acid-Base Management: Metabolic Alkalosis
Acid-Base Management: Respiratory
    Acidosis
Acid-Base Management: Respiratory
    Alkalosis
Acid-Base Monitoring
Airway Management
Cardiac Care
Cardiac Care: Acute
Cardiac Care: Rehabilitative
Circulatory Care: Arterial Insufficiency
Circulatory Care: Mechanical Assist Devices
Circulatory Care: Venous Insufficiency
Code Management
Electrolyte Management
Electrolyte Management: Hypercalcemia
Electrolyte Management: Hyperkalemia
Electrolyte Management: Hypermagnesemia
Electrolyte Management: Hypernatremia
Electrolyte Management: Hyperphosphatemia
Electrolyte Management: Hypocalcemia
Electrolyte Management: Hypokalemia
Electrolyte Management: Hypomagnesemia

Electrolyte Management: Hyponatremia
Electrolyte Management:
    Hypophosphatemia
Electrolyte Monitoring
Electronic Fetal Monitoring: Intrapartum
Energy Management
Fluid/Electrolyte Management
Fluid Management
Fluid Monitoring
Hemodialysis Therapy
Hemodynamic Regulation
Medication Administration
Medication Management
Neurologic Monitoring
Oxygen Therapy
Peripherally Inserted Central (PIC)
    Catheter Care
Respiratory Monitoring
Resuscitation
Resuscitation: Fetus
Resuscitation: Neonate
Shock Management
Shock Management: Cardiac
Shock Prevention
Vital Signs Monitoring

ADDITIONAL OPTIONAL INTERVENTIONS:

Anxiety Reduction
Bleeding Precautions
Bleeding Reduction
Bleeding Reduction: Antepartum Uterus
Bleeding Reduction: Gastrointestinal
Bleeding Reduction: Nasal
Bleeding Reduction: Postpartum Uterus
Bleeding Reduction: Wound
Blood Products Administration
Cardiac Precautions
Cerebral Edema Management
Dying Care
Dysrhythmia Management
Emergency Care
Invasive Hemodynamic Monitoring
Intravenous (IV) Insertion
Intravenous (IV) Therapy

Malignant Hyperthermia Precautions
Nutrition Management
Pain Management
Patient Rights Protection
Peritoneal Dialysis Therapy
Phlebotomy: Arterial Blood Sample
Phlebotomy: Cannulated Vessel
Phlebotomy: Venous Blood Sample
Positioning
Sleep Enhancement
Skin Surveillance
Surveillance
Temporary Pacemaker Management
Total Parenteral Nutrition (TPN)
    Administration
Visitation Facilitation
Weight Management

Caregiver Role Strain

DEFINITION: Difficulty in performing caregiver role.

SUGGESTED NURSING INTERVENTIONS FOR PROBLEM RESOLUTION:
Abuse Protection Support: Child
Abuse Protection Support: Domestic Partner
Abuse Protection Support: Elder
Caregiver Support
Home Maintenance Assistance
Parent Education: Adolescent
Parent Education: Childrearing Family
Parent Education: Infant
Parenting Promotion
Respite Care
Role Enhancement

ADDITIONAL OPTIONAL INTERVENTIONS:
Behavior Management: Overactivity/
  Inattention
Counseling
Family Integrity Promotion
Family Involvement Promotion
Family Mobilization
Family Process Maintenance
Family Support
Family Therapy
Guilt Work Facilitation
Kangaroo Care
Referral
Support Group
Support System Enhancement
Teaching: Infant Nutrition
Teaching: Infant Safety
Teaching: Infant Stimulation
Teaching: Toddler Nutrition
Teaching: Toddler Safety
Teaching: Toilet Training

Caregiver Role Strain, Risk for

DEFINITION: Caregiver is vulnerable for felt difficulty in performing the family caregiver role.

SUGGESTED NURSING INTERVENTIONS FOR PROBLEM RESOLUTION:
Caregiver Support
Family Support
Home Maintenance Assistance
Kangaroo Care
Normalization Promotion
Parent Education: Adolescent
Parent Education: Childrearing Family
Parent Education: Infant
Parenting Promotion
Respite Care
Support Group

ADDITIONAL OPTIONAL INTERVENTIONS:
Behavior Management: Overactivity/
  Inattention
Counseling
FamilyIntegrity Promotion
Family Involvement Promotion
Family Mobilization
Family Process Maintenance
Family Therapy
Guilt Work Facilitation
Referral
Role Enhancement
Support System Enhancement
Teaching: Infant Nutrition
Teaching: Infant Safety
Teaching: Infant Stimulation
Teaching: Toddler Nutrition
Teaching: Toddler Safety
Teaching: Toilet Training

Communication, Impaired Verbal

DEFINITION: Decreased, delayed, or absent ability to receive, process, transmit, and use a system of symbols.

SUGGESTED NURSING INTERVENTIONS FOR PROBLEM RESOLUTION:

Active Listening
Anxiety Reduction
Communication Enhancement: Hearing Deficit
Communication Enhancement: Speech Deficit
Communication Enhancement: Visual Deficit

Environmental Management
Presence
Self-Care Assistance: IADL
Surveillance: Safety
Touch

ADDITIONAL OPTIONAL INTERVENTIONS:

Art Therapy
Culture Brokerage
Decision-Making Support
Ear Care
Energy Management

Learning Facilitation
Referral
Relocation Stress Reduction
Support System Enhancement

Community Coping, Ineffective

DEFINITION: Pattern of community activities (for adaptation and problem solving) that is unsatisfactory for meeting the demands or needs of the community.

SUGGESTED NURSING INTERVENTIONS FOR PROBLEM RESOLUTION:

Bioterrorism Preparedness
Communicable Disease Management
Community Disaster Preparedness
Community Health Development
Environmental Management: Community
Environmental Management: Safety
Environmental Management: Violence
   Prevention
Environmental Risk Protection

Fiscal Resource Management
Health Education
Health Policy Monitoring
Health Screening
Immunization/Vaccination Management
Program Development
Risk Identification
Surveillance: Community

ADDITIONAL OPTIONAL INTERVENTIONS:

Documentation
Infection Control
Multidisciplinary Care Conference
Referral

Resiliency Promotion
Sustenance Support
Triage: Disaster
Vehicle Safety Promotion

Community Coping, Readiness for Enhanced

DEFINITION: Pattern of community activities for adaptation and problem solving that is satisfactory for meeting the demands or needs of the community but can be improved for management of current and future problems/stressors.

SUGGESTED NURSING INTERVENTIONS FOR PROBLEM RESOLUTION:

Bioterrorism Preparedness
Environmental Management: Community
Environmental Management: Violence
    Prevention
Environmental Management: Worker Safety
Environmental Risk Protection

Fiscal Resource Management
Health Education
Health Policy Monitoring
Program Development
Surveillance: Community
Vehicle Safety Promotion

ADDITIONAL OPTIONAL INTERVENTIONS:

Anticipatory Guidance
Communicable Disease Management
Community Disaster Preparedness
Community Health Development

Health Screening
Immunization/Vaccination Management
Resiliency Promotion
Risk Identification

Community Therapeutic Regimen Management, Ineffective

DEFINITION: Pattern of regulating and integrating into community processes programs for treatment of illness and the sequelae of illness that are unsatisfactory for meeting health-related goals.

SUGGESTED NURSING INTERVENTIONS FOR PROBLEM RESOLUTION:

Bioterrorism Preparedness
Communicable Disease Management
Community Health Development
Environmental Management: Community
Environmental Management: Safety
Fiscal Resource Management

Health Education
Health Policy Monitoring
Health Screening
Program Development
Risk Identification
Surveillance: Community

ADDITIONAL OPTIONAL INTERVENTIONS:

Community Disaster Preparedness
Environmental Management: Worker Safety
Immunization/Vaccination Management

Resiliency Promotion
Surveillance: Safety
Vehicle Safety Promotion

Confusion, Acute

DEFINITION: Abrupt onset of a cluster of global, transient changes and disturbances in attention, cognition, psychomotor activity, level of consciousness, and/or sleep/wake cycle.

SUGGESTED NURSING INTERVENTIONS FOR PROBLEM RESOLUTION:

Acid-Base Management	Medication Management
Analgesic Administration	Pain Management
Anxiety Reduction	Physical Restraint
Delirium Management	Reality Orientation
Delusion Management	Seclusion
Environmental Management: Safety	Sleep Enhancement
Fall Prevention	Surveillance: Safety
Hallucination Management	Vital Signs Monitoring
Medication Administration	

ADDITIONAL OPTIONAL INTERVENTIONS:

Calming Technique	Self-Care Assistance
Presence	Touch

Confusion, Chronic

DEFINITION: Irreversible, long-standing, and/or progressive deterioration of intellect and personality characterized by decreased ability to interpret environmental stimuli; decreased capacity for intellectual thought processes; and manifested by disturbances of memory, orientation, and behavior.

SUGGESTED NURSING INTERVENTIONS FOR PROBLEM RESOLUTION:

Anxiety Reduction
Area Restriction
Calming Technique
Chemical Restraint
Cognitive Stimulation
Dementia Management
Dementia Management: Bathing
Emotional Support
Energy Management
Environmental Management
Environmental Management: Safety
Family Involvement Promotion

Family Support
Humor
Milieu Therapy
Mood Management
Music Therapy
Physical Restraints
Presence
Risk Identification
Sleep Enhancement
Surveillance
Surveillance: Safety

ADDITIONAL OPTIONAL INTERVENTIONS:

Activity Therapy
Animal-Assisted Therapy
Art Therapy
Exercise Promotion
Fall Prevention
Health System Guidance

Immunization/Vaccination Management
Patient Rights Protection
Recreation Therapy
Relocation Stress Reduction
Reminiscence Therapy
Medication Management

Constipation

DEFINITION: Decrease in normal frequency of defecation accompanied by difficult or incomplete passage of stool and/or passage of excessively hard, dry stool.

SUGGESTED NURSING INTERVENTIONS FOR PROBLEM RESOLUTION:

Bowel Irrigation	Fluid Management
Bowel Management	Fluid Monitoring
Bowel Training	Medication Prescribing
Constipation/Impaction Management	Nutrition Management
Diet Staging	Rectal Prolapse Management

ADDITIONAL OPTIONAL INTERVENTIONS:

Anxiety Reduction	Medication Management
Exercise Promotion	Ostomy Care
Exercise Therapy: Ambulation	Pain Management
Exercise Therapy: Joint Mobility	Self-Care Assistance: Toileting
Flatulence Reduction	Simple Relaxation Therapy
Gastrointestinal Intubation	Skin Surveillance
Medication Administration: Oral	Teaching: Toilet Training
Medication Administration: Rectal	Tube Care: Gastrointestinal

Constipation, Perceived

DEFINITION: Self-diagnosis of constipation and abuse of laxatives, enemas, and suppositories to ensure a daily bowel movement.

SUGGESTED NURSING INTERVENTIONS FOR PROBLEM RESOLUTION:

Bowel Management	Fluid Monitoring
Counseling	Medication Management
Fluid Management	Teaching: Individual

ADDITIONAL OPTIONAL INTERVENTIONS:

Distraction	Simple Relaxation Therapy
Exercise Promotion	Teaching: Toilet Training
Nutrition Management	

Constipation, Risk for

DEFINITION: At risk for a decrease in normal frequency of defecation accompanied by difficult or incomplete passage of stool and/or passage of excessive hard, dry stool.

SUGGESTED NURSING INTERVENTIONS FOR PROBLEM RESOLUTION:

Bowel Management
Bowel Training
Constipation/Impaction Management
Diet Staging
Fluid Management

Fluid Monitoring
Medication Management
Medication Prescribing
Nutrition Management

ADDITIONAL OPTIONAL INTERVENTIONS:

Anxiety Reduction
Exercise Promotion
Exercise Therapy: Ambulation
Exercise Therapy: Joint Mobility
Flatulence Reduction
Medication Administration: Oral

Ostomy Care
Pain Management
Rectal Prolapse Management
Self-Care Assistance: Toileting
Simple Relaxation Therapy
Teaching: Toilet Training

Coping, Defensive

DEFINITION: Rejected projection of falsely positive self-evaluation based on a self-protective pattern that defends against underlying perceived threats to positive self regard.

SUGGESTED NURSING INTERVENTIONS FOR PROBLEM RESOLUTION:

Complex Relationship Building
Coping Enhancement
Patient Contracting

Self-Awareness Enhancement
Socialization Enhancement
Surveillance: Safety

ADDITIONAL OPTIONAL INTERVENTIONS:

Cognitive Restructuring
Counseling
Emotional Support
Environmental Management

Reminiscence Therapy
Truth Telling
Values Clarification

Coping, Ineffective

DEFINITION: Inability to form a valid appraisal of the stressors, inadequate choices of practiced responses, and/or inability to use available resources.

SUGGESTED NURSING INTERVENTIONS FOR PROBLEM RESOLUTION:

Anger Control Assistance
Anxiety Reduction
Behavior Management: Self-Harm
Behavior Management: Sexual
Calming Technique
Complex Relationship Building
Coping Enhancement
Counseling
Crisis Intervention
Decision-Making Support
Delusion Management
Dementia Management
Distraction
Emotional Support
Environmental Management

Fire-Setting Precautions
Impulse Control Training
Meditation Facilitation
Mood Management
Pass Facilitation
Presence
Progressive Muscle Relaxation
Reminiscence Therapy
Sleep Enhancement
Substance Use Prevention
Support Group
Support System Enhancement
Teaching: Individual
Therapy Group

ADDITIONAL OPTIONAL INTERVENTIONS:

Abuse Protection Support
Activity Therapy
Animal-Assisted Therapy
Art Therapy
Autogenic Training
Behavior Management
Biofeedback
Cognitive Restructuring
Environmental Management: Violence
    Prevention
Family Therapy
Hypnosis
Learning Facilitation
Learning Readiness Enhancement
Limit Setting

Medication Administration
Medication Management
Mutual Goal Setting
Patient Contracting
Seclusion
Self-Esteem Enhancement
Self-Modification Assistance
Self-Responsibility Facilitation
Substance Use Treatment
Substance Use Treatment: Alcohol
    Withdrawal
Substance Use Treatment: Drug Withdrawal
Substance Use Treatment: Overdose
Sustenance Support
Weight Management

Death Anxiety

DEFINITION: Apprehension, worry, or fear related to death or dying.

SUGGESTED NURSING INTERVENTIONS FOR PROBLEM RESOLUTION:

Anxiety Reduction
Caregiver Support
Decision-Making Support
Dying Care
Forgiveness Facilitation
Grief Work Facilitation
Medication Management

Mutual Goal Setting
Patient-Controlled Analgesia (PCA) Assistance
Referral
Simple Guided Imagery
Simple Relaxation Therapy
Spiritual Support
Values Clarification

ADDITIONAL OPTIONAL INTERVENTIONS:

Active Listening
Animal-Assisted Therapy
Bibliotherapy
Culture Brokerage
Family Integrity Promotion
Family Process Maintenance

Family Support
Music Therapy
Patient Rights Protection
Reminiscence Therapy
Visitation Facilitation

Decisional Conflict (Specify)

DEFINITION: Uncertainty about course of action to be taken when choice among competing actions involves risk, loss, or challenge to personal life values.

SUGGESTED NURSING INTERVENTIONS FOR PROBLEM RESOLUTION:

Coping Enhancement
Counseling
Decision-Making Support
Mutual Goal Setting
Preconception Counseling

Self-Awareness Enhancement
Support System Enhancement
Teaching: Individual
Telephone Consultation

ADDITIONAL OPTIONAL INTERVENTIONS:

Autogenic Training
Dementia Management
Grief Work Facilitation: Perinatal Death
Meditation Facilitation
Music Therapy
Pass Facilitation
Patient Contracting

Preparatory Sensory Information
Progressive Muscle Relaxation
Reminiscence Therapy
Simple Guided Imagery
Simple Relaxation Therapy
Teaching: Sexuality
Values Clarification

Denial, Ineffective

DEFINITION: Conscious or unconscious attempt to disavow the knowledge or meaning of an event to reduce anxiety/fear, but leading to the detriment of health.

SUGGESTED NURSING INTERVENTIONS FOR PROBLEM RESOLUTION:

Anxiety Reduction
Complex Relationship Building
Coping Enhancement

Counseling
Reality Orientation
Truth Telling

ADDITIONAL OPTIONAL INTERVENTIONS:

Cognitive Restructuring
Decision-Making Support
Family Therapy
Milieu Therapy
Mutual Goal Setting

Reminiscence Therapy
Security Enhancement
Spiritual Support
Therapeutic Play
Therapy Group

Dentition, Impaired

DEFINITION: Disruption in tooth development/eruption patterns or structural integrity of individual teeth.

SUGGESTED NURSING INTERVENTIONS FOR PROBLEM RESOLUTION:

Medication Management
Nutrition Management
Oral Health Maintenance

Oral Health Restoration
Pain Management
Referral

ADDITIONAL OPTIONAL INTERVENTIONS:

Health System Guidance
Insurance Authorization

Teaching: Psychomotor Skill

Development, Risk for Delayed

DEFINITION: At risk for delay of 25% or more in one or more of the areas of social or self-regulatory behavior, or cognitive, language, gross or fine motor skills.

SUGGESTED NURSING INTERVENTIONS FOR PROBLEM RESOLUTION:

Anticipatory Guidance
Attachment Promotion
Behavior Management
Behavior Management: Overactivity/
    Inattention
Behavior Modification
Behavior Modification: Social Skills
Bowel Incontinence Care: Encopresis
Caregiver Support
Counseling
Developmental Care

Developmental Enhancement: Adolescent
Developmental Enhancement: Child
Family Therapy
High-Risk Pregnancy Care
Impulse Control Training
Risk Identification: Genetic
Self-Responsibility Facilitation
Support Group
Support System Enhancement
Urinary Incontinence Care: Enuresis

ADDITIONAL OPTIONAL INTERVENTIONS:

Abuse Protection Support: Child
Behavior Management: Sexual
Coping Enhancement
Decision-Making Support
Fire-Setting Precautions
Respite Care
Surveillance: Safety

Teaching: Infant Nutrition
Teaching: Infant Safety
Teaching: Infant Stimulation
Teaching: Toddler Nutrition
Teaching: Toddler Safety
Teaching: Toilet Training

Diarrhea

DEFINITION: Passage of loose, unformed stools.

SUGGESTED NURSING INTERVENTIONS FOR PROBLEM RESOLUTION:

Bowel Incontinence Care: Encopresis
Bowel Management
Diarrhea Management
Electrolyte Monitoring
Fluid/Electrolyte Management
Fluid Management
Fluid Monitoring

Medication Management
Medication Prescribing
Nutrition Management
Perineal Care
Skin Surveillance
Weight Management

ADDITIONAL OPTIONAL INTERVENTIONS:

Anxiety Reduction
Bathing
Enteral Tube Feeding
Environmental Management
Intravenous (IV) Insertion
Intravenous (IV) Therapy
Peripherally Inserted Central (PIC)
   Catheter Care

Self-Care Assistance: Toileting
Skin Care: Topical Treatment
Surveillance
Total Parenteral Nutrition (TPN)
   Administration
Tube Care: Gastrointestinal

Disuse Syndrome, Risk for

DEFINITION: At risk for deterioration of body systems as the result of prescribed or unavoidable musculoskeletal inactivity.

SUGGESTED NURSING INTERVENTIONS FOR PROBLEM RESOLUTION:

Bowel Management
Energy Management
Environmental Management
Exercise Promotion: Stretching
Exercise Therapy: Ambulation
Exercise Therapy: Balance
Exercise Therapy: Joint Mobility

Exercise Therapy: Muscle Control
Fluid Management
Fluid Monitoring
Medication Administration
Medication Management
Pneumatic Tourniquet Precautions
Positioning: Intraoperative

ADDITIONAL OPTIONAL INTERVENTIONS:

Exercise Promotion
Exercise Promotion: Strength Training
Nutrition Management
Pain Management
Physical Restraint
Positioning

Progressive Muscle Relaxation
Reality Orientation
Simple Relaxation Therapy
Surveillance
Vital Signs Monitoring

Diversional Activity, Deficient

DEFINITION: Decreased stimulation from (or interest or engagement in) recreational or leisure activities.

SUGGESTED NURSING INTERVENTIONS FOR PROBLEM RESOLUTION:

Activity Therapy
Animal-Assisted Therapy
Art Therapy
Milieu Therapy
Music Therapy
Mutual Goal Setting

Recreation Therapy
Reminiscence Therapy
Self-Esteem Enhancement
Self-Responsibility Facilitation
Therapeutic Play
Visitation Facilitation

ADDITIONAL OPTIONAL INTERVENTIONS:

Energy Management
Environmental Management
Exercise Promotion
High-Risk Pregnancy Care
Labor Induction
Pain Management

Pass Facilitation
Patient Contracting
Support Group
Surveillance: Safety
Teaching: Individual

Energy Field, Disturbed

DEFINITION: Disruption in the flow of energy surrounding a person's being that results in a disharmony of the body, mind and/or spirit.

SUGGESTED NURSING INTERVENTIONS FOR PROBLEM RESOLUTION:

Acupressure
Energy Management
Meditation Facilitation
Pain Management
Simple Guided Imagery

Spiritual Support
Temperature Regulation
Therapeutic Touch
Vital Signs Monitoring

ADDITIONAL OPTIONAL INTERVENTIONS:

Aromatherapy
Communication Enhancement: Hearing Deficit
Communication Enhancement: Visual Deficit

Environmental Management
Fever Treatment

Environmental Interpretation Syndrome, Impaired

DEFINITION: Consistent lack of orientation to person, place, time, or circumstances over more than 3 to 6 months necessitating a protective environment.

SUGGESTED NURSING INTERVENTIONS FOR PROBLEM RESOLUTION:

Anxiety Reduction
Communication Enhancement: Speech Deficit
Dementia Management
Dementia Management: Bathing
Emotional Support
Energy Management
Environmental Management
Environmental Management: Safety
Milieu Therapy

Mood Management
Music Therapy
Reality Orientation
Reminiscence Therapy
Security Enhancement
Sleep Enhancement
Surveillance
Surveillance: Safety

ADDITIONAL OPTIONAL INTERVENTIONS:

Area Restriction
Behavior Management
Calming Technique
Cognitive Stimulation
Feeding
Medication Management

Patient Rights Protection
Self-Care Assistance
Self-Care Assistance: IADL
Therapeutic Play
Touch

Failure to Thrive, Adult

DEFINITION: Progressive functional deterioration of a physical and cognitive nature. The individual's ability to live with multisystem diseases, cope with ensuing problems, and manage his/her care are remarkably diminished.

SUGGESTED NURSING INTERVENTIONS FOR PROBLEM RESOLUTION:

Caregiver Support
Case Management
Coping Enhancement
Diet Staging
Energy Management
Environmental Management: Comfort
Feeding
Financial Resource Assistance
Hope Instillation
Medication Management
Mood Management
Nutrition Management

Nutrition Therapy
Nutritional Monitoring
Patient Rights Protection
Relocation Stress Reduction
Self-Care Assistance
Self-Care Assistance: Bathing/Hygiene
Self-Care Assistance: Dressing/Grooming
Self-Care Assistance: Feeding
Self-Care Assistance: IADL
Self-Care Assistance: Toileting
Spiritual Support

ADDITIONAL OPTIONAL INTERVENTIONS:

Animal-Assisted Therapy
Bathing
Dressing
Dying Care
Family Involvement

Family Mobilization
Family Process Maintenance
Foot Care
Hair Care
Nail Care

Falls, Risk for

DEFINITION: Increased susceptibility to falling that may cause physical harm.

SUGGESTED NURSING INTERVENTIONS FOR PROBLEM RESOLUTION:

Area Restriction

Body Mechanics Promotion

Dementia Management

Dementia Management: Bathing

Environmental Management: Safety

Exercise Therapy: Balance

Exercise Therapy: Muscle Control

Fall Prevention

Medication Management

Positioning

Positioning: Wheelchair

Seizure Precautions

Self-Care Assistance: Toileting

Self-Care Assistance: Transfer

Teaching: Infant Safety

Teaching: Toddler Safety

Transport

Urinary Elimination Management

Vital Signs Monitoring

ADDITIONAL OPTIONAL INTERVENTIONS:

Exercise Promotion

Exercise Promotion: Strength Training

Exercise Promotion: Stretching

Pain Management

Self-Care Assistance

Surveillance: Safety

Family Coping: Compromised

DEFINITION: Usually supportive primary person (family member or close friend) provides insufficient, ineffective, or compromised support, comfort, assistance, or encouragement that may be needed by the client to manage or master adaptive tasks related to his/her health challenge.

SUGGESTED NURSING INTERVENTIONS FOR PROBLEM RESOLUTION:

Abuse Protection Support: Child
Abuse Protection Support: Domestic Partner
Abuse Protection Support: Elder
Bowel Incontinence Care: Encopresis
Complex Relationship Building
Coping Enhancement
Family Integrity Promotion
Family Involvement Promotion
Family Mobilization

Family Presence Facilitation
Family Process Maintenance
Family Support
Grief Work Facilitation: Perinatal Death
Normalization Promotion
Spiritual Support
Sustenance Support
Urinary Incontinence Care: Enuresis

ADDITIONAL OPTIONAL INTERVENTIONS:

Abuse Protection Support
Anger Control Assistance
Anxiety Reduction
Behavior Management: Overactivity/
    Inattention
Calming Technique
Caregiver Support
Counseling
Crisis Intervention
Decision-Making Support
Environmental Management: Attachment
    Process
Environmental Management: Comfort

Environmental Management: Violence
    Prevention
Family Therapy
Mutual Goal Setting
Organ Procurement
Pass Facilitation
Relocation Stress Reduction
Reminiscence Therapy
Respite Care
Role Enhancement
Sibling Support
Trauma Therapy: Child

Family Coping: Disabled

DEFINITION: Behavior of significant person (family member or other primary person) that disables his/her own capacities and the client's capacities to effectively address tasks essential to either person's adaptation to the health challenge.

SUGGESTED NURSING INTERVENTIONS FOR PROBLEM RESOLUTION:

Abuse Protection Support: Child
Abuse Protection Support: Domestic Partner
Abuse Protection Support: Elder
Complex Relationship Building
Coping Enhancement
Counseling
Family Involvement Promotion
Family Integrity Promotion

Family Mobilization
Family Process Maintenance
Family Support
Family Therapy
Normalization Promotion
Spiritual Support
Sustenance Support

ADDITIONAL OPTIONAL INTERVENTIONS:

Abuse Protection Support
Anger Control Assistance
Anxiety Reduction
Calming Technique
Crisis Intervention
Decision-Making Support

Environmental Management: Comfort
Environmental Management: Violence
    Prevention
Mutual Goal Setting
Relocation Stress Reduction
Trauma Therapy: Child

Family Coping: Readiness for Enhanced

DEFINITION: Effective management of adaptive tasks by family member involved with the client's health challenge, who now exhibits desire and readiness for enhanced health and growth in regard to self and in relation to the client.

SUGGESTED NURSING INTERVENTIONS FOR PROBLEM RESOLUTION:

Anticipatory Guidance
Counseling
Developmental Care
Developmental Enhancement: Adolescent
Developmental Enhancement: Child
Family Involvement Promotion
Family Mobilization
Family Support

High-Risk Pregnancy Care
Normalization Promotion
Parent Education: Adolescent
Parent Education: Infant
Pass Facilitation
Preconception Counseling
Sibling Support

ADDITIONAL OPTIONAL INTERVENTIONS:

Family Integrity Promotion
Family Planning: Contraception
Family Therapy
Grief Work Facilitation: Perinatal Death
Labor Suppression
Mutual Goal Setting
Organ Procurement
Prenatal Care
Reproductive Technology Management

Risk Identification: Genetic
Role Enhancement
Teaching: Individual
Teaching: Infant Nutrition
Teaching: Infant Stimulation
Teaching: Safety
Teaching: Toddler Nutrition
Teaching: Toddler Safety
Teaching: Toilet Training

Family Processes, Dysfunctional: Alcoholism

DEFINITION: Psychosocial, spiritual, and physiological functions of the family unit are chronically disorganized, which leads to conflict, denial of problems, resistance to change, ineffective problem-solving, and a series of self-perpetuating crises.

SUGGESTED NURSING INTERVENTIONS FOR PROBLEM RESOLUTION:

Abuse Protection Support
Abuse Protection Support: Child
Abuse Protection Support: Domestic Partner
Abuse Protection Support: Elder
Anger Control Assistance
Anxiety Reduction
Behavior Management
Body Image Enhancement
Crisis Intervention
Counseling
Emotional Support
Family Integrity Promotion
Family Process Maintenance
Family Support

Family Therapy
Impulse Control Training
Limit Setting
Mutual Goal Setting
Normalization Promotion
Self-Awareness Enhancement
Self-Responsibility Facilitation
Spiritual Support
Substance Use Prevention
Substance Use Treatment
Support Group
Teaching: Disease Process
Therapy Group

ADDITIONAL OPTIONAL INTERVENTIONS:

Calming Technique
Decision-Making Support

Referral

Family Processes, Interrupted

DEFINITION: Change in family relationships and/or functioning.

SUGGESTED NURSING INTERVENTIONS FOR PROBLEM RESOLUTION:

Counseling
Developmental Enhancement: Adolescent
Developmental Enhancement: Child
Emotional Support
Family Integrity Promotion
Family Mobilization
Family Process Maintenance
Family Support

Family Therapy
Financial Resource Assistance
Labor Suppression
Normalization Promotion
Reproductive Technology Management
Role Enhancement
Support System Enhancement

ADDITIONAL OPTIONAL INTERVENTIONS:

Art Therapy
Assertiveness Training
Attachment Promotion
Behavior Management
Behavior Modification
Caregiver Support
Conflict Mediation
Coping Enhancement
Decision-Making Support
Dementia Management
Family Integrity Promotion: Childbearing
    Family
Family Involvement Promotion
Family Planning: Contraception
Family Planning: Infertility

Family Planning: Unplanned Pregnancy
Grief Work Facilitation
Guilt Work Facilitation
Home Maintenance Assistance
Mutual Goal Setting
Newborn Care
Parent Education: Adolescent
Parent Education: Childrearing Family
Prenatal Care
Respite Care
Self-Esteem Enhancement
Support Group
Visitation Facilitation

Family Therapeutic Regimen Management, Ineffective

DEFINITION: Pattern of regulating and integrating into family processes a program for treatment of illness and the sequelae of illness that is unsatisfactory for meeting specific health goals.

SUGGESTED NURSING INTERVENTIONS FOR PROBLEM RESOLUTION:

Case Management
Counseling
Family Integrity Promotion
Family Involvement Promotion
Family Mobilization
Family Process Maintenance
Family Support
Family Therapy

Health System Guidance
Normalization Promotion
Risk Identification
Role Enhancement
Sibling Support
Sustenance Support
Teaching: Disease Process

ADDITIONAL OPTIONAL INTERVENTIONS:

Abuse Protection Support
Caregiver Support
Culture Brokerage
Home Maintenance Assistance
Referral

Relocation Stress Reduction
Respite Care
Support Group
Support System Enhancement

Fatigue

DEFINITION: An overwhelming sustained sense of exhaustion and decreased capacity for physical and mental work at usual level.

SUGGESTED NURSING INTERVENTIONS FOR PROBLEM RESOLUTION:

Energy Management
Exercise Promotion
Mood Management

Mutual Goal Setting
Nutrition Management
Sleep Enhancement

ADDITIONAL OPTIONAL INTERVENTIONS:

Asthma Management
Crisis Intervention
Decision-Making Support
Dementia Management
Dying Care
Exercise Promotion: Strength Training
Exercise Promotion: Stretching
Exercise Therapy: Ambulation

Exercise Therapy: Balance
Exercise Therapy: Joint Mobility
Exercise Therapy: Muscle Control
Simple Guided Imagery
Simple Massage
Simple Relaxation Therapy
Support System Enhancement

Fear

DEFINITION: Response to perceived threat that is consciously recognized as a danger.

SUGGESTED NURSING INTERVENTIONS FOR PROBLEM RESOLUTION:

Anxiety Reduction
Cognitive Restructuring
Coping Enhancement
Counseling
Crisis Intervention
Decision-Making Support
Emotional Support
Environmental Management

Examination Assistance
Preparatory Sensory Information
Presence
Security Enhancement
Support System Enhancement
Telephone Consultation
Touch

ADDITIONAL OPTIONAL INTERVENTIONS:

Anger Control Assistance
Art Therapy
Autogenic Training
Biofeedback
Childbirth Preparation
Communication Enhancement: Hearing Deficit
Communication Enhancement: Visual Deficit
Family Presence Facilitation
Grief Work Facilitation: Perinatal Death
High-Risk Pregnancy Care
Hypnosis
Labor Suppression
Meditation Facilitation

Progressive Muscle Relaxation
Reminiscence Therapy
Resuscitation: Fetus
Self-Esteem Enhancement
Simple Guided Imagery
Simple Relaxation Therapy
Spiritual Support
Support Group
Teaching: Preoperative
Teaching: Procedure/Treatment
Therapy Group
Vital Signs Monitoring

Fluid Volume, Deficient

DEFINITION: Decreased intravascular, interstitial, and/or intracellular fluid. This refers to dehydration, water loss alone without change in sodium.

SUGGESTED NURSING INTERVENTIONS FOR PROBLEM RESOLUTION:

Amnioinfusion
Bleeding Precautions
Bleeding Reduction
Bleeding Reduction: Antepartum Uterus
Bleeding Reduction: Gastrointestinal
Bleeding Reduction: Postpartum Uterus
Blood Products Administration
Cardiac Care: Acute
Electrolyte Management
Electrolyte Management: Hypercalcemia
Electrolyte Management: Hyperkalemia
Electrolyte Management: Hypermagnesemia
Electrolyte Management: Hypernatremia
Electrolyte Management: Hyperphosphatemia
Electrolyte Management: Hypocalcemia
Electrolyte Management: Hypokalemia
Electrolyte Management: Hypomagnesemia
Electrolyte Management: Hyponatremia
Electrolyte Management: Hypophosphatemia
Electrolyte Monitoring
Fluid/Electrolyte Management
Fluid Management
Fluid Monitoring
Hypovolemia Management
Intravenous (IV) Insertion
Intravenous (IV) Therapy
Resuscitation: Fetus
Shock Management
Shock Management: Volume
Shock Prevention
Surveillance
Venous Access Devices (VAD)
  Maintenance
Vital Signs Monitoring

ADDITIONAL OPTIONAL INTERVENTIONS:

Capillary Blood Sample
Cerebral Edema Management
Dysrhythmia Management
Feeding
Fever Treatment
Gastrointestinal Intubation
Hemodynamic Regulation
Invasive Hemodynamic Monitoring
Labor Suppression
Medication Management
Neurologic Monitoring
Nutrition Management
Peripherally Inserted Central (PIC)
  Catheter Care
Phlebotomy: Arterial Blood Sample
Phlebotomy: Cannulated Vessel
Phlebotomy: Venous Blood Sample
Temperature Regulation
Total Parenteral Nutrition (TPN) Administration
Tube Care: Chest
Tube Care: Gastrointestinal
Urinary Catheterization
Weight Management
Wound Care

Fluid Volume, Excess

DEFINITION: Increased isotonic fluid retention.

SUGGESTED NURSING INTERVENTIONS FOR PROBLEM RESOLUTION:

Electrolyte Management
Electrolyte Management: Hypercalcemia
Electrolyte Management: Hyperkalemia
Electrolyte Management: Hypermagnesemia
Electrolyte Management: Hypernatremia
Electrolyte Management: Hyperphosphatemia
Electrolyte Management: Hypocalcemia
Electrolyte Management: Hypokalemia
Electrolyte Management: Hypomagnesemia
Electrolyte Management: Hyponatremia

Electrolyte Management: Hypophosphatemia
Electrolyte Monitoring
Fluid/Electrolyte Management
Fluid Management
Fluid Monitoring
Hypervolemia Management
Intravenous (IV) Insertion
Intravenous (IV) Therapy
Temperature Regulation
Vital Signs Monitoring

ADDITIONAL OPTIONAL INTERVENTIONS:

Capillary Blood Sample
Cerebral Edema Management
Dysrhythmia Management
Feeding
Gastrointestinal Intubation
Hemodialysis Therapy
Hemodynamic Regulation
Invasive Hemodynamic Monitoring
Labor Suppression
Medication Management
Neurologic Monitoring
Nutrition Management
Peripherally Inserted Central (PIC)
    Catheter Care

Peritoneal Dialysis Therapy
Phlebotomy: Arterial Blood Sample
Phlebotomy: Cannulated Vessel
Phlebotomy: Venous Blood Sample
Positioning
Skin Surveillance
Total Parenteral Nutrition (TPN)
    Administration
Tube Care: Gastrointestinal
Urinary Catheterization
Weight Management
Wound Care

Fluid Volume, Risk for Deficient

DEFINITION: At risk for experiencing vascular, cellular, or intracellular dehydration.

SUGGESTED NURSING INTERVENTIONS FOR PROBLEM RESOLUTION:

Autotransfusion
Bleeding Precautions
Bleeding Reduction
Bleeding Reduction: Gastrointestinal
Blood Products Administration
Cardiac Care: Acute
Electrolyte Management
Electrolyte Management: Hypercalcemia
Electrolyte Management: Hyperkalemia
Electrolyte Management: Hypermagnesemia
Electrolyte Management: Hypernatremia
Electrolyte Management: Hyperphosphatemia
Electrolyte Management: Hypocalcemia
Electrolyte Management: Hypokalemia
Electrolyte Management: Hypomagnesemia
Electrolyte Management: Hyponatremia

Electrolyte Management: Hypophosphatemia
Electrolyte Monitoring
Fluid/Electrolyte Management
Fluid Management
Fluid Monitoring
Hypovolemia Management
Intrapartal Care: High-Risk Delivery
Intravenous (IV) Insertion
Intravenous (IV) Therapy
Resuscitation: Neonate
Shock Management
Shock Management: Volume
Shock Prevention
Surveillance
Venous Access Devices (VAD) Maintenance
Vital Signs Monitoring

ADDITIONAL OPTIONAL INTERVENTIONS:

Capillary Blood Sample
Cerebral Edema Management
Dysrhythmia Management
Electronic Fetal Monitoring: Intrapartum
Feeding
Fever Treatment
Gastrointestinal Intubation
Hemodynamic Regulation
Invasive Hemodynamic Monitoring
Medication Management
Neurologic Monitoring
Nutrition Management

Peripherally Inserted Central (PIC) Catheter
    Care
Phlebotomy: Arterial Blood Sample
Phlebotomy: Cannulated Vessel
Phlebotomy: Venous Blood Sample
Temperature Regulation
Total Parenteral Nutrition (TPN) Administration
Tube Care: Chest
Tube Care: Gastrointestinal
Urinary Catheterization
Weight Management
Wound Care

Fluid Volume, Risk for Imbalanced

DEFINITION: At risk for a decrease, increase, or rapid shift from one to the other of intravascular, interstitial, and/or intracellular fluid. This refers to body fluid loss, gain, or both.

SUGGESTED NURSING INTERVENTIONS FOR PROBLEM RESOLUTION:

Autotransfusion
Bleeding Precautions
Bleeding Reduction
Bleeding Reduction: Gastrointestinal
Blood Products Administration
Electrolyte Management
Electrolyte Management: Hypercalcemia
Electrolyte Management: Hyperkalemia
Electrolyte Management: Hypermagnesemia
Electrolyte Management: Hypernatremia
Electrolyte Management: Hyperphosphatemia
Electrolyte Management: Hypocalcemia
Electrolyte Management: Hypokalemia
Electrolyte Management: Hypomagnesemia
Electrolyte Management: Hyponatremia

Electrolyte Management: Hypophosphatemia
Electrolyte Monitoring
Fluid/Electrolyte Management
Fluid Management
Fluid Monitoring
Hypovolemia Management
Intravenous (IV) Insertion
Intravenous (IV) Therapy
Shock Management
Shock Management: Volume
Shock Prevention
Surveillance
Venous Access Devices (VAD) Maintenance
Vital Signs Monitoring

ADDITIONAL OPTIONAL INTERVENTIONS:

Capillary Blood Sample
Cerebral Edema Management
Dysrhythmia Management
Fever Treatment
Gastrointestinal Intubation
Hemodynamic Regulation
Invasive Hemodynamic
    Monitoring
Medication Management
Neurologic Monitoring
Nutrition Management

Peripherally Inserted Central (PIC)
    Catheter Care
Phlebotomy: Arterial Blood Sample
Phlebotomy: Cannulated Vessel
Phlebotomy: Venous Blood Sample
Temperature Regulation
Total Parenteral Nutrition (TPN) Administration
Tube Care: Chest
Tube Care: Gastrointestinal
Urinary Catheterization
Wound Care

Gas Exchange, Impaired

DEFINITION: Excess or deficit in oxygenation and/or carbon dioxide elimination at the alveolar-capillary membrane.

SUGGESTED NURSING INTERVENTIONS FOR PROBLEM RESOLUTION:

Acid-Base Management
Acid-Base Management: Metabolic Acidosis
Acid-Base Management: Metabolic Alkalosis
Acid-Base Management: Respiratory Acidosis
Acid-Base Management: Respiratory Alkalosis
Acid-Base Monitoring
Airway Management
Bedside Laboratory Testing
Cough Enhancement

Exercise Promotion
Intrapartal Care: High-Risk Delivery
Laboratory Data Interpretation
Oxygen Therapy
Postanesthesia Care
Respiratory Monitoring
Resuscitation: Neonate
Vital Signs Monitoring

ADDITIONAL OPTIONAL INTERVENTIONS:

Airway Suctioning
Allergy Management
Anxiety Reduction
Artificial Airway Management
Aspiration Precautions
Asthma Management
Chest Physiotherapy
Coping Enhancement
Dysrhythmia Management
Embolus Care: Pulmonary
Energy Management
Exercise Therapy: Ambulation
Fluid Management
Fluid Monitoring
Hemodynamic Regulation
Intravenous (IV) Insertion
Intravenous (IV) Therapy

Invasive Hemodynamic Regulation
Malignant Hyperthermia Precautions
Mechanical Ventilation
Mechanical Ventilatory Weaning
Nutrition Management
Pain Management
Peripherally Inserted Central (PIC)
    Catheter Care
Phlebotomy: Arterial Blood Sample
Positioning
Resuscitation
Shock Management
Smoking Cessation Assistance
Surveillance
Total Parenteral Nutrition (TPN) Administration
Tube Care: Chest
Ventilation Assistance

Grieving, Anticipatory

DEFINITION: Intellectual and emotional responses and behaviors by which individuals, families, and communities work through the process of modifying self-concept based on the perception of potential loss.

SUGGESTED NURSING INTERVENTIONS FOR PROBLEM RESOLUTION:

Active Listening
Anger Control Assistance
Counseling
Dying Care
Emotional Support
Family Integrity Promotion
Family Support
Grief Work Facilitation

Grief Work Facilitation: Perinatal Death
Hope Instillation
Presence
Reminiscence Therapy
Support System Enhancement
Truth Telling
Touch

ADDITIONAL OPTIONAL INTERVENTIONS:

Bioterrorism Preparedness
Community Disaster Preparedness
Environmental Management
Environmental Management: Comfort
Family Therapy
Normalization Promotion

Organ Procurement
Reproductive Technology Management
Spiritual Support
Support Group
Surveillance: Safety

Grieving, Dysfunctional

DEFINITION: Extended, unsuccessful use of intellectual and emotional responses by which individuals, families, and communities attempt to work through the process of modifying self-concept based upon the perception of loss.

SUGGESTED NURSING INTERVENTIONS FOR PROBLEM RESOLUTION:

Active Listening
Anger Control Assistance
Anxiety Reduction
Community Health Development
Coping Enhancement
Counseling
Crisis Intervention
Culture Brokerage

Emotional Support
Family Integrity Promotion
Family Support
Family Therapy
Grief Work Facilitation
Grief Work Facilitation: Perinatal Death
Presence
Spiritual Support

ADDITIONAL OPTIONAL INTERVENTIONS:

Art Therapy
Guilt Work Facilitation
Hope Instillation
Mutual Goal Setting
Normalization Promotion
Nutrition Management

Reminiscence Therapy
Simple Relaxation Therapy
Suicide Prevention
Support Group
Support System Enhancement
Values Clarification

Growth and Development, Delayed

DEFINITION: Deviations from age-group norms.

SUGGESTED NURSING INTERVENTIONS FOR PROBLEM RESOLUTION:

Anticipatory Guidance
Attachment Promotion
Behavior Management
Behavior Management: Overactivity/
   Inattention
Behavior Modification
Behavior Modification: Social Skills
Bowel Incontinence Care: Encopresis
Caregiver Support
Counseling
Developmental Care
Developmental Enhancement: Adolescent

Developmental Enhancement: Child
Family Therapy
High-Risk Pregnancy Care
Impulse Control Training
Nutrition Management
Nutrition Therapy
Nutritional Monitoring
Self-Responsibility Facilitation
Support Group
Support System Enhancement
Urinary Incontinence Care: Enuresis

ADDITIONAL OPTIONAL INTERVENTIONS:

Abuse Protection Support: Child
Behavior Management: Sexual
Coping Enhancement
Decision Making Support
Fire-Setting Precautions
Presence
Reproductive Technology Management
Respite Care

Surveillance: Safety
Teaching: Infant Nutrition
Teaching: Infant Safety
Teaching: Infant Stimulation
Teaching: Toddler Safety
Teaching: Toilet Training
Weight Management

Growth, Risk for Disproportionate

DEFINITION: At risk for growth above the 97th percentile or below the 3rd percentile for age, crossing two percentile channels; disproportionate growth.

SUGGESTED NURSING INTERVENTIONS FOR PROBLEM RESOLUTION:

Attachment Promotion

Behavior Modification

Bottle Feeding

Caregiver Support

Counseling

Eating Disorders Management

Family Therapy

Kangaroo Care

Lactation Counseling

Nutrition Management

Nutrition Therapy

Nutritional Monitoring

Parent Education: Childrearing Family

Teaching: Infant Nutrition

Teaching: Prescribed Diet

Teaching: Toddler Nutrition

Weight Gain Assistance

Weight Management

Weight Reduction Assistance

ADDITIONAL OPTIONAL INTERVENTIONS:

Abuse Protection Support: Child

Coping Enhancement

Enteral Tube Feeding

Parent Education: Infant

Risk Identification: Genetic

Sibling Support

Swallowing Therapy

Total Parenteral Nutrition (TPN) Administration

Health Maintenance, Ineffective

DEFINITION: Inability to identify, manage, and/or seek out help to maintain health.

SUGGESTED NURSING INTERVENTIONS FOR PROBLEM RESOLUTION:

Anticipatory Guidance
Cognitive Restructuring
Coping Enhancement
Counseling
Decision-Making Support
Discharge Planning
Exercise Promotion
Financial Resource Assistance
Health Education

Health Screening
Health System Guidance
Physician Support
Referral
Risk Identification
Risk Identification: Childbearing Family
Self-Responsibility Facilitation
Support System Enhancement
Teaching: Disease Process

ADDITIONAL OPTIONAL INTERVENTIONS:

Environmental Management: Community
Environmental Management: Worker Safety
Family Mobilization
Family Process Maintenance
Medication Management
Nutrition Management
Pass Facilitation

Patient Contracting
Self-Modification Assistance
Smoking Cessation Assistance
Substance Use Prevention
Values Clarification
Weight Management

Health Seeking Behaviors (Specify)

DEFINITION: Active seeking (by a person in stable health) of ways to alter personal health habits and/or the environment in order to move toward a higher level of health.

SUGGESTED NURSING INTERVENTIONS FOR PROBLEM RESOLUTION:

Coping Enhancement
Emotional Support
Exercise Promotion
Exercise Promotion: Stretching
Family Integrity Promotion: Childbearing
  Family
Fertility Preservation
Health Education
Health System Guidance

Immunization/Vaccination Management
Nutrition Management
Preconception Counseling
Self-Modification Assistance
Smoking Cessation Assistance
Spiritual Growth Facilitation
Spiritual Support
Teaching: Sexuality
Weight Management

ADDITIONAL OPTIONAL INTERVENTIONS:

Activity Therapy
Aromatherapy
Decision-Making Support
Environmental Management: Community
Environmental Management: Worker Safety
Examination Assistance
Health Screening
Meditation Facilitation
Mutual Goal Setting

Reminiscence Therapy
Risk Identification
Sexual Counseling
Simple Guided Imagery
Simple Relaxation Therapy
Socialization Enhancement
Surveillance: Safety
Teaching: Individual

Home Maintenance, Impaired

DEFINITION: Inability to independently maintain a safe growth-promoting immediate environment.

SUGGESTED NURSING INTERVENTIONS FOR PROBLEM RESOLUTION:

Discharge Planning
Family Support
Home Maintenance Assistance
Pass Facilitation

Self-Care Assistance: IADL
Support System Enhancement
Sustenance Support

ADDITIONAL OPTIONAL INTERVENTIONS:

Caregiver Support
Counseling
Energy Management
Environmental Management

Environmental Management: Home Preparation
Mutual Goal Setting
Referral
Teaching: Individual

Hopelessness

DEFINITION: Subjective state in which an individual sees limited or no alternatives or personal choices available and is unable to mobilize energy on own behalf.

SUGGESTED NURSING INTERVENTIONS FOR PROBLEM RESOLUTION:

Complex Relationship Building
Decision-Making Support
Emotional Support
Energy Management
Hope Instillation
Mood Management
Presence

Reminiscence Therapy
Sleep Enhancement
Socialization Enhancement
Spiritual Growth Facilitation
Support Group
Support System Enhancement

ADDITIONAL OPTIONAL INTERVENTIONS:

Activity Therapy
Anger Control Assistance
Animal-Assisted Therapy
Cognitive Stimulation
Counseling
Crisis Intervention
Distraction
Electroconvulsive (ECT) Therapy Management
Exercise Promotion
Exercise Therapy: Ambulation

Grief Work Facilitation
Grief Work Facilitation: Perinatal Death
Music Therapy
Mutual Goal Setting
Patient Contracting
Phototherapy: Mood/Sleep Regulation
Self-Care Assistance
Spiritual Support
Suicide Prevention
Therapeutic Play

Hyperthermia

DEFINITION: Body temperature elevated above normal range.

SUGGESTED NURSING INTERVENTIONS FOR PROBLEM RESOLUTION:

Bathing
Environmental Management
Fever Treatment
Fluid Management
Heat Exposure Treatment
Hemodynamic Regulation
Infection Control
Infection Protection

Malignant Hyperthermia Precautions
Medication Management
Medication Prescribing
Shock Management
Skin Surveillance
Temperature Regulation
Temperature Regulation: Intraoperative
Vital Signs Monitoring

ADDITIONAL OPTIONAL INTERVENTIONS:

Heat/Cold Application
Nutrition Management
Oxygen Therapy
Peripherally Inserted Central (PIC)
    Catheter Care

Seizure Management
Seizure Precautions
Total Parenteral Nutrition (TPN) Administration

Hypothermia

DEFINITION: Body temperature below normal range.

SUGGESTED NURSING INTERVENTIONS FOR PROBLEM RESOLUTION:

Circulatory Precautions
Electrolyte Monitoring
Environmental Management
Fluid/Electrolyte Management
Fluid Management
Fluid Monitoring
Hemodynamic Regulation
Hypothermia Treatment
Oxygen Therapy

Respiratory Monitoring
Shock Management
Shock Prevention
Skin Surveillance
Surveillance: Safety
Temperature Regulation
Temperature Regulation: Intraoperative
Vital Signs Monitoring

ADDITIONAL OPTIONAL INTERVENTIONS:

Circulatory Care: Arterial Insufficiency
Circulatory Care: Venous Insufficiency
Heat/Cold Application
Shock Management: Cardiac

Shock Management: Vasogenic
Peripherally Inserted Central (PIC)
    Catheter Care
Total Parenteral Nutrition (TPN) Administration

Infant Behavior, Disorganized

DEFINITION: Disintegrated physiological and neurobehavioral response to the environment.

SUGGESTED NURSING INTERVENTIONS FOR PROBLEM RESOLUTION:

Attachment Promotion
Breastfeeding Assistance
Developmental Care
Energy Management
Environmental Management
Environmental Management: Attachment
  Process
Environmental Management: Comfort
Infant Care
Kangaroo Care
Lactation Counseling

Neurologic Monitoring
Newborn Care
Newborn Monitoring
Nonnutritive Sucking
Nutritional Monitoring
Pain Management
Positioning
Respiratory Monitoring
Sleep Enhancement
Temperature Regulation
Vital Signs Monitoring

ADDITIONAL OPTIONAL INTERVENTIONS:

Bottle Feeding
Circumcision Care
Cutaneous Stimulation
Parent Education: Infant
Risk Identification: Genetic

Teaching: Infant Nutrition
Teaching: Infant Safety
Teaching: Infant Stimulation
Touch
Visitation Facilitation

Infant Behavior, Organized, Readiness for Enhanced

DEFINITION: A pattern of modulation of the physiologic and behavioral systems of functioning (i.e., autonomic, motor, state, organizational, self-regulators, and attentional-interactional systems) that is satisfactory but that can be improved, resulting in higher levels of integration in response to environmental stimuli.

SUGGESTED NURSING INTERVENTIONS FOR PROBLEM RESOLUTION:

Attachment Promotion
Developmental Care
Energy Management
Environmental Management
Environmental Management: Attachment Process
Family Integrity Promotion: Childbearing Family

Family Mobilization
Infant Care
Kangaroo Care
Nonnutritive Sucking
Pain Management
Sleep Enhancement
Touch

ADDITIONAL OPTIONAL INTERVENTIONS:

Circumcision Care
Cutaneous Stimulation
Developmental Enhancement: Child
Lactation Counseling
Music Therapy
Newborn Care
Newborn Monitoring

Surveillance
Teaching: Infant Nutrition
Teaching: Infant Safety
Teaching: Infant Stimulation
Visitation Facilitation
Vital Signs Monitoring

Infant Behavior, Risk for Disorganized

Definition: Risk for alteration in integration and modulation of the physiological and behavioral systems of functioning (i.e., autonomic, motor, state, organizational, self-regulatory, and attentional-interactional systems).

Suggested Nursing Interventions for Problem Resolution:

Developmental Care
Environmental Management
Environmental Management: Comfort
Infant Care
Kangaroo Care
Lactation Counseling
Neurologic Monitoring
Newborn Monitoring

Nonnutritive Sucking
Nutritional Monitoring
Pain Management
Positioning
Respiratory Monitoring
Surveillance
Vital Signs Monitoring

Additional Optional Interventions:

Bottle Feeding
Circumcision Care
Teaching: Infant Nutrition

Teaching: Infant Safety
Teaching: Infant Stimulation
Temperature Regulation

Infant Feeding Pattern, Ineffective

Definition: Impaired ability to suck or coordinate the suck-swallow response.

Suggested Nursing Interventions for Problem Resolution:

Aspiration Precautions
Bottle Feeding
Breastfeeding Assistance
Energy Management
Enteral Tube Feeding
Environmental Management
Fluid Management
Fluid Monitoring

Kangaroo Care
Lactation Counseling
Nonnutritive Sucking
Nutrition Management
Nutritional Monitoring
Swallowing Therapy
Tube Care: Umbilical Line
Weight Management

Additional Optional Interventions:

Gastrointestinal Intubation
Infant Care
Parent Education: Infant
Referral

Teaching: Infant Nutrition
Teaching: Infant Safety
Teaching: Infant Stimulation

Infection, Risk for

DEFINITION: At increased risk for being invaded by pathogenic organisms.

SUGGESTED NURSING INTERVENTIONS FOR PROBLEM RESOLUTION:

Amnioinfusion
Bathing
Communicable Disease Management
Cough Enhancement
Electrolyte Monitoring
Environmental Management
Exercise Promotion
Fertility Preservation
Fluid/Electrolyte Management
High-Risk Pregnancy Care
Immunization/Vaccination Management
Infection Control

Infection Control: Intraoperative
Infection Protection
Labor Induction
Medication Prescribing
Nutrition Management
Perineal Care
Positioning
Skin Surveillance
Surveillance
Tube Care: Umbilical Line
Wound Care
Wound Care: Closed Drainage

ADDITIONAL OPTIONAL INTERVENTIONS:

Airway Management
Birthing
Cesarean Section Care
Electronic Fetal Monitoring: Intrapartum
Exercise Promotion: Stretching
Exercise Therapy: Ambulation
Exercise Therapy: Balance
Exercise Therapy: Joint Mobility
Exercise Therapy: Muscle Control
Home Maintenance Assistance
Incision Site Care
Intrapartal Care
Intrapartal Care: High-Risk Delivery
Medication Management
Newborn Care

Postpartal Care
Pregnancy Termination Care
Rectal Prolapse Management
Respiratory Monitoring
Resuscitation: Fetus
Resuscitation: Neonate
Shock Management
Teaching: Disease Process
Teaching: Sexuality
Tube Care
Tube Care: Chest
Tube Care: Gastrointestinal
Tube Care: Urinary
Tube Care: Ventriculostomy/Lumbar Drain
Vital Signs Monitoring

Injury, Risk for

DEFINITION: At risk of injury as a result of environmental conditions interacting with the individual's adaptive and defensive resources.

SUGGESTED NURSING INTERVENTIONS FOR PROBLEM RESOLUTION:

Allergy Management
Artificial Airway Management
Asthma Management
Anger Control Assistance
Bleeding Precautions
Bleeding Reduction
Delusion Management
Dementia Management
Dementia Management: Bathing
Electroconvulsive (ECT) Therapy Management
Electronic Fetal Monitoring: Antepartum
Electronic Fetal Monitoring: Intrapartum
Elopement Precautions
Environmental Management
Environmental Management: Safety
Environmental Management: Violence
  Prevention
Fall Prevention
Feeding
Fire-Setting Precautions
Health Education
High-Risk Pregnancy Care
Home Maintenance Assistance
Impulse Control Training
Intrapartal Care
Intrapartal Care: High-Risk Delivery
Labor Induction

Labor Suppression
Laser Precautions
Latex Precautions
Malignant Hyperthermia Precautions
Phototherapy: Neonate
Physical Restraint
Pneumatic Tourniquet Precautions
Positioning: Intraoperative
Postanesthesia Care
Reality Orientation
Resuscitation: Fetus
Resuscitation: Neonate
Risk Identification
Seclusion
Security Enhancement
Sedation Management
Seizure Management
Seizure Precautions
Sports-Injury Prevention: Youth
Surgical Precautions
Surveillance
Surveillance: Safety
Teaching: Disease Process
Tube Care: Umbilical Line
Ultrasonography: Limited
  Obstetric

ADDITIONAL OPTIONAL INTERVENTIONS:

Airway Management
Airway Suctioning
Cerebral Edema Management
Infection Control
Infection Protection
Medication Administration

Medication Management
Neurologic Monitoring
Presence
Referral
Respite Care
Visitation Facilitation

Intracranial Adaptive Capacity, Decreased

DEFINITION: Intracranial fluid dynamic mechanisms that normally compensate for increases in intracranial volumes are compromised, resulting in repeated disproportionate increases in intracranial pressure (ICP) in response to a variety of noxious and non-noxious stimuli.

SUGGESTED NURSING INTERVENTIONS FOR PROBLEM RESOLUTION:

Cerebral Edema Management
Cerebral Perfusion Promotion
Fluid/Electrolyte Management
Fluid Management
Fluid Monitoring
Intracranial Pressure (ICP) Monitoring
Intravenous (IV) Insertion
Intravenous (IV) Therapy
Laboratory Data Interpretation

Medication Administration
Medication Management
Neurologic Monitoring
Peripheral Sensation Management
Positioning: Neurologic
Surveillance
Surveillance: Safety
Tube Care: Ventriculostomy/Lumbar Drain
Vital Signs Monitoring

ADDITIONAL OPTIONAL INTERVENTIONS:

Acid-Base Management
Airway Management
Anxiety Reduction
Infection Protection

Patient Rights Protection
Positioning
Presence
Touch

Knowledge Deficient (Specify)

DEFINITION: Absence or deficiency of cognitive information related to specific topic.

SUGGESTED NURSING INTERVENTIONS FOR PROBLEM RESOLUTION:

Breastfeeding Assistance
Health Education
Health System Guidance
Lactation Counseling
Learning Facilitation
Learning Readiness Enhancement
Parent Education: Adolescent
Parent Education: Childrearing Family
Parent Education: Infant
Patient Rights Protection
Preconception Counseling
Preparatory Sensory Information
Teaching: Disease Process
Teaching: Foot Care
Teaching: Individual

Teaching: Infant Nutrition
Teaching: Infant Safety
Teaching: Infant Stimulation
Teaching: Preoperative
Teaching: Prescribed Activity/Exercise
Teaching: Prescribed Diet
Teaching: Prescribed Medication
Teaching: Procedure/Treatment
Teaching: Psychomotor Skill
Teaching: Safe Sex
Teaching: Sexuality
Teaching: Toddler Nutrition
Teaching: Toddler Safety
Teaching: Toilet Training

ADDITIONAL OPTIONAL INTERVENTIONS:

Admission Care
Allergy Management
Analgesia Administration
Anxiety Reduction
Asthma Management
Behavior Modification
Behavior Modification: Social Skills
Counseling
Decision-Making Support
Developmental Enhancement: Child
Discharge Planning
Examination Assistance
Family Support
Genetic Counseling
Home Maintenance Assistance
Immunization/Vaccination Management

Labor Induction
Medication Management
Nutrition Management
Pain Management
Parenting Promotion
Prenatal Care
Referral
Self-Modification Assistance
Staff Development
Support Group
Teaching: Group
Therapeutic Play
Values Clarification
Vehicle Safety Promotion
Weight Management

Latex Allergy Response

DEFINITION: An allergic response to natural latex rubber products.

SUGGESTED NURSING INTERVENTIONS FOR PROBLEM RESOLUTION:

Allergy Management
Environmental Management
Environmental Risk Protection
Latex Precautions
Medication Administration
Medication Administration: Nasal

Medication Administration: Skin
Respiratory Monitoring
Risk Identification
Shock Prevention
Teaching: Individual
Vital Signs Monitoring

ADDITIONAL OPTIONAL INTERVENTIONS:

Anaphylaxis Management
Code Management
Fluid Management
Intravenous (IV) Insertion

Intravenous (IV) Therapy
Shock Prevention
Surveillance

Latex Allergy Response, Risk for

DEFINITION: At risk for allergic response to natural latex rubber products.

SUGGESTED NURSING INTERVENTIONS FOR PROBLEM RESOLUTION:

Allergy Management
Environmental Management
Health System Guidance

Latex Precautions
Risk Identification
Teaching: Individual

ADDITIONAL OPTIONAL INTERVENTIONS:

Environmental Management: Worker Safety
Health Care Information Exchange

Surveillance

Loneliness, Risk for

DEFINITION: At risk of experiencing vague dysphoria.

SUGGESTED NURSING INTERVENTIONS FOR PROBLEM RESOLUTION:

Activity Therapy
Anxiety Reduction
Assertiveness Training
Complex Relationship Building
Coping Enhancement
Counseling
Emotional Support
Energy Management
Environmental Management
Family Integrity Promotion
Family Involvement Promotion

Family Mobilization
Hope Instillation
Mood Management
Presence
Relocation Stress Reduction
Self-Awareness Enhancement
Self-Esteem Enhancement
Socialization Enhancement
Support System Enhancement
Visitation Facilitation

ADDITIONAL OPTIONAL INTERVENTIONS:

Animal-Assisted Therapy
Art Therapy
Body Image Enhancement
Exercise Promotion
Family Therapy

Recreation Therapy
Reminiscence Therapy
Support Group
Therapy Group

Memory, Impaired

DEFINITION: Inability to remember or recall bits of information or behavioral skills (impaired memory may be attributed to pathophysiological or situational causes that are either temporary or permanent).

SUGGESTED NURSING INTERVENTIONS FOR PROBLEM RESOLUTION:

Anxiety Reduction
Cardiac Care
Dementia Management
Electrolyte Monitoring
Environmental Management
Environmental Management: Safety
Fluid/Electrolyte Management
Fluid Management

Fluid Monitoring
Medication Management
Memory Training
Neurologic Monitoring
Oxygen Therapy
Reality Orientation
Surveillance
Surveillance: Safety

ADDITIONAL OPTIONAL INTERVENTIONS:

Area Restriction
Calming Technique
Emotional Support
Family Support

Milieu Therapy
Patient Rights Protection
Reminiscence Therapy

Mobility: Bed, Impaired

DEFINITION: Limitation of independent movement from one bed position to another.

SUGGESTED NURSING INTERVENTIONS FOR PROBLEM RESOLUTION:

Bed Rest Care
Body Mechanics Promotion
Exercise Promotion: Stretching
Exercise Therapy: Muscle Control

Positioning
Positioning: Neurologic
Teaching: Prescribed Activity/Exercise

ADDITIONAL OPTIONAL INTERVENTIONS:

Bowel Management
Medication Management
Mutual Goal Setting
Nutrition Management
Pain Management
Self-Care Assistance
Self-Care Assistance: Bathing/Hygiene
Self-Care Assistance: Dressing/Grooming

Self-Care Assistance: Feeding
Self-Care Assistance: IADL
Self-Care Assistance: Toileting
Self-Care Assistance: Transfer
Sleep Enhancement
Traction/Immobilization Care
Urinary Elimination Management

Mobility: Physical, Impaired

DEFINITION: Limitation in independent, purposeful physical movement of the body or of one or more extremities.

SUGGESTED NURSING INTERVENTIONS FOR PROBLEM RESOLUTION:

Bed Rest Care
Cerebral Perfusion Promotion
Energy Management
Environmental Management
Exercise Promotion
Exercise Promotion: Strength Training
Exercise Promotion: Stretching
Exercise Therapy: Ambulation
Exercise Therapy: Balance
Exercise Therapy: Joint Mobility

Exercise Therapy: Muscle Control
Positioning
Positioning: Intraoperative
Positioning: Neurologic
Positioning: Wheelchair
Self-Care Assistance
Self-Care Assistance: IADL
Self-Care Assistance: Transfer
Teaching: Prescribed Activity/Exercise
Traction/Immobilization Care

ADDITIONAL OPTIONAL INTERVENTIONS:

Activity Therapy
Autogenic Training
Body Mechanics Promotion
Biofeedback
Cast Care: Maintenance
Cast Care: Wet
Circulatory Care: Arterial Insufficiency
Circulatory Care: Venous Insufficiency
Circulatory Precautions
Distraction
Fall Prevention
Foot Care
Hypnosis
Labor Suppression
Medication Management
Meditation Facilitation

Neurologic Monitoring
Pain Management
Pass Facilitation
Peripheral Sensation Management
Phototherapy: Neonate
Physical Restraint
Pressure Management
Progressive Muscle Relaxation
Prosthesis Care
Simple Massage
Skin Surveillance
Splinting
Surveillance: Safety
Therapeutic Touch
Weight Management

Mobility: Wheelchair, Impaired

DEFINITION: Limitation of independent operation of wheelchair within environment.

SUGGESTED NURSING INTERVENTIONS FOR PROBLEM RESOLUTION:

Body Mechanics Promotion
Energy Management
Exercise Promotion
Exercise Promotion: Strength Training
Exercise Promotion: Stretching
Exercise Therapy: Balance
Exercise Therapy: Muscle Control
Positioning

Positioning: Neurologic
Positioning: Wheelchair
Self-Care Assistance
Self-Care Assistance: IADL
Self-Care Assistance: Transfer
Teaching: Prescribed Activity/Exercise
Transport

ADDITIONAL OPTIONAL INTERVENTIONS:

Medication Management
Mutual Goal Setting
Nutrition Management

Pain Management
Sleep Enhancement
Weight Management

Nausea

DEFINITION: Unpleasant, wavelike sensation in the back of the throat, epigastrium, or throughout the abdomen that may or may not lead to vomiting.

SUGGESTED NURSING INTERVENTIONS FOR PROBLEM RESOLUTION:

Calming Technique
Diet Staging
Distraction
Fluid/Electrolyte Management
Fluid Monitoring

Medication Administration
Medication Management
Nausea Management
Pain Management
Simple Relaxation Therapy

ADDITIONAL OPTIONAL INTERVENTIONS:

Accupressure
Aspiration Precautions
Intravenous (IV) Insertion
Intravenous (IV) Therapy

Temperature Regulation
Venous Access Devices (VAD) Maintenance
Vomiting Management

Noncompliance

DEFINITION: Behavior of person and/or caregiver that fails to coincide with a health-promoting or therapeutic plan agreed on by the person (and/or family and/or community) and health care professional. In the presence of an agreed-on, health-promoting or therapeutic plan, person's or caregiver's behavior is fully or partially nonadherent and may lead to clinically ineffective or partially ineffective outcomes.

SUGGESTED NURSING INTERVENTIONS FOR PROBLEM RESOLUTION:

Coping Enhancement
Counseling
Culture Brokerage
Decision-Making Support
Discharge Planning
Elopement Precautions
Financial Resource Assistance
Health Education
Health System Guidance
Mutual Goal Setting
Patient Contracting
Patient Rights Protection

Self-Modification Assistance
Support System Enhancement
Teaching: Disease Process
Teaching: Individual
Teaching: Prescribed Activity/Exercise
Teaching: Prescribed Diet
Teaching: Prescribed Medication
Teaching: Procedure/Treatment
Teaching: Psychomotor Skill
Telephone Consultation
Values Clarification

ADDITIONAL OPTIONAL INTERVENTIONS:

Case Management
Home Maintenance Assistance
Medication Management
Prenatal Care
Referral
Smoking Cessation Assistance
Support Group

Teaching: Infant Nutrition
Teaching: Infant Safety
Teaching: Infant Stimulation
Teaching: Safe Sex
Teaching: Toddler Nutrition
Teaching: Toddler Safety
Truth Telling

Nutrition: Imbalanced, Less Than Body Requirements

DEFINITION: Intake of nutrients insufficient to meet metabolic needs.

SUGGESTED NURSING INTERVENTIONS FOR PROBLEM RESOLUTION:

Diet Staging
Eating Disorders Management
Fluid/Electrolyte Management
Fluid Management
Fluid Monitoring
Lactation Counseling
Nutrition Management
Nutrition Therapy

Nutritional Counseling
Nutritional Monitoring
Self-Care Assistance: Feeding
Swallowing Therapy
Vital Signs Monitoring
Weight Gain Assistance
Weight Management

ADDITIONAL OPTIONAL INTERVENTIONS:

Allergy Management
Bottle Feeding
Bowel Management
Dementia Management
Energy Management
Enteral Tube Feeding
Exercise Promotion
Feeding
Gastrointestinal Intubation
Hyperglycemia Management
Hypoglycemia Management
Infant Care

Intravenous (IV) Insertion
Intravenous (IV) Therapy
Medication Management
Mutual Goal Setting
Newborn Care
Phlebotomy: Venous Blood Sample
Positioning
Referral
Teaching: Individual
Teaching: Prescribed Diet
Total Parenteral Nutrition (TPN) Administration
Venous Access Devices (VAD) Maintenance

Nutrition: Imbalanced, More Than Body Requirements

DEFINITION: Intake of nutrients that exceeds metabolic needs.

SUGGESTED NURSING INTERVENTIONS FOR PROBLEM RESOLUTION:

Behavior Modification

Eating Disorders Management

Exercise Promotion

Fluid Management

Nutrition Management

Nutritional Counseling

Nutritional Monitoring

Weight Management

Weight Reduction Assistance

ADDITIONAL OPTIONAL INTERVENTIONS:

Anxiety Reduction

Behavior Management

Bottle Feeding

Coping Enhancement

Enteral Tube Feeding

Exercise Therapy: Ambulation

Feeding

Fluid Monitoring

Hyperglycemia Management

Hypoglycemia Management

Infant Care

Limit Setting

Mutual Goal Setting

Newborn Care

Nutrition Therapy

Patient Contracting

Referral

Self-Responsibility Facilitation

Skin Surveillance

Teaching: Individual

Teaching: Prescribed Diet

Nutrition: Imbalanced, Risk for More Than Body Requirements

DEFINITION: At risk for an intake of nutrients that exceeds metabolic needs.

SUGGESTED NURSING INTERVENTIONS FOR PROBLEM RESOLUTION:

Eating Disorders Management
Exercise Promotion
Nutrition Management
Nutrition Therapy

Nutritional Counseling
Nutritional Monitoring
Weight Management

ADDITIONAL OPTIONAL INTERVENTIONS:

Bottle Feeding
Enteral Tube Feeding
Infant Care
Mutual Goal Setting

Newborn Care
Teaching: Individual
Teaching: Prescribed Diet
Weight Gain Assistance

Oral Mucous Membrane, Impaired

DEFINITION: Disruptions of the lips and soft tissue of the oral cavity.

SUGGESTED NURSING INTERVENTIONS FOR PROBLEM RESOLUTION:

Nutrition Management
Oral Health Maintenance

Oral Health Promotion
Oral Health Restoration

ADDITIONAL OPTIONAL INTERVENTIONS:

Airway Insertion and Stabilization
Airway Suctioning
Artificial Airway Management
Diet Staging
Dying Care

Exercise Therapy: Joint Mobility
Medication Management
Pain Management
Wound Irrigation

Pain, Acute

DEFINITION: Unpleasant sensory and emotional experience arising from actual or potential tissue damage or described in terms of such damage (International Association for the Study of Pain); sudden or slow onset of any intensity from mild to severe with an anticipated or predictable end and a duration of less than 6 months.

SUGGESTED NURSING INTERVENTIONS FOR PROBLEM RESOLUTION:

Acupressure
Analgesic Administration
Analgesic Administration: Intraspinal
Anesthesia Administration
Anxiety Reduction
Cutaneous Stimulation
Environmental Management: Comfort
Flatulence Reduction
Heat/Cold Application
Intrapartal Care: High-Risk Delivery
Medication Administration

Medication Administration: Intramuscular (IM)
Medication Administration: Intravenous (IV)
Medication Administration: Oral
Medication Management
Medication Prescribing
Pain Management
Patient-Controlled Analgesia (PCA) Assistance
Rectal Prolapse Management
Sedation Management
Transcutaneous Electrical Nerve Stimulation (TENS)

ADDITIONAL OPTIONAL INTERVENTIONS:

Active Listening
Animal-Assisted Therapy
Autogenic Training
Bathing
Biofeedback
Body Mechanics Promotion
Bowel Management
Coping Enhancement
Distraction
Emotional Support
Energy Management
Environmental Management
Exercise Promotion
Exercise Promotion: Stretching
Exercise Therapy: Ambulation
Exercise Therapy: Balance
Exercise Therapy: Joint Mobility
Exercise Therapy: Muscle Control
Hope Instillation
Humor
Hypnosis

Lactation Suppression
Meditation Facilitation
Music Therapy
Oral Health Restoration
Oxygen Therapy
Positioning
Postanesthesia Care
Preparatory Sensory Information
Presence
Progressive Muscle Relaxation
Security Enhancement
Self-Hypnosis Facilitation
Simple Guided Imagery
Simple Massage
Simple Relaxation Therapy
Sleep Enhancement
Therapeutic Play
Therapeutic Touch
Touch
Vital Signs Monitoring

Pain, Chronic

DEFINITION: Unpleasant sensory and emotional experience arising from actual or potential tissue damage or described in terms of such damage (International Association for the Study of Pain); sudden or slow onset of any intensity from mild to severe, constant or recurring without an anticipated or predictable end and a duration of greater than 6 months.

SUGGESTED NURSING INTERVENTIONS FOR PROBLEM RESOLUTION:

Acupressure

Analgesic Administration

Analgesic Administration: Intraspinal

Cutaneous Stimulation

Heat/Cold Application

Medication Administration

Medication Management

Medication Prescribing

Pain Management

Patient-Controlled Analgesia (PCA) Assistance

Progressive Muscle Relaxation

Simple Massage

Transcutaneous Electrical Nerve Stimulation (TENS)

ADDITIONAL OPTIONAL INTERVENTIONS:

Active Listening

Autogenic Training

Biofeedback

Distraction

Environmental Management: Comfort

Exercise Promotion: Stretching

Exercise Therapy: Ambulation

Exercise Therapy: Joint Mobility

Exercise Therapy: Muscle Control

Humor

Hypnosis

Meditation Facilitation

Self-Hypnosis Facilitation

Simple Relaxation Therapy

Touch

Vital Signs Monitoring

Parental Role Conflict

DEFINITION: Parent experience of role confusion and conflict in response to crisis.

SUGGESTED NURSING INTERVENTIONS FOR PROBLEM RESOLUTION:

Abuse Protection Support: Child
Caregiver Support
Childbirth Preparation
Counseling
Crisis Intervention
Decision-Making Support
Family Integrity Promotion
Family Integrity Promotion: Childbearing
    Family
Family Presence Facilitation

Family Process Maintenance
Family Support
Family Therapy
Grief Work Facilitation: Perinatal Death
High-Risk Pregnancy Care
Parenting Promotion
Role Enhancement
Self-Esteem Enhancement
Socialization Enhancement

ADDITIONAL OPTIONAL INTERVENTIONS:

Environmental Management: Attachment
    Process
Health System Guidance
Limit Setting
Mutual Goal Setting

Respite Care
Trauma Therapy: Child
Values Clarification
Visitation Facilitation

Parent/Infant/Child Attachment, Risk for Impaired

DEFINITION: Disruption of the interactive process between parent/significant other and infant that fosters the development of a protective and nurturing reciprocal relationship.

SUGGESTED NURSING INTERVENTIONS FOR PROBLEM RESOLUTION:

Anxiety Reduction
Anticipatory Guidance
Attachment Promotion
Coping Enhancement
Developmental Enhancement: Child
Environmental Management
Environmental Management:
    Attachment Process
Normalization Promotion
Parent Education: Infant

Parenting Promotion
Role Enhancement
Self-Awareness Enhancement
Self-Esteem Enhancement
Self-Responsibility Facilitation
Socialization Enhancement
Substance Use Prevention
Substance Use Treatment
Support System Enhancement
Therapy Group

ADDITIONAL OPTIONAL INTERVENTIONS:

Behavior Management
Behavior Management: Overactivity/
    Inattention
Behavior Modification
Family Involvement Promotion
Family Mobilization
Family Process Maintenance
Family Support

Family Therapy
Parent Education: Childrearing Family
Sibling Support
Support Group
Teaching: Infant Nutrition
Teaching: Infant Safety
Teaching: Infant Stimulation
Trauma Therapy: Child

Parenting, Impaired

DEFINITION: Inability of the primary caretaker to create, maintain, or regain an environment that promotes the optimum growth and development of the child.

SUGGESTED NURSING INTERVENTIONS FOR PROBLEM RESOLUTION:

Abuse Protection Support: Child
Anticipatory Guidance
Anxiety Reduction
Attachment Promotion
Caregiver Support
Coping Enhancement
Counseling
Developmental Enhancement: Adolescent
Developmental Enhancement: Child
Environmental Management: Attachment
　　Process
Family Integrity Promotion

Family Support
Family Therapy
Guilt Work Facilitation
Mutual Goal Setting
Normalization Promotion
Parenting Promotion
Risk Identification: Childbearing Family
Role Enhancement
Security Enhancement
Self-Esteem Enhancement
Support Group
Teaching: Individual

ADDITIONAL OPTIONAL INTERVENTIONS:

Behavior Management: Overactivity/
　　Inattention
Childbirth Preparation
Family Integrity Promotion: Childbearing
　　Family
Family Involvement Promotion
Family Process Maintenance
Financial Resource Assistance
Health Education
Home Maintenance Assistance
Infant Care

Intrapartal Care
Newborn Care
Parent Education: Adolescent
Parent Education: Childrearing Family
Parent Education: Infant
Patient Contracting
Postpartal Care
Prenatal Care
Respite Care
Surveillance

Parenting, Risk for Impaired

DEFINITION: Risk for inability of the primary caretaker to create, maintain, or regain an environment that promotes the optimum growth and development of the child.

SUGGESTED NURSING INTERVENTIONS FOR PROBLEM RESOLUTION:

Abuse Protection Support: Child
Anticipatory Guidance
Attachment Promotion
Caregiver Support
Coping Enhancement
Developmental Enhancement: Adolescent
Developmental Enhancement: Child
Environmental Management:
   Attachment Process
Family Integrity Promotion

High-Risk Pregnancy Care
Normalization Promotion
Parenting Promotion
Resiliency Promotion
Role Enhancement
Self-Esteem Enhancement
Support System Enhancement
Sibling Support
Teaching: Sexuality

ADDITIONAL OPTIONAL INTERVENTIONS:

Childbirth Preparation
Energy Management
Family Integrity Promotion: Childbearing
   Family
Family Involvement Promotion
Family Process Maintenance
Family Therapy
Financial Resource Assistance
Health Education
Home Maintenance Assistance
Infant Care
Intrapartal Care

Newborn Care
Parent Education: Adolescent
Parent Education: Childrearing
   Family
Parent Education: Infant
Patient Contracting
Postpartal Care
Prenatal Care
Respite Care
Support Group
Surveillance

Perioperative Positioning Injury, Risk for

DEFINITION: At risk for injury as a result of the environmental conditions found in the perioperative setting.

SUGGESTED NURSING INTERVENTIONS FOR PROBLEM RESOLUTION:

Aspiration Precautions
Bleeding Reduction: Wound
Cerebral Perfusion Promotion
Circulatory Care: Arterial Insufficiency
Circulatory Care: Venous Insufficiency
Circulatory Precautions

Incision Site Care
Peripheral Sensation Management
Positioning: Intraoperative
Skin Surveillance
Surgical Precautions
Temperature Regulation: Intraoperative

ADDITIONAL OPTIONAL INTERVENTIONS:

Cast Care: Wet
Embolus Care: Peripheral
Embolus Care: Pulmonary

Embolus Precautions
Infection Control: Intraoperative
Pressure Management

Peripheral Neurovascular Dysfunction, Risk for

DEFINITION: At risk for disruption in circulation, sensation, or motion of an extremity.

SUGGESTED NURSING INTERVENTIONS FOR PROBLEM RESOLUTION:

Cardiac Care
Circulatory Care: Arterial Insufficiency
Circulatory Care: Venous Insufficiency
Circulatory Precautions
Exercise Therapy: Joint Mobility
Fluid Management

Lower Extremity Monitoring
Neurologic Monitoring
Peripheral Sensation Management
Pneumatic Tourniquet Precautions
Positioning: Neurologic
Skin Surveillance

ADDITIONAL OPTIONAL INTERVENTIONS:

Bed Rest Care
Bleeding Precautions
Body Mechanics Promotion
Cast Care: Maintenance
Cast Care: Wet
Cutaneous Stimulation
Embolus Care: Peripheral
Embolus Precautions
Exercise Promotion
Exercise Therapy: Ambulation
Heat/Cold Application

Pain Management
Physical Restraint
Positioning
Positioning: Wheelchair
Pressure Management
Pressure Ulcer Prevention
Splinting
Teaching: Prescribed Activity/Exercise
Traction/Immobilization Care
Transport
Vital Signs Monitoring

Personal Identity, Disturbed

DEFINITION: Inability to distinguish between self and nonself.

SUGGESTED NURSING INTERVENTIONS FOR PROBLEM RESOLUTION:

Anticipatory Guidance
Counseling
Decision-Making Support
Mutual Goal Setting
Self-Awareness Enhancement

Self-Esteem Enhancement
Self-Responsibility Facilitation
Sexual Counseling
Substance Use Prevention

ADDITIONAL OPTIONAL INTERVENTIONS:

Anxiety Reduction
Art Therapy
Assertiveness Training
Behavior Management: Self-Harm
Bibliotherapy
Calming Technique
Cognitive Restructuring
Complex Relationship Building
Coping Enhancement
Delirium Management
Delusion Management
Dementia Management
Developmental Enhancement: Adolescent

Developmental Enhancement: Child
Emotional Support
Hallucination Management
Hypnosis
Security Enhancement
Self-Care Assistance
Substance Use Treatment
Substance Use Treatment: Alcohol Withdrawal
Substance Use Treatment: Drug Withdrawal
Substance Use Treatment: Overdose
Therapy Group
Values Clarification

Poisoning, Risk for

DEFINITION: At accentuated risk of accidental exposure to, or ingestion of, drugs or dangerous products in doses sufficient to cause poisoning.

SUGGESTED NURSING INTERVENTIONS FOR PROBLEM RESOLUTION:

Environmental Management: Safety
First Aid
Health Education
Medication Management

Surveillance
Surveillance: Safety
Vital Signs Monitoring

ADDITIONAL OPTIONAL INTERVENTIONS:

Bioterrorism Preparedness
Chemotherapy Management

Environmental Risk Protection
Fluid/Electrolyte Management

Post-Trauma Syndrome

DEFINITION: Sustained maladaptive response to a traumatic, overwhelming event.

SUGGESTED NURSING INTERVENTIONS FOR PROBLEM RESOLUTION:

Anger Control Assistance
Anxiety Reduction
Coping Enhancement
Counseling
Forgiveness Facilitation

Mood Management
Simple Relaxation Therapy
Substance Use Prevention
Support System Enhancement
Trauma Therapy: Child

ADDITIONAL OPTIONAL INTERVENTIONS:

Environmental Management
Mutual Goal Setting
Progressive Muscle Relaxation
Reality Orientation

Reminiscence Therapy
Socialization Enhancement
Suicide Prevention
Support Group

Post-Trauma Syndrome, Risk for

DEFINITION: A risk for sustained maladaptive response to traumatic, overwhelming event.

SUGGESTED NURSING INTERVENTIONS FOR PROBLEM RESOLUTION:

Active Listening
Anxiety Reduction
Coping Enhancement
Counseling
Crisis Intervention
Decision-Making Support
Forgiveness Facilitation
Guilt Work Facilitation

Hope Instillation
Presence
Simple Relaxation Therapy
Spiritual Support
Support Group
Support System Enhancement
Telephone Follow-up
Trauma Therapy: Child

ADDITIONAL OPTIONAL INTERVENTIONS:

Animal-Assisted Therapy
Environmental Management
Family Involvement
Family Mobilization
Mutual Goal Setting

Progressive Muscle Relaxation
Reality Orientation
Reminiscence Therapy
Socialization Enhancement
Suicide Prevention

Powerlessness

DEFINITION: Perception that one's own action will not significantly affect an outcome; a perceived lack of control over a current situation or immediate happening.

SUGGESTED NURSING INTERVENTIONS FOR PROBLEM RESOLUTION:

Cognitive Restructuring
Complex Relationship Building
Crisis Intervention
Decision-Making Support
Emotional Support
Health System Guidance
Learning Facilitation

Mutual Goal Setting
Presence
Relocation Stress Reduction
Self-Esteem Enhancement
Self-Responsibility Facilitation
Values Clarification

ADDITIONAL OPTIONAL INTERVENTIONS:

Abuse Protection Support
Activity Therapy
Animal-Assisted Therapy
Anticipatory Guidance
Anxiety Reduction
Art Therapy
Assertiveness Training
Environmental Management
Family Presence Facilitation

Meditation Facilitation
Patient Contracting
Progressive Muscle Relaxation
Rape-Trauma Treatment
Reminiscence Therapy
Self-Care Assistance
Support Group
Teaching: Individual
Weight Management

Powerlessness, Risk for

DEFINITION: At risk for perceived lack of control over a situation and/or one's ability to significantly affect an outcome

SUGGESTED NURSING INTERVENTIONS FOR PROBLEM RESOLUTION:

Assertiveness Training
Cognitive Restructuring
Complex Relationship Building
Crisis Intervention
Decision-Making Support
Emotional Support
Health System Guidance

Learning Facilitation
Mutual Goal Setting
Presence
Relocation Stress Reduction
Self-Esteem Enhancement
Self-Responsibility Facilitation
Values Clarification

ADDITIONAL OPTIONAL INTERVENTIONS:

Abuse Protection Support
Activity Therapy
Animal-Assisted Therapy
Anticipatory Guidance
Anxiety Reduction
Art Therapy

Bioterrorism Preparedness
Environmental Management
Family Presence Facilitation
Meditation Facilitation
Rape-Trauma Treatment

Protection, Ineffective

DEFINITION: Decrease in the ability to guard self from internal or external threats such as illness or injury.

SUGGESTED NURSING INTERVENTIONS FOR PROBLEM RESOLUTION:

Bleeding Precautions
Chemotherapy Management
Coping Enhancement
Electronic Fetal Monitoring: Antepartum
Electronic Fetal Monitoring: Intrapartum
Environmental Management: Violence
   Prevention
Emergency Care
Infection Control
Infection Protection
Intrapartal Care: High-Risk Delivery
Labor Induction

Latex Precautions
Phototherapy: Neonate
Postanesthesia Care
Risk Identification
Self-Care Assistance
Surgical Precautions
Surveillance
Surveillance: Late Pregnancy
Surveillance: Remote Electronic
Surveillance: Safety
Ultrasonography: Limited Obstetric

ADDITIONAL OPTIONAL INTERVENTIONS:

Autotransfusion
Bioterrorism Preparedness
Dementia Management
Energy Management
Nutrition Management
Nutrition Therapy
Nutritional Counseling
Positioning
Pressure Management

Pressure Ulcer Prevention
Pruritus Management
Seclusion
Sleep Enhancement
Substance Use Treatment
Support Group
Teaching: Individual
Wound Care

Rape-Trauma Syndrome

DEFINITION: Sustained maladaptive response to a forced, violent sexual penetration against the victim's will and consent.

SUGGESTED NURSING INTERVENTIONS FOR PROBLEM RESOLUTION:

Anger Control Assistance
Anxiety Reduction
Crisis Intervention
Counseling
Calming Technique
Decision-Making Support
Emotional Support
Hope Instillation
Presence
Rape-Trauma Treatment

Referral
Self-Esteem Enhancement
Sexual Counseling
Specimen Management
Support Group
Support System Enhancement
Trauma Therapy: Child
Vital Signs Monitoring
Wound Care

ADDITIONAL OPTIONAL INTERVENTIONS:

Anticipatory Guidance
Art Therapy
Coping Enhancement
Family Planning: Contraception
Grief Work Facilitation

Pain Management
Security Enhancement
Spiritual Support
Substance Use Prevention
Therapeutic Play

Rape-Trauma Syndrome: Compound Reaction

DEFINITION: Forced, violent sexual penetration against the victim's will and consent. The trauma syndrome that develops from this attack or attempted attack includes an acute phase of disorganization of the victim's life-style and a long-term process or reorganization of life-style.

SUGGESTED NURSING INTERVENTIONS FOR PROBLEM RESOLUTION:

Anger Control Assistance
Anticipatory Guidance
Anxiety Reduction
Calming Technique
Counseling
Crisis Intervention
Decision-Making Support
Emotional Support
Forgiveness Facilitation
Hope Instillation
Mood Management

Pain Management
Presence
Rape-Trauma Treatment
Referral
Sexual Counseling
Substance Use Prevention
Support Group
Support System Enhancement
Trauma Therapy: Child
Vital Signs Monitoring

ADDITIONAL OPTIONAL INTERVENTIONS:

Abuse Protection Support
Art Therapy
Coping Enhancement

Grief Work Facilitation
Spiritual Support
Therapeutic Play

Rape-Trauma Syndrome: Silent Reaction

DEFINITION: Forced, violent sexual penetration against the victim's will and consent. The trauma syndrome that develops from this attack or attempted attack includes an acute phase of disorganization of the victim's life-style and a long-term process of reorganization of life-style.

SUGGESTED NURSING INTERVENTIONS FOR PROBLEM RESOLUTION:

Anger Control Assistance
Anticipatory Guidance
Anxiety Reduction
Art Therapy
Crisis Intervention
Counseling
Calming Technique
Decision-Making Support
Emotional Support
Hope Instillation

Presence
Rape-Trauma Treatment
Referral
Security Enhancement
Sexual Counseling
Support Group
Support System Enhancement
Therapy Group
Trauma Therapy: Child

ADDITIONAL OPTIONAL INTERVENTIONS:

Abuse Protection Support
Coping Enhancement
Grief Work Facilitation

Spiritual Support
Therapeutic Play

Relocation Stress Syndrome

DEFINITION: Physiological and/or psychosocial disturbance as a result of transfer from one environment to another.

SUGGESTED NURSING INTERVENTIONS FOR PROBLEM RESOLUTION:

Active Listening
Anger Control Assistance
Coping Enhancement
Counseling
Delirium Management
Discharge Planning
Emotional Support
Family Involvement Promotion
Family Mobilization
Family Support
Hope Instillation

Mutual Goal Setting
Patient Rights Protection
Relocation Stress Reduction
Security Enhancement
Self-Responsibility Facilitation
Sleep Enhancement
Socialization Enhancement
Spiritual Support
Support System Enhancement
Visitation Facilitation

ADDITIONAL OPTIONAL INTERVENTIONS:

Activity Therapy
Admission Care
Animal-Assisted Therapy
Anticipatory Guidance
Anxiety Reduction
Art Therapy
Dementia Management
Humor

Music Therapy
Nutritional Monitoring
Nutrition Therapy
Presence
Recreation Therapy
Reminiscence Therapy
Risk Identification
Touch

Relocation Stress Syndrome, Risk for

DEFINITION: At risk for physiological and/or psychosocial disturbance following transfer from one environment to another.

SUGGESTED NURSING INTERVENTIONS FOR PROBLEM RESOLUTION:

Active Listening
Anger Control Assistance
Coping Enhancement
Counseling
Delirium Management
Discharge Planning
Emotional Support
Family Involvement Promotion
Family Mobilization
Family Support
Hope Instillation

Mutual Goal Setting
Patient Rights Protection
Relocation Stress Reduction
Security Enhancement
Self-Responsibility Facilitation
Sleep Enhancement
Socialization Enhancement
Spiritual Support
Support System Enhancement
Visitation Facilitation

ADDITIONAL OPTIONAL INTERVENTIONS:

Activity Therapy
Admission Care
Animal-Assisted Therapy
Anticipatory Guidance
Anxiety Reduction
Art Therapy
Dementia Management
Humor

Music Therapy
Nutritional Monitoring
Nutrition Therapy
Presence
Recreation Therapy
Reminiscence Therapy
Risk Identification
Touch

Role Performance, Ineffective

DEFINITION: Patterns of behavior and self-expression that do not match the environmental context, norms, and expectations.

SUGGESTED NURSING INTERVENTIONS FOR PROBLEM RESOLUTION:

Caregiver Support
Complex Relationship Building
Normalization Promotion
Parent Education: Adolescent
Parent Education: Childrearing Family

Parent Education: Infant Care
Parenting Promotion
Role Enhancement
Self-Awareness Enhancement
Self-Esteem Enhancement

ADDITIONAL OPTIONAL INTERVENTIONS:

Body Image Enhancement
Coping Enhancement
Counseling
Family Therapy
Labor Suppression
Mood Management

Mutual Goal Setting
Reproductive Technology Management
Support Group
Teaching: Individual
Teaching: Sexuality
Values Clarification

Self Care Deficit: Bathing/Hygiene

Definition: Impaired ability to perform or complete bathing/hygiene activities for oneself.

SUGGESTED NURSING INTERVENTIONS FOR PROBLEM RESOLUTION:

Bathing
Contact Lens Care
Dementia Management: Bathing
Ear Care
Eye Care
Foot Care
Hair Care

Infant Care
Nail Care
Oral Health Maintenance
Perineal Care
Self-Care Assistance: Bathing/Hygiene
Self-Responsibility Facilitation
Teaching: Individual

ADDITIONAL OPTIONAL INTERVENTIONS:

Behavior Management
Behavior Modification
Body Image Enhancement
Decision-Making Support
Discharge Planning
Emotional Support
Energy Management
Exercise Promotion
Exercise Promotion: Stretching
Exercise Therapy: Ambulation
Exercise Therapy: Balance

Exercise Therapy: Joint Mobility
Exercise Therapy: Muscle Control
Fall Prevention
Mutual Goal Setting
Patient Contracting
Positioning
Self-Care Assistance
Self-Care Assistance: IADL
Self-Esteem Enhancement
Surveillance: Safety

Self Care Deficit: Dressing/Grooming

DEFINITION: Impaired ability to perform or complete dressing and grooming activities for self.

SUGGESTED NURSING INTERVENTIONS FOR PROBLEM RESOLUTION:

Dressing

Energy Management

Environmental Management

Exercise Promotion

Hair Care

Nail Care

Self-Care Assistance: Dressing/Grooming

ADDITIONAL OPTIONAL INTERVENTIONS:

Body Image Enhancement

Discharge Planning

Exercise Promotion: Stretching

Exercise Therapy: Ambulation

Exercise Therapy: Balance

Exercise Therapy: Joint Mobility

Exercise Therapy: Muscle Control

Pain Management

Patient Contracting

Self-Care Assistance

Self-Care Assistance: IADL

Skin Surveillance

Teaching: Individual

Self Care Deficit: Feeding

DEFINITION: Impaired ability to perform or complete feeding activities.

SUGGESTED NURSING INTERVENTIONS FOR PROBLEM RESOLUTION:

Bottle Feeding

Environmental Management

Feeding

Nutrition Management

Oral Health Maintenance

Positioning

Self-Care Assistance: Feeding

Swallowing Therapy

ADDITIONAL OPTIONAL INTERVENTIONS:

Communication Enhancement: Hearing Deficit

Communication Enhancement: Visual Deficit

Discharge Planning

Pain Management

Patient Contracting

Self-Care Assistance

Self-Care Assistance: IADL

Socialization Enhancement

Teaching: Individual

Self Care Deficit: Toileting

DEFINITION: Impaired ability to perform or complete own toileting activities.

SUGGESTED NURSING INTERVENTIONS FOR PROBLEM RESOLUTION:

Bowel Incontinence Care: Encopresis
Bowel Management
Environmental Management
Fluid Management
Medication Management

Nutrition Management
Patient Contracting
Self-Care Assistance: Toileting
Teaching: Individual
Urinary Elimination Management

ADDITIONAL OPTIONAL INTERVENTIONS:

Bathing
Bowel Irrigation
Constipation/Impaction Management
Discharge Planning
Exercise Promotion
Exercise Promotion: Stretching
Exercise Therapy: Ambulation
Exercise Therapy: Balance
Exercise Therapy: Joint Mobility

Exercise Therapy: Muscle Control
Fluid Monitoring
Ostomy Care
Pain Management
Perineal Care
Self-Care Assistance
Self-Care Assistance: IADL
Skin Surveillance

Self-Esteem, Chronic Low

DEFINITION: Long-standing negative self evaluation/feelings about self or self capabilities.

SUGGESTED NURSING INTERVENTIONS FOR PROBLEM RESOLUTION:

Body Image Enhancement
Cognitive Restructuring
Counseling
Emotional Support

Self-Esteem Enhancement
Socialization Enhancement
Support System Enhancement

ADDITIONAL OPTIONAL INTERVENTIONS:

Active Listening
Anxiety Reduction
Complex Relationship Building
Coping Enhancement
Crisis Intervention
Decision-Making Support
Grief Work Facilitation
Mutual Goal Setting
Pain Management

Presence
Role Enhancement
Suicide Prevention
Support Group
Surveillance: Safety
Therapeutic Touch
Values Clarification
Wound Care

Self-Esteem, Situational Low

DEFINITION: Development of a negative perception of self-worth in response to a current situation (specify).

SUGGESTED NURSING INTERVENTIONS FOR PROBLEM RESOLUTION:

Assertiveness Training
Body Image Enhancement
Coping Enhancement
Decision-Making Support
Grief Work Facilitation

Mood Management
Role Enhancement
Self-Esteem Enhancement
Socialization Enhancement

ADDITIONAL OPTIONAL INTERVENTIONS:

Abuse Protection Support
Animal-Assisted Therapy
Art Therapy
Bowel Incontinence Care: Encopresis
Complex Relationship Building
Counseling

Emotional Support
Guilt Work Facilitation
Hormone Replacement Therapy
Support System Enhancement
Urinary Incontinence Care: Enuresis

Self-Esteem, Situational Low, Risk for

DEFINITION: At risk for developing negative perception of self-worth in response to a current situation (specify).

SUGGESTED NURSING INTERVENTIONS FOR PROBLEM RESOLUTION:

Body Image Enhancement
Childbirth Preparation
Counseling
Emotional Support
Mood Management
Reproductive Technology Management
Self-Esteem Enhancement
Substance Use Prevention

Substance Use Treatment
Substance Use Treatment: Alcohol Withdrawal
Substance Use Treatment: Drug Withdrawal
Substance Use Treatment: Overdose
Support Group
Therapy Group
Weight Management

ADDITIONAL OPTIONAL INTERVENTIONS:

Abuse Protection Support
Animal-Assisted Therapy
Art Therapy
Bowel Incontinence Care: Encopresis
Cognitive Restructuring
Complex Relationship Building
Decision-Making Support
Developmental Enhancement: Adolescent

Developmental Enhancement: Child
Hormone Replacement Therapy
Lactation Counseling
Mutual Goal Setting
Prenatal Care
Reminiscence Therapy
Urinary Incontinence Care: Enuresis

Self-Mutilation

DEFINITION: Deliberate self-injurious behavior causing tissue damage with the intent of causing nonfatal injury to attain relief of tension.

SUGGESTED NURSING INTERVENTIONS FOR PROBLEM RESOLUTION:

Active Listening
Activity Therapy
Anger Control Assistance
Area Restriction
Behavior Management
Behavior Management: Self-Harm
Behavior Modification
Body Image Enhancement
Calming Technique
Chemical Restraint
Counseling
Environmental Management: Safety
Environmental Management: Violence
   Prevention
Impulse Control Training

Limit Setting
Mood Management
Mutual Goal Setting
Physical Restraint
Presence
Risk Identification
Seclusion
Self-Awareness Enhancement
Self-Esteem Enhancement
Self-Modification Assistance
Self-Responsibility Facilitation
Socialization Enhancement
Suicide Prevention
Surveillance: Safety
Wound Care

ADDITIONAL OPTIONAL INTERVENTIONS:

Animal Assisted Therapy
Anticipatory Guidance
Anxiety Reduction
Art Therapy
Assertiveness Training
Bibliotherapy
Cognitive Restructuring
Emotional Support

Family Therapy
Grief Work Facilitation
Hallucination Management
Medication Administration
Milieu Therapy
Patient Contracting
Security Enhancement
Therapy Group

Self-Mutilation, Risk for

DEFINITION: At risk for deliberate self-injurious behavior causing tissue damage with the intent of causing nonfatal injury to attain relief of tension.

SUGGESTED NURSING INTERVENTIONS FOR PROBLEM RESOLUTION:

Active Listening
Activity Therapy
Anger Control Assistance
Area Restriction
Behavior Management
Behavior Management: Self-Harm
Behavior Modification
Body Image Enhancement
Calming Technique
Counseling
Environmental Management: Safety
Environmental Management: Violence
    Prevention
Limit Setting

Mood Management
Mutual Goal Setting
Physical Restraint
Presence
Risk Identification
Self-Awareness Enhancement
Self-Esteem Enhancement
Self-Modification Assistance
Self-Responsibility Facilitation
Socialization Enhancement
Suicide Prevention
Surveillance: Safety

ADDITIONAL OPTIONAL INTERVENTIONS:

Animal-Assisted Therapy
Anticipatory Guidance
Anxiety Reduction
Art Therapy
Assertiveness Training
Bibliotherapy
Cognitive Restructuring
Emotional Support
Family Therapy

Grief Work Facilitation
Hallucination Management
Impulse Control Training
Medication Administration
Milieu Therapy
Patient Contracting
Security Enhancement
Therapy Group

Sensory/Perceptual: Auditory, Disturbed

DEFINITION: Change in the amount or patterning of incoming stimuli accompanied by a diminished, exaggerated, distorted, or impaired response to such stimuli.

SUGGESTED NURSING INTERVENTIONS FOR PROBLEM RESOLUTION:

Activity Therapy
Cerebral Perfusion Promotion
Cognitive Restructuring
Cognitive Stimulation
Communication Enhancement: Hearing
   Deficit
Communication Enhancement: Speech Deficit
Delusion Management
Dementia Management

Emotional Support
Environmental Management
Exercise Therapy: Balance
Fall Prevention
Hallucination Management
Reality Orientation
Sleep Enhancement
Surveillance: Safety

ADDITIONAL OPTIONAL INTERVENTIONS:

Developmental Enhancement: Child
Ear Care
Exercise Therapy: Ambulation
Feeding
Fluid Management
Fluid Monitoring

Intracranial Pressure (ICP) Monitoring
Medication Management
Neurologic Monitoring
Nutrition Management
Positioning
Self-Esteem Enhancement

Sensory/Perceptual: Gustatory, Disturbed

DEFINITION: Change in the amount or patterning of incoming stimuli accompanied by a diminished, exaggerated, distorted, or impaired response to such stimuli.

SUGGESTED NURSING INTERVENTIONS FOR PROBLEM RESOLUTION:

Cerebral Perfusion Promotion
Delusion Management
Dementia Management
Electrolyte Monitoring
Environmental Management
Feeding
Fluid Management

Fluid Monitoring
Nausea Management
Nutrition Management
Reality Orientation
Sleep Enhancement
Surveillance: Safety
Vomiting Management

ADDITIONAL OPTIONAL INTERVENTIONS:

Developmental Enhancement: Child
Exercise Therapy: Muscle Control
Medication Management
Neurologic Monitoring
Self-Esteem Enhancement

Swallowing Therapy
Teaching: Infant Nutrition
Teaching: Toddler Nutrition
Weight Gain Assistance

Sensory/Perceptual: Kinesthetic, Disturbed

DEFINITION: Change in the amount or patterning of incoming stimuli accompanied by a diminished, exaggerated, distorted, or impaired response to such stimuli.

SUGGESTED NURSING INTERVENTIONS FOR PROBLEM RESOLUTION:

Activity Therapy
Body Mechanics Promotion
Cerebral Perfusion Promotion
Delusion Management
Dementia Management
Environmental Management
Exercise Promotion
Exercise Promotion: Strength Training

Exercise Therapy: Ambulation
Exercise Therapy: Balance
Exercise Therapy: Muscle Control
Positioning
Reality Orientation
Sleep Enhancement
Surveillance: Safety

ADDITIONAL OPTIONAL INTERVENTIONS:

Cognitive Restructuring
Cognitive Stimulation
Developmental Enhancement: Child
Exercise Promotion: Stretching
Feeding
Fluid Management

Fluid Monitoring
Neurologic Monitoring
Nutrition Management
Medication Management
Self-Esteem Enhancement

Sensory/Perceptual: Olfactory, Disturbed

DEFINITION: Change in the amount or patterning of incoming stimuli accompanied by a diminished, exaggerated, distorted, or impaired response to such stimuli.

SUGGESTED NURSING INTERVENTIONS FOR PROBLEM RESOLUTION:

Cerebral Perfusion Promotion
Delusion Management
Dementia Management
Environmental Management
Feeding

Nutrition Management
Nausea Management
Reality Orientation
Weight Management

ADDITIONAL OPTIONAL INTERVENTIONS:

Developmental Enhancement: Child
Fluid Management
Fluid Monitoring
Hallucination Management
Medication Management

Neurologic Monitoring
Self-Esteem Enhancement
Sleep Enhancement
Surveillance: Safety
Vomiting Management

Sensory/Perceptual: Tactile, Disturbed

DEFINITION: Change in the amount or patterning of incoming stimuli accompanied by a diminished, exaggerated, distorted, or impaired response to such stimuli.

SUGGESTED NURSING INTERVENTIONS FOR PROBLEM RESOLUTION:

Activity Therapy
Cerebral Perfusion Promotion
Delusion Management
Dementia Management
Environmental Management
Environmental Management: Attachment
  Process
Exercise Therapy: Ambulation
Exercise Therapy: Balance
Feeding

Lower Extremity Monitoring
Peripheral Sensation Management
Positioning
Pressure Management
Reality Orientation
Sleep Enhancement
Surveillance: Safety
Teaching: Foot Care
Touch

ADDITIONAL OPTIONAL INTERVENTIONS:

Cerebral Edema Management
Developmental Enhancement: Child
Fluid Management
Fluid Monitoring

Medication Management
Neurologic Monitoring
Nutrition Management
Self-Esteem Enhancement

Sensory/Perceptual: Visual, Disturbed

DEFINITION: Change in the amount or patterning of incoming stimuli accompanied by a diminished, exaggerated, distorted, or impaired response to such stimuli.

SUGGESTED NURSING INTERVENTIONS FOR PROBLEM RESOLUTION:

Activity Therapy
Cerebral Perfusion Promotion
Cognitive Restructuring
Cognitive Stimulation
Communication Enhancement: Visual Deficit
Delusion Management
Dementia Management
Emotional Support

Environmental Management
Exercise Therapy: Balance
Fall Prevention
Feeding
Hallucination Management
Reality Orientation
Sleep Enhancement
Surveillance: Safety

ADDITIONAL OPTIONAL INTERVENTIONS:

Cerebral Edema Management
Contact Lens Care
Developmental Enhancement: Child
Eye Care
Exercise Therapy: Ambulation
Fluid Management
Fluid Monitoring

Intracranial Pressure (ICP) Monitoring
Medication Management
Neurologic Monitoring
Nutrition Management
Positioning
Self-Esteem Enhancement

Sexual Dysfunction

DEFINITION: Change in sexual function that is viewed as unsatisfying, unrewarding, inadequate.

SUGGESTED NURSING INTERVENTIONS FOR PROBLEM RESOLUTION:

Anxiety Reduction
Behavior Management: Sexual
Childbirth Preparation
Prenatal Care
Reproductive Technology Management

Role Enhancement
Self-Awareness Enhancement
Self-Esteem Enhancement
Sexual Counseling
Teaching: Sexuality

ADDITIONAL OPTIONAL INTERVENTIONS:

Abuse Protection Support
Circulatory Care: Arterial Insufficiency
Counseling
Decision-Making Support
Energy Management
Family Planning: Contraception
Family Planning: Infertility
Family Process Maintenance
Fertility Preservation
Hormone Replacement Therapy

Premenstrual Syndrome Management
Medication Management
Pain Management
Simple Relaxation Therapy
Substance Use Treatment
Substance Use Treatment: Alcohol Withdrawal
Teaching: Individual
Teaching: Safe Sex
Values Clarification

Sexuality Patterns, Ineffective

DEFINITION: Expressions of concern regarding own sexuality.

SUGGESTED NURSING INTERVENTIONS FOR PROBLEM RESOLUTION:

Anticipatory Guidance
Anxiety Reduction
Body Image Enhancement
Coping Enhancement
Counseling
Family Planning: Contraception
Family Planning: Infertility

Fertility Preservation
Reproductive Technology Management
Self-Awareness Enhancement
Sexual Counseling
Teaching: Safe Sex
Teaching: Sexuality

ADDITIONAL OPTIONAL INTERVENTIONS:

Behavior Management: Sexual
Decision-Making Support
Hormone Replacement Therapy
Premenstrual Syndrome Management

Postpartal Care
Self-Esteem Enhancement
Support Group
Support System Enhancement

Skin Integrity, Impaired

DEFINITION: Altered epidermis and/or dermis.

SUGGESTED NURSING INTERVENTIONS FOR PROBLEM RESOLUTION:

Amputation Care
Bathing
Bleeding Reduction
Bleeding Reduction: Wound
Cast Care: Maintenance
Cast Care: Wet
Circulatory Precautions
Electrolyte Monitoring
Exercise Promotion
Fluid/Electrolyte Management
Foot Care
Incision Site Care
Latex Precautions
Lower Extremity Monitoring
Medication Administration: Skin
Medication Management
Ostomy Care

Perineal Care
Positioning
Pressure Management
Pressure Ulcer Care
Pressure Ulcer Prevention
Prosthesis Care
Skin Care: Donor Site
Skin Care: Graft Site
Skin Care: Topical Treatments
Skin Surveillance
Splinting
Suturing
Teaching: Foot Care
Traction/Immobilization Care
Wound Care
Wound Care: Closed Drainage
Wound Irrigation

ADDITIONAL OPTIONAL INTERVENTIONS:

Bed Rest Care
Cutaneous Stimulation
Exercise Promotion: Stretching
Exercise Therapy: Ambulation
Exercise Therapy: Balance
Exercise Therapy: Joint Mobility
Exercise Therapy: Muscle Control
Infection Control
Infection Protection
Leech Therapy

Nutrition Management
Nutrition Therapy
Peripherally Inserted Central (PIC)
    Catheter Care
Surveillance
Total Parenteral Nutrition (TPN) Administration
Transcutaneous Electrical Nerve Stimulation
    (TENS)
Vital Signs Monitoring

Skin Integrity, Risk for Impaired

DEFINITION: At risk for skin being adversely altered.

SUGGESTED NURSING INTERVENTIONS FOR PROBLEM RESOLUTION:

Amputation Care
Cast Care: Maintenance
Cast Care: Wet
Circulatory Precautions
Exercise Promotion
Exercise Promotion: Strength Training
Exercise Therapy: Ambulation
Exercise Therapy: Balance
Exercise Therapy: Joint Mobility
Exercise Therapy: Muscle Control
Foot Care
Incision Site Care
Infection Control
Infection Protection
Lactation Counseling
Latex Precautions

Lower Extremity Monitoring
Medication Administration: Skin
Ostomy Care
Positioning
Positioning: Intraoperative
Pressure Management
Pressure Ulcer Prevention
Skin Care: Topical Treatments
Skin Surveillance
Splinting
Surveillance
Teaching: Foot Care
Traction/Immobilization Care
Tube Care: Umbilical Line
Wound Care

ADDITIONAL OPTIONAL INTERVENTIONS:

Bathing
Bed Rest Care
Bleeding Precautions
Bowel Incontinence Care
Electrolyte Monitoring
Exercise Promotion: Stretching
Fluid/Electrolyte Management
Medication Management
Nail Care

Nutrition Management
Nutrition Therapy
Perineal Care
Pneumatic Tourniquet Precautions
Rectal Prolapse Management
Vital Signs Monitoring
Total Parenteral Nutrition (TPN) Administration
Transcutaneous Electrical Nerve
    Stimulation (TENS)

Sleep Deprivation

DEFINITION: Prolonged periods of time without sleep (sustained natural, periodic suspension of relative consciousness).

SUGGESTED NURSING INTERVENTIONS FOR PROBLEM RESOLUTION:

Anxiety Reduction
Coping Enhancement
Dementia Management
Energy Management
Environmental Management: Comfort
Medication Management
Meditation Facilitation

Pain Management
Phototherapy: Mood Sleep Regulation
Progressive Muscle Relaxation
Simple Guided Imagery
Sleep Enhancement
Surveillance: Safety

ADDITIONAL OPTIONAL INTERVENTIONS:

Animal-Assisted Therapy
Art Therapy
Music Therapy
Nausea Management
Reminiscence Therapy

Simple Massage
Sustenance Support
Urinary Incontinence Care: Enuresis
Vomiting Management

Sleep Pattern, Disturbed

DEFINITION: Time-limited disruption of sleep (natural, periodic suspension of consciousness) amount and quality.

SUGGESTED NURSING INTERVENTIONS FOR PROBLEM RESOLUTION:

Dementia Management
Environmental Management
Environmental Management: Comfort
Hormone Replacement Therapy
Medication Administration
Medication Management

Medication Prescribing
Phototherapy: Mood/Sleep Regulation
Security Enhancement
Simple Relaxation Therapy
Sleep Enhancement
Touch

ADDITIONAL OPTIONAL INTERVENTIONS:

Anxiety Reduction
Autogenic Training
Bathing
Calming Technique
Coping Enhancement
Energy Management
Exercise Promotion
Exercise Therapy: Ambulation
Kangaroo Care

Meditation Facilitation
Music Therapy
Nutrition Management
Pain Management
Positioning
Progressive Muscle Relaxation
Self-Care Assistance: Toileting
Simple Massage
Urinary Incontinence Care: Enuresis

Social Interaction, Impaired

DEFINITION: Insufficient or excessive quantity or ineffective quality of social exchange.

SUGGESTED NURSING INTERVENTIONS FOR PROBLEM RESOLUTION:

Behavior Management: Overactivity/
    Inattention
Behavior Management: Sexual
Behavior Modification: Social Skills
Complex Relationship Building
Dementia Management
Normalization Promotion
Reminiscence Therapy
Resiliency Promotion

Self-Awareness Enhancement
Self-Esteem Enhancement
Socialization Enhancement
Substance Use Treatment
Support Group
Support System Enhancement
Therapy Group
Values Clarification

ADDITIONAL OPTIONAL INTERVENTIONS:

Abuse Protection Support
Active Listening
Anger Control Assistance
Animal-Assisted Therapy
Anxiety Reduction
Assertiveness Training
Cognitive Stimulation
Coping Enhancement
Family Support
Family Therapy
Humor

Mutual Goal Setting
Pass Facilitation
Recreation Therapy
Relocation Stress Reduction
Substance Use Treatment: Alcohol Withdrawal
Substance Use Treatment: Drug Withdrawal
Substance Use Treatment: Overdose
Suicide Prevention
Teaching: Individual
Therapeutic Play
Truth Telling

Social Isolation

DEFINITION: Aloneness experienced by the individual and perceived as imposed by others and as a negative or threatening state.

SUGGESTED NURSING INTERVENTIONS FOR PROBLEM RESOLUTION:

Abuse Protection Support: Child
Abuse Protection Support: Domestic Partner
Abuse Protection Support: Elder
Activity Therapy
Complex Relationship Building
Counseling
Emotional Support
Environmental Management
Hope Instillation

Normalization Promotion
Presence
Relocation Stress Reduction
Self-Awareness Enhancement
Self-Esteem Enhancement
Socialization Enhancement
Support System Enhancement
Visitation Facilitation

ADDITIONAL OPTIONAL INTERVENTIONS:

Animal-Assisted Therapy
Art Therapy
Bowel Incontinence Care: Encopresis
Exercise Promotion
Family Therapy
Grief Work Facilitation
Mood Management

Mutual Goal Setting
Pass Facilitation
Reminiscence Therapy
Support Group
Therapy Group
Urinary Elimination Management
Weight Management

Sorrow: Chronic

DEFINITION: Cyclical, recurring, and potentially progressive pattern of pervasive sadness that is experienced (by a parent, caregiver, individual with chronic illness or disability) in response to continual loss, throughout the trajectory of an illness or disability.

SUGGESTED NURSING INTERVENTIONS FOR PROBLEM RESOLUTION:

Coping Enhancement
Counseling
Decision-Making Support
Emotional Support
Energy Management
Genetic Counseling

Grief Work Facilitation
Hope Instillation
Mood Management
Socialization Enhancement
Spiritual Support
Support Group

ADDITIONAL OPTIONAL INTERVENTIONS:

Activity Therapy
Anger Control Assistance
Animal-Assisted Therapy
Dying Care
Exercise Promotion

Forgiveness Facilitation
Humor
Music Therapy
Sleep Enhancement
Substance Use Prevention

Spiritual Distress

DEFINITION: Disruption in the life principle that pervades a person's entire being and that integrates and transcends one's biological and psychosocial nature.

SUGGESTED NURSING INTERVENTIONS FOR PROBLEM RESOLUTION:

Anticipatory Guidance
Coping Enhancement
Counseling
Crisis Intervention
Decision-Making Support
Dying Care
Emotional Support
Forgiveness Facilitation
Grief Work Facilitation

Guilt Work Facilitation
Hope Instillation
Presence
Resiliency Promotion
Spiritual Growth Facilitation
Spiritual Support
Support Group
Values Clarification

ADDITIONAL OPTIONAL INTERVENTIONS:

Abuse Protection Support: Religious
Active Listening
Activity Therapy
Animal-Assisted Therapy
Anxiety Reduction
Art Therapy
Caregiver Support
Distraction
Family Planning: Unplanned Pregnancy
Family Support

Mood Management
Music Therapy
Referral
Religious Addiction Prevention
Reminiscence Therapy
Security Enhancement
Socialization Enhancement
Touch
Truth Telling

Spiritual Distress, Risk for

DEFINITION: At risk for an altered sense of harmonious connectedness with all of life and the universe in which dimensions that transcend and empower the self may be disrupted.

SUGGESTED NURSING INTERVENTIONS FOR PROBLEM RESOLUTION:

Active Listening
Anticipatory Guidance
Anxiety Reduction
Coping Enhancement
Counseling
Decision-Making Support
Emotional Support
Forgiveness Facilitation

Grief Work Facilitation
Hope Instillation
Mood Management
Resiliency Promotion
Spiritual Growth Facilitation
Spiritual Support
Support Group
Values Clarification

ADDITIONAL OPTIONAL INTERVENTIONS:

Abuse Protection Support: Religious
Animal-Assisted Therapy
Caregiver Support
Family Support
Music Therapy
Referral

Religious Addiction Prevention
Religious Ritual Enhancement
Reminiscence Therapy
Socialization Enhancement
Truth Telling

Spiritual Well-Being, Readiness for Enhanced

DEFINITION: Process of developing/unfolding of mystery through harmonious interconnectedness that springs from inner strengths.

SUGGESTED NURSING INTERVENTIONS FOR PROBLEM RESOLUTION:

Bibliotherapy
Meditation Facilitation
Religious Ritual Enhancement
Resiliency Promotion
Role Enhancement
Self-Awareness Enhancement

Self-Esteem Enhancement
Self-Modification Assistance
Self-Responsibility Facilitation
Spiritual Growth Facilitation
Spiritual Support

ADDITIONAL OPTIONAL INTERVENTIONS:

Autogenic Training
Body Image Enhancement
Hope Instillation
Music Therapy

Religious Addiction Prevention
Reminiscence Therapy
Simple Guided Imagery
Values Clarification

Suffocation, Risk for

DEFINITION: Accentuated risk of accidental suffocation (inadequate air available for inhalation).

SUGGESTED NURSING INTERVENTIONS FOR PROBLEM RESOLUTION:

Airway Management
Artificial Airway Management
Aspiration Precautions
Environmental Management: Safety
Respiratory Monitoring

Security Enhancement
Surveillance
Surveillance: Safety
Teaching: Infant Safety
Vital Signs Monitoring

ADDITIONAL OPTIONAL INTERVENTIONS:

Infant Care
Parent Education: Infant

Positioning

Suicide, Risk for

DEFINITION: At risk for self-inflicted, life-threatening injury.

SUGGESTED NURSING INTERVENTIONS FOR PROBLEM RESOLUTION:

Anger Control Assistance
Anxiety Reduction
Area Restriction
Behavior Management: Self-Harm
Behavior Modification
Calming Technique
Coping Enhancement
Counseling
Crisis Intervention
Delusion Management
Environmental Management: Safety

Grief Work Facilitation
Impulse Control Training
Limit Setting
Mood Management
Patient Contracting
Presence
Substance Use Treatment
Suicide Prevention
Support Group
Surveillance: Safety
Therapy Group

ADDITIONAL OPTIONAL INTERVENTIONS:

Assertiveness Training
Behavior Modification: Social Skills
Cognitive Restructuring
Family Involvement Promotion
Family Therapy
Forgiveness Facilitation
Grief Work Facilitation

Hallucination Management
Medication Management
Phototherapy: Mood/Sleep Regulation
Self-Awareness Enhancement
Self-Esteem Enhancement
Self-Modification Assistance
Self-Responsibility Enhancement

Surgical Recovery, Delayed

DEFINITION: Extension of the number of postoperative days required to initiate and perform activities that maintain life, health, and well-being.

SUGGESTED NURSING INTERVENTIONS FOR PROBLEM RESOLUTION:

Case Management
Diet Staging
Energy Management
Exercise Therapy: Ambulation
Fever Treatment
Fluid/Electrolyte Management
Incision Site Care
Infection Control
Medication Administration
Medication Management

Nausea Management
Nutrition Management
Nutrition Therapy
Pain Management
Self-Care Assistance
Sleep Enhancement
Temperature Regulation
Vital Signs Monitoring
Wound Care

ADDITIONAL OPTIONAL INTERVENTIONS:

Airway Management
Bed Rest Care
Bowel Management
Caregiver Support
Cough Enhancement
Discharge Planning
Enteral Tube Feeding
Environmental Management: Home
    Preparation
Health Care Information Exchange
Health System Guidance

Home Maintenance Assistance
Insurance Authorization
Multidisciplinary Care Conference
Oral Health Maintenance
Positioning
Respiratory Monitoring
Sleep Enhancement
Telephone Consultation
Urinary Elimination Management
Wound Irrigation

Swallowing, Impaired

DEFINITION: Abnormal functioning of the swallowing mechanism associated with deficits in oral, pharyngeal, or esophageal structure or function.

SUGGESTED NURSING INTERVENTIONS FOR PROBLEM RESOLUTION:

Airway Suctioning
Aspiration Precautions
Progressive Muscle Relaxation

Surveillance
Swallowing Therapy

ADDITIONAL OPTIONAL INTERVENTIONS:

Anxiety Reduction
Emotional Support
Enteral Tube Feeding
Feeding

Medication Management
Nutrition Management
Positioning
Referral

Therapeutic Regimen Management, Effective

DEFINITION: Pattern of regulating and integrating into daily living a program for treatment of illness and its sequelae that is satisfactory for meeting specific health goals.

SUGGESTED NURSING INTERVENTIONS FOR PROBLEM RESOLUTIONS:

Anticipatory Guidance
Health Education
Health Screening
Health System Guidance
Learning Facilitation

Learning Readiness Enhancement
Risk Identification
Self-Modification Assistance
Surveillance

ADDITIONAL OPTIONAL INTERVENTIONS:

Cultural Brokerage

Referral

Therapeutic Regimen Management, Ineffective

DEFINITION: Pattern of regulating and integrating into daily living a program for treatment of illness and the sequelae of illness that is unsatisfactory for meeting specific health goals.

SUGGESTED NURSING INTERVENTIONS FOR PROBLEM RESOLUTION:

Active Listening
Behavior Modification
Cognitive Restructuring
Complex Relationship Building
Coping Enhancement
Counseling
Crisis Intervention
Culture Brokerage
Emotional Support
Family Support
Financial Resource Assistance

Health System Guidance
Labor Suppression
Mutual Goal Setting
Nutritional Counseling
Patient Contracting
Risk Identification
Self-Modification Assistance
Teaching: Disease Process
Teaching: Prescribed Diet
Telephone Consultation
Telephone Follow-up

ADDITIONAL OPTIONAL INTERVENTIONS:

Bibliotherapy
Decision-Making Support
Exercise Promotion
Family Integrity Promotion
Family Mobilization
High-Risk Pregnancy Care
Humor
Learning Facilitation
Presence
Referral

Self-Awareness Enhancement
Self-Esteem Enhancement
Self-Responsibility Facilitation
Smoking Cessation Assistance
Support Group
Support System Enhancement
Touch
Truth Telling
Values Clarification

Thermoregulation, Ineffective

DEFINITION: Temperature fluctuation between hypothermia and hyperthermia.

SUGGESTED NURSING INTERVENTIONS FOR PROBLEM RESOLUTION:

Bathing
Environmental Management
Fever Treatment
Fluid Management
Fluid Monitoring

Hemodynamic Regulation
Temperature Regulation
Temperature Regulation: Intraoperative
Vital Signs Monitoring

ADDITIONAL OPTIONAL INTERVENTIONS:

Anxiety Reduction
Blood Products Administration
Medication Administration

Peripherally Inserted Central (PIC)
    Catheter Care
Phlebotomy: Arterial Blood Sample

Thought Processes, Disturbed

DEFINITION: Disruption in cognitive operations and activities.

SUGGESTED NURSING INTERVENTIONS FOR PROBLEM RESOLUTION:

Anxiety Reduction
Behavior Management
Behavior Management: Overactivity/
    Inattention
Cerebral Perfusion Promotion
Delusion Management
Dementia Management

Elopement Precautions
Environmental Management
Environmental Management: Safety
Self-Care Assistance: IADL
Surveillance
Surveillance: Safety

ADDITIONAL OPTIONAL INTERVENTIONS:

Area Restriction
Behavior Modification
Calming Technique
Cerebral Edema Management
Cognitive Restructuring
Cognitive Stimulation
Delirium Management
Emotional Support
Energy Management
Family Support
Feeding
Hallucination Management
Intracranial Pressure (ICP) Monitoring
Medication Administration
Medication Administration: Oral
Medication Management
Memory Training

Milieu Therapy
Mood Management
Music Therapy
Neurologic Monitoring
Pain Management
Patient Rights Protection
Physical Restraint
Reality Orientation
Relocation Stress Reduction
Reminiscence Therapy
Security Enhancement
Self-Esteem Enhancement
Sleep Enhancement
Temperature Regulation
Therapeutic Touch
Touch

Tissue Integrity, Impaired

DEFINITION: Damage to mucous membrane, corneal, integumentary, or subcutaneous tissue.

SUGGESTED NURSING INTERVENTIONS FOR PROBLEM RESOLUTION:

Bleeding Reduction: Gastrointestinal
Bleeding Reduction: Nasal
Bleeding Reduction: Postpartum Uterus
Blood Products Administration
Electrolyte Monitoring
Fluid Management
Fluid Monitoring
Hemorrhage Control
Incision Site Care
Infection Protection
Latex Precautions
Medication Administration: Ear
Medication Administration: Eye
Medication Administration: Rectal
Medication Administration: Vaginal

Nutrition Management
Oral Health Maintenance
Positioning
Pressure Ulcer Care
Pressure Ulcer Prevention
Rectal Prolapse Management
Skin-Care: Donor Site
Skin-Care: Graft Site
Skin Surveillance
Splinting
Suturing
Traction/Immobilization Care
Wound Care
Wound Irrigation

ADDITIONAL OPTIONAL INTERVENTIONS:

Bathing
Infection Control
Intrapartal Care: High-Risk Delivery
Leech Therapy
Lower Extremity Monitoring
Medication Administration

Medication Management
Pressure Management
Simple Massage
Teaching: Foot Care
Tube Care: Urinary
Vital Signs Monitoring

Tissue Perfusion: Cardiopulmonary, Ineffective

DEFINITION: Decrease in oxygen resulting in the failure to nourish the tissues at the capillary level.

SUGGESTED NURSING INTERVENTIONS FOR PROBLEM RESOLUTION:

Acid-Base Management
Acid-Base Management: Metabolic Acidosis
Acid-Base Management: Metabolic Alkalosis
Acid-Base Management: Respiratory Acidosis
Acid-Base Management: Respiratory Alkalosis
Acid-Base Monitoring
Bleeding Reduction: Antepartum Uterus
Bedside Laboratory Testing
Cardiac Care
Cardiac Care: Acute
Cardiac Precautions
Circulatory Care: Arterial Insufficiency
Circulatory Care: Mechanical Assist Device
Circulatory Care: Venous Insufficiency
Circulatory Precautions
Dysrhythmia Management
Electronic Fetal Monitoring: Intrapartum

Emergency Care
Fluid/Electrolyte Management
Fluid Management
Fluid Monitoring
Hemodynamic Regulation
Hypovolemia Management
Invasive Hemodynamic Monitoring
Laboratory Data Interpretation
Oxygen Therapy
Respiratory Monitoring
Resuscitation
Resuscitation: Neonate
Shock Management
Shock Management: Cardiac
Shock Management: Vasogenic
Temporary Pacemaker Management
Vital Signs Monitoring

ADDITIONAL OPTIONAL INTERVENTIONS:

Embolus Care: Pulmonary
Embolus Precautions
Intracranial Pressure (ICP) Monitoring
Intravenous (IV) Insertion
Intravenous (IV) Therapy
Medication Administration
Medication Administration: Intraosseous
Medication Management
Neurologic Monitoring
Pain Management
Peripherally Inserted Central (PIC)
    Catheter Care

Phlebotomy: Arterial Blood Sample
Phlebotomy: Cannulated Vessel
Phlebotomy: Venous Blood Sample
Seizure Management
Seizure Precautions
Smoking Cessation Assistance
Substance Use Treatment
Surveillance
Temperature Regulation
Total Parenteral Nutrition (TPN) Administration

Tissue Perfusion: Cerebral, Ineffective

DEFINITION: Decrease in oxygen resulting in the failure to nourish the tissues at the capillary level.

SUGGESTED NURSING INTERVENTIONS FOR PROBLEM RESOLUTION:

Acid-Base Management
Acid-Base Management: Metabolic Acidosis
Acid-Base Management: Metabolic Alkalosis
Acid-Base Management: Respiratory Acidosis
Acid-Base Management: Respiratory Alkalosis
Acid-Base Monitoring
Bedside Laboratory Testing
Cerebral Perfusion Promotion
Circulatory Care: Arterial Insufficiency
Circulatory Care: Mechanical Assist Device
Circulatory Care: Venous Insufficiency
Circulatory Precautions
Electronic Fetal Monitoring: Intrapartum
Emergency Care
Fluid/Electrolyte Management
Fluid Management
Fluid Monitoring

Hemodynamic Regulation
Hypovolemia Management
Intracranial Pressure (ICP) Monitoring
Invasive Hemodynamic Monitoring
Laboratory Data Interpretation
Neurologic Monitoring
Nutrition Management
Oxygen Therapy
Peripheral Sensation Management
Resuscitation
Resuscitation: Fetus
Resuscitation: Neonate
Seizure Management
Seizure Precautions
Shock Management
Vital Signs Monitoring

ADDITIONAL OPTIONAL INTERVENTIONS:

Amnioinfusion
Embolus Care: Peripheral
Embolus Precautions
Enteral Tube Feeding
Intravenous (IV) Insertion
Intravenous (IV) Therapy
Medication Administration
Medication Administration: Intraosseous
Medication Management

Pain Management
Peripherally Inserted Central (PIC)
    Catheter Care
Phlebotomy: Arterial Blood Sample
Phlebotomy: Cannulated Vessel
Phlebotomy: Venous Blood Sample
Surveillance
Temperature Regulation
Total Parenteral Nutrition (TPN) Administration

Tissue Perfusion: Gastrointestinal, Ineffective

DEFINITION: Decrease in oxygen resulting in the failure to nourish the tissues at the capillary level.

SUGGESTED NURSING INTERVENTIONS FOR PROBLEM RESOLUTION:

Acid-Base Management
Acid-Base Monitoring
Bedside Laboratory Testing
Emergency Care
Flatulence Reduction
Fluid/Electrolyte Management
Fluid Management
Fluid Monitoring
Gastrointestinal Intubation
Hemodynamic Regulation
Hypovolemia Management
Invasive Hemodynamic Monitoring

Laboratory Data Interpretation
Medication Administration: Enteral
Nausea Management
Nutrition Management
Nutrition Therapy
Nutritional Monitoring
Oxygen Therapy
Resuscitation
Shock Management
Tube Care: Gastrointestinal
Vital Signs Monitoring

ADDITIONAL OPTIONAL INTERVENTIONS:

Bowel Management
Enteral Tube Feeding
Intravenous (IV) Insertion
Intravenous (IV) Therapy
Medication Administration
Medication Administration: Intraosseous
Medication Management
Peripherally Inserted Central (PIC)
    Catheter Care

Phlebotomy: Arterial Blood Sample
Phlebotomy: Cannulated Vessel
Phlebotomy: Venous Blood Sample
Surveillance
Temperature Regulation
Total Parenteral Nutrition (TPN)
    Administration

Tissue Perfusion: Peripheral, Ineffective

DEFINITION: Decrease in oxygen resulting in the failure to nourish the tissues at the capillary level.

SUGGESTED NURSING INTERVENTIONS FOR PROBLEM RESOLUTION:

Acid-Base Management
Acid-Base Monitoring
Bedside Laboratory Testing
Circulatory Care: Arterial Insufficiency
Circulatory Care: Mechanical Assist Device
Circulatory Care: Venous Insufficiency
Circulatory Precautions
Emergency Care
Fluid/Electrolyte Management
Fluid Management
Fluid Monitoring
Foot Care
Hemodynamic Regulation
Hypovolemia Management
Invasive Hemodynamic Monitoring
Laboratory Data Interpretation

Lower Extremity Monitoring
Neurologic Monitoring
Nutrition Management
Oxygen Therapy
Peripheral Sensation Management
Pneumatic Tourniquet Precautions
Positioning
Pressure Ulcer Prevention
Resuscitation
Resuscitation: Neonate
Shock Management
Shock Management: Cardiac
Shock Management: Vasogenic
Skin Surveillance
Vital Signs Monitoring

ADDITIONAL OPTIONAL INTERVENTIONS:

Embolus Care: Peripheral
Embolus Precautions
Exercise Promotion
Exercise Therapy: Ambulation
Exercise Therapy: Balance
Exercise Therapy: Joint Mobility
Exercise Therapy: Muscle Control
Intravenous (IV) Insertion
Intravenous (IV) Therapy
Medication Administration
Medication Administration: Intraosseous

Medication Management
Pain Management
Peripherally Inserted Central (PIC)
    Catheter Care
Phlebotomy: Arterial Blood Sample
Phlebotomy: Cannulated Vessel
Phlebotomy: Venous Blood Sample
Surveillance
Temperature Regulation
Total Parenteral Nutrition (TPN)
    Administration

Tissue Perfusion: Renal, Ineffective

DEFINITION: Decrease in oxygen resulting in the failure to nourish the tissues at the capillary level.

SUGGESTED NURSING INTERVENTIONS FOR PROBLEM RESOLUTION:

Acid-Base Management
Acid-Base Management: Metabolic Acidosis
Acid-Base Management: Metabolic Alkalosis
Acid-Base Management: Respiratory Acidosis
Acid-Base Management: Respiratory Alkalosis
Acid-Base Monitoring
Bedside Laboratory Testing
Dialysis Access Maintenance
Emergency Care
Fluid/Electrolyte Management
Fluid Management
Fluid Monitoring

Hemodialysis Therapy
Hemodynamic Regulation
Hemofiltration Therapy
Hypovolemia Management
Invasive Hemodynamic Monitoring
Laboratory Data Interpretation
Nutrition Management
Oxygen Therapy
Peritoneal Dialysis Therapy
Resuscitation
Shock Management
Vital Signs Monitoring

ADDITIONAL OPTIONAL INTERVENTIONS:

Intravenous (IV) Insertion
Intravenous (IV) Therapy
Medication Administration
Medication Administration: Intraosseous
Medication Management
Pain Management
Peripherally Inserted Central (PIC)
 Catheter Care

Phlebotomy: Arterial Blood Sample
Phlebotomy: Cannulated Vessel
Phlebotomy: Venous Blood Sample
Surveillance
Temperature Regulation
Total Parenteral Nutrition (TPN) Administration

Transfer Ability, Impaired

DEFINITION: Limitation of independent movement between two nearby surfaces.

SUGGESTED NURSING INTERVENTIONS FOR PROBLEM RESOLUTION:

Body Mechanics Promotion
Energy Management
Exercise Promotion
Exercise Promotion: Stretching
Exercise Promotion: Strength Training
Exercise Therapy: Balance
Exercise Therapy: Muscle Control

Positioning
Positioning: Neurologic
Positioning: Wheelchair
Self-Care Assistance: Transfer
Teaching: Prescribed Activity/Exercise
Transport

ADDITIONAL OPTIONAL INTERVENTIONS:

Medication Management
Mutual Goal Setting
Nutrition Management
Pain Management
Self-Care Assistance
Self-Care Assistance: Bathing/Hygiene

Self-Care Assistance: Dressing/Grooming
Self-Care Assistance: Feeding
Self-Care Assistance: Toileting
Sleep Enhancement
Weight Management

Trauma, Risk for

DEFINITION: Accentuated risk of accidental tissue injury (e.g., wound, burn, fracture).

SUGGESTED NURSING INTERVENTIONS FOR PROBLEM RESOLUTION:

Community Health Development
Environmental Management: Safety
Environmental Management: Worker Safety
Fall Prevention
Health Education
Laser Precautions
Peripheral Sensation Management
Physical Restraint
Positioning
Pressure Management
Radiation Therapy Management
Seizure Precautions

Skin Surveillance
Sports-Injury Prevention: Youth
Surgical Precautions
Surveillance
Surveillance: Safety
Teaching: Disease Process
Teaching: Individual
Teaching: Infant Safety
Teaching: Toddler Safety
Vehicle Safety Promotion
Vital Signs Monitoring

ADDITIONAL OPTIONAL INTERVENTIONS:

Embolus Precautions
Parent Education: Adolescent
Parent Education: Childrearing Family
Parent Education: Infant

Perineal Care
Positioning: Neurologic
Positioning: Wheelchair
Self-Care Assistance: Transfer

Unilateral Neglect

DEFINITION: Lack of awareness and attention to one side of the body.

SUGGESTED NURSING INTERVENTIONS FOR PROBLEM RESOLUTION:

Amputation Care

Body Image Enhancement

Coping Enhancement

Communication Enhancement: Visual Deficit

Environmental Management: Safety

Positioning

Touch

Unilateral Neglect Management

ADDITIONAL OPTIONAL INTERVENTIONS:

Cerebral Perfusion Promotion

Caregiver Support

Exercise Promotion

Exercise Promotion: Stretching

Exercise Therapy: Ambulation

Exercise Therapy: Balance

Exercise Therapy: Joint Mobility

Exercise Therapy: Muscle Control

Lower Extremity Monitoring

Mutual Goal Setting

Support System Enhancement

Teaching: Individual

Urinary Elimination, Impaired

DEFINITION: Disturbance in urine elimination.

SUGGESTED NURSING INTERVENTIONS FOR PROBLEM RESOLUTION:

Bladder Irrigation

Fluid Management

Fluid Monitoring

Medication Management

Medication Prescribing

Pelvic Muscle Management

Pessary Management

Urinary Catheterization

Urinary Catheterization: Intermittent

Urinary Elimination Management

Urinary Incontinence Care

Urinary Incontinence Care: Enuresis

Urinary Retention Care

ADDITIONAL OPTIONAL INTERVENTIONS:

Anxiety Reduction

Hemodialysis Therapy

Infection Control

Infection Protection

Pain Management

Perineal Care

Postpartal Care

Skin Surveillance

Teaching: Toilet Training

Tube Care: Urinary

Weight Management

Urinary Incontinence: Functional

DEFINITION: Inability of usually continent persons to reach toilet in time to avoid unintentional loss of urine.

SUGGESTED NURSING INTERVENTIONS FOR PROBLEM RESOLUTION:

Environmental Management
Pelvic Muscle Exercise
Prompted Voiding
Self-Care Assistance: Toileting

Urinary Elimination Management
Urinary Habit Training
Urinary Incontinence Care

ADDITIONAL OPTIONAL INTERVENTIONS:

Bathing
Communication Enhancement: Visual
Dressing
Exercise Promotion

Exercise Therapy: Ambulation
Perineal Care
Self-Awareness Enhancement
Surveillance: Safety

Urinary Incontinence: Reflex

DEFINITION: Involuntary loss of urine at somewhat predictable intervals when a specific bladder volume is reached.

SUGGESTED NURSING INTERVENTIONS FOR PROBLEM RESOLUTION:

Pelvic Muscle Exercise
Tube Care: Urinary
Urinary Bladder Training
Urinary Catheterization

Urinary Catheterization: Intermittent
Urinary Elimination Management
Urinary Incontinence Care
Urinary Retention Care

ADDITIONAL OPTIONAL INTERVENTIONS:

Bathing
Perineal Care

Self-Care Assistance: Toileting
Teaching: Toilet Training

Urinary Incontinence: Stress

DEFINITION: Loss of less than 50 ml of urine occurring with increased abdominal pressure.

SUGGESTED NURSING INTERVENTIONS FOR PROBLEM RESOLUTION:

Biofeedback
Medication Management
Pelvic Muscle Exercise
Pessary Management
Teaching: Individual

Teaching: Prescribed Medication
Urinary Elimination Management
Urinary Habit Training
Urinary Incontinence Care
Weight Management

ADDITIONAL OPTIONAL INTERVENTIONS:

Perineal Care
Respiratory Monitoring

Self-Care Assistance: Toileting

Urinary Incontinence: Total

DEFINITION: Continuous and unpredictable loss of urine.

SUGGESTED NURSING INTERVENTIONS FOR PROBLEM RESOLUTION:

Environmental Management
Perineal Care
Self-Care Assistance: Toileting

Urinary Catheterization
Urinary Incontinence Care

ADDITIONAL OPTIONAL INTERVENTIONS:

Bathing
Fluid Management

Fluid Monitoring
Urinary Elimination Management

Urinary Incontinence: Urge

DEFINITION: Involuntary passage of urine occurring soon after a strong sense of urgency to void.

SUGGESTED NURSING INTERVENTIONS FOR PROBLEM RESOLUTION:

Environmental Management
Fluid Management
Fluid Monitoring
Medication Management

Urinary Elimination Management
Urinary Habit Training
Urinary Incontinence Care

ADDITIONAL OPTIONAL INTERVENTIONS:

Bathing
Perineal Care
Self-Care Assistance: Toileting
Teaching: Toilet Training

Tube Care: Urinary
Urinary Catheterization
Urinary Catheterization: Intermittent

Urinary Incontinence: Urge, Risk for

DEFINITION: At risk for involuntary loss of urine associated with a sudden, strong sensation or urinary urgency.

SUGGESTED NURSING INTERVENTIONS FOR PROBLEM RESOLUTION:

Environmental Management
Fluid Management
Fluid Monitoring
Medication Management

Urinary Elimination Management
Urinary Habit Training
Self-Care Assistance: Toileting

ADDITIONAL OPTIONAL INTERVENTIONS:

Exercise Promotion
Pelvic Muscle Exercise
Perineal Care
Pessary Management
Prompted Voiding

Teaching: Toilet Training
Tube Care: Urinary
Urinary Catheterization
Weight Management

Urinary Retention

DEFINITION: Incomplete emptying of the bladder.

SUGGESTED NURSING INTERVENTIONS FOR PROBLEM RESOLUTION:

Bladder Irrigation
Fluid Management
Fluid Monitoring
Medication Management
Tube Care: Urinary

Urinary Catheterization
Urinary Catheterization: Intermittent
Urinary Elimination Management
Urinary Retention Care

ADDITIONAL OPTIONAL INTERVENTIONS:

Distraction
Exercise Promotion
Exercise Therapy: Ambulation
Exercise Therapy: Balance
Exercise Therapy: Joint Mobility

Exercise Therapy: Muscle Control
Perineal Care
Simple Massage
Simple Relaxation Therapy

Ventilation, Impaired Spontaneous

DEFINITION: Decreased energy reserves result in an individual's inability to maintain breathing adequate to support life.

SUGGESTED NURSING INTERVENTIONS FOR PROBLEM RESOLUTION:

Acid-Base Management
Acid-Base Management: Respiratory Acidosis
Acid-Base Management: Respiratory Alkalosis
Acid-Base Monitoring
Airway Management
Airway Suctioning
Anxiety Reduction
Artificial Airway Management
Aspiration Precautions
Calming Technique
Chest Physiotherapy
Emotional Support
Energy Management
Environmental Management
Environmental Management: Comfort
Environmental Management: Safety

Fluid/Electrolyte Management
Fluid Management
Fluid Monitoring
Fluid Resuscitation
Infection Control
Infection Protection
Mechanical Ventilation
Mechanical Ventilatory Weaning
Oral Health Maintenance
Oxygen Therapy
Positioning
Respiratory Monitoring
Resuscitation: Neonate
Skin Surveillance
Ventilation Assistance
Vital Signs Monitoring

ADDITIONAL OPTIONAL INTERVENTIONS:

Active Listening
Bed Rest Care
Body Image Enhancement
Coping Enhancement
Decision-Making Support
Distraction
Emergency Care
Endotracheal Extubation
Hope Instillation
Humor
Intravenous (IV) Insertion
Intravenous (IV) Therapy
Patient Rights Protection
Phlebotomy: Arterial Blood Sample
Physical Restraint

Presence
Pressure Management
Pressure Ulcer Prevention
Security Enhancement
Self-Care Assistance
Spiritual Support
Surveillance
Surveillance: Safety
Technology Management
Touch
Tube Care
Tube Care: Chest
Tube Care: Gastrointestinal
Tube Care: Urinary

Ventilatory Weaning Response, Dysfunctional

DEFINITION: Inability to adjust to lowered levels of mechanical ventilator support that interrupts and prolongs the weaning process.

SUGGESTED NURSING INTERVENTIONS FOR PROBLEM RESOLUTION:

Acid-Base Management	Environmental Management: Safety
Airway Management	Mechanical Ventilation
Artificial Airway Management	Mechanical Ventilatory Weaning
Aspiration Precautions	Ventilation Assistance

ADDITIONAL OPTIONAL INTERVENTIONS:

Anxiety Reduction	Phlebotomy: Arterial Blood Sample
Calming Technique	Presence
Communication Enhancement: Speech Deficit	Simple Relaxation Therapy
Coping Enhancement	Sleep Enhancement
Distraction	Support System Enhancement
Emotional Support	Surveillance
Energy Management	Teaching: Procedure/Treatment
Environmental Management: Comfort	Technology Management
Hope Instillation	Touch

Violence: Other-Directed, Risk for

DEFINITION: At risk for behaviors in which an individual demonstrates that he/she can be physically, emotionally, and/or sexually harmful to others.

SUGGESTED NURSING INTERVENTIONS FOR PROBLEM RESOLUTION:

Abuse Protection Support
Abuse Protection Support: Child
Abuse Protection Support: Domestic
 Partner
Abuse Protection Support: Elder
Anger Control Assistance
Anxiety Reduction
Area Restriction
Art Therapy
Behavior Management
Behavior Modification
Calming Technique
Coping Enhancement
Crisis Intervention
Delusion Management
Dementia Management
Dementia Management: Bathing

Distraction
Environmental Management: Violence
 Prevention
Fire-Setting Precautions
Medication Administration
Mood Management
Physical Restraint
Seclusion
Security Enhancement
Substance Use Prevention
Substance Use Treatment
Substance Use Treatment: Alcohol Withdrawal
Substance Use Treatment: Drug Withdrawal
Support System Enhancement
Surveillance
Surveillance: Safety

ADDITIONAL OPTIONAL INTERVENTIONS:

Animal-Assisted Therapy
Behavior Modification: Social Skills
Family Involvement Promotion
Family Support
Guilt Work Facilitation
Impulse Control Training
Medication Management
Mutual Goal Setting

Presence
Reality Orientation
Self-Esteem Enhancement
Support Group
Therapeutic Play
Triage: Emergency Center
Triage: Telephone

Violence: Self-Directed, Risk for

DEFINITION: At risk for behaviors in which an individual demonstrates that he/she can be physically, emotionally, and/or sexually harmful to self.

SUGGESTED NURSING INTERVENTIONS FOR PROBLEM RESOLUTION:

Anger Control Assistance
Anxiety Reduction
Area Restriction
Behavior Management: Self-Harm
Behavior Modification
Calming Technique
Coping Enhancement
Counseling
Crisis Intervention
Delusion Management
Environmental Management: Safety
Environmental Management: Violence
    Prevention
Impulse Control Training
Limit Setting
Mood Management

Patient Contracting
Physical Restraint
Seclusion
Security Enhancement
Self-Awareness Enhancement
Self-Esteem Enhancement
Self-Modification Assistance
Self-Responsibility Enhancement
Substance Use Treatment
Substance Use Treatment: Alcohol
    Withdrawal
Substance Use Treatment: Drug Withdrawal
Substance Use Treatment: Overdose
Suicide Prevention
Surveillance: Safety

ADDITIONAL OPTIONAL INTERVENTIONS:

Animal-Assisted Therapy
Assertiveness Training
Behavior Modification: Social Skills
Cognitive Restructuring
Family Involvement Promotion
Family Therapy
Grief Work Facilitation

Guilt Work Facilitation
Hallucination Management
Medication Management
Phototherapy: Mood/Sleep Regulation
Support Group
Therapy Group

Walking, Impaired

DEFINITION: Limitation of independent movement within the environment on foot.

SUGGESTED NURSING INTERVENTIONS FOR PROBLEM RESOLUTION:

Body Mechanics Promotion

Energy Management

Environmental Management

Exercise Promotion

Exercise Promotion: Strength Training

Exercise Promotion: Stretching

Exercise Therapy: Ambulation

Exercise Therapy: Balance

Exercise Therapy: Muscle Control

Pain Management

Positioning

Teaching: Prescribed Activity/Exercise

Transport

ADDITIONAL OPTIONAL INTERVENTIONS:

Lower Extremity Monitoring

Medication Management

Mutual Goal Setting

Nutrition Management

Sleep Enhancement

Weight Management

Wandering

DEFINITION: Meandering, aimless or repetitive locomotion that exposes the individual to harm; frequently incongruent with boundaries, limits, or obstacles.

SUGGESTED NURSING INTERVENTIONS FOR PROBLEM RESOLUTION:

Area Restriction

Behavior Management

Behavior Management: Overactivity/
   Inattention

Dementia Management

Elopement Precautions

Environmental Management: Safety

Fall Prevention

Limit Setting

Medication Management

Pain Management

Reality Orientation

Self-Care Assistance

Surveillance: Safety

Teaching: Toddler Safety

ADDITIONAL OPTIONAL INTERVENTIONS:

Anxiety Reduction

Calming Technique

Caregiver Support

Distraction

Family Involvement

Health System Guidance

Patient Rights Protection

Respite Care

PART FIVE

Core Interventions for Nursing Specialty Areas

Core Interventions for Nursing Speciality Areas

In this section we have listed alphabetically the core interventions for 43 specialty areas. Core interventions are defined as a limited, central set of interventions that define the nature of the specialty. A person reading the list of core interventions would be able to determine the area of specialty practice. The core set of interventions does not include all the interventions used by nurses in the specialty but, rather, includes those interventions that are used most often by nurses in the specialty, are used predominately by nurses in the specialty, or are critical to the role of the specialty nurse.

These lists of specialty core interventions initially resulted from a survey that was sent to specialty organizations in 1995 and 1996; the research and an initial list of core interventions for 39 specialty areas were published in the third edition of *Nursing Interventions Classification (NIC)*. The results of the survey are also published in an article: McCloskey, J. C., Bulechek, G., & Donahue, W. (1998). Nursing interventions core to specialty practice. *Nursing Outlook, 46,* 67-76.

For this edition, the core lists in the previous edition were updated to include interventions new to the third and fourth editions, and four new specialties were added: College Health Nursing, Community Health Nursing, Correctional Nursing, and Parish Nursing. The entire list of 43 specialties for which care interventions are identified follows:

1. Addictions Nursing
2. Ambulatory Nursing
3. Anesthesia Nursing
4. Chemical Dependency Nursing
5. Child & Adolescent Psychiatric Nursing
6. College Health Nursing
7. Community/Public Health Nursing
8. Correctional Nursing
9. Critical Care Nursing
10. Dermatology Nursing
11. Developmental Disability Nursing
12. Emergency Nursing
13. Flight Nursing
14. Gastroenterological Nursing
15. Genetics Nursing
16. Gerontological Nursing
17. Holistic Nursing
18. Infection Control and Epidemiological Nursing
19. Intravenous Nursing
20. Medical-Surgical Nursing
21. Midwifery Nursing
22. Neonatal Nursing
23. Nephrology Nursing
24. Neuroscience Nursing

25. Obstetric Nursing
26. Occupational Health Nursing
27. Oncology Nursing
28. Ophthalmic Nursing
29. Orthopedic Nursing
30. Otorhinolaryngology and Head/Neck Nursing
31. Pain Management Nursing
32. Parish Nursing
33. Pediatric Nursing
34. Pediatric Oncology Nursing
35. Perioperative Nursing
36. Psychiatric/Mental Health Nursing
37. Radiological Nursing
38. Rehabilitation Nursing
39. School Nursing
40. Spinal Cord Injury Nursing
41. Urologic Nursing
42. Vascular Nursing
43. Women's Health Nursing

The identification of core interventions by specialty is an initial step to communicate the nature of nursing in different practice areas. The listing of core interventions by specialty areas of practice is very useful in the development of nursing information systems, staff education programs and competency evaluation, referral networks, certification and licensing examinations, nursing school curricula, and research and theory construction. We encourage members of specialty organizations who are interested in building clinical databases to use the interventions contained in NIC so that nurses can achieve the benefits inherent in a standardized language. We welcome the submission of new interventions as users see the need.

Addictions Nursing

- Anticipatory Guidance
- Behavior Management
- Behavior Modification
- Conflict Mediation
- Coping Enhancement
- Counseling
- Discharge Planning
- Documentation
- Eating Disorders Management
- Environmental Management: Safety
- Family Therapy
- Fluid/Electrolyte Management
- Forgiveness Facilitation
- Health Education
- Health Screening
- Medication Administration

- Nutrition Management
- Referral
- Risk Identification
- Self-Awareness Enhancement
- Self-Responsibility Facilitation
- Smoking Cessation Assistance
- Spiritual Support
- Substance Use Prevention
- Substance Use Treatment
- Substance Use Treatment: Alcohol Withdrawal
- Substance Use Treatment: Drug Withdrawal
- Substance Use Treatment: Overdose
- Teaching: Group
- Teaching: Safe Sex
- Therapy Group
- Vital Signs Monitoring

Ambulatory Nursing

- Anxiety Reduction
- Bedside Laboratory Testing
- Behavior Modification
- Capillary Blood Sample
- Coping Enhancement
- Decision-Making Support
- Delegation
- Documentation
- Emotional Support
- Examination Assistance
- Health Education
- Health Screening
- Health System Guidance
- Immunization/Vaccination Administration
- Medication Administration: Intradermal
- Medication Administration: Intramuscular
- Medication Administration: Intravenous

- Medication Administration: Oral
- Medication Management
- Nutritional Counseling
- Physician Support
- Referral
- Risk Identification
- Staff Supervision
- Teaching: Disease Process
- Teaching Individual
- Teaching: Prescribed Diet
- Teaching: Prescribed Medication
- Teaching: Procedure/Treatment
- Telephone Follow-Up
- Triage: Disaster
- Triage: Telephone
- Vital Signs Monitoring

Anesthesia Nursing

- Acid-Base Management
- Acid-Base Management: Metabolic Acidosis
- Acid-Base Management: Metabolic Alkalosis
- Acid-Base Management: Respiratory Acidosis
- Acid-Base Management: Respiratory Alkalosis
- Acid-Base Monitoring
- Airway Insertion and Stabilization
- Airway Management
- Airway Suctioning
- Analgesic Administration
- Analgesic Administration: Intraspinal
- Anaphylaxis Management
- Anesthesia Administration
- Artificial Airway Management
- Autotransfusion
- Blood Products Administration
- Circulatory Care: Mechanical Assist Device
- Code Management
- Controlled Substance Checking
- Documentation
- Dysrhythmia Management
- Electrolyte Management
- Electrolyte Management: Hypercalcemia
- Electrolyte Management: Hyperkalemia
- Electrolyte Management: Hypermagnesemia
- Electrolyte Management: Hypernatremia
- Electrolyte Management: Hyperphosphatemia
- Electrolyte Management: Hypocalcemia
- Electrolyte Management: Hypokalemia
- Electrolyte Management: Hypomagnesemia
- Electrolyte Management: Hyponatremia
- Electrolyte Management: Hypophosphatemia
- Electrolyte Monitoring
- Emergency Care
- Endotracheal Extubation
- Eye Care
- Fluid Management
- Fluid Monitoring
- Fluid/Electrolyte Management
- Fluid Resuscitation
- Hyperglycemia Management
- Hypervolemia Management
- Hypoglycemia Management
- Hypothermia Treatment
- Hypovolemia Management
- Incident Reporting
- Infection Control
- Infection Control: Intraoperative
- Intracranial Pressure (ICP) Monitoring
- Intravenous (IV) Insertion
- Laboratory Data Interpretation
- Laser Precautions
- Latex Precautions
- Learning Facilitation
- Malignant Hyperthermia Precautions
- Mechanical Ventilation
- Medication Administration
- Medication Administration: Intramuscular
- Medication Administration: Intraspinal
- Medication Administration: Intravenous
- Medication Administration: Oral
- Medication Management
- Medication Prescribing
- Nausea Management
- Oxygen Therapy
- Pain Management
- Patient Controlled Analgesia (PCA) Assistance
- Peer Review
- Peripherally Inserted Central (PIC) Catheter Care
- Phlebotomy: Arterial Blood Sample
- Phlebotomy: Blood Unit Acquisition
- Phlebotomy: Cannulated Vessel
- Phlebotomy: Venous Blood Sample
- Physician Support
- Pneumatic Tourniquet Precautions
- Positioning
- Positioning: Intraoperative
- Positioning: Neurologic
- Postanesthesia Care
- Preoperative Coordination
- Product Evaluation
- Prosthesis Care
- Quality Monitoring
- Referral
- Respiratory Monitoring
- Resuscitation
- Resuscitation: Fetus
- Resuscitation: Neonate
- Sedation Management
- Shock Management
- Shock Management: Cardiac
- Shock Management: Vasogenic
- Shock Management: Volume
- Surgical Precautions
- Surgical Preparation
- Teaching: Preoperative
- Temporary Pacemaker Management
- Transcutaneous Electrical Nerve Stimulation (TENS)
- Triage: Emergency Center
- Ventilation Assistance
- Vital Signs Monitoring

Chemical Dependency Nursing

- Active Listening
- Anger Control Assistance
- Assertiveness Training
- Behavior Management
- Behavior Modification
- Behavior Modification: Social Skills
- Bibliotherapy
- Capillary Blood Sample
- Chemical Restraint
- Conflict Mediation
- Coping Enhancement
- Counseling
- Delirium Management
- Elopement Precautions
- Family Therapy
- Forgiveness Facilitation
- Guilt Work Facilitation
- Hope Instillation
- Impulse Control Training
- Limit Setting
- Medication Management
- Patient Contracting
- Recreational Therapy
- Seizure Management
- Self-Awareness Enhancement
- Self-Esteem Enhancement
- Self-Responsibility Facilitation
- Socialization Enhancement
- Substance Use Prevention
- Substance Use Treatment
- Substance Use Treatment: Alcohol Withdrawal
- Substance Use Treatment: Drug Withdrawal
- Substance Use Treatment: Overdose
- Support Group
- Teaching: Disease Process
- Teaching: Safe Sex
- Therapy Group

Child and Adolescent Psychiatric Nursing

- Abuse Protection Support: Child
- Behavior Management: Overactivity/Inattention
- Behavior Management: Self-Harm
- Behavior Management: Sexual
- Behavior Modification: Social Skills
- Bowel Incontinence Care: Encopresis
- Case Management
- Complex Relationship Building
- Conflict Mediation
- Delusion Management
- Developmental Enhancement
- Elopement Precautions
- Environmental Management: Community
- Exercise Promotion: Stretching
- Family Involvement Promotion
- Family Therapy
- Health Education
- Impulse Control Training
- Medication Management
- Medication Prescribing
- Mood Management
- Multidisciplinary Care Conference
- Normalization Promotion
- Parenting Promotion
- Peer Review
- Product Evaluation
- Research Data Collection
- Resiliency Promotion
- Staff Supervision
- Teaching: Prescribed Medication
- Telephone Consultation
- Trauma Therapy: Child
- Urinary Bladder Training

College Health Nursing

- Active Listening
- Asthma Management
- Anxiety Reduction
- Communicable Disease Management
- Coping Enhancement
- Counseling
- Crisis Intervention
- Decision-Making Support
- Eating Disorders Management
- Emotional Support
- First Aid
- Health Education
- Health System Guidance
- Immunization/Vaccination Management
- Medication Administration: Subcutaneous
- Medication Management
- Medication Prescribing
- Nutrition Management
- Rape-Trauma Treatment
- Referral
- Self-Esteem Enhancement
- Sexual Counseling
- Sleep Enhancement
- Smoking Cessation Assistance
- Sports-Injury Prevention: Youth
- Substance Use Prevention
- Suicide Prevention
- Teaching: Individual
- Teaching: Safe Sex
- Teaching: Sexuality
- Vehicle Safety Promotion
- Weight Management

Community/Public Health Nursing

- Abuse Protection Support
- Bioterrorism Preparedness
- Case Management
- Community Disaster Preparedness
- Community Health Development
- Consultation
- Culture Brokerage
- Environmental Management: Community
- Environmental Management: Home Preparation
- Environmental Management: Worker Safety
- Environmental Risk Protection
- Family Planning: Contraception
- Fiscal Resource Management
- Health Care Information Exchange
- Health Education
- Health Policy Monitoring
- Health Screening
- Health System Guidance
- Home Maintenance Assistance
- Immunization/Vaccination Management
- Medication Administration: Subcutaneous
- Parenting Promotion
- Program Development
- Referral
- Risk Identification
- Surveillance: Community
- Sustenance Support
- Teaching: Group
- Teaching: Infant Nutrition
- Teaching: Infant Safety
- Teaching: Safe Sex
- Teaching: Toddler Nutrition
- Teaching: Toddler Safety
- Vehicle Safety Promotion

Correctional Nursing

- Active Listening
- Area Restriction
- Complex Relationship Building
- Coping Enhancement
- Counseling
- Culture Brokerage
- Emergency Care
- Emotional Support
- Environmental Management: Violence Prevention
- Environmental Risk Protection
- First Aid
- Forgiveness Facilitation
- Health Care Information Exchange
- Health Policy Monitoring
- Health Screening
- Humor
- Limit Setting
- Medication Administration
- Medication Management
- Nutrition Management
- Patient Contracting
- Presence
- Program Development
- Referral
- Skin Surveillance
- Substance Use Prevention
- Substance Use Treatment
- Substance Use Treatment: Alcohol Withdrawal
- Substance Use Treatment: Drug Withdrawal
- Substance Use Treatment: Overdose
- Suicide Prevention
- Surveillance
- Surveillance: Safety
- Teaching: Group
- Teaching: Individual
- Teaching: Prescribed Medication
- Teaching: Safe Sex
- Wound Care

Critical Care Nursing

- Acid-Base Monitoring
- Airway Management
- Airway Suctioning
- Analgesic Administration
- Anaphylaxis Management
- Anxiety Reduction
- Artificial Airway Management
- Cardiac Care
- Cardiac Care: Acute
- Cardiac Precautions
- Caregiver Support
- Circulatory Care: Mechanical Assist Device
- Code Management
- Critical Path Development
- Decision-Making Support
- Delegation
- Discharge Planning
- Documentation
- Electrolyte Management
- Electrolyte Management: Hyperkalemia
- Electrolyte Management: Hypokalemia
- Electrolyte Monitoring
- Emergency Care
- Emotional Support
- Family Involvement Promotion
- Family Presence Facilitation
- Fluid Management
- Fluid Monitoring
- Fluid/Electrolyte Management
- Hemodynamic Regulation
- Intravenous (IV) Therapy
- Invasive Hemodynamic Monitoring
- Mechanical Ventilation
- Mechanical Ventilatory Weaning
- Medication Administration
- Medication Administration: Intravenous
- Medication Administration: Oral
- Medication Management: Intramuscular
- Multidisciplinary Care Conference
- Nausea Management
- Neurologic Monitoring
- Oxygen Therapy
- Pain Management
- Patient Rights Protection
- Physician Support
- Positioning
- Respiratory Monitoring
- Sedation Management
- Teaching: Procedure/Treatment
- Technology Management
- Temporary Pacemaker Management
- Visitation Facilitation
- Vital Signs Monitoring
- Vomiting Management

Dermatology Nursing

- Behavior Modification
- Body Image Enhancement
- Coping Enhancement
- Decision-Making Support
- Documentation
- Emotional Support
- Environmental Management: Community
- Examination Assistance
- Health Education
- Health Screening
- Incision Site Care
- Infection Control
- Laser Precautions
- Learning Facilitation
- Medication Administration: Skin
- Physician Support
- Pressure Ulcer Care
- Pruritus Management
- Self-Responsibility Facilitation
- Skin Care: Donor Site
- Skin Care: Graft Site
- Skin Care: Topical Treatments
- Skin Surveillance
- Support System Enhancement
- Surgical Assistance
- Teaching: Disease Process
- Teaching: Prescribed Medication
- Teaching: Procedure/Treatment
- Telephone Consultation
- Wound Care
- Wound Irrigation

Developmental Disability Nursing

- Abuse Protection Support
- Anxiety Reduction
- Aspiration Precautions
- Behavior Management
- Behavior Management: Self-Harm
- Behavior Management: Social Skills
- Bowel Management
- Case Management
- Communication Enhancement: Hearing Deficit
- Communication Enhancement: Speech Deficit
- Communication Enhancement: Visual Deficit
- Developmental Enhancement: Adolescent
- Developmental Enhancement: Child
- Documentation
- Environmental Management: Safety
- Family Involvement Promotion
- Financial Resource Assistance
- Health Education
- Health Screening
- Incident Reporting
- Infection Control
- Medication Administration
- Medication Management
- Multidisciplinary Care Conference
- Normalization Promotion
- Nutrition Management
- Patient Rights Protection
- Relocation Stress Reduction
- Risk Identification: Genetic
- Seizure Management
- Seizure Precautions
- Self-Care Assistance
- Self-Care Assistance: IADL
- Staff Supervision
- Teaching: Prescribed Medication
- Teaching: Safe Sex
- Telephone Consultation
- Telephone Follow-up
- Weight Management

Emergency Nursing

- Abuse Protection Support: Child
- Abuse Protection Support: Domestic Partner
- Airway Management
- Anaphylaxis Management
- Bioterrorism Preparedness
- Blood Products Administration
- Cardiac Care: Acute
- Circulatory Care: Arterial Insufficiency
- Circulatory Care: Venous Insufficiency
- Code Management
- Crisis Intervention
- Documentation
- Dysrhythmia Management
- Electrolyte Management
- Emergency Care
- Family Presence Facilitation
- First Aid
- Fluid/Electrolyte Management
- Fluid Resuscitation
- Heat Exposure Treatment
- Hypovolemia Management
- Intravenous (IV) Insertion
- Intravenous (IV) Therapy
- Medication Administration
- Medication Administration: Intramuscular
- Medication Administration: Intravenous
- Neurologic Monitoring
- Oxygen Therapy
- Pain Management
- Phlebotomy: Venous Blood Sample
- Rape-Trauma Treatment
- Respiratory Monitoring
- Resuscitation
- Seizure Management
- Shock Management
- Teaching: Individual
- Temporary Pacemaker Management
- Triage: Emergency Center
- Triage: Telephone
- Vital Signs Monitoring
- Wound Care

Flight Nursing

- Anaphylaxis Management
- Artificial Airway Management
- Blood Products Administration
- Cardiac Care
- Cardiac Care: Acute
- Cardiac Precautions
- Caregiver Support
- Code Management
- Emergency Care
- Family Presence Facilitation
- Hemorrhage Control
- Hypovolemia Management
- Intravenous (IV) Insertion
- Intravenous (IV) Therapy
- Invasive Hemodynamic Monitoring
- Laboratory Data Interpretation
- Mechanical Ventilation
- Medication Administration: Intramuscular
- Medication Administration: Intravenous
- Newborn Care
- Newborn Monitoring
- Oxygen Therapy
- Respiratory Monitoring
- Resuscitation
- Sedation Management
- Shock Management
- Shock Management: Cardiac
- Shock Management: Vasogenic
- Shock Management: Volume
- Shock Prevention
- Technology Management
- Telephone Consultation
- Transport
- Triage: Disaster
- Ventilation Assistance
- Vital Signs Monitoring
- Wound Care

Gastroenterological Nursing

- Airway Management
- Airway Suctioning
- Anesthesia Administration
- Aspiration Precautions
- Bowel Incontinence Care: Encopresis
- Bowel Irrigation
- Bowel Management
- Calming Technique
- Constipation/Impaction Management
- Diarrhea Management
- Distraction
- Emotional Support
- Flatulence Reduction
- Gastrointestinal Intubation
- Infection Control
- Intravenous (IV) Insertion
- Medication Administration: Intramuscular (IM)
- Medication Administration: Intravenous (IV)
- Medication Administration: Oral
- Medication Administration: Rectal
- Nausea Management
- Nutritional Counseling
- Ostomy Care
- Sedation Management
- Specimen Management
- Surveillance
- Technology Management
- Tube Care: Gastrointestinal
- Vital Signs Monitoring
- Vomiting Management

Genetics Nursing

- Active Listening
- Anticipatory Guidance
- Anxiety Reduction
- Coping Enhancement
- Counseling
- Crisis Intervention
- Documentation
- Emotional Support
- Environmental Management: Community
- Environmental Risk Protection
- Family Integrity Promotion
- Family Mobilization
- Family Support
- Genetic Counseling
- Grief Work Facilitation
- Health Care Information Exchange
- Health Policy Monitoring
- Health Screening
- Laboratory Data Interpretation
- Multidisciplinary Care Conference
- Normalization Promotion
- Parent Education: Infant
- Parent Education: Childrearing Family
- Patient Rights Protection
- Preconception Counseling
- Pregnancy Termination Care
- Referral
- Risk Identification: Genetic
- Support Group
- Teaching: Disease Process
- Values Clarification

Gerontological Nursing

- Abuse Protection Support: Elder
- Active Listening
- Activity Therapy
- Behavior Management
- Bowel Incontinence Care
- Bowel Training
- Caregiver Support
- Case Management
- Communication Enhancement: Hearing Deficit
- Constipation/Impaction Management
- Coping Enhancement
- Delirium Management
- Dementia Management
- Dementia Management: Bathing
- Dressing
- Dying Care
- Emotional Support
- Environmental Management: Comfort
- Environmental Management: Home Preparation
- Exercise Promotion
- Exercise Therapy: Ambulation
- Family Involvement Promotion
- Financial Resource Assistance
- Fluid/Electrolyte Management
- Foot Care
- Grief Work Facilitation
- Hair Care
- Insurance Authorization
- Lower Extremity Monitoring
- Medication Administration
- Nutrition Management
- Patient Rights Protection
- Positioning
- Pressure Management
- Prompted Voiding
- Rectal Prolapse Management
- Reminiscence Therapy
- Respite Care
- Self-Care Assistance
- Self-Care Assistance: IADL
- Telephone Follow-up
- Urinary Habit Training
- Urinary Incontinence Care

Holistic Nursing

- Active Listening
- Acupressure
- Animal-Assisted Therapy
- Anticipatory Guidance
- Anxiety Reduction
- Aromatherapy
- Art Therapy
- Autogenic Training
- Bibliotherapy
- Body Image Enhancement
- Calming Technique
- Caregiver Support
- Cognitive Restructuring
- Coping Enhancement
- Counseling
- Decision-Making Support
- Diet Staging
- Discharge Planning
- Documentation
- Emotional Support
- Energy Management
- Environmental Management
- Exercise Promotion
- Family Involvement Promotion
- Health Education
- Health Screening
- Hope Instillation
- Humor
- Meditation
- Music Therapy
- Mutual Goal Setting
- Nutritional Counseling
- Presence
- Progressive Muscle Relaxation
- Self-Awareness Enhancement
- Self-Esteem Enhancement
- Self-Modification Assistance
- Self-Responsibility Facilitation
- Simple Guided Imagery
- Simple Massage
- Simple Relaxation Therapy
- Spiritual Growth Facilitation
- Spiritual Support
- Teaching: Group
- Teaching: Individual
- Therapeutic Touch
- Touch
- Truth Telling
- Values Clarification

Infection Control and Epidemiological Nursing

- Bioterrorism Preparedness
- Environmental Management: Safety
- Environmental Risk Protection
- Health Education
- Health Policy Monitoring
- Immunization/Vaccination Administration
- Infection Control
- Infection Control: Intraoperative
- Infection Protection
- Latex Precautions
- Learning Facilitation
- Product Evaluation
- Quality Monitoring
- Research Data Collection
- Risk Identification
- Surveillance
- Teaching: Safe Sex

Intravenous Nursing

- Acid-Base Management
- Acid-Base Management: Metabolic Acidosis
- Acid-Base Management: Metabolic Alkalosis
- Acid-Base Management: Respiratory Acidosis
- Acid-Base Management: Respiratory Alkalosis
- Acid-Base Monitoring
- Allergy Management
- Analgesic Administration: Intraspinal
- Blood Products Administration
- Capillary Blood Sample
- Caregiver Support
- Chemotherapy Management
- Dialysis Access Maintenance
- Electrolyte Management
- Electrolyte Management: Hypercalcemia
- Electrolyte Management: Hyperkalemia
- Electrolyte Management: Hypermagnesemia
- Electrolyte Management: Hypernatremia
- Electrolyte Management: Hyperphosphatemia
- Electrolyte Management: Hypocalcemia
- Electrolyte Management: Hypokalemia
- Electrolyte Management: Hypomagnesemia
- Electrolyte Management: Hyponatremia
- Electrolyte Management: Hypophosphatemia
- Electrolyte Monitoring
- Environmental Management: Safety
- Fluid/Electrolyte Management
- Fluid Management
- Fluid Monitoring
- Health Care Information Exchange
- Health Education
- Hyperglycemia Management
- Hypervolemia Management
- Hypothermia Treatment
- Hypovolemia Management
- Incident Reporting
- Infection Control
- Infection Protection
- Intravenous (IV) Insertion
- Intravenous (IV) Therapy
- Invasive Hemodynamic Monitoring
- Laboratory Data Interpretation
- Medication Administration: Enteral
- Medication Administration: Intraosseous
- Medication Administration: Intraspinal
- Medication Administration: Intravenous
- Medication Administration: Ventricular Reservoir
- Nutrition Management
- Nutrition Therapy
- Nutritional Monitoring
- Pain Management
- Patient-Controlled Analgesia (PCA) Assistance
- Peripherally Inserted Central (PIC) Catheter Care
- Peritoneal Dialysis Therapy
- Phlebotomy: Arterial Blood Sample
- Phlebotomy: Blood Unit Acquisition
- Phlebotomy: Cannulated Vessel
- Phlebotomy: Venous Blood Sample
- Product Evaluation
- Quality Monitoring
- Risk Identification
- Supply Management
- Teaching: Prescribed Medication
- Teaching: Procedure/Treatment
- Technology Management
- Total Parenteral Nutrition (TPN) Administration
- Tube Care: Umbilical Line
- Tube Care: Ventriculostomy/Lumbar Drain
- Venous Access Devices (VAD) Maintenance

Medical-Surgical Nursing

- Acid-Base Management
- Airway Suctioning
- Artificial Airway Management
- Aspiration Precautions
- Asthma Management
- Bed Rest Care
- Bleeding Reduction: Gastrointestinal
- Blood Products Administration
- Bowel Incontinence Care
- Bowel Training
- Capillary Blood Sample
- Chemical Restraint
- Chemotherapy Management
- Circulatory Care: Arterial Insufficiency
- Circulatory Care: Venous Insufficiency
- Code Management
- Critical Path Development
- Discharge Planning
- Documentation
- Electrolyte Management
- Emotional Support
- Enteral Tube Feeding
- Fall Prevention
- Family Involvement Promotion
- Family Presence Facilitation
- Fluid/Electrolyte Management
- Gastrointestinal Intubation
- Hyperglycemia Management
- Hypoglycemia Management
- Incision Site Care
- Infection Control
- Intravenous (IV) Insertion
- Intravenous (IV) Therapy
- Laboratory Data Interpretation
- Medication Administration
- Medication Administration: Ear
- Medication Administration: Enteral
- Medication Administration: Eye
- Medication Administration: Nasal
- Medication Administration: Oral
- Medication Administration: Rectal
- Medication Administration: Vaginal
- Medication Management
- Multidisciplinary Care Conference
- Nausea Management
- Neurologic Monitoring
- Nutrition Management
- Ostomy Care
- Oxygen Therapy
- Pain Management
- Patient-Controlled Analgesia (PCA) Assistance
- Patient Rights Protection
- Physical Restraint
- Postmortem Care
- Pressure Management
- Pressure Ulcer Care
- Pressure Ulcer Prevention
- Quality Monitoring
- Respiratory Monitoring
- Seizure Management
- Seizure Precautions
- Self-Care Assistance
- Shock Management
- Shock Prevention
- Skin Surveillance
- Staff Supervision
- Teaching: Disease Process
- Teaching: Individual
- Teaching: Prescribed Medication
- Teaching: Procedure/Treatment
- Total Parenteral Nutrition (TPN) Administration
- Traction/Immobilization Care
- Tube Care: Chest
- Tube Care: Gastrointestinal
- Tube Care: Urinary
- Urinary Elimination Management
- Urinary Incontinence Care
- Vital Signs Monitoring
- Vomiting Management
- Wound Care

Midwifery Nursing

- Abuse Protection Support
- Active Listening
- Admission Care
- Amnioinfusion
- Anticipatory Guidance
- Attachment Promotion
- Birthing
- Breast Examination
- Breastfeeding Assistance
- Childbirth Preparation
- Decision-Making Support
- Delegation
- Discharge Planning
- Documentation
- Emotional Support
- Environmental Management
- Family Integrity Promotion: Childbearing Family
- Family Planning: Contraception
- Family Planning: Unplanned Pregnancy
- Fertility Preservation
- Health Education
- Health Screening
- High-Risk Pregnancy Care
- Hormone Replacement Therapy
- Intrapartal Care
- Lactation Counseling
- Lactation Suppression
- Medication Administration: Intraspinal
- Medication Management
- Medication Prescribing
- Newborn Care
- Nutrition Counseling
- Pain Management
- Parent Education: Infant
- Premenstrual Syndrome Management
- Physician Support
- Postpartal Care
- Referral
- Risk Identification: Childbearing Family
- Sexual Counseling
- Suturing
- Teaching: Individual
- Telephone Consultation

Neonatal Nursing

- Acid-Base Management
- Airway Insertion and Stabilization
- Airway Management
- Airway Suctioning
- Analgesic Administration
- Artificial Airway Management
- Attachment Promotion
- Blood Products Administration
- Bottle Feeding
- Breastfeeding Assistance
- Caregiver Support
- Circumcision Care
- Critical Path Development
- Discharge Planning
- Documentation
- Electrolyte Management
- Electrolyte Management: Hypercalcemia
- Electrolyte Management: Hyperkalemia
- Electrolyte Management: Hypermagnesemia
- Electrolyte Management: Hypernatremia
- Electrolyte Management: Hyperphosphatemia
- Electrolyte Management: Hypocalcemia
- Electrolyte Management: Hypokalemia
- Electrolyte Management: Hypomagnesemia
- Electrolyte Management: Hyponatremia
- Electrolyte Management: Hypophosphatemia
- Endotracheal Extubation
- Enteral Tube Feeding
- Environmental Management
- Environmental Management: Attachment Process
- Environmental Management: Comfort
- Eye Care
- Family Involvement Promotion
- Family Support
- Feeding
- Fluid Management
- Fluid Monitoring
- Health Care Information Exchange
- Hypovolemia Management
- Infant Care
- Infection Protection
- Intravenous (IV) Insertion
- Intravenous (IV) Therapy
- Kangaroo Care
- Laboratory Data Interpretation
- Mechanical Ventilation
- Mechanical Ventilatory Weaning
- Medication Administration
- Medication Administration: Enteral
- Medication Administration: Eye
- Medication Administration: Intramuscular (IM)
- Medication Administration: Intravenous (IV)
- Medication Administration: Oral
- Medication Management
- Multidisciplinary Care Conference
- Newborn Care
- Newborn Monitoring
- Nonnutritive Sucking
- Nutrition Management
- Nutrition Therapy
- Nutritional Monitoring
- Ostomy Care
- Oxygen Therapy
- Pain Management
- Parent Education: Infant
- Phototherapy: Neonate
- Positioning
- Respiratory Monitoring
- Resuscitation
- Resuscitation: Neonate
- Shock Management: Volume
- Sibling Support
- Skin Care: Topical Treatments
- Skin Surveillance
- Sleep Enhancement
- Surveillance
- Technology Management
- Temperature Regulation
- Total Parenteral Nutrition (TPN) Administration
- Transport
- Tube Care: Chest
- Tube Care: Gastrointestinal
- Tube Care: Urinary
- Tube Care: Umbilical Line
- Urinary Catheterization
- Urinary Catheterization: Intermittent
- Venous Access Devices (VAD) Maintenance
- Ventilation Assistance
- Visitation Facilitation
- Vital Signs Monitoring
- Wound Care

Nephrology Nursing

- Acid-Base Management
- Bedside Laboratory Testing
- Bleeding Reduction: Wound
- Capillary Blood Sample
- Case Management
- Constipation/Impaction Management
- Culture Brokerage
- Decision-Making Support
- Delegation
- Dialysis Access Maintenance
- Electrolyte Management
- Electrolyte Monitoring
- Emotional Support
- Environmental Management: Comfort
- Environmental Management: Safety
- Family Involvement Promotion
- Financial Resource Assistance
- Fluid/Electrolyte Management
- Fluid Management
- Fluid Monitoring
- Hemodialysis Therapy
- Hyperglycemia Management
- Hypervolemia Management
- Hypoglycemia Management

- Hypovolemia Management
- Infection Control
- Infection Protection
- Laboratory Data Interpretation
- Medication Administration
- Medication Management
- Multidisciplinary Care Conference
- Nausea Management
- Nutritional Monitoring
- Organ Procurement
- Peritoneal Dialysis Therapy
- Phlebotomy: Cannulated Vessel
- Physician Support
- Pruritus Management
- Specimen Management
- Teaching: Disease Process
- Teaching: Individual
- Teaching: Prescribed Medication
- Teaching: Procedure/Treatment
- Teaching: Psychomotor Skill
- Technology Management
- Telephone Consultation
- Vital Signs Monitoring
- Vomiting Management

Neuroscience Nursing

- Airway Management
- Anxiety Reduction
- Behavior Management
- Body Image Enhancement
- Bowel Management
- Cerebral Edema Management
- Cerebral Perfusion Promotion
- Chemical Restraint
- Cognitive Stimulation
- Communication Enhancement: Speech Deficit
- Communication Enhancement: Visual Deficit
- Delirium Management
- Delusion Management
- Dementia Management
- Dysreflexia Management
- Energy Management
- Environmental Management: Safety
- Fall Prevention
- Intracranial Pressure (ICP) Monitoring

- Medication Administration
- Medication Management
- Neurologic Monitoring
- Pain Management
- Positioning: Neurologic
- Seizure Management
- Seizure Precautions
- Sleep Enhancement
- Subarachnoid Hemorrhage Precautions
- Surveillance
- Swallowing Therapy
- Temperature Regulation
- Transcutaneous Electrical Nerve Stimulation (TENS)
- Tube Care: Ventriculostomy/Lumbar Drain
- Unilateral Neglect Management
- Urinary Catheterization: Intermittent
- Urinary Elimination Management
- Vehicle Safety Promotion

Obstetric Nursing

- Birthing
- Bleeding Reduction: Antepartum Uterus
- Bleeding Reduction: Postpartum Uterus
- Bottle Feeding
- Breastfeeding Assistance
- Cesarean Section Care
- Childbirth Preparation
- Circumcision Care
- Electronic Fetal Monitoring: Antepartum
- Electronic Fetal Monitoring: Intrapartum
- Environmental Management: Attachment Process
- Family Integrity Promotion: Childbearing Family
- Family Planning: Contraception
- Grief Work Facilitation: Perinatal Death
- High-Risk Pregnancy Care
- Intrapartal Care
- Intrapartal Care: High-Risk Delivery
- Invasive Hemodynamic Monitoring
- Labor Induction
- Labor Suppression
- Lactation Counseling
- Medication Administration
- Medication Administration: Intraspinal
- Newborn Care
- Newborn Monitoring
- Pain Management
- Parent Education: Infant
- Parenting Promotion
- Postpartal Care
- Pregnancy Termination Care
- Prenatal Care
- Resuscitation: Fetus
- Resuscitation: Neonate
- Risk Identification: Childbearing Family
- Surveillance: Late Pregnancy

Occupational Health Nursing

- Active Listening
- Allergy Management
- Anticipatory Guidance
- Anxiety Reduction
- Asthma Management
- Bioterrorism Preparedness
- Cardiac Care: Rehabilitative
- Case Management
- Communicable Disease Management
- Counseling
- Crisis Intervention
- Decision-Making Support
- Ear Care
- Emergency Care
- Emotional Support
- Environmental Management: Community
- Environmental Management: Safety
- Environmental Management: Violence Prevention
- Environmental Management: Worker Safety
- Environmental Risk Protection
- Exercise Promotion
- Fall Prevention
- Family Support
- Health Education
- Health Screening
- Health System Guidance
- Immunization/Vaccination Management
- Infection Protection
- Nutritional Counseling
- Parent Education: Adolescent
- Parent Education: Childrearing Family
- Prenatal Care
- Referral
- Respiratory Monitoring
- Risk Identification
- Smoking Cessation Assistance
- Substance Use Prevention
- Substance Use Treatment
- Surveillance: Safety
- Teaching: Group
- Teaching: Individual
- Technology Management
- Telephone Consultation
- Telephone Follow-up
- Transport
- Triage: Disaster
- Vehicle Safety Promotion
- Weight Management
- Weight Reduction Assistance
- Wound Care

Oncology Nursing

- Analgesic Administration
- Anxiety Reduction
- Bleeding Precautions
- Bowel Management
- Caregiver Support
- Chemotherapy Management
- Coping Enhancement
- Dying Care
- Energy Management
- Environmental Management: Comfort
- Family Involvement Promotion
- Fever Treatment
- Financial Resource Assistance
- Fluid Management
- Infection Control
- Infection Protection
- Intravenous (IV) Insertion
- Laboratory Data Interpretation
- Medication Administration
- Medication Management
- Nausea Management
- Nutrition Management
- Nutritional Monitoring
- Pain Management
- Peripheral Sensation Management
- Phlebotomy: Cannulated Vessel
- Preparatory Sensory Information
- Radiation Therapy Management
- Spiritual Support
- Support Group
- Teaching: Disease Process
- Teaching: Procedure/Treatment
- Telephone Follow-up
- Therapeutic Touch
- Urinary Elimination Management
- Venous Access Devices (VAD) Maintenance
- Vomiting Management

Ophthalmic Nursing

- Active Listening
- Communication Enhancement: Visual Deficit
- Consultation
- Contact Lens Care
- Discharge Planning
- Emotional Support
- Eye Care
- Fall Prevention
- Family Involvement Promotion
- Hypoglycemia Management
- Incision Site Care
- Infection Control
- Infection Control: Intraoperative
- Intravenous (IV) Insertion
- Intravenous (IV) Therapy
- Laser Precautions
- Medication Administration
- Medication Administration: Eye
- Medication Administration: Intramuscular
- Medication Administration: Oral
- Preoperative Coordination
- Prosthesis Care
- Sedation Management
- Self-Care Assistance: IADL
- Surgical Assistance
- Surgical Preparation
- Surveillance
- Teaching: Disease Process
- Teaching: Individual
- Teaching: Preoperative
- Teaching: Prescribed Medication
- Teaching: Procedure/Treatment
- Teaching: Psychomotor Skill
- Telephone Follow-up
- Vital Signs Monitoring

Orthopedic Nursing

- Analgesic Administration
- Autotransfusion
- Bathing
- Bed Rest Care
- Blood Products Administration
- Cast Care: Maintenance
- Cast Care: Wet
- Constipation/Impaction Management
- Controlled Substance Checking
- Cough Enhancement
- Critical Path Development
- Delirium Management
- Discharge Planning
- Embolus Care: Peripheral
- Exercise Promotion
- Exercise Therapy: Ambulation
- Exercise Therapy: Joint Mobility
- Fall Prevention
- Heat/Cold Application
- Incision Site Care
- Infection Control
- Intravenous (IV) Insertion
- Intravenous (IV) Therapy
- Lower Extremity Monitoring
- Medication Administration
- Medication Administration: Intramuscular (IM)
- Medication Administration: Intravenous (IV)
- Medication Administration: Oral
- Pain Management
- Patient-Controlled Analgesia (PCA) Assistance
- Physical Restraint
- Positioning
- Preparatory Sensory Information
- Pressure Management
- Prosthesis Care
- Self-Care Assistance
- Self-Care Assistance: IADL
- Self-Care Assistance: Transfer
- Skin Care: Topical Treatments
- Skin Surveillance
- Splinting
- Teaching: Individual
- Teaching: Preoperative
- Teaching: Prescribed Activity/Exercise
- Teaching: Prescribed Medications
- Teaching: Procedure/Treatment
- Traction/Immobilization Care
- Tube Care: Urinary
- Urinary Retention Care
- Wound Care
- Wound Care: Closed Drainage

Otorhinolaryngology and Head/Neck Nursing

- Airway Insertion and Stabilization
- Airway Management
- Airway Suctioning
- Allergy Management
- Analgesic Administration
- Anxiety Reduction
- Artificial Airway Management
- Aspiration Precautions
- Asthma Management
- Bleeding Reduction: Nasal
- Body Image Enhancement
- Chemotherapy Management
- Communication Enhancement: Hearing Deficit
- Communication Enhancement: Speech Deficit
- Critical Path Development
- Discharge Planning
- Ear Care
- Exercise Therapy: Balance
- Infection Control: Intraoperative
- Intracranial Pressure (ICP) Monitoring
- Medication Administration
- Medication Administration: Inhalation
- Medication Administration: Nasal
- Oral Health Maintenance
- Oral Health Promotion
- Oral Health Restoration
- Positioning: Intraoperative
- Postanesthesia Care
- Preoperative Coordination
- Radiation Therapy Management
- Smoking Cessation Assistance
- Surgical Assistance
- Surgical Precautions
- Surgical Preparation
- Swallowing Therapy
- Teaching: Preoperative
- Teaching: Prescribed Activity/Exercise
- Teaching: Prescribed Diet
- Teaching: Prescribed Medication
- Teaching: Procedure/Treatment
- Telephone Consultation
- Tube Care

Pain Management Nursing

- Analgesic Administration
- Analgesic Administration: Intraspinal
- Case Management
- Controlled Substance Checking
- Coping Enhancement
- Decision-Making Support
- Discharge Planning
- Distraction
- Dying Care
- Energy Management
- Environmental Management: Comfort
- Exercise Promotion
- Health Care Information Exchange
- Health Education
- Health Policy Monitoring
- Heat/Cold Application
- Humor
- Infection Control
- Insurance Authorization
- Limit Setting
- Medication Administration
- Medication Administration: Enteral
- Medication Administration: Interpleural
- Medication Administration: Intramuscular (IM)
- Medication Administration: Intraspinal
- Medication Administration: Intravenous (IV)
- Medication Administration: Oral
- Medication Administration: Skin
- Medication Management
- Meditation Facilitation
- Multidisciplinary Care Conference
- Music Therapy
- Mutual Goal Setting
- Pain Management
- Patient Contracting
- Patient-Controlled Analgesia (PCA) Assistance
- Physician Support
- Product Evaluation
- Progressive Muscle Relaxation
- Quality Monitoring
- Referral
- Research Data Collection
- Sedation Management
- Self-Esteem Enhancement
- Simple Guided Imagery
- Simple Massage
- Simple Relaxation Therapy
- Spiritual Support
- Support Group
- Surgical Assistance
- Surgical Preparation
- Surveillance
- Teaching: Prescribed Medication
- Teaching: Procedure/Treatment
- Therapeutic Touch
- Touch
- Transcutaneous Electrical Nerve Stimulation (TENS)
- Venous Access Devices (VAD) Maintenance

Parish Nursing

- Abuse Protection Support: Religious
- Active Listening
- Anticipatory Guidance
- Caregiver Support
- Coping Enhancement
- Crisis Intervention
- Culture Brokerage
- Decision-Making Support
- Emotional Support
- Environmental Management-Community
- Family Integrity Promotion
- Family Support
- Forgiveness Facilitation
- Grief Work Facilitation
- Guilt Work Facilitation
- Health Education
- Health Information Exchange
- Health System Guidance
- Hope Instillation
- Humor
- Presence
- Referral
- Religious Addiction Prevention
- Religious Ritual Enhancement
- Relocation Stress Reduction
- Socialization Enhancement
- Self-Care Assistance: IADL
- Spiritual Growth Facilitation
- Spiritual Support
- Surveillance
- Sustenance Support
- Teaching: Group
- Teaching: Individual
- Telephone Consultation
- Touch
- Values Clarification

Pediatric Nursing

- Abuse Protection Support: Child
- Asthma Management
- Breastfeeding Assistance
- Caregiver Support
- Developmental Care
- Developmental Enhancement: Child
- Discharge Planning
- Documentation
- Emotional Support
- Environmental Management: Safety
- Family Involvement Promotion
- Family Presence Facilitation
- Feeding
- Fever Treatment
- Fluid/Electrolyte Management
- Health Education
- Immunization/Vaccination Management
- Infant Care
- Intravenous (IV) Therapy
- Medication Administration
- Multidisciplinary Care Conference
- Normalization Promotion
- Nutrition Management
- Oxygen Therapy
- Pain Management
- Parent Education: Adolescent
- Parent Education: Childbearing Family
- Parent Education: Infant
- Parenting Promotion
- Respiratory Monitoring
- Risk Identification
- Risk Identification: Genetic
- Sports-Injury Prevention: Youth
- Surveillance
- Teaching: Infant Stimulation
- Teaching: Toilet Training
- Technology Management
- Therapeutic Play
- Total Parenteral Nutrition (TPN) Administration
- Trauma Therapy: Child
- Vehicle Safety Promotion
- Vital Signs Monitoring

Pediatric Oncology Nursing

- Active Listening
- Analgesic Administration
- Anxiety Reduction
- Bleeding Precautions
- Blood Products Administration
- Calming Technique
- Caregiver Support
- Case Management
- Chemotherapy Management
- Coping Enhancement
- Decision-Making Support
- Developmental Enhancement: Child
- Dying Care
- Family Integrity Promotion
- Family Involvement Promotion
- Family Mobilization
- Family Presence Facilitation
- Family Process Maintenance
- Fever Treatment
- Fluid/Electrolyte Management
- Grief Work Facilitation
- Hope Instillation
- Infection Protection
- Medication Administration: Intramuscular (IM)
- Medication Administration: Intravenous (IV)
- Medication Administration: Oral
- Multidisciplinary Care Conference
- Nausea Management
- Normalization Promotion
- Pain Management
- Parent Education: Childrearing Family
- Radiation Therapy Management
- Sedation Management
- Sibling Support
- Teaching: Disease Process
- Teaching: Prescribed Medication
- Therapeutic Play
- Total Parenteral Nutrition (TPN) Administration
- Trauma Therapy: Child
- Venous Access Device (VAD) Maintenance
- Vomiting Management

Perioperative Nursing

- Active Listening
- Anaphylaxis Management
- Anxiety Reduction
- Autotransfusion
- Blood Products Administration
- Critical Path Development
- Delegation
- Discharge Planning
- Documentation
- Electrolyte Management
- Emotional Support
- Environmental Management: Comfort
- Environmental Management: Safety
- Environmental Management: Worker Safety
- Fluid Monitoring
- Infection Control: Intraoperative
- Laser Precautions
- Latex Precautions
- Malignant Hyperthermia Precautions
- Patient Rights Protection
- Physician Support
- Pneumatic Tourniquet Precautions
- Positioning: Intraoperative
- Postanesthesia Care
- Preceptor: Employee
- Preoperative Coordination
- Presence
- Pressure Management
- Product Evaluation
- Quality Monitoring
- Sedation Management
- Self-Care Assistance: Transfer
- Skin Care: Donor Site
- Skin Care: Graft Site
- Skin Surveillance
- Specimen Management
- Supply Management
- Surgical Assistance
- Surgical Precautions
- Surgical Preparation
- Surveillance: Safety
- Suturing
- Teaching: Preoperative
- Technology Management
- Temperature Regulation: Intraoperative
- Touch
- Transport
- Vital Signs Monitoring
- Wound Care

Psychiatric/Mental Health Nursing

- Abuse Protection Support
- Active Listening
- Anger Control Assistance
- Anxiety Reduction
- Area Restriction
- Assertiveness Training
- Behavior Management: Overactivity/Inattention
- Behavior Management: Self-Harm
- Behavior Management: Sexual
- Behavior Modification
- Behavior Modification: Social Skills
- Body Image Enhancement
- Calming Technique
- Case Management
- Chemical Restraint
- Cognitive Restructuring
- Complex Relationship Building
- Consultation
- Coping Enhancement
- Counseling
- Crisis Intervention
- Delusion Management
- Dementia Management
- Dementia Management: Bathing
- Eating Disorders Management
- Electroconvulsive Therapy Management
- Elopement Precautions
- Environmental Management: Violence Prevention
- Family Involvement Promotion
- Family Therapy
- Fire Safety Precautions
- Grief Work Facilitation
- Guilt Work Facilitation
- Hallucination Management
- Impulse Control Training
- Limit Setting
- Medication Administration
- Medication Management
- Milieu Therapy
- Mood Management
- Phototherapy: Mood/Sleep Regulation
- Physical Restraint
- Reality Orientation
- Reminiscence Therapy
- Seclusion
- Self-Awareness Enhancement
- Self-Care Assistance: IADL
- Self-Esteem Enhancement
- Substance Use Prevention
- Substance Use Treatment: Alcohol Withdrawal
- Substance Use Treatment: Drug Withdrawal
- Suicide Prevention
- Support Group
- Therapeutic Play
- Therapy Group

Radiological Nursing

- Airway Management
- Airway Suctioning
- Allergy Management
- Analgesic Administration
- Anxiety Reduction
- Aspiration Precautions
- Bleeding Precautions
- Bleeding Reduction
- Blood Products Administration
- Calming Technique
- Cardiac Precautions
- Cerebral Perfusion Promotion
- Circulatory Precautions
- Code Management
- Discharge Planning
- Dysrhythmia Management
- Embolus Care: Peripheral
- Embolus Care: Pulmonary
- Embolus Precautions
- Emergency Care
- Emergency Cart Checking
- Emotional Support
- Environmental Management: Safety
- Examination Assistance
- Fluid/Electrolyte Management
- Fluid Management
- Fluid Monitoring
- Fluid Resuscitation
- Health Care Information Exchange
- Health Screening
- Hemorrhage Control
- Incident Reporting
- Infection Control
- Infection Protection
- Intravenous (IV) Insertion
- Intravenous (IV) Therapy
- Laser Precautions
- Latex Precautions
- Medication Administration
- Medication Administration: Intravenous (IV)
- Neurologic Monitoring
- Oxygen Therapy
- Pain Management
- Preparatory Sensory Information
- Quality Monitoring
- Radiation Therapy Management
- Referral
- Research Data Collection
- Respiratory Monitoring
- Resuscitation
- Security Enhancement
- Sedation Management
- Shock Prevention
- Simple Relaxation Therapy
- Smoking Cessation Assistance
- Staff Supervision
- Teaching: Individual
- Teaching: Procedure/Treatment
- Technology Management
- Telephone Consultation
- Touch
- Transport
- Tube Care
- Tube Care: Chest
- Tube Care: Gastrointestinal
- Tube Care: Urinary
- Urinary Catheterization
- Ventilation Assistance
- Vital Signs Monitoring

Rehabilitation Nursing

- Amputation Care
- Behavior Management
- Body Image Enhancement
- Body Mechanics Promotion
- Bowel Management
- Case Management
- Communication Enhancement: Speech Deficit
- Coping Enhancement
- Decision-Making Support
- Discharge Planning
- Dressing
- Embolus Precautions
- Emotional Support
- Energy Management
- Environmental Management: Safety
- Environmental Management: Home Preparation
- Exercise Promotion: Strength Training
- Family Involvement Promotion
- Family Support
- Financial Resource Assistance
- Health Education
- Learning Facilitation
- Medication Management
- Memory Training
- Multidisciplinary Care Conference
- Mutual Goal Setting
- Normalization Promotion
- Nutrition Management
- Pain Management
- Positioning
- Pressure Ulcer Care
- Pressure Ulcer Prevention
- Relocation Stress Reduction
- Self-Care Assistance
- Self-Care Assistance: IADL
- Self-Responsibility Facilitation
- Socialization Enhancement
- Swallowing Therapy
- Teaching: Individual
- Unilateral Neglect Management
- Urinary Elimination Management

School Nursing

- Abuse Protection Support: Child
- Active Listening
- Allergy Management
- Analgesic Administration
- Anger Control Assistance
- Anticipatory Guidance
- Anxiety Reduction
- Asthma Management
- Bleeding Reduction
- Bleeding Reduction: Wound
- Calming Technique
- Caregiver Support
- Contact Lens Care
- Coping Enhancement
- Counseling
- Crisis Intervention
- Decision-Making Support
- Delegation
- Documentation
- Emergency Care
- Emotional Support
- Eye Care
- Family Integrity Promotion
- Family Involvement Promotion
- Family Support
- Fever Treatment
- First Aid
- Grief Work Facilitation
- Health Care Information Exchange
- Health Education
- Health Screening
- Health System Guidance
- Heat/Cold Application
- Humor
- Infection Control
- Learning Facilitation
- Learning Readiness Enhancement
- Medication Administration: Oral
- Medication Management
- Multidisciplinary Care Conference
- Nutritional Counseling
- Pain Management
- Parent Education: Adolescent
- Parent Education: Childrearing Family
- Patient Rights Protection
- Referral
- Resiliency Promotion
- Self-Esteem Enhancement
- Skin Surveillance
- Socialization Enhancement
- Spiritual Support
- Sports-Injury Prevention: Youth
- Substance Use Prevention
- Suicide Prevention
- Support Group
- Teaching: Individual
- Telephone Consultation
- Touch
- Values Clarification
- Vehicle Safety Promotion
- Vital Signs Monitoring
- Wound Care

Spinal Cord Injury Nursing

- Active Listening
- Airway Suctioning
- Artificial Airway Management
- Behavior Management
- Body Image Enhancement
- Bowel Management
- Bowel Training
- Caregiver Support
- Case Management
- Chest Physiotherapy
- Circulatory Care
- Coping Enhancement
- Discharge Planning
- Dysreflexia Management
- Emotional Support
- Family Involvement Promotion
- Financial Resource Assistance
- Fluid Management
- Health Care Information Exchange
- Infection Protection
- Lower Extremity Monitoring
- Mechanical Ventilation
- Medication Management
- Multidisciplinary Care Conference
- Mutual Goal Setting
- Nutrition Management
- Pain Management
- Pass Facilitation
- Peripheral Sensation Management
- Positioning
- Positioning: Wheelchair
- Pressure Ulcer Care
- Pressure Ulcer Prevention
- Relocation Stress Reduction
- Self-Care Assistance: Bathing/Hygiene
- Self-Care Assistance: Dressing/Grooming
- Self-Care Assistance: Feeding
- Self-Care Assistance: IADL
- Self-Care Assistance: Toileting
- Self-Care Assistance: Transfer
- Teaching: Disease Process
- Teaching: Group
- Teaching: Individual
- Teaching: Prescribed Medication
- Teaching: Psychomotor Skill
- Traction/Immobilization Care
- Tube Care: Urinary
- Urinary Bladder Training
- Urinary Catheterization
- Urinary Catheterization: Intermittent

Urologic Nursing

- Active Listening
- Analgesic Administration
- Behavior Modification
- Biofeedback
- Bladder Irrigation
- Body Image Enhancement
- Caregiver Support
- Case Management
- Chemotherapy Management
- Dialysis Access Maintenance
- Fluid/Electrolyte Management
- Infection Control: Intraoperative
- Intravenous (IV) Therapy
- Latex Precautions
- Medication Administration
- Medication Management
- Ostomy Care
- Pelvic Muscle Exercise
- Pessary Management
- Positioning: Intraoperative
- Preoperative Coordination
- Preparatory Sensory Information
- Prompted Voiding
- Specimen Management
- Surgical Assistance
- Surgical Precautions
- Surgical Preparation
- Teaching: Disease Process
- Teaching: Individual
- Teaching: Preoperative
- Teaching: Prescribed Medication
- Teaching: Procedure/Treatment
- Temperature Regulation: Intraoperative
- Tube Care
- Tube Care: Urinary
- Urinary Bladder Training
- Urinary Catheterization
- Urinary Catheterization: Intermittent
- Urinary Elimination Management
- Urinary Habit Training
- Urinary Incontinence Care
- Urinary Retention Care

Vascular Nursing

- Amputation Care
- Circulatory Care: Arterial Insufficiency
- Circulatory Care: Venous Insufficiency
- Circulatory Precautions
- Discharge Planning
- Embolus Care: Peripheral
- Embolus Care: Pulmonary
- Embolus Precautions
- Exercise Promotion: Strength Training
- Exercise Therapy: Ambulation
- Exercise Therapy: Joint Mobility
- Exercise Therapy: Muscle Control
- Foot Care
- Grief Work Facilitation
- Health Screening
- Incision Site Care
- Infection Protection
- Leech Therapy
- Lower Extremity Monitoring
- Medication Management
- Nail Care
- Nutrition Management
- Pain Management
- Peripheral Sensation Management
- Pressure Ulcer Care
- Pressure Ulcer Prevention
- Prosthesis Care
- Risk Identification
- Self-Care Assistance
- Skin Care: Donor Site
- Skin Care: Graft Site
- Skin Care: Topical Treatments
- Smoking Cessation Assistance
- Teaching: Foot Care
- Teaching: Individual
- Teaching: Prescribed Activity/Exercise
- Unilateral Neglect Management
- Wound Care

Women's Health Nursing

- Abuse Protection Support
- Abuse Protection Support: Domestic Partner
- Anticipatory Guidance
- Behavior Modification
- Body Image Enhancement
- Breast Examination
- Coping Enhancement
- Counseling
- Decision-Making Support
- Emotional Support
- Exercise Promotion
- Family Planning: Contraception
- Family Planning: Infertility
- Family Planning: Unplanned Pregnancy
- Fertility Preservation
- Health Education
- Health Screening
- Health System Guidance
- Hormone Replacement Therapy
- Medication Management
- Nutritional Counseling
- Pelvic Muscle Exercise
- Pessary Management
- Preconception Counseling
- Pregnancy Termination Care
- Premenstrual Syndrome Management
- Risk Identification
- Teaching: Disease Process
- Teaching: Individual
- Teaching: Safe Sex
- Telephone Consultation
- Urinary Bladder Training
- Weight Management
- Weight Reduction Assistance

PART SIX

Estimated Time and Education Level Necessary to Perform NIC Interventions

Estimated Time and Education Level Necessary to Perform NIC Interventions

In this section we list the estimated time to perform and type of personnel required to deliver each of the 514 interventions. The material included here is an update of a previously prepared monograph entitled, *Estimated Time and Educational Requirements to Perform 486 Nursing Interventions*,[2] published by the Center for Nursing Classification and Clinical Effectiveness at the College of Nursing, the University of Iowa. An earlier draft of portions of the monograph was published in *Nursing Economic$* ("Determining Cost of Nursing Interventions: A Beginning").[3]

METHODOLOGY

Step One: The 433 interventions included in the second edition of *Nursing Interventions Classification (NIC)* were rated in 1999 in response to a request from a user who was incorporating NIC into a coding/reimbursement manual.[1] Small groups of research team members rated selected interventions in their area of expertise on (1) education needed for each intervention and (2) time needed for each intervention. Rating group members referred to the second edition of NIC[4] for intervention definitions and activities. Each group of raters returned their work to the principal investigators who, with two other members of the research team, reviewed all of the ratings for all interventions for overall consistency.

Step Two: In fall 2000, ratings were done by using the same method for the 53 interventions new to the third edition of NIC published in 2000.[5] Changes in interventions from the second to third edition were also examined for their impact on the ratings. Following this, all 486 intervention ratings were reviewed together, and a few of these were modified to be consistent with others in the same class. This information was published in monograph form.[2]

Step Three: In 2002, during the manuscript preparation for this edition, we estimated the time and education for each of the 29 new interventions in this edition and revised the tables, adding the new interventions and deleting one old intervention, and we also made some other minor modifications.

An example of the instructions and rating form are included in Figures 1 and 2.

Education needed was defined as the *minimal* educational level necessary to perform the intervention in most cases in most states and rated as (a) nursing assistant/LPN/LVN/technician; (b) RN (basic education, whether baccalaureate, AD, or diploma); or (c) RN with post-basic education or certification. Post-basic education was defined as specialized education or training beyond the RN basic education, including master's degree with or without certification or short course leading to certificate or certification. These categories were arrived at after thorough discussion. They were chosen over other possibilities because it was believed that the categories allowed raters to discriminate among them but were not so fine that raters could not be consistent. The basic types of RN preparation were grouped in one category because this reflects the reality of the practice situation, which does not usually differentiate job responsibilities by educational preparation of the RN.

Time needed was defined as the average time needed to perform the intervention. Raters were asked to identify an average time that could be used to determine reimbursement rates—long

Check only one box in each area.

Education Needed: What is the *minimal* educational level necessary to perform the intervention? (This means that all or the vast majority of the activities can be done by the person indicated.) RN license includes associate's degree, diploma, baccalaureate. Post-basic means specialized education or training beyond any one of these educational preparations. This could include a master's degree with or without certification or a short course that leads to a certificate or certification. The indication of only 3 categories is not a very sensitive measure but it is not possible (or desirable) at this time to make any finer judgment. Also, think "in most cases in most states." There may be regional or state differences but that will be up to the insurance people to determine.

Time Needed: Think about the average time needed to perform the intervention—when you do the intervention how long, on average, does it take each time? While time may vary by patients and nurses and the specialty, these differences are unknown for now and averages will be used. We need some starting point—an average time that can be used to determine reimbursement rates. We want to make it long enough so that it can be done but not so long that it prices the intervention too high. The more time that is checked will result in a higher price for the insurance company/client.

Fig. 1 Instructions for education and time needed for each intervention.

enough that the intervention could be done but not so long that it would price the intervention unreasonably high for insurance or client payment. Raters selected one of five possible time estimates: (a) 15 minutes or less; (b) 16 to 30 minutes; (c) 31 to 45 minutes; (d) 46 to 60 minutes; and (e) more than 1 hour.

RESULTS

Table 1 lists time and education requirements as judged by raters for all 514 interventions listed alphabetically. This table can be used to look up the time or education requirements for any one of the interventions.

Tables 2 and 3 focus on education requirements. Table 2 lists the interventions appropriate for delegation to a nursing assistant (depending on the patient, setting, and care provider), and Table 3 lists interventions that are appropriate for RNs with post-basic education. These tables are organized by the seven NIC domains and classes.

Tables 4, 5, 6, 7, and 8 focus on the time requirements and list interventions according to each of the five time periods: 15 minutes or less (Table 4), 16 to 30 minutes (Table 5), 31 to 45 minutes (Table 6), 46 to 60 minutes (Table 7), and more than 1 hour (Table 8). Table 9 provides a summary of the number of interventions in each of the time periods and demonstrates that each category has a good number of interventions. Nearly 21% of the 514 interventions were judged to take less than 15 minutes to perform and 21% were judged to take more than 1 hour to perform.

SUMMARY

This part lists beginning estimates of time and education level necessary to perform the 514 interventions included in this edition of the Classification. It is emphasized that the estimates are based on judgments of those who are familiar with the intervention and the specialty practice area. The ratings included here may differ by practice facility and provider. The estimates provide a starting point for estimating time required, level of provider education needed, and cost of nursing care.

PHYSIOLOGICAL BASIC: Activity and Exercise Enhancement

Body Mechanics Promotion
   Education Needed (check one)   **Time Needed (check one)**
   Nursing assistant/LPN/LVN/technician   15 minutes or less
                                        16-30 minutes
   RN (basic education either bacc., AD, dip.)   31-45 minutes
                                        46-60 minutes
   RN with post-basic education or certification Over 1 hour

Energy Management
   Education Needed (check one)   **Time Needed (check one)**
   Nursing assistant/LPN/LVN/technician   15 minutes or less
                                        16-30 minutes
   RN (basic education either bacc., AD, dip.)   31-45 minutes
                                        46-60 minutes
   RN with post-basic education or certification Over 1 hour

Exercise Promotion
   Education Needed (check one)   **Time Needed (check one)**
   Nursing assistant/LPN/LVN/technician   15 minutes or less
                                        16-30 minutes
   RN (basic education either bacc., AD, dip.)   31-45 minutes
                                        46-60 minutes
   RN with post-basic education or certification Over 1 hour

Exercise Therapy: Ambulation
   Education Needed (check one)   **Time Needed (check one)**
   Nursing assistant/LPN/LVN/technician   15 minutes or less
                                        16-30 minutes
   RN (basic education either bacc., AD, dip.)   31-45 minutes
                                        46-60 minutes
   RN with post-basic education or certification Over 1 hour

© Center for Nursing Classification, 2000

Fig. 2 Example of rating form. (Estimates were made on this form for NIC interventions within the Activity and Exercise Enhancement taxonomic class of the Physiological: Basic domain).*(Copyright-Center for Nursing Classification and Clinical Effectiveness, 2000. Used with permission.)*

References

1. Alternative Link, Inc. *CAM and Nursing Coding Manual©*. (2001). Las Cruces, NM: Author.
2. Center for Nursing Classification. (2001). *Estimated time and educational requirements to perform 486 nursing interventions*. Iowa City, IA: Author.
3. Iowa Intervention Project. (2001). Determining cost of nursing interventions: A beginning, *Nursing Economic$, 19(4)*, 146-160.
4. McCloskey, J. C., & Bulechek, G. M. (Eds.). (1996). *Nursing interventions classification (NIC)* (2nd ed.). St. Louis, MO: Mosby.
5. McCloskey, J. C., & Bulechek, G. M. (Eds.). (2000). *Nursing interventions classification (NIC)* (3rd ed.). St. Louis, MO: Mosby.

Table 1	TIME AND EDUCATION FOR **514 NIC** INTERVENTIONS LISTED ALPHABETICALLY		
Intervention	**Code No.**	**Educational Level**	**Time Required**
Abuse Protection Support	6400	RN basic	More than 1 hr
Abuse Protection Support: Child	6402	RN basic	More than 1 hr
Abuse Protection Support: Domestic Partner	6403	RN basic	More than 1 hr
Abuse Protection Support: Elder	6404	RN basic	More than 1 hr
Abuse Protection Support: Religious	6408	RN basic	More than 1 hr
Acid-Base Management	1910	RN basic	More than 1 hr
Acid-Base Management: Metabolic Acidosis	1911	RN basic	31-45 min
Acid-Base Management: Metabolic Alkalosis	1912	RN basic	31-45 min
Acid-Base Management: Respiratory Acidosis	1913	RN basic	31-45 min
Acid-Base Management: Respiratory Alkalosis	1914	RN basic	31-45 min
Acid-Base Monitoring	1920	RN basic	15 min or less
Active Listening	4920	RN basic	16-30 min
Activity Therapy	4310	RN basic	46-60 min
Acupressure	1320	RN post basic	16-30 min
Admission Care	7310	RN basic	16-30 min
Airway Insertion and Stabilization	3120	RN basic	16-30 min
Airway Management	3140	RN basic	16-30 min
Airway Suctioning	3160	RN basic	15 min or less
Allergy Management	6410	RN basic	31-45 min
Amnioinfusion	6700	RN post basic	31-45 min
Amputation Care	3420	RN basic	31-45 min
Analgesic Administration	2210	RN basic	16-30 min
Analgesic Administration: Intraspinal	2214	RN post basic	16-30 min
Anaphylaxis Management	6412	RN basic	46-60 min
Anesthesia Administration	2840	RN post basic	More than 1 hr
Anger Control Assistance	4640	RN post basic	16-30 min
Animal-Assisted Therapy	4320	Nursing assistant	16-30 min
Anticipatory Guidance	5210	RN basic	31-45 min

Table 1	TIME AND EDUCATION FOR 514 NIC INTERVENTIONS LISTED ALPHABETICALLY—CONT'D		
Intervention	**Code No.**	**Educational Level**	**Time Required**
Anxiety Reduction	5820	Nursing assistant	31-45 min
Area Restriction	6420	Nursing assistant	More than 1 hr
Aromatherapy	1330	RN basic	15 min or less
Art Therapy	4330	RN post basic	46-60 min
Artificial Airway Management	3180	RN basic	15 min or less
Aspiration Precautions	3200	Nursing assistant	15 min or less
Assertiveness Training	4340	RN basic	46-60 min
Asthma Management	3210	RN basic	16-30 min
Attachment Promotion	6710	RN basic	More than 1 hr
Autogenic Training	5840	RN post basic	46-60 min
Autotransfusion	2860	RN basic	46-60 min
Bathing	1610	Nursing assistant	16-30 min
Bed Rest Care	740	Nursing assistant	16-30 min
Bedside Laboratory Testing	7610	Nursing assistant	15 min or less
Behavior Management	4350	RN basic	46-60 min
Behavior Management: Overactivity/Inattention	4352	RN basic	31-45 min
Behavior Management: Self-Harm	4354	RN basic	31-45 min
Behavior Management: Sexual	4356	RN basic	31-45 min
Behavior Modification	4360	RN basic	More than 1 hr
Behavior Modification: Social Skills	4362	RN basic	More than 1 hr
Bibliotherapy	4680	RN post basic	46-60 min
Biofeedback	5860	RN post basic	46-60 min
Bioterrorism Preparedness	8810	RN post basic	More than 1 hr
Birthing	6720	RN post basic	More than 1 hr
Bladder Irrigation	550	RN basic	16-30 min
Bleeding Precautions	4010	RN basic	31-45 min
Bleeding Reduction	4020	RN basic	46-60 min
Bleeding Reduction: Antepartum Uterus	4021	RN basic	46-60 minutes

Continued

Table 1	TIME AND EDUCATION FOR 514 NIC INTERVENTIONS LISTED ALPHABETICALLY—CONT'D		
Intervention	**Code No.**	**Educational Level**	**Time Required**
Bleeding Reduction: Gastrointestinal	4022	RN basic	46-60 min
Bleeding Reduction: Nasal	4024	RN basic	16-30 min
Bleeding Reduction: Postpartum Uterus	4026	RN basic	46-60 min
Bleeding Reduction: Wound	4028	RN basic	46-60 min
Blood Products Administration	4030	RN basic	More than 1 hr
Body Image Enhancement	5220	RN basic	31-45 min
Body Mechanics Promotion	140	RN basic	16-30 min
Bottle Feeding	1052	Nursing assistant	31-45 min
Bowel Incontinence Care	410	RN basic	16-30 min
Bowel Incontinence Care: Encopresis	412	RN basic	16-30 min
Bowel Irrigation	420	RN basic	16-30 min
Bowel Management	430	RN basic	31-45 min
Bowel Training	440	RN basic	16-30 min
Breast Examination	6522	RN basic	15 min or less
Breastfeeding Assistance	1054	RN basic	16-30 min
Calming Technique	5880	Nursing assistant	31-45 min
Capillary Blood Sample	4035	RN basic	15 min or less
Cardiac Care	4040	RN basic	31-45 min
Cardiac Care: Acute	4044	RN basic	31-45 min
Cardiac Care: Rehabilitative	4046	RN basic	More than 1 hr
Cardiac Precautions	4050	RN basic	31-45 min
Caregiver Support	7040	RN basic	More than 1 hr
Case Management	7320	RN post basic	More than 1 hr
Cast Care: Maintenance	762	Nursing assistant	15 min or less
Cast Care: Wet	764	RN basic	16-30 min
Cerebral Edema Management	2540	RN basic	More than 1 hr
Cerebral Perfusion Promotion	2550	RN basic	31-45 min
Cesarean Section Care	6750	RN basic	31-45 min

Table 1	TIME AND EDUCATION FOR 514 NIC INTERVENTIONS LISTED ALPHABETICALLY—CONT'D		
Intervention	**Code No.**	**Educational Level**	**Time Required**
Chemical Restraint	6430	RN basic	15 min or less
Chemotherapy Management	2240	RN post basic	46-60 min
Chest Physiotherapy	3230	RN basic	16-30 min
Childbirth Preparation	6760	RN basic	More than 1 hr
Circulatory Care: Arterial Insufficiency	4062	RN basic	15 min or less
Circulatory Care: Mechanical Assist Device	4064	RN basic	31-45 min
Circulatory Care: Venous Insufficiency	4066	RN basic	15 min or less
Circulatory Precautions	4070	RN basic	16-30 min
Circumcision Care	3000	RN basic	46-60 min
Code Management	6140	RN basic	31-45 min
Cognitive Restructuring	4700	RN post basic	16-30 min
Cognitive Stimulation	4720	RN post basic	16-30 min
Communicable Disease Management	8820	RN basic	46-60 min
Communication Enhancement: Hearing	4974	Nursing assistant	16-30 min
Communication Enhancement: Speech Deficit	4976	RN basic	31-45 min
Communication Enhancement: Visual Deficit	4978	Nursing assistant	16-30 min
Community Disaster Preparedness	8840	RN basic	More than 1 hr
Community Health Development	8500	RN basic	More than 1 hr
Complex Relationship Building	5000	RN basic	More than 1 hr
Conflict Mediation	5020	RN post basic	46-60 min
Constipation/Impaction Management	450	RN basic	16-30 min
Consultation	7910	RN basic	46-60 min
Contact Lens Care	1620	Nursing assistant	15 min or less
Controlled Substance Checking	7620	RN basic	15 min or less
Coping Enhancement	5230	RN basic	31-45 min
Cost Containment	7630	RN basic	31-45 min
Cough Enhancement	3250	Nursing assistant	15 min or less

Continued

Table 1	TIME AND EDUCATION FOR 514 NIC INTERVENTIONS LISTED ALPHABETICALLY—CONT'D		
Intervention	Code No.	Educational Level	Time Required
Counseling	5240	RN post basic	46-60 min
Crisis Intervention	6160	RN post basic	46-60 min
Critical Path Development	7640	RN basic	More than 1 hr
Culture Brokerage	7330	RN basic	16-30 min
Cutaneous Stimulation	1340	RN basic	16-30 min
Decision-Making Support	5250	RN basic	16-30 min
Delegation	7650	RN basic	15 min or less
Delirium Management	6440	RN basic	More than 1 hr
Delusion Management	6450	RN basic	More than 1 hr
Dementia Management	6460	RN basic	More than 1 hr
Dementia Management: Bathing	6462	Nursing assistant	31-45 min
Deposition/Testimony	7930	RN basic	More than 1 hr
Developmental Care	8250	RN basic	46-60 min
Developmental Enhancement: Adolescent	8272	RN basic	46-60 min
Developmental Enhancement: Child	8274	RN basic	46-60 min
Dialysis Access Maintenance	4240	RN basic	15 min or less
Diarrhea Management	460	RN basic	15 min or less
Diet Staging	1020	RN basic	15 min or less
Discharge Planning	7370	RN basic	46-60 min
Distraction	5900	Nursing assistant	31-45 min
Documentation	7920	RN basic	15 min or less
Dressing	1630	Nursing assistant	15 min or less
Dying Care	5260	RN basic	16-30 min
Dysreflexia Management	2560	RN basic	16-30 min
Dysrhythmia Management	4090	RN basic	16-30 min
Ear Care	1640	RN basic	16-30 min
Eating Disorders Management	1030	RN post basic	31-45 min
Electroconvulsive Therapy (ECT) Management	2570	RN basic	More than 1 hr

Table 1	TIME AND EDUCATION FOR 514 NIC INTERVENTIONS LISTED ALPHABETICALLY—CONT'D		
Intervention	**Code No.**	**Educational Level**	**Time Required**
Electrolyte Management	2000	RN basic	31-45 min
Electrolyte Management: Hypercalcemia	2001	RN basic	16-30 min
Electrolyte Management: Hyperkalemia	2002	RN basic	16-30 min
Electrolyte Management: Hypermagnesemia	2003	RN basic	16-30 min
Electrolyte Management: Hypernatremia	2004	RN basic	16-30 min
Electrolyte Management: Hyperphosphatemia	2005	RN basic	16-30 min
Electrolyte Management: Hypocalcemia	2006	RN basic	16-30 min
Electrolyte Management: Hypokalemia	2007	RN basic	16-30 min
Electrolyte Management: Hypomagnesemia	2008	RN basic	16-30 min
Electrolyte Management: Hyponatremia	2009	RN basic	16-30 min
Electrolyte Management: Hypophosphatemia	2010	RN basic	16-30 min
Electrolyte Monitoring	2020	RN basic	15 min or less
Electronic Fetal Monitoring: Antepartum	6771	RN post basic	More than 1 hr
Electronic Fetal Monitoring: Intrapartum	6772	RN post basic	More than 1 hr
Elopement Precautions	6470	Nursing assistant	More than 1 hr
Embolus Care: Peripheral	4104	RN basic	16-30 min
Embolus Care: Pulmonary	4106	RN basic	16-30 min
Embolus Precautions	4110	RN basic	16-30 min
Emergency Care	6200	Nursing assistant	16-30 min
Emergency Cart Checking	7660	Nursing assistant	15 min or less
Emotional Support	5270	RN basic	16-30 min
Endotracheal Extubation	3270	RN basic	15 min or less
Energy Management	180	RN basic	16-30 min
Enteral Tube Feeding	1056	RN basic	16-30 min
Environmental Management	6480	Nursing assistant	31-45 min
Environmental Management: Attachment Process	6481	Nursing assistant	16-30 min
Environmental Management: Comfort	6482	Nursing assistant	15 min or less

Continued

Table 1		TIME AND EDUCATION FOR **514 NIC** INTERVENTIONS LISTED ALPHABETICALLY—CONT'D	
Intervention	Code No.	Educational Level	Time Required
Environmental Management: Community	6484	RN basic	More than 1 hr
Environmental Management: Home Preparation	6485	RN basic	More than 1 hr
Environmental Management: Safety	6486	RN basic	31-45 min
Environmental Management: Violence Prevention	6487	Nursing assistant	More than 1 hr
Environmental Management: Worker Safety	6489	RN basic	More than 1 hr
Environmental Risk Protection	8880	RN basic	46-60 min
Examination Assistance	7680	Nursing assistant	16-30 min
Exercise Promotion	200	RN basic	31-45 min
Exercise Promotion: Strength Training	201	RN basic	31-45 min
Exercise Promotion: Stretching	202	RN basic	31-45 min
Exercise Therapy: Ambulation	221	Nursing assistant	15 min or less
Exercise Therapy: Balance	222	RN basic	16-30 min
Exercise Therapy: Joint Mobility	224	RN basic	16-30 min
Exercise Therapy: Muscle Control	226	RN post basic	16-30 min
Eye Care	1650	RN basic	15 min or less
Fall Prevention	6490	RN basic	More than 1 hr
Family Integrity Promotion	7100	RN basic	More than 1 hr
Family Integrity Promotion: Childbearing Family	7104	RN basic	More than 1 hr
Family Involvement Promotion	7110	RN basic	More than 1 hr
Family Mobilization	7120	RN basic	More than 1 hr
Family Planning: Contraception	6784	RN basic	31-45 min
Family Planning: Infertility	6786	RN post basic	46-60 min
Family Planning: Unplanned Pregnancy	6788	RN basic	46-60 min
Family Presence Facilitation	7170	RN basic	More than 1 hr
Family Process Maintenance	7130	RN basic	More than 1 hr
Family Support	7140	RN basic	More than 1 hr
Family Therapy	7150	RN post basic	More than 1 hr
Feeding	1050	Nursing assistant	16-30 min

Table 1   TIME AND EDUCATION FOR 514 NIC INTERVENTIONS LISTED ALPHABETICALLY—CONT'D

Intervention	Code No.	Educational Level	Time Required
Fertility Preservation	7160	RN post basic	31-45 min
Fever Treatment	3740	RN basic	16-30 min
Financial Resource Assistance	7380	RN basic	46-60 min
Fire-Setting Precautions	6500	Nursing assistant	More than 1 hr
First Aid	6240	Nursing assistant	16-30 min
Fiscal Resource Management	8550	RN post basic	More than 1 hr
Flatulence Reduction	470	RN basic	15 min or less
Fluid/Electrolyte Management	2080	RN basic	15 min or less
Fluid Management	4120	RN basic	31-45 min
Fluid Monitoring	4130	RN basic	16-30 min
Fluid Resuscitation	4140	RN basic	15 min or less
Foot Care	1660	RN basic	16-30 min
Forgiveness Facilitation	5280	RN basic	16-30 min
Gastrointestinal Intubation	1080	RN basic	15 min or less
Genetic Counseling	5242	RN post basic	46-60 min
Grief Work Facilitation	5290	RN basic	31-45 min
Grief Work Facilitation: Perinatal Death	5294	RN basic	31-45 min
Guilt Work Facilitation	5300	RN basic	31-45 min
Hair Care	1670	Nursing assistant	16-30 min
Hallucination Management	6510	RN basic	More than 1 hr
Health Care Information Exchange	7960	RN basic	15 min or less
Health Education	5510	RN basic	16-30 min
Health Policy Monitoring	7970	RN basic	More than 1 hr
Health Screening	6520	RN basic	46-60 min
Health System Guidance	7400	RN basic	16-30 min
Heat/Cold Application	1380	RN basic	15 min or less
Heat Exposure Treatment	3780	RN basic	16-30 min
Hemodialysis Therapy	2100	RN post basic	More than 1 hr

Continued

Table 1	TIME AND EDUCATION FOR 514 NIC INTERVENTIONS LISTED ALPHABETICALLY—CONT'D		
Intervention	**Code No.**	**Educational Level**	**Time Required**
Hemodynamic Regulation	4150	RN basic	16-30 min
Hemofiltration Therapy	2110	RN basic	More than 1 hr
Hemorrhage Control	4160	RN basic	15 min or less
High-Risk Pregnancy Care	6800	RN post basic	More than 1 hr
Home Maintenance Assistance	7180	RN basic	31-45 min
Hope Instillation	5310	RN basic	16-30 min
Hormone Replacement Therapy	2280	RN post basic	16-30 min
Humor	5320	Nursing assistant	15 min or less
Hyperglycemia Management	2120	RN basic	More than 1 hr
Hypervolemia Management	4170	RN basic	16-30 min
Hypnosis	5920	RN post basic	46-60 min
Hypoglycemia Management	2130	RN basic	More than 1 hr
Hypothermia Treatment	3800	RN basic	More than 1 hr
Hypovolemia Management	4180	RN basic	16-30 min
Immunization/Vaccination Management	6530	RN basic	16-30 min
Impulse Control Training	4370	RN post basic	More than 1 hr
Incident Reporting	7980	RN basic	16-30 min
Incision Site Care	3440	RN basic	31-45 min
Infant Care	6820	RN basic	More than 1 hr
Infection Control	6540	RN basic	31-45 min
Infection Control: Intraoperative	6545	RN basic	More than 1 hr
Infection Protection	6550	RN basic	31-45 min
Insurance Authorization	7410	RN basic	16-30 min
Intracranial Pressure (ICP) Monitoring	2590	RN basic	More than 1 hr
Intrapartal Care	6830	RN basic	More than 1 hr
Intrapartal Care: High-Risk Delivery	6834	RN post basic	More than 1 hr
Intravenous (IV) Insertion	4190	RN basic	15 min or less
Intravenous (IV) Therapy	4200	RN basic	15 min or less

Table 1   TIME AND EDUCATION FOR **514 NIC** INTERVENTIONS LISTED ALPHABETICALLY—CONT'D

Intervention	Code No.	Educational Level	Time Required
Invasive Hemodynamic Monitoring	4210	RN basic	46-60 min
Kangaroo Care	6840	RN basic	46-60 min
Labor Induction	6850	RN post basic	More than 1 hr
Labor Suppression	6860	RN post basic	More than 1 hr
Laboratory Data Interpretation	7690	RN basic	15 min or less
Lactation Counseling	5244	RN basic	31-45 min
Lactation Suppression	6870	RN basic	16-30 min
Laser Precautions	6560	RN post basic	31-45 min
Latex Precautions	6570	RN basic	31-45 min
Learning Facilitation	5520	RN basic	16-30 min
Learning Readiness Enhancement	5540	RN basic	15 min or less
Leech Therapy	3460	RN basic	46-60 min
Limit Setting	4380	RN basic	16-30 min
Lower Extremity Monitoring	3480	RN basic	15 min or less
Malignant Hyperthermia Precautions	3840	RN basic	More than 1 hr
Mechanical Ventilatory Weaning	3310	RN basic	More than 1 hr
Mechanical Ventilation	3300	RN basic	More than 1 hr
Medication Administration	2300	RN basic	15 min or less
Medication Administration: Ear	2308	Nursing assistant	15 min or less
Medication Administration: Enteral	2301	Nursing assistant	15 min or less
Medication Administration: Eye	2310	Nursing assistant	15 min or less
Medication Administration: Inhalation	2311	Nursing assistant	15 min or less
Medication Administration: Interpleural	2302	RN post basic	15 min or less
Medication Administration: Intradermal	2312	RN basic	15 min or less
Medication Administration: Intramuscular (IM)	2313	RN basic	15 min or less
Medication Administration: Intraosseous	2303	RN post basic	15 min or less
Medication Administration: Intraspinal	2319	RN basic	15 min or less
Medication Administration: Intravenous (IV)	2314	RN basic	15 min or less

Continued

Table 1	TIME AND EDUCATION FOR 514 NIC INTERVENTIONS LISTED ALPHABETICALLY—CONT'D		
Intervention	Code No.	Educational Level	Time Required
Medication Administration: Nasal	2320	Nursing assistant	15 min or less
Medication Administration: Oral	2304	Nursing assistant	15 min or less
Medication Administration: Rectal	2315	Nursing assistant	15 min or less
Medication Administration: Skin	2316	Nursing assistant	15 min or less
Medication Administration: Subcutaneous	2317	RN basic	15 min or less
Medication Administration: Vaginal	2318	Nursing assistant	15 min or less
Medication Administration: Ventricular Reservoir	2307	RN post basic	15 min or less
Medication Management	2380	RN basic	16-30 min
Medication Prescribing	2390	RN post basic	15 min or less
Meditation Facilitation	5960	RN basic	16-30 min
Memory Training	4760	RN post basic	31-45 min
Milieu Therapy	4390	RN basic	More than 1 hr
Mood Management	5330	RN basic	31-45 min
Multidisciplinary Care Conference	8020	RN basic	More than 1 hr
Music Therapy	4400	RN basic	15 min or less
Mutual Goal Setting	4410	RN basic	46-60 min
Nail Care	1680	Nursing assistant	16-30 min
Nausea Management	1450	RN basic	16-30 min
Neurologic Monitoring	2620	RN basic	16-30 min
Newborn Care	6880	RN basic	More than 1 hr
Newborn Monitoring	6890	RN basic	More than 1 hr
Nonnutritive Sucking	6900	Nursing assistant	16-30 min
Normalization Promotion	7200	RN basic	More than 1 hr
Nutrition Management	1100	RN post basic	31-45 min
Nutrition Therapy	1120	RN basic	16-30 min
Nutritional Counseling	5246	RN basic	16-30 min
Nutritional Monitoring	1160	RN basic	15 min or less

Table 1	TIME AND EDUCATION FOR 514 NIC INTERVENTIONS LISTED ALPHABETICALLY—CONT'D		

Intervention	Code No.	Educational Level	Time Required
Oral Health Maintenance	1710	RN basic	15 min or less
Oral Health Promotion	1720	RN basic	15 min or less
Oral Health Restoration	1730	RN basic	15 min or less
Order Transcription	8060	RN basic	15 min or less
Organ Procurement	6260	RN basic	46-60 min
Ostomy Care	480	RN post basic	16-30 min
Oxygen Therapy	3320	RN basic	15 min or less
Pain Management	1400	RN basic	More than 1 hr
Parent Education: Adolescent	5562	RN basic	16-30 min
Parent Education: Childrearing Family	5566	RN basic	16-30 min
Parent Education: Infant	5568	RN basic	31-45 min
Parenting Promotion	8300	RN basic	31-45 min
Pass Facilitation	7440	RN basic	15 min or less
Patient Contracting	4420	RN basic	46-60 min
Patient Rights Protection	7460	Nursing assistant	15 min or less
Patient-Controlled Analgesia	2400	RN basic	16-30 min
Peer Review	7700	RN basic	More than 1 hr
Pelvic Muscle Exercise	560	RN post basic	16-30 min
Perineal Care	1750	Nursing assistant	15 min or less
Peripheral Sensation Management	2660	RN basic	15 min or less
Peripherally Inserted Central (PIC) Catheter	4220	RN post basic	16-30 min
Peritoneal Dialysis Therapy	2150	RN basic	More than 1 hr
Pessary Management	630	RN basic	16-30 min
Phlebotomy: Arterial Blood Sample	4232	RN basic	15 min or less
Phlebotomy: Blood Unit Acquisition	4234	RN basic	More than 1 hr
Phlebotomy: Cannulated Vessel	4235	RN basic	15 min or less
Phlebotomy: Venous Blood Sample	4238	RN basic	15 min or less
Phototherapy: Mood/Sleep Regulation	6926	RN basic	31-45 min

Continued

Table 1   TIME AND EDUCATION FOR 514 NIC INTERVENTIONS LISTED ALPHABETICALLY—CONT'D

Intervention	Code No.	Educational Level	Time Required
Phototherapy: Neonate	6924	RN basic	More than 1 hr
Physical Restraint	6580	RN basic	15 min or less
Physician Support	7710	RN basic	16-30 min
Pneumatic Tourniquet Precautions	6590	RN post basic	More than 1 hr
Positioning	840	Nursing assistant	16-30 min
Positioning: Intraoperative	842	RN basic	16-30 min
Positioning: Neurologic	844	Nursing assistant	16-30 min
Positioning: Wheelchair	846	RN basic	15 min or less
Postanesthesia Care	2870	RN basic	46-60 min
Postmortem Care	1770	Nursing assistant	16-30 min
Postpartal Care	6930	RN basic	More than 1 hr
Preceptor: Employee	7722	RN basic	More than 1 hr
Preceptor: Student	7726	RN basic	More than 1 hr
Preconception Counseling	5247	RN post basic	More than 1 hr
Pregnancy Termination Care	6950	RN post basic	More than 1 hr
Premenstrual Syndrome Management	1440	RN post basic	16-30 min
Prenatal Care	6960	RN basic	More than 1 hr
Preoperative Coordination	2880	RN basic	31-45 min
Preparatory Sensory Information	5580	RN basic	31-45 min
Presence	5340	Nursing assistant	16-30 min
Pressure Management	3500	RN basic	16-30 min
Pressure Ulcer Care	3520	Nursing assistant	16-30 min
Pressure Ulcer Prevention	3540	RN basic	16-30 min
Product Evaluation	7760	RN basic	More than 1 hr
Program Development	8700	RN post basic	More than 1 hr
Progressive Muscle Relaxation	1460	RN post basic	16-30 min
Prompted Voiding	640	Nursing assistant	15 min or less
Prosthesis Care	1780	Nursing assistant	15 min or less

Table 1	TIME AND EDUCATION FOR 514 NIC INTERVENTIONS LISTED ALPHABETICALLY—CONT'D		
Intervention	**Code No.**	**Educational Level**	**Time Required**
Pruritus Management	3550	RN basic	16-30 min
Quality Monitoring	7800	RN basic	More than 1 hr
Radiation Therapy Management	6600	RN basic	46-60 min
Rape-Trauma Treatment	6300	RN basic	More than 1 hr
Reality Orientation	4820	Nursing assistant	15 min or less
Recreation Therapy	5360	Nursing assistant	16-30 min
Rectal Prolapse Management	490	RN post basic	16-30 min
Referral	8100	RN basic	16-30 min
Religious Addiction Prevention	5422	RN basic	46-60 min
Religious Ritual Enhancement	5424	RN basic	31-45 min
Relocation Stress Reduction	5350	RN basic	16-30 min
Reminiscence Therapy	4860	RN post basic	46-60 min
Reproductive Technology Management	7886	RN post basic	More than 1 hr
Research Data Collection	8120	RN basic	16-30 min
Resiliency Promotion	8340	RN basic	More than 1 hr
Respiratory Monitoring	3350	RN basic	15 min or less
Respite Care	7260	RN basic	More than 1 hr
Resuscitation	6320	RN basic	16-30 min
Resuscitation: Fetus	6972	RN post basic	More than 1 hr
Resuscitation: Neonate	6974	RN post basic	46-60 min
Risk Identification	6610	RN basic	46-60 min
Risk Identification: Childbearing Family	6612	RN basic	More than 1 hr
Risk Identification: Genetic	6614	RN post basic	More than 1 hr
Role Enhancement	5370	RN basic	16-30 min
Seclusion	6630	RN basic	More than 1 hr
Security Enhancement	5380	RN basic	16-30 min
Sedation Management	2260	RN post basic	More than 1 hr
Seizure Management	2680	RN basic	16-30 min

Continued

Table 1	TIME AND EDUCATION FOR 514 NIC INTERVENTIONS LISTED ALPHABETICALLY—CONT'D		
Intervention	**Code No.**	**Educational Level**	**Time Required**
Seizure Precautions	2690	RN basic	15 min or less
Self-Awareness Enhancement	5390	RN basic	16-30 min
Self-Care Assistance	1800	Nursing assistant	16-30 min
Self-Care Assistance: Bathing/Hygiene	1801	Nursing assistant	15 min or less
Self-Care Assistance: Dressing/Grooming	1802	Nursing assistant	15 min or less
Self-Care Assistance: Feeding	1803	Nursing assistant	16-30 min
Self-Care Assistance: IADL	1805	RN basic	46-60 min
Self-Care Assistance: Toileting	1804	Nursing assistant	15 min or less
Self-Care Assistance: Transfer	1806	Nursing assistant	15 min or less
Self-Esteem Enhancement	5400	RN basic	16-30 min
Self-Hypnosis Facilitation	5922	RN post basic	46-60 min
Self-Modification Assistance	4470	RN basic	46-60 min
Self-Responsibility Facilitation	4480	RN basic	46-60 min
Sexual Counseling	5248	RN post basic	46-60 min
Shift Report	8140	RN basic	31-45 min
Shock Management	4250	RN basic	16-30 min
Shock Management: Cardiac	4254	RN basic	16-30 min
Shock Management: Vasogenic	4256	RN basic	31-45 min
Shock Management: Volume	4258	RN basic	31-45 min
Shock Prevention	4260	RN basic	16-30 min
Sibling Support	7280	RN basic	16-30 min
Simple Guided Imagery	6000	RN basic	31-45 min
Simple Massage	1480	RN basic	15 min or less
Simple Relaxation Therapy	6040	RN basic	31-45 min
Skin Care: Donor Site	3582	RN basic	16-30 min
Skin Care: Graft Site	3583	RN basic	16-30 min
Skin Care: Topical Treatment	3584	RN basic	16-30 min
Skin Surveillance	3590	RN basic	16-30 min

Table 1   TIME AND EDUCATION FOR **514 NIC** INTERVENTIONS LISTED ALPHABETICALLY—CONT'D

Intervention	Code No.	Educational Level	Time Required
Sleep Enhancement	1850	RN basic	16-30 min
Smoking Cessation Assistance	4490	RN basic	46-60 min
Socialization Enhancement	5100	RN basic	31-45 min
Specimen Management	7820	Nursing assistant	15 min or less
Spiritual Growth Facilitation	6426	RN basic	31-45 min
Spiritual Support	5420	RN basic	16-30 min
Splinting	910	RN basic	15 min or less
Sports-Injury Prevention: Youth	6648	RN basic	46-60 min
Staff Development	7850	RN basic	More than 1 hr
Staff Supervision	7830	RN basic	More than 1 hr
Subarachnoid Hemorrhage Precautions	2720	RN basic	15 min or less
Substance Use Prevention	4500	RN basic	46-60 min
Substance Use Treatment	4510	RN basic	46-60 min
Substance Use Treatment: Alcohol Withdrawal	4512	RN post basic	More than 1 hr
Substance Use Treatment: Drug Withdrawal	4514	RN post basic	More than 1 hr
Substance Use Treatment: Overdose	4516	RN post basic	More than 1 hr
Suicide Prevention	6340	RN basic	More than 1 hr
Supply Management	7840	Nursing assistant	16-30 min
Support Group	5430	RN post basic	46 60 min
Support System Enhancement	5440	RN basic	31-45 min
Surgical Assistance	2900	Nursing assistant	More than 1 hr
Surgical Precautions	2920	RN basic	More than 1 hr
Surgical Preparation	2930	RN basic	46-60 min
Surveillance	6650	RN basic	More than 1 hr
Surveillance: Community	6652	RN basic	More than 1 hr
Surveillance: Late Pregnancy	6656	RN post basic	More than 1 hr
Surveillance: Remote Electronic	6658	RN basic	31-45 min
Surveillance: Safety	6654	RN basic	31-45 min

Continued

Table 1	TIME AND EDUCATION FOR 514 NIC INTERVENTIONS LISTED ALPHABETICALLY—CONT'D			

Intervention	Code No.	Educational Level	Time Required
Sustenance Support	7500	RN basic	31-45 min
Suturing	3620	RN basic	16-30 min
Swallowing Therapy	1860	RN basic	31-45 min
Teaching: Disease Process	5602	RN basic	16-30 min
Teaching: Foot Care	5603	RN basic	16-30 min
Teaching: Group	5604	RN basic	More than 1 hr
Teaching: Individual	5606	RN basic	31-45 min
Teaching: Infant Nutrition	5626	RN basic	16-30 min
Teaching: Infant Safety	5628	RN basic	16-30 min
Teaching: Infant Stimulation	5605	RN basic	16-30 min
Teaching: Preoperative	5610	RN basic	16-30 min
Teaching: Prescribed Activity/Exercise	5612	RN basic	16-30 min
Teaching: Prescribed Diet	5614	RN basic	16-30 min
Teaching: Prescribed Medication	5616	RN basic	16-30 min
Teaching: Procedure/Treatment	5618	RN basic	16-30 min
Teaching: Psychomotor Skill	5620	RN basic	16-30 min
Teaching: Safe Sex	5622	RN basic	16-30 min
Teaching: Sexuality	5624	RN basic	16-30 min
Teaching: Toddler Nutrition	5630	RN basic	16-30 min
Teaching: Toddler Safety	5630	RN basic	16-30 min
Teaching: Toilet Training	5634	RN basic	16-30 min
Technology Management	7880	RN basic	15 min or less
Telephone Consultation	8180	RN basic	16-30 min
Telephone Follow-up	8190	RN basic	15 min or less
Temperature Regulation	3900	RN basic	31-45 min
Temperature Regulation: Intraoperative	3902	RN basic	More than 1 hr
Temporary Pacemaker Management	4092	RN basic	16-30 min

Table 1	TIME AND EDUCATION FOR 514 NIC INTERVENTIONS LISTED ALPHABETICALLY—CONT'D		
Intervention	**Code No.**	**Educational Level**	**Time Required**
Therapeutic Play	4430	RN basic	46-60 min
Therapeutic Touch	5465	RN post basic	46-60 min
Therapy Group	5450	RN post basic	46-60 min
Total Parenteral Nutrition (TPN) Administration	1200	RN basic	16-30 min
Touch	5460	Nursing assistant	15 min or less
Traction/Immobilization Care	940	RN basic	15 min or less
Transcutaneous Electrical Nerve Stimulation	1540	RN post basic	16-30 min
Transport	960	Nursing assistant	15 min or less
Trauma Therapy: Child	5410	RN post basic	46-60 min
Triage: Disaster	6360	RN basic	15 min or less
Triage: Emergency Center	6364	RN basic	15 min or less
Triage: Telephone	6366	RN basic	15 min or less
Truth Telling	5470	RN basic	16-30 min
Tube Care	1870	Nursing assistant	15 min or less
Tube Care: Chest	1872	RN basic	15 min or less
Tube Care: Gastrointestinal	1874	RN basic	15 min or less
Tube Care: Umbilical Line	1875	RN post basic	46-60 min
Tube Care: Urinary	1876	Nursing assistant	15 min or less
Tube Care: Ventriculostomy/Lumbar Drain	1878	RN basic	15 min or less
Ultrasonography: Limited Obstetric	6982	RN post basic	31-45 min
Unilateral Neglect Management	2760	RN basic	31-45 min
Urinary Bladder Training	570	RN post basic	16-30 min
Urinary Catheterization	580	Nursing assistant	15 min or less
Urinary Catheterization: Intermittent	582	Nursing assistant	15 min or less
Urinary Elimination Management	590	RN post basic	31-45 min
Urinary Habit Training	600	RN post basic	31-45 min
Urinary Incontinence Care	610	RN basic	31-45 min

Continued

Table 1	TIME AND EDUCATION FOR 514 NIC INTERVENTIONS LISTED ALPHABETICALLY—CONT'D		
Intervention	**Code No.**	**Educational Level**	**Time Required**
Urinary Incontinence Care: Enuresis	612	RN basic	16-30 min
Urinary Retention Care	620	RN basic	15 min or less
Values Clarification	5480	RN basic	16-30 min
Vehicle Safety Promotion	9050	RN basic	More than 1 hr
Venous Access Devices (VAD) Maintenance	2440	RN post basic	31-45 min
Ventilation Assistance	3390	RN basic	15 min or less
Visitation Facilitation	7560	Nursing assistant	15 min or less
Vital Signs Monitoring	6680	RN basic	15 min or less
Vomiting Management	1570	RN basic	16-30 min
Weight Gain Assistance	1240	RN basic	16-30 min
Weight Management	1260	RN basic	31-45 min
Weight Reduction Assistance	1280	RN basic	16-30 min
Wound Care	3660	RN basic	31-45 min
Wound Care: Closed Drainage	3662	RN basic	31-45 min
Wound Irrigation	3680	RN basic	31-45 min

Table 2	INTERVENTIONS APPROPRIATE FOR NURSING ASSISTANTS

Physiological: Basic Domain
Bathing
Bed Rest Care
Cast Care: Maintenance
Contact Lens Care
Dressing
Environmental Management: Comfort
Exercise Therapy: Ambulation
Feeding
Hair Care
Nail Care
Perineal Care
Positioning
Postmortem Care
Prompted Voiding
Prosthesis Care
Self-Care Assistance
Self-Care Assistance: Bathing/Hygiene
Self-Care Assistance: Dressing/Grooming
Self-Care Assistance: Feeding
Self-Care Assistance: Toileting
Self-Care Assistance: Transfer
Transport
Tube Care
Tube Care: Urinary
Urinary Catheterization
Urinary Catheterization: Intermittent

Physiological: Complex Domain
Aspiration Precautions
Cough Enhancement
Medication Administration: Ear
Medication Administration: Enteral
Medication Administration: Eye
Medication Administration: Inhalation
Medication Administration: Nasal
Medication Administration: Rectal
Medication Administration: Skin
Medication Administration: Vaginal
Medication Administration: Oral

Positioning: Neurologic
Pressure Ulcer Care
Surgical Assistance

Behavioral Domain
Animal-Assisted Therapy
Anxiety Reduction
Calming Technique
Communication Enhancement: Hearing
Communication Enhancement: Visual Deficit
Distraction
Humor
Presence
Reality Orientation
Recreation Therapy
Touch

Safety Domain
Area Restriction
Dementia Management: Bathing
Elopement Precautions
Emergency Care
Environmental Management
Environmental Management: Violence Prevention
Fire-Setting Precautions
First Aid

Family Domain
Bottle Feeding
Environmental Management: Attachment Process
Nonnutritive Sucking

Health System Domain
Bedside Laboratory Testing
Emergency Cart Checking
Examination Assistance
Patient Rights Protection
Specimen Management
Supply Management
Visitation Facilitation

Table 3	INTERVENTIONS APPROPRIATE FOR RNs WITH POST-BASIC EDUCATION

Physiological: Basic Domain
Acupressure
Eating Disorders Management
Exercise Therapy: Muscle Control
Nutrition Management
Ostomy Care
Pelvic Muscle Exercise
Premenstrual Syndrome Management
Progressive Muscle Relaxation
Rectal Prolapse Management
Therapeutic Touch
Transcutaneous Electrical Nerve Stimulation
Urinary Bladder Training
Urinary Elimination Management
Urinary Habit Training

Physiological: Complex Domain
Analgesic Administration: Intraspinal
Anesthesia Administration
Chemotherapy Management
Hemodialysis Therapy
Hormone Replacement Therapy
Medication Administration: Interpleural
Medication Administration: Intraosseous
Medication Administration: Ventricular Reservoir
Medication Prescribing
Peripherally Inserted Central (PIC) Catheter
Sedation Management
Venous Access Devices (VAD) Maintenance

Behavioral Domain
Anger Control Assistance
Art Therapy
Autogenic Training
Bibliotherapy
Biofeedback
Cognitive Restructuring
Cognitive Stimulation
Conflict Mediation
Counseling
Crisis Intervention
Genetic Counseling
Hypnosis
Impulse Control Training

Memory Training
Reminiscence Therapy
Self-Hypnosis Facilitation
Sexual Counseling
Substance Use Treatment: Alcohol Withdrawal
Substance Use Treatment: Drug Withdrawal
Substance Use Treatment: Overdose
Support Group
Therapy Group
Trauma Therapy: Child

Safety Domain
Laser Precautions
Pneumatic Tourniquet Precautions

Family Domain
Amnioinfusion
Birthing
Electronic Fetal Monitoring: Antepartum
Electronic Fetal Monitoring: Intrapartum
Family Planning: Infertility
Family Therapy
Fertility Preservation
High-Risk Pregnancy Care
Intrapartal Care: High-Risk Delivery
Labor Induction
Labor Suppression
Preconception Counseling
Pregnancy Termination Care
Reproductive Technology Management
Resuscitation: Fetus
Resuscitation: Neonate
Risk Identification: Genetic
Surveillance: Late Pregnancy
Tube Care: Umbilical Line
Ultrasonography: Limited Obstetric

Health System Domain
Case Management

Community
Bioterrorism Preparedness
Fiscal Resource Management
Program Development

Table 4	INTERVENTIONS THAT TAKE 15 MINUTES OR LESS

Acid-Base Monitoring
Airway Suctioning
Aromatherapy
Artificial Airway Management
Aspiration Precautions
Bedside Laboratory Testing
Breast Examination
Capillary Blood Sample
Cast Care: Maintenance
Chemical Restraint
Circulatory Care: Arterial Insufficiency
Circulatory Care: Venous Insufficiency
Contact Lens Care
Controlled Substance Checking
Cough Enhancement
Delegation
Dialysis Access Maintenance
Diarrhea Management
Diet Staging
Documentation
Dressing
Electrolyte Monitoring
Emergency Cart Checking
Endotrachial Extubation
Environmental Management: Comfort
Exercise Therapy: Ambulation
Eye Care
Flatulence Reduction
Fluid/Electrolyte Management
Fluid Resuscitation
Gastrointestinal Intubation
Health Care Information Exchange
Heat/Cold Application
Hemorrhage Control
Humor
Intravenous (IV) Therapy
Intravenous (IV) Insertion
Laboratory Data Interpretation
Learning Readiness Enhancement
Lower Extremity Monitoring
Medication Administration
Medication Administration: Ear
Medication Administration: Enteral
Medication Administration: Eye
Medication Administration: Inhalation
Medication Administration: Interpleural
Medication Administration: Intradermal
Medication Administration: Intramuscular (IM)
Medication Administration: Intraosseous
Medication Administration: Intraspinal
Medication Administration: Intravenous (IV)
Medication Administration: Nasal
Medication Administration: Oral
Medication Administration: Rectal

Medication Administration: Skin
Medication Administration: Subcutaneous
Medication Administration: Vaginal
Medication Administration: Ventricular
    Reservoir
Medication Prescribing
Music Therapy
Nutritional Monitoring
Oral Health Maintenance
Oral Health Promotion
Oral Health Restoration
Order Transcription
Oxygen Therapy
Pass Facilitation
Patient Rights Protection
Perineal Care
Peripheral Sensation Management
Phlebotomy: Arterial Blood Sample
Phlebotomy: Cannulated Vessel
Phlebotomy: Venous Blood Sample
Physical Restraint
Positioning: Wheelchair
Prompted Voiding
Prosthesis Care
Reality Orientation
Respiratory Monitoring
Seizure Precautions
Self-Care Assistance: Bathing/Hygiene
Self-Care Assistance: Dressing/Grooming
Self-Care Assistance: Toileting
Self-Care Assistance: Transfer
Simple Massage
Specimen Management
Splinting
Subarachnoid Hemorrhage Precautions
Technology Management
Telephone Follow-up
Touch
Traction/Immobilization Care
Transport
Triage: Disaster
Triage: Emergency Center
Triage: Telephone
Tube Care
Tube Care: Chest
Tube Care: Gastrointestinal
Tube Care: Urinary
Tube Care: Ventriculostomy/Lumbar Drain
Urinary Catheterization
Urinary Catheterization: Intermittent
Urinary Retention Care
Ventilation Assistance
Visitation Facilitation
Vital Signs Monitoring

Table 5	INTERVENTIONS THAT TAKE 16 TO 30 MINUTES

Active Listening
Acupressure
Admission Care
Airway Insertion and Stabilization
Airway Management
Analgesic Administration
Analgesic Administration: Intraspinal
Anger Control Assistance
Animal-Assisted Therapy
Asthma Management
Bathing
Bed Rest Care
Bladder Irrigation
Bleeding Reduction: Nasal
Body Mechanics Promotion
Bowel Incontinence Care
Bowel Incontinence Care: Encopresis
Bowel Irrigation
Bowel Training
Breastfeeding Assistance
Cast Care: Wet
Chest Physiotherapy
Circulatory Precautions
Cognitive Restructuring
Cognitive Stimulation
Communication Enhancement: Hearing
Communication Enhancement: Visual Deficit
Constipation/Impaction Management
Culture Brokerage
Cutaneous Stimulation
Decision-Making Support
Dying Care
Dysreflexia Management
Dysrhythmia Management
Ear Care
Electrolyte Management: Hypercalcemia
Electrolyte Management: Hyperkalemia
Electrolyte Management: Hypermagnesemia
Electrolyte Management: Hypernatremia
Electrolyte Management: Hyperphosphatemia
Electrolyte Management: Hypocalcemia
Electrolyte Management: Hypokalemia
Electrolyte Management: Hypomagnesemia
Electrolyte Management: Hyponatremia
Electrolyte Management: Hypophosphatemia
Embolus Care: Peripheral
Embolus Care: Pulmonary
Embolus Precautions
Emergency Care
Emotional Support
Energy Management
Enteral Tube Feeding
Environmental Management: Attachment Process

Examination Assistance
Exercise Therapy: Balance
Exercise Therapy: Joint Mobility
Exercise Therapy: Muscle Control
Feeding
Fever Treatment
First Aid
Fluid Monitoring
Foot Care
Forgiveness Facilitation
Hair Care
Health Education
Health System Guidance
Heat Exposure Treatment
Hemodynamic Regulation
Hope Instillation
Hormone Replacement Therapy
Hypervolemia Management
Hypovolemia Management
Immunization/Vaccination Management
Incident Reporting
Insurance Authorization
Lactation Suppression
Learning Facilitation
Limit Setting
Medication Management
Meditation Facilitation
Nail Care
Nausea Management
Neurologic Monitoring
Nonnutritive Sucking
Nutrition Therapy
Nutritional Counseling
Ostomy Care
Parent Education: Adolescent
Parent Education: Childrearing Family
Patient-Controlled Analgesia
Pelvic Muscle Exercise
Peripherally Inserted Central (PIC)
    Catheter
Pessary Management
Physician Support
Positioning
Positioning: Intraoperative
Positioning: Neurologic
Postmortem Care
Premenstrual Syndrome Management
Presence
Pressure Management
Pressure Ulcer Care
Pressure Ulcer Prevention
Progressive Muscle Relaxation
Pruritus Management

Table 5	INTERVENTIONS THAT TAKE 16 TO 30 MINUTES—CONT'D

Recreation Therapy	Teaching: Foot Care
Rectal Prolapse Management	Teaching: Infant Nutrition
Referral	Teaching: Infant Safety
Relocation Stress Reduction	Teaching: Infant Stimulation
Research Data Collection	Teaching: Preoperative
Resuscitation	Teaching: Prescribed Activity/Exercise
Role Enhancement	Teaching: Prescribed Diet
Security Enhancement	Teaching: Prescribed Medication
Seizure Management	Teaching: Procedure/Treatment
Self-Awareness Enhancement	Teaching: Psychomotor Skill
Self-Care Assistance	Teaching: Safe Sex
Self-Care Assistance: Feeding	Teaching: Sexuality
Self-Esteem Enhancement	Teaching: Toddler Nutrition
Shock Management	Teaching: Toddler Safety
Shock Management: Cardiac	Teaching: Toilet Training
Shock Prevention	Telephone Consultation
Sibling Support	Temporary Pacemaker Management
Skin Care: Donor Site	Total Parenteral Nutrition (TPN) Administration
Skin Care: Graft Site	Transcutaneous Electrical Nerve Stimulation
Skin Care: Topical Treatment	Truth Telling
Skin Surveillance	Urinary Bladder Training
Sleep Enhancement	Urinary Incontinence Care: Enuresis
Spiritual Support	Values Clarification
Supply Management	Vomiting Management
Suturing	Weight Gain Assistance
Teaching: Disease Process	Weight Reduction Assistance

Table 6	INTERVENTIONS THAT TAKE 31 TO 45 MINUTES

Acid-Base Management: Metabolic Acidosis	Cerebral Perfusion Promotion
Acid-Base Management: Metabolic Alkalosis	Cesarean Section Care
Acid-Base Management: Respiratory Acidosis	Circulatory Care: Mechanical Assist Device
Acid-Base Management: Respiratory Alkalosis	Code Management
Allergy Management	Communication Enhancement: Speech Deficit
Amnioinfusion	Coping Enhancement
Amputation Care	Cost Containment
Anticipatory Guidance	Dementia Management: Bathing
Anxiety Reduction	Distraction
Behavior Management: Overactivity/Inattention	Eating Disorders Management
Behavior Management: Self-Harm	Electrolyte Management
Behavior Management: Sexual	Environmental Management
Bleeding Precautions	Environmental Management: Safety
Body Image Enhancement	Exercise Promotion
Bottle Feeding	Exercise Promotion: Strength Training
Bowel Management	Exercise Promotion: Stretching
Calming Technique	Family Planning: Contraception
Cardiac Care	Fertility Preservation
Cardiac Care: Acute	Fluid Management
Cardiac Precautions	Grief Work Facilitation

Continued

Table 6	INTERVENTIONS THAT TAKE 31 TO 45 MINUTES—CONT'D

Grief Work Facilitation: Perinatal Death	Simple Guided Imagery
Guilt Work Facilitation	Simple Relaxation Therapy
Home Maintenance Assistance	Socialization Enhancement
Incision Site Care	Spiritual Growth Facilitation
Infection Control	Support System Enhancement
Infection Protection	Surveillance: Remote Electronic
Lactation Counseling	Surveillance: Safety
Laser Precautions	Sustenance Support
Latex Precautions	Swallowing Therapy
Memory Training	Teaching: Individual
Mood Management	Temperature Regulation
Nutrition Management	Ultrasonography: Limited Obstetric
Parent Education: Infant	Unilateral Neglect Management
Parenting Promotion	Urinary Elimination Management
Phototherapy: Mood/Sleep Regulation	Urinary Habit Training
Preoperative Coordination	Urinary Incontinence Care
Preparatory Sensory Information	Venous Access Devices (VAD) Maintenance
Religious Ritual Enhancement	Weight Management
Shift Report	Wound Care
Shock Management: Vasogenic	Wound Care: Closed Drainage
Shock Management: Volume	Wound Irrigation

Table 7	INTERVENTIONS THAT TAKE 46 TO 60 MINUTES

Activity Therapy	Discharge Planning
Anaphylaxis Management	Environmental Risk Protection
Art Therapy	Family Planning: Infertility
Assertiveness Training	Family Planning: Unplanned Pregnancy
Autogenic Training	Financial Resource Assistance
Autotransfusion	Genetic Counseling
Behavior Management	Health Screening
Bibliotherapy	Hypnosis
Biofeedback	Invasive Hemodynamic Monitoring
Bleeding Reduction	Kangaroo Care
Bleeding Reduction: Antepartum Uterus	Leech Therapy
Bleeding Reduction: Gastrointestinal	Mutual Goal Setting
Bleeding Reduction: Postpartum Uterus	Organ Procurement
Bleeding Reduction: Wound	Patient Contracting
Chemotherapy Management	Postanesthesia Care
Circumcision Care	Radiation Therapy Management
Communicable Disease Management	Religious Addiction Prevention
Conflict Mediation	Reminiscence Therapy
Consultation	Resuscitation: Neonate
Counseling	Risk Identification
Crisis Intervention	Self-Care Assistance: IADL
Developmental Care	Self-Hypnosis Facilitation
Developmental Enhancement: Adolescent	Self-Modification Assistance
Developmental Enhancement: Child	Self-Responsibility Facilitation

Table 7	INTERVENTIONS THAT TAKE 46 TO 60 MINUTES—CONT'D

Sexual Counseling	Surgical Preparation
Smoking Cessation Assistance	Therapeutic Touch
Sports-Injury Prevention: Youth	Therapy Group
Substance Use Prevention	Trauma Therapy: Child
Substance Use Treatment	Tube Care: Umbilical Line
Support Group	

Table 8	INTERVENTIONS THAT TAKE MORE THAN 1 HOUR

Abuse Protection Support	Family Presence Facilitation
Abuse Protection Support: Child	Family Process Maintenance
Abuse Protection Support: Domestic Partner	Family Support
Abuse Protection Support: Elder	Family Therapy
Abuse Protection Support: Religious	Fire-Setting Precautions
Acid-Base Management	Fiscal Resource Management
Anesthesia Administration	Hallucination Management
Area Restriction	Health Policy Monitoring
Attachment Promotion	Hemodialysis Therapy
Behavior Modification	Hemofiltration Therapy
Behavior Modification: Social Skills	High-Risk Pregnancy Care
Bioterrorism Preparedness	Hyperglycemia Management
Birthing	Hypoglycemia Management
Blood Products Administration	Hypothermia Treatment
Cardiac Care: Rehabilitative	Impulse Control Training
Caregiver Support	Infant Care
Case Management	Infection Control: Intraoperative
Cerebral Edema Management	Intracranial Pressure (ICP) Monitoring
Childbirth Preparation	Intrapartal Care
Community Disaster Preparedness	Intrapartal Care: High-Risk Delivery
Community Health Development	Labor Induction
Complex Relationship Building	Labor Suppression
Critical Path Development	Malignant Hyperthermia Precautions
Delirium Management	Mechanical Ventilatory Weaning
Delusion Management	Mechanical Ventilation
Dementia Management	Milieu Therapy
Deposition/Testimony	Multidisciplinary Care Conference
Electroconvulsive Therapy Management	Newborn Care
Electronic Fetal Monitoring: Antepartum	Newborn Monitoring
Electronic Fetal Monitoring: Intrapartum	Normalization Promotion
Elopement Precautions	Pain Management
Environmental Management: Community	Peer Review
Environmental Management: Home Preparation	Peritoneal Dialysis Therapy
Environmental Management: Violence Prevention	Phlebotomy: Blood Unit Acquisition
Environmental Management: Worker Safety	Phototherapy: Neonate
Fall Prevention	Pneumatic Tourniquet Precautions
Family Integrity Promotion	Postpartal Care
Family Integrity Promotion: Childbearing Family	Preceptor: Employee
Family Involvement Promotion	Preceptor: Student
Family Mobilization	Preconception Counseling

Continued

Table 8	INTERVENTIONS THAT TAKE MORE THAN **1** HOUR—CONT'D

Pregnancy Termination Care	Staff Development
Prenatal Care	Staff Supervision
Product Evaluation	Substance Use Treatment: Alcohol Withdrawal
Program Development	Substance Use Treatment: Drug Withdrawal
Quality Monitoring	Substance Use Treatment: Overdose
Rape-Trauma Treatment	Suicide Prevention
Reproductive Technology Management	Surgical Assistance
Resiliency Promotion	Surgical Precautions
Respite Care	Surveillance
Resuscitation: Fetus	Surveillance: Community
Risk Identification: Childbearing Family	Surveillance: Late Pregnancy
Risk Identification: Genetic	Teaching: Group
Seclusion	Temperature Regulation: Intraoperative
Sedation Management	Vehicle Safety Promotion

Table 9	ESTIMATED TIME TO COMPLETE **514 NIC** INTERVENTIONS BY TIME INTERVALS

Time Interval	Frequency	Percent
15 min or less	107	20.8
16-30 min	157	30.5
31-45 min	82	16.0
46-60 min	60	11.7
More than 1 hr	108	21.0
Total	514	100.0

PART SEVEN

Appendixes

APPENDIX A

Interventions: New, Revised, and Deleted Since the Third Edition

INTERVENTIONS NEW TO THE FOURTH EDITION (n = 29)

Aromatherapy
Asthma Management
Bioterrorism Preparedness
Capillary Blood Sample
Chemical Restraint
Circumcision Care
Dementia Management: Bathing
Deposition/Testimony
Dialysis Access Maintenance
Electroconvulsive Therapy Management
Family Presence Facilitation
Hormone Replacement Therapy
Lower Extremity Monitoring
Medication Administration: Intraspinal
Medication Administration: Nasal
Phlebotomy: Cannulated Vessel
Phototherapy: Mood/Sleep Regulation
Premenstrual Syndrome Management
Relocation Stress Reduction
Self-Care Assistance: IADL
Self-Care Assistance: Transfer
Self-Hypnosis Facilitation
Skin Care: Donor Site
Skin Care: Graft Site
Teaching: Foot Care
Teaching: Infant Stimulation
Teaching: Toilet Training
Temporary Pacemaker Management
Trauma Therapy: Child

INTERVENTIONS REVISED FOR THE FOURTH EDITION
Label Name Changes (n = 1)

Sedation Management (previously *Conscious Sedation*)

Substantive Intervention Changes: Major (n = 23)

Interventions in this category have substantive changes in definition or addition/revision of multiple activities that further explicate the nursing actions associated with the intervention.

Amputation Care
Anaphylaxis Management
Caregiver Support

Cognitive Restructuring
Distraction
Enteral Tube Feeding
Environmental Management
Exercise Promotion
Fall Prevention
Family Involvement Promotion
Health Care Information Exchange
Health System Guidance
Medication Administration: Enteral
Medication Management
Peripherally Inserted Central (PIC) Catheter Care
Phlebotomy: Blood Unit Acquisition
Postanesthesia Care
Reminiscence Therapy
Shock Management
Smoking Cessation Assistance
Spiritual Support
Suicide Prevention
Wound Care

Substantive Intervention Changes: Minor (n = 70)

Interventions in this category have addition or revision of a few activities that enhance the clinical application of the intervention.

Abuse Protection Support
Abuse Protection Support: Domestic Partner
Abuse Protection Support: Elder
Acid-Base Management: Metabolic Alkalosis
Acid-Base Management: Respiratory Acidosis
Active Listening
Admission Care
Airway Management
Amnioinfusion
Anxiety Reduction
Blood Products Administration
Cerebral Edema Management
Circulatory Care: Arterial Insufficiency
Circulatory Care: Venous Insufficiency
Complex Relationship Building
Constipation/Impaction Management
Cough Enhancement
Dementia Management
Diarrhea Management
Emotional Support
Family Mobilization
Foot Care
Grief Work Facilitation
Hemodialysis Therapy
Home Maintenance Assistance
Hyperglycemia Management
Immunization/Vaccination Management

Intravenous (IV) Therapy
Invasive Hemodynamic Monitoring
Latex Precautions
Learning Readiness Enhancement
Leech Therapy
Medication Administration: Ear
Medication Administration: Inhalation
Medication Administration: Intramuscular
Medication Administration: Intraosseous
Medication Administration: Intravenous
Medication Administration: Oral
Medication Administration: Rectal
Medication Administration: Subcutaneous
Medication Administration: Vaginal
Medication Administration: Ventricular Reservoir
Medication Prescribing
Memory Training
Music Therapy
Nail Care
Nutrition Therapy
Oral Health Maintenance
Ostomy Care
Pain Management
Patient Contracting
Patient Rights Protection
Pelvic Muscle Exercise
Peritoneal Dialysis Therapy
Phlebotomy: Arterial Blood Sample
Pressure Ulcer Care
Pressure Ulcer Prevention
Religious Ritual Enhancement
Self-Awareness Enhancement
Self-Esteem Enhancement
Sleep Enhancement
Socialization Enhancement
Surveillance
Sustenance Support
Teaching: Disease Process
Teaching: Prescribed Medication
Urinary Bladder Training
Urinary Elimination Management
Vital Signs Monitoring
Weight Gain Assistance
Weight Management

INTERVENTIONS IN THE THIRD EDITION THAT WERE DELETED IN THIS EDITION

Medication Administration: Epideral (Expanded to become Medication Administration: Intraspinal)

Guidelines for Submission of a New or Revised Intervention

This appendix contains materials to assist you in preparing an intervention to submit for review or to suggest a change for an existing intervention. It is important that a submitter be familiar with NIC and with the Principles for Intervention Development and Refinement (included in this Appendix) before developing or revising an intervention.

THE MATERIALS NEEDED

All submissions should be typed and formatted in the same style as appears in NIC. *Three copies* of all materials should be submitted. Background readings/references should be typed in APA format. Materials that are too difficult to read or incomplete will be sent back to the submitter without being reviewed.

Each submission of a **proposed new intervention** should include a label, a definition, activities listed in logical order, and a short list of background readings that support the intervention. In addition, *a rationale for inclusion* should also be attached and the submitter *should note how the proposed new intervention differs from existing interventions.* If a new intervention would call for changes in existing interventions, these changes should also be submitted. The Demographic Information Form should be filled out and included.

Each submission for a **revised intervention** should indicate how the proposed changes relate to the existing intervention. In most instances a copy of the intervention from the NIC book with additions, deletions, and modifications made on the copy will be the best way to clearly indicate changes. If changes are substantial, however, the revised intervention should be retyped with the current intervention attached. A rationale must also be included. The Demographic Information Form should be filled out and included.

THE REVIEW PROCESS

1. Submitted materials for proposed new or revised interventions are assigned to two or three reviewers who have expertise in the content area and who are familiar with NIC.
2. The reviewers receive a copy of what has been submitted and a review form.
3. The reviewers are asked to return their comments and their recommendations within 1 month. The initial submission and the reviewers' comments are then reviewed by the research team and a decision is made.
4. Approximately 2 to 6 months after submission, the submitter will receive a letter stating the outcome of the process. If the decision is for inclusion in NIC, the submitter will be acknowledged in the next edition.

PRINCIPLES FOR INTERVENTION DEVELOPMENT AND REFINEMENT

A set of guiding principles is necessary in forming intervention labels, definitions, and activities. Such principles, used to maintain consistency and cohesion within the Classification, can help the user to understand the Classification's language and form.

General Principles for Intervention Labels

Intervention labels are concepts. The following principles should be used when selecting names for concepts:

1. They should be noun statements; no verbs.
2. They should, preferably, be three words or less; no more than five words.
3. When a two-part label is required, use a colon to separate the words (e.g., Bleeding Reduction: Nasal). Guidelines for use of the colon are: (1) avoid unless it is indicated and desired by clinical practice and (2) use to indicate a more specialized area of practice only when there are different activities that require a new intervention.
4. Capitalize each word.
5. Labels will include modifiers to represent the nurse's actions. Choose modifiers to represent the nurse's actions (e.g., Administration, Assistance, Management, Promotion). The modifier should be selected based on its meaning, how it sounds in relationship to the other words in the label, and its acceptability in general practice. Some of the possible modifiers are listed here:

Administration—directing the movement or behavior of, having charge of; see also Management

Assistance—helping

Care—paying close attention, giving protection, being concerned about

Enhancement—making greater, augmenting, increasing; see also Promotion

Maintenance—continuing or carrying on, supporting

Management—directing the movement or behavior of, having charge of; see also Administration

Monitoring—watching and checking

Precaution—taking care beforehand against a possible danger; see also Protection

Promotion—advancing; see also Enhancement

Protection—shielding from injury; see also Precaution

Reduction—lessening, diminishing

Restoration—reinstating, bringing back to normal or unimpaired state

Therapy—having a therapeutic nature, healing

NOTE: Some of these terms mean the same thing; a choice of which one to use will depend upon which sounds better in context and whether one is already more familiar and more accepted in practice.

General Principles for Definitions of Interventions

A definition for an intervention label is a phrase that defines the concept. It is a summary of the most distinguishing characteristics. The definition, together with the defining activities, delineates the boundaries of nurse behavior circumscribed by the label.

1. Use phrases (not complete sentences) that describe the behavior of the nurse and can stand alone without examples.
2. Avoid using terms for the patient and nurse, but when a term must be used, *patient* or *person* is preferred rather than *client*.
3. For those phrases that begin with a verb form, consider the situation and choose either the -ion form (e.g., limitation) or the -ing form (e.g., limiting).

General Principles for Activities

Activities are actions that a nurse does to implement the intervention. The following principles relate to activities:

1. Begin each activity with a verb. Possible verbs include *assist, administer, explain, avoid,*

inspect, facilitate, monitor, and *use.* Use the most active verb that is appropriate for the situation. Use the term *monitor* rather than *assess.* Monitoring is a type of assessment but is done postdiagnosis as part of an intervention rather than as preparation for making a diagnosis. Avoid the terms *observe* and *evaluate.*

2. Keep the activities as generic as possible (e.g., instead of saying, "Place on Kinair bed" or "Place on circlelectric bed," say "Place on therapeutic bed"). Eliminate brand names.

3. Avoid combining two different ideas in one activity unless they illustrate the same point.

4. Avoid repeating an idea; when two activities are saying the same thing, even in different words, eliminate one.

5. Focus on the critical activities; do not worry about including all supporting activities. The number of activities depends on the intervention, but, on average, use a one-page list.

6. Word similar activities modifying different interventions the same for each intervention.

7. Word activities so they are clear without referring to the patient or the nurse. If the patient must be referred to, use the term *patient* or *person* in preference to *client* or other terms. Use the terms *family member(s)* or *significant other(s)* rather than *spouse.*

8. Add the phrase "as appropriate," "as necessary," or "as needed" to the end of those activities that are important but used only on some occasions.

9. Check for consistency between the activities and the label's definition.

10. Arrange the activities in the order in which they are usually carried out, when appropriate.

Demographic Information Form

(Please complete and submit with new/revised intervention[s].)
Please complete the following:

1. Are you currently employed as an RN?
   _____ (1) Yes _____(2) No, am an RN but not currently employed as an RN
   _____ (3) No, am studying to be an RN _____(4) No, am not an RN

2. How long have you practiced as an RN?
   _____ (0) Not practiced as an RN
   _____ (1) One Year or Less
   _____ (2) 1 to 3 Years
   _____ (3) 3 to 5 Years
   _____ (4) 5 to 10 Years
   _____ (5) Over 10 Years

3. Which of the following *best* describes the setting in which you are employed? (Check only *ONE* area.)
   _____ (1) Hospital
   _____ (2) Long-Term Care
   _____ (3) Public/Community Health
   _____ (4) Occupational Health
   _____ (5) Office Nursing
   _____ (6) School Nursing
   _____ (7) Outpatient Setting
   _____ (8) Nursing Education
   _____ (9) Other (specify) _____

4. Which of the following *best* describes the type of unit/specialty area in which you practice? (Check only *ONE* area)
   _____ (1) General Medicine
   _____ (2) General Surgery
   _____ (3) Intensive Care
   _____ (4) OB/GYN/Pediatrics
   _____ (5) Specialty Medicine
   _____ (6) Specialty Surgery
   _____ (7) Psychiatric (adult or child)
   _____ (8) Ambulatory Care/Outpatient
   _____ (9) General Long-term Care/Rehabilitation
   _____ (10) Other

5. What is your *highest* level of educational preparation?
   _____ (1) Associate Degree
   _____ (2) Diploma

_____ (3) Baccalaureate
_____ (4) Master's
_____ (5) Doctorate

6. Are you currently certified by any professional organizations?
_____ (1) Yes _____ (2) No

7. How have you used the Classification?
_____ Clinical Practice
_____ Teaching
_____ Research
_____ Administration
_____ Other (please specify)

Please elaborate on how you have used the Classification:

General comments about the Classification:

If your suggestions are included in NIC, we would like to acknowledge your help in the next edition. Please sign here if you will permit us to include your name as a contributor.

Print your name: _____

Employment title: _____

Place of employment: _____

Street: _____

City, State, and ZIP Code: _____

Telephone: _____

E-mail address: _____

Please mail, e-mail, or fax this form along with your proposed new or revised interventions(s) to:

Center for Nursing Classification and Clinical Effectiveness:
NIC Review
The University of Iowa College of Nursing:
Iowa City, Iowa 52242-1121:

Fax: (319) 335-6820 or (319) 335-7129
Phone: (319) 335-7051
Email: sharon-sweeney@uiowa.edu

APPENDIX C

Timeline and Highlights: Nursing Interventions Classification (NIC)

1985
Nursing Interventions: Treatments for Nursing Diagnoses, edited by Bulechek and McCloskey and published by Saunders, is one of the first two books to define independent nursing interventions.

1987
Intervention research team is formed by Joanne McCloskey and Gloria Bulechek at the University of Iowa.

1990
The Iowa Research Team, led by Joanne McCloskey and Gloria Bulechek, is funded by a research grant from the National Institute of Nursing Research (NINR) (1990-1993).

First publication about Nursing Interventions Classification (NIC) appears in print in the *Journal of Professional Nursing.*

1991
American Nurses Association (ANA) recognizes NIC.

1992
The first edition of *Nursing Interventions Classification (NIC)* is published by Mosby.

The Nursing Clinics of North America publishes an entire volume (*Nursing Interventions,* 27[2]. Philadelphia: W. B. Saunders) on the initial survey research on the interventions in the first edition of NIC.

Nursing Interventions: Essential Nursing Treatments, edited by Bulechek and McCloskey, is published by W. B. Saunders Company.

1993
NIC is added to the National Library of Medicine's Unified Medical Language System Metathesaurus.

The second NIC intervention grant is funded by NINR (June 1993-1997; extended to 1998), with Joanne McCloskey and Gloria Bulechek as the co-principal investigators.

NIC is included in the International Council of Nurses (ICN) *International Classification for Nursing Practice (Alpha Version).*

Publication of *The NIC Letter* begins at the University of Iowa.

1994

Cumulative Index to Nursing and Health Care Literature (CINAHL) and Silver Platter add NIC to their indexes.

The Joint Commission on Accreditation of Healthcare Organizations (JCAHO) includes NIC as a means to meet the standard on uniform data collection.

The National League for Nursing (NLN) makes a video describing the development and testing of NIC.

An institutional effectiveness grant for preparing PhD candidates and postdoctoral students is funded at the University of Iowa, with Joanne McCloskey and Meridean Maas as directors.

The Nursing Classifications Fund is established at The University of Iowa to provide ongoing financial support for the continued development and use of NIC and NOC.

1995

The Center for Nursing Classification at the University of Iowa is approved (December 13) by the Iowa Board of Regents (without funding) to facilitate the ongoing research and implementation of NIC and NOC. A fundraising advisory board for the Center is established and members are appointed.

1996

Mosby publishes the second edition of *Nursing Interventions Classification (NIC)*.

The first meeting of the Center for Nursing Classification's fundraising advisory board is held.

The ANA's *Social Policy Statement* includes the NIC definition of an intervention.

The first vendor signs a licensing agreement for NIC and NOC.

NIC is linked to the Omaha Classification and distributed in a monograph published by the Center for Nursing Classification.

1997

The NIC Letter becomes *The NIC/NOC Letter*.

The first joint international North American Nursing Diagnosis Association (NANDA), NIC, and NOC Conference is held in St. Charles, Illinois.

1998

NIC submits information to the American National Standards Institute Health Informatics Standards Board (ANSI HISB) for the Inventory of Clinical Information Standards.

The NIC/ NOC Letter is sponsored by Mosby–Year Book.

Multiple translations of NIC are processed (Dutch, Korean, Chinese, French, Japanese, German, and Spanish).

The Center for Nursing Classification receives 3 years of support from the College of Nursing at the University of Iowa (1998-2001) and is allocated space on the fourth floor of the College of Nursing, and Joanne McCloskey is appointed director.

NIC interventions are linked to NOC outcomes in a monograph published by the Center for Nursing Classification at the University of Iowa.

1999
NIC is included in Alternative Link *ABC Codes* for reimbursement.

The First Institute on Informatics and Classification is held at the University of Iowa.

Nursing Interventions: Effective Nursing Treatments, edited by Bulechek and McCloskey, is published by W. B. Saunders Company.

2000
Mosby publishes the third edition of *Nursing Interventions Classification (NIC)*.

The NNN Alliance is created, with Dorothy Jones and Joanne McCloskey Dochterman as co-chairs.

NIC and NOC are linked with Resident Assessment Protocols (RAP) and the Outcome and Assessment Information Set (OASIS).

Second Institute on Informatics and Classification is held.

2001
The book that links the three languages—*Nursing Diagnoses, Outcomes, Interventions: NANDA, NOC, and NIC Linkages*—is authored by the NIC and NOC principal investigators and published by Mosby.

An NNN Invitational Common Structure Conference is funded by the National Library of Medicine (Joanne Dochterman and Dorothy Jones, principal investigators) and held in Utica, Illinois, in August.

An effectiveness grant is funded (NINR and Agency for Healthcare Research and Quality [AHRQ]) for large database research with the use of NIC (Marita Titler and Joanne Dochterman). This is likely the first such grant to fund nursing effectiveness research in which a clinical database with nursing standardized language is used.

NIC is registered in Health Level 7 (HL 7).

Third Institute on Informatics and Classification is held.

2002
The NNN Alliance holds an international conference on nursing language, classification, and informatics in Chicago. This is a replacemnt for NANDA's biennial conference. A White Paper on the development of a common structure for NANDA, NIC, and NOC is presented to conference participants.

SNOMED (Systematized Nomenclature of Medicine) licenses NIC for inclusion in its database.

The Center for Nursing Classification expands its name to Center for Nursing Classification and Clinical Effectiveness; endowment reaches $600,000.

Fourth Institute on Informatics and Classification is held.

A 4-hour web course on standardized languages—NANDA, NIC, and NOC—is offered by the Center for Nursing Classification and Clinical Effectiveness at the University of Iowa.

A second institutional training grant for PhD candidates and postdoctoral students in effectiveness research is funded at the University of Iowa by NINR, with Joanne Dochterman and Martha Craft-Rosenberg as directors.

The position of Center Fellow is established (to assist in the ongoing development of NIC and NOC), and about 30 people are appointed for 3-year terms.

2003
ANA publishes the "Common Taxonomy of Nursing Practice" in a monograph, *Unifying Nursing Languages: The Harmonization of NANDA, NIC and NOC* (Edited by Joanne Dochterman and Dorothy Jones).

A NANDA, NIC, and NOC software program, based on the linkage book, is produced by Mosby.

Fifth Institute on Informatics and Classification is held.

In addition to the events listed in the timeline, NIC was presented over the years at numerous national and international conferences. Other countries in which NIC was presented include Australia, Brazil, Canada, Denmark, England, France, Iceland, Italy, Japan, Korea, Netherlands, Spain, Switzerland, and Turkey.

APPENDIX D

NIC Interventions Placed in Taxonomy of Nursing Practice

In 2001 a collaborative effort resulted in a common organizing structure for use by NANDA, NIC, and NOC and other nursing classifications as desired (NNN August 2001 Conference Group). The purpose of the initiative was to create a structure that could be used for all classifications to enhance efficiency and promote linkages among diagnoses, interventions, and outcomes. The structure was recently published by the American Nurses Association in a monograph that includes other supporting material (Dochterman & Jones, 2003). Consisting of four domains and 28 classes, this structure is somewhat similar to but has several differences from the NIC taxonomy contained in the front of this book.

In this appendix we have placed the 514 interventions in this common structure, the Taxonomy of Nursing Practice. Each intervention has been placed in only one class, the one judged to be the primary class. At the bottom of some of the classes, there are notes (e.g., "see also Knowledge class") indicating another class where additional interventions are located. All of the teaching interventions were put in the class called *Knowledge*, even when they had content related to another class (e.g., Teaching: Safe Sex and Teaching: Sexuality are in the Knowledge class but are also interventions that are appropriate for the Sexuality class).

The purpose of this exercise was to test the structure for a fit with interventions. All NIC interventions could be placed in this structure and all classes were used. Some of the classes have many more interventions than others; some of the shorter classes might indicate that they should be combined with others in future versions. The developers of NANDA and NOC are also committed to testing the structure for a fit with diagnoses and outcomes. At this time, each group is publishing the placement of their concepts within this structure in their own books; in the future, with perhaps some adjustment of the classes and domains, we hope that this work will lead to one structure in which diagnoses, interventions, and outcomes can be placed together. We hope that this will facilitate the teaching and clinical use of the classifications. Persons who want to use the Taxonomy of Nursing Practice structure may do so freely because it is in the public domain; as always, permission to use NIC in a nursing information system or to produce multiple copies of NIC interventions placed in this structure must be requested from Mosby.

References

Dochterman, J., & Jones, D. (Eds.). (2003). *Harmonization in nursing language classification*. Washington, DC: American Nurses Association.

NNN August 2001 Conference Group. (2003). Collaboration in nursing classification—The creation of a common unifying structure for NANDA, NIC, and NOC. In J. Dochterman & D. Jones (Eds.), *Harmonization in nursing language classification*. Washington, DC: American Nurses Association.

Level 1 Domains	I. FUNCTIONAL DOMAIN		
	Includes diagnoses, outcomes, and interventions to promote basic needs		
Level 2 Classes	**Activity/Exercise** Physical activity, including energy conservation and expenditure	**Comfort** A sense of emotional, physical, and spiritual well-being and relative freedom from distress	**Growth and Development** Physical, emotional, and social growth and development milestones

Level 3 Interventions	4310 Activity Therapy
	0740 Bed Rest Care
	0140 Body Mechanics
	        Promotion
	0762 Cast Care: Maintenance
	0764 Cast Care: Wet
	0180 Energy Management
	0200 Exercise Promotion
	0201 Exercise Promotion:
	        Strength Training
	0202 Exercise Promotion:
	        Stretching
	0221 Exercise Therapy:
	        Ambulation
	0222 Exercise Therapy: Balance
	0224 Exercise Therapy: Joint
	        Mobility
	0226 Exercise Therapy: Muscle
	        Control
	0840 Positioning
	0842 Positioning: Intraoperative
	0846 Positioning: Wheelchair
	0910 Splinting
	0940 Traction/Immobilization
	        Care
	0960 Transport
	
	[see also Knowledge class]
		1320 Acupressure
		5820 Anxiety Reduction
		5840 Autogenic Training
		5860 Biofeedback
		5880 Calming Technique
		1340 Cutaneous Stimulation
		5900 Distraction
		5260 Dying Care
		6482 Environmental
		        Management: Comfort
		1380 Heat/Cold Application
		5920 Hypnosis
		5960 Meditation Facilitation
		1450 Nausea Management
		1400 Pain Management
		1440 Premenstrual Syndrome
		        Management
		3550 Pruritus Management
		5465 Therapeutic Touch
		1540 Transcutaneous Electrical
		        Nerve Stimulation (TENS)
		1570 Vomiting Management
			5210 Anticipatory Guidance
			6710 Attachment Promotion
			1052 Bottle Feeding
			8250 Developmental Care
			8272 Developmental
			        Enhancement: Adolescent
			8274 Developmental
			        Enhancement: Child
			6820 Infant Care
			5244 Lactation Counseling
			7200 Normalization Promotion
			8300 Parenting Promotion
			8340 Resiliency Promotion
			6614 Risk Identification:
			        Genetic
			7280 Sibling Support
			
			[see also Knowledge class]

Level 1 Domains	I. FUNCTIONAL DOMAIN—cont'd		
	Includes diagnoses, outcomes, and interventions to promote basic needs		
Level 2 Classes	**Nutrition** Processes related to taking in, assimilating, and using nutrients	**Self-Care** Ability to accomplish basic and instrumental activities of daily living	**Sexuality** Maintenance or modification of sexual identity and patterns
Level 3 Interventions	1020 Diet Staging 1030 Eating Disorders Management 1056 Enteral Tube Feeding 1050 Feeding 1080 Gastrointestinal Intubation 1100 Nutrition Management 1120 Nutrition Therapy 5246 Nutritional Counseling 1160 Nutritional Monitoring 1860 Swallowing Therapy 1200 Total Parenteral Nutrition (TPN) Administration 1874 Tube Care: Gastrointestinal 1240 Weight Gain Assistance 1260 Weight Management 1280 Weight Reduction Assistance [see also Knowledge class]	1610 Bathing 1620 Contact Lens Care 6462 Dementia Management: Bathing 1630 Dressing 1640 Ear Care 1650 Eye Care 1660 Foot Care 1670 Hair Care 1680 Nail Care 1710 Oral Health Maintenance 1720 Oral Health Promotion 1730 Oral Health Restoration 1750 Perineal Care 1770 Postmortem Care 1780 Prosthesis Care 1800 Self-Care Assistance 1801 Self-Care Assistance: Bathing/Hygiene 1802 Self-Care Assistance: Dressing/Grooming 1803 Self-Care Assistance: Feeding 1805 Self-Care Assistance: IADL 1804 Self-Care Assistance: Toileting 1806 Self-Care Assistance: Transfer [see also Knowledge class]	4356 Behavior Management: Sexual 6300 Rape-Trauma Treatment 5248 Sexual Counseling [see also Knowledge class]

Continued

Level 1 Domains	I. FUNCTIONAL DOMAIN—cont'd	
	Includes diagnoses, outcomes, and interventions to promote basic needs	
Level 2 Classes	**Sleep/Rest** The quantity and quality of sleep, rest, and relaxation patterns	**Values/Beliefs** Ideas, goals, perceptions, and spiritual and other beliefs that influence choices or decisions
Level 3 Interventions	6926 Phototherapy: Mood/Sleep Regulation 1460 Progressive Muscle Relaxation 6000 Simple Guided Imagery 6040 Simple Relaxation Therapy 1850 Sleep Enhancement	5250 Decision-Making Support 7140 Family Support 5280 Forgiveness Facilitation 5422 Religious Addiction Prevention 5424 Religious Ritual Enhancement 5426 Spiritual Growth Facilitation 5420 Spiritual Support 5470 Truth Telling 5480 Values Clarification

Level 1 Domains	**II. Physiological Domain** Includes diagnoses, outcomes, and interventions to promote optimal biophysical health		
Level 2 Classes	**Cardiac Function** Cardiac mechanisms used to maintain tissue perfusion	**Elimination** Processes related to secretion and excretion of body wastes	**Fluid and Electrolyte** Regulation of fluid/electrolytes and acid-base balance
Level 3 Interventions	2860 Autotransfusion 4010 Bleeding Precautions 4020 Bleeding Reduction 4030 Blood Products Administration 4035 Capillary Blood Sample 4040 Cardiac Care 4044 Cardiac Care: Acute 4046 Cardiac Care: Rehabilitative 4050 Cardiac Precautions 4062 Circulatory Care: Arterial Insufficiency 4064 Circulatory Care: Mechanical Assist Device 4066 Circulatory Care: Venous Insufficiency 4070 Circulatory Precautions 4240 Dialysis Access Maintenance 4090 Dysrhythmia Management 4104 Embolus Care: Peripheral 4106 Embolus Care: Pulmonary 4110 Embolus Precautions 4150 Hemodynamic Regulation 4160 Hemorrhage Control 4210 Invasive Hemodynamic Monitoring 4220 Peripherally Inserted Central (PIC) Catheter Care 4232 Phlebotomy: Arterial Blood Sample 4234 Phlebotomy: Blood Unit Acquisition 4235 Phlebotomy: Cannulated Vessel 4238 Phlebotomy: Venous Blood Sample 4250 Shock Management 4254 Shock Management: Cardiac 4256 Shock Management: Vasogenic 4258 Shock Management: Volume 4260 Shock Prevention 4092 Temporary Pacemaker Management 2440 Venous Access Devices (VAD) Maintenance	0550 Bladder Irrigation 0410 Bowel Incontinence Care 0412 Bowel Incontinence Care: Encopresis 0420 Bowel Irrigation 0430 Bowel Management 0440 Bowel Training 0450 Constipation/Impaction Management 0460 Diarrhea Management 0470 Flatulence Reduction 0480 Ostomy Care 0560 Pelvic Muscle Exercise 0630 Pessary Management 0640 Prompted Voiding 0490 Rectal Prolapse Management 1870 Tube Care 1876 Tube Care: Urinary 0570 Urinary Bladder Training 0580 Urinary Catheterization 0582 Urinary Catheterization: Intermittent 0590 Urinary Elimination Management 0600 Urinary Habit Training 0610 Urinary Incontinence Care 0612 Urinary Incontinence Care: Enuresis 0620 Urinary Retention Care	1910 Acid-Base Management 1911 Acid-Base Management: Metabolic Acidosis 1912 Acid-Base Management: Metabolic Alkalosis 1920 Acid-Base Monitoring 2000 Electrolyte Management 2001 Electrolyte Management: Hypercalcemia 2002 Electrolyte Management: Hyperkalemia 2003 Electrolyte Management: Hypermagnesemia 2004 Electrolyte Management: Hypernatremia 2005 Electrolyte Management: Hyperphosphatemia 2006 Electrolyte Management: Hypocalcemia 2007 Electrolyte Management: Hypokalemia 2008 Electrolyte Management: Hypomagnesemia 2009 Electrolyte Management: Hyponatremia 2010 Electrolyte Management: Hypophosphatemia 2020 Electrolyte Monitoring 4120 Fluid Management 2080 Fluid/Electrolyte Management 4130 Fluid Monitoring 4140 Fluid Resuscitation 2100 Hemodialysis Therapy 2110 Hemofiltration Therapy 2120 Hyperglycemia Management 2130 Hypoglycemia Management 4170 Hypervolemia Management 4180 Hypovolemia Management 4190 Intravenous (IV) Insertion 4200 Intravenous (IV) Therapy 2150 Peritoneal Dialysis Therapy 6590 Pneumatic Tourniquet Precautions

Continued

Level 1 Domains	**II. PHYSIOLOGICAL DOMAIN—cont'd** **Includes diagnoses, outcomes, and interventions to promote optimal biophysical health**		
Level 2 Classes	**Neurocognition** Mechanisms related to the nervous system and neurocognitive functioning including memory, thinking, and judgment	**Pharmacological Function** Effects (therapeutic and adverse) of medications or drugs and other pharmacologically active products	**Physical Regulation** Body temperature and endocrine and immune system responses to regulate cellular processes
Level 3 Interventions	2540 Cerebral Edema Management 2550 Cerebral Profusion Promotion 6440 Delirium Management 6450 Delusion Management 6460 Dementia Management 2560 Dysreflexia Management 2570 Electroconvulsive Therapy Management 6510 Hallucination Management 2590 Intracranial Pressure (ICP) Monitoring 4760 Memory Training 2620 Neurologic Monitoring 2660 Peripheral Sensation Management 0844 Positioning: Neurologic 4820 Reality Orientation 4860 Reminiscence Therapy 2680 Seizure Management 2690 Seizure Precautions 2720 Subarachnoid Hemorrhage Precautions 1878 Tube Care: Ventriculostomy/ Lumbar Drain 2760 Unilateral Neglect Management	2210 Analgesic Administration 2214 Analgesic Administration: Intraspinal 2840 Anesthesia Administration 6430 Chemical Restraint 2240 Chemotherapy Management 2280 Hormone Replacement Therapy 2300 Medication Administration 2308 Medication Administration: Ear 2301 Medication Administration: Enteral 2310 Medication Administration: Eye 2311 Medication Administration: Inhalation 2302 Medication Administration: Interpleural 2312 Medication Administration: Intradermal 2313 Medication Administration: Intramuscular 2303 Medication Administration: Intraosseous 2319 Medication Administration: Intraspinal 2314 Medication Administration: Intravenous 2320 Medication Administration: Nasal 2304 Medication Administration: Oral 2315 Medication Administration: Rectal 2316 Medication Administration: Skin 2317 Medication Administration: Subcutaneous 2318 Medication Administration: Vaginal 2307 Medication Administration: Ventricular Reservoir 2380 Medication Management 2390 Medication Prescribing 2400 Patient-Controlled Analgesia (PCA) Assistance 2260 Sedation Management [see also Knowledge class]	6410 Allergy Management 3740 Fever Treatment 3780 Heat Exposure Treatment 3800 Hypothermia Treatment 3840 Malignant Hyperthermia Precautions 2870 Postanesthesia Care 3900 Temperature Regulation 3902 Temperature Regulation: Intraoperative

Level 1 Domains	**II. PHYSIOLOGICAL DOMAIN—cont'd** Includes diagnoses, outcomes, and interventions to promote optimal biophysical health	
Level 2 Classes	**Reproduction** Processes related to human procreation and birth	**Respiratory Function** Ventilation adequate to maintain arterial blood gases within normal limits
Level 3 Interventions	6700 Amnioinfusion 6720 Birthing 4021 Bleeding Reduction: Antepartum Uterus 4026 Bleeding Reduction: Postpartum Uterus 1054 Breastfeeding Assistance 6750 Cesarean Section Care 6760 Childbirth Preparation 3000 Circumcision Care 6771 Electronic Fetal Monitoring: Antepartum 6772 Electronic Fetal Monitoring: Intrapartum 6784 Family Planning: Contraception 6786 Family Planning: Infertility 6788 Family Planning: Unplanned Pregnancy 7160 Fertility Preservation 6800 High-Risk Pregnancy Care 6830 Intrapartal Care 6834 Intrapartal Care: High-Risk Delivery 6850 Labor Induction 6860 Labor Suppression 6870 Lactation Suppression 6880 Newborn Care 6890 Newborn Monitoring 6900 Nonnutritive Sucking 6924 Phototherapy: Neonate 6930 Postpartal Care 5247 Preconception Counseling 6950 Pregnancy Termination Care 6960 Prenatal Care 7886 Reproductive Technology Management 6972 Resuscitation: Fetus 6974 Resuscitation: Neonate 6656 Surveillance: Late Pregnancy 1875 Tube Care: Umbilical Line 6982 Ultrasonography: Limited Obstetric	1913 Acid-Base Management: Respiratory Acidosis 1914 Acid-Base Management: Respiratory Alkalosis 3120 Airway Insertion and Stabilization 3140 Airway Management 3460 Airway Suctioning 6412 Anaphylaxis Management 3180 Artificial Airway Management 3200 Aspiration Precautions 3210 Asthma Management 3230 Chest Physiotherapy 3250 Cough Enhancement 3270 Endotracheal Extubation 3300 Mechanical Ventilation 3310 Mechanical Ventilatory Weaning 3320 Oxygen Therapy 3350 Respiratory Monitoring 1872 Tube Care: Chest 3390 Ventilation Assistance

Continued

Level 1 *Domains*	**II. PHYSIOLOGICAL DOMAIN—cont'd** Includes diagnoses, outcomes, and interventions to promote optimal biophysical health	
Level 2 *Classes*	**Sensation/Perception** Intake and interpretation of information through the senses including seeing, hearing, touching, tasting, and smelling	**Tissue Integrity** Skin and mucous membrane protection to support secretion, excretion, and healing
Level 3 *Interventions*	1330 Aromatherapy 4974 Communication Enhancement: Hearing Deficit 4976 Communication Enhancement: Speech Deficit 4978 Communication Enhancement: Visual Deficit 6840 Kangaroo Care 1480 Simple Massage 5460 Touch [see also Communication class]	3420 Amputation Care 4022 Bleeding Reduction: Gastrointestinal 4024 Bleeding Reduction: Nasal 4028 Bleeding Reduction: Wound 3440 Incision Site Care 3460 Leech Therapy 3480 Lower Extremity Monitoring 3500 Pressure Management 3520 Pressure Ulcer Care 3540 Pressure Ulcer Prevention 3582 Skin Care: Donor Site 3583 Skin Care: Graft Site 3584 Skin Care: Topical Treatments 3590 Skin Surveillance 3620 Suturing 3660 Wound Care 3662 Wound Care: Closed Drainage 3680 Wound Irrigation

Level 1 *Domains*	**III. PSYCHOSOCIAL DOMAIN** Includes diagnoses, outcomes, and interventions to promote optimal mental and emotional health and social functioning		
Level 2 *Classes*	**Behavior** Actions that promote, maintain, or restore health	**Communication** Receiving, interpreting, and expressing spoken, written, and nonverbal messages	**Coping** Adjusting or adapting to stressful events
Level 3 *Interventions*	4320 Animal-Assisted Therapy 6420 Area Restriction 4340 Assertiveness Training 4350 Behavior Management 4352 Behavior Management: Overactivity/Inattention 4360 Behavior Modification 4362 Behavior Modification: Social Skills 4370 Impulse Control Training 4380 Limit Setting 4400 Music Therapy 4410 Mutual Goal Setting 4420 Patient Contracting 6630 Seclusion 4470 Self-Modification Assistance 4480 Self-Responsibility Facilitation 4490 Smoking Cessation Assistance 4500 Substance Use Prevention 4510 Substance Use Treatment 4512 Substance Use Treatment: Alcohol Withdrawal 4514 Substance Use Treatment: Drug Withdrawal 4516 Substance Use Treatment: Overdose 4430 Therapeutic Play	4920 Active Listening 4330 Art Therapy 5000 Complex Relationship Building 5020 Conflict Mediation 5320 Humor 5100 Socialization Enhancement 6658 Surveillance: Remote Electronic 8180 Telephone Consultation 8190 Telephone Follow-up **[see also Sensation/Perception class]**	5230 Coping Enhancement 5240 Counseling 5242 Genetic Counseling 6460 Crisis Intervention 5290 Grief Work Facilitation 5294 Grief Work Facilitation: Perinatal Death 5300 Guilt Work Facilitation 6260 Organ Procurement 5340 Presence 5360 Recreation Therapy 5350 Relocation Stress Reduction 5430 Support Group 5440 Support System Enhancement 5450 Therapy Group 5410 Trauma Therapy: Child

Continued

Level 1 Domains	**III. PSYCHOSOCIAL DOMAIN—cont'd** Includes diagnoses, outcomes, and interventions to promote optimal mental and emotional health and social functioning		
Level 2 Classes	**Emotional** A mental state or feeling that may influence perceptions of the world	**Knowledge** Understanding and skill in applying information to promote, maintain, and restore health	**Roles/Relationships** Maintenance and/or modification of expected social behaviors and emotional connectedness with others

Level 3
Interventions
	4640 Anger Control
	     Assistance
	4680 Bibliotherapy
	5270 Emotional Support
	7110 Family Involvement
	     Promotion
	7170 Family Presence
	     Facilitation
	5310 Hope Instillation
	5330 Mood Management
		5520 Learning Facilitation
		5540 Learning Readiness
		     Enhancement
		5562 Parent Education:
		     Adolescent
		5566 Parent Education:
		     Childrearing Family
		5568 Parent Education: Infant
		5580 Preparatory Sensory
		     Information
		5602 Teaching: Disease Process
		5603 Teaching: Foot Care
		5604 Teaching: Group
		5606 Teaching: Individual
		5626 Teaching: Infant Nutrition
		5628 Teaching: Infant Safety
		5605 Teaching: Infant
		     Stimulation
		5610 Teaching: Preoperative
		5612 Teaching: Prescribed
		     Activity/Exercise
		5614 Teaching: Prescribed Diet
		5616 Teaching: Prescribed
		     Medication
		5618 Teaching: Procedure/
		     Treatment
		5620 Teaching: Psychomotor
		     Skill
		5622 Teaching: Safe Sex
		5624 Teaching: Sexuality
		5630 Teaching: Toddler
		     Nutrition
		5632 Teaching: Toddler Safety
		5634 Teaching: Toilet Training
			7040 Caregiver Support
			6481 Environmental
			     Management: Attachment
			     Process
			7100 Family Integrity
			     Promotion
			7104 Family Integrity
			     Promotion: Childbearing
			     Family
			7120 Family Mobilization
			7130 Family Process
			     Maintenance
			7150 Family Therapy
			7180 Home Maintenance
			     Assistance
			4390 Milieu Therapy
			7260 Respite Care
			6612 Risk Identification:
			     Childbearing Family
			5370 Role Enhancement
			7560 Visitation Facilitation

Level 1 *Domains*	**III. PSYCHOSOCIAL DOMAIN—cont'd** **Includes diagnoses, outcomes, and interventions to promote optimal mental and emotional health and social functioning**
Level 2 *Classes*	**Self-Perception** Awareness of one's body and personal identity
Level 3 *Interventions*	4354 Behavior Management: Self-Harm 5220 Body Image Enhancement 4700 Cognitive Restructuring 4720 Cognitive Stimulation 5390 Self-Awareness Enhancement 5400 Self-Esteem Enhancement

Level 1 Domains	**IV. ENVIRONMENTAL DOMAIN** Includes diagnoses, outcomes, and interventions to promote and protect the environmental health and safety of individuals, systems, and communities		
Level 2 Classes	**Health Care System** Social, political, and economic structures and processes for the delivery of health care services	**Populations** Aggregates of individuals or communities having characteristics in common	**Risk Management** Avoidance or control of identifiable health threats
Level 3 Interventions	7310 Admission Care 7610 Bedside Laboratory Testing 7910 Consultation 7620 Controlled Substance Checking 7630 Cost Containment 7640 Critical Path Development 7330 Culture Brokerage 7650 Delegation 7930 Deposition/Testimony 7370 Discharge Planning 7920 Documentation 7660 Emergency Cart Checking 6485 Environmental Management: Home Preparation 7680 Examination Assistance 7380 Financial Resource Assistance 7960 Health Care Information Exchange 7400 Health System Guidance 7980 Incident Reporting 7410 Insurance Authorization 7690 Laboratory Data Interpretation 8020 Multidisciplinary Care Conference 8060 Order Transcription 7440 Pass Facilitation 7460 Patient Rights Protection 7700 Peer Review 7710 Physician Support 7722 Preceptor: Employee 7726 Preceptor: Student 2880 Preoperative Coordination 7760 Product Evaluation 7800 Quality Monitoring 8100 Referral 8120 Research Data Collection 8140 Shift Report 7820 Specimen Management 7830 Staff Supervision 7850 Staff Development 7840 Supply Management 7500 Sustenance Support 7880 Technology Management	8810 Bioterrorism Preparedness 7320 Case Management 8820 Communicable Disease Management 8840 Community Disaster Preparedness 8500 Community Health Development 6484 Environmental Management: Community 6489 Environmental Management: Worker Safety 8880 Environmental Risk Protection 8550 Fiscal Resource Management 5510 Health Education 7970 Health Policy Monitoring 8700 Program Development 6652 Surveillance: Community	6400 Abuse Protection Support 6402 Abuse Protection Support: Child 6403 Abuse Protection Support: Domestic Partner 6404 Abuse Protection Support: Elder 6408 Abuse Protection Support: Religious 6522 Breast Examination 6140 Code Management 6470 Elopement Precautions 6200 Emergency Care 6480 Environmental Management 6486 Environmental Management: Safety 6487 Environmental Management: Violence Prevention 6490 Fall Prevention 6500 Fire-Setting Precautions 6240 First Aid 6520 Health Screening 6530 Immunization/Vaccination Management 6540 Infection Control 6545 Infection Control: Intraoperative 6550 Infection Protection 6560 Laser Precautions 6570 Latex Precautions 6580 Physical Restraint 6600 Radiation Therapy Management 6320 Resuscitation 6610 Risk Identification 6648 Sports-Injury Prevention: Youth 6340 Suicide Prevention 2920 Surgical Precautions 2930 Surgical Preparation 6650 Surveillance 6654 Surveillance: Safety 6362 Triage: Disaster 6364 Triage: Emergency Center 6366 Triage: Telephone 6660 Vehicle Safety Promotion 6680 Vital Signs Monitoring

APPENDIX E

Selected Publications

A. Previous editions of the NIC classification:

McCloskey, J.C., & Bulechek, G.M. (Eds.) (1992). *Nursing interventions classification (NIC)*. St. Louis: Mosby–Year Book. (336 Interventions)
　　-Translated into French, 1996: Decarie Editeur Inc.

McCloskey, J.C., & Bulechek, G.M. (Eds.) (1996). *Nursing interventions classification (NIC)* (2nd ed). St. Louis: Mosby–Year Book. (433 Interventions)
　　-Translated into Dutch, 1997: De Tijdstroom, Utrecht.
　　-Translated into Korean, 1998: Hung Moon Sa.
　　-Translated into Chinese, 2000: Farseeing.
　　-Translated into French, 2000: Masson.
　　-Translated into Spanish, 2000: Sintesis.
　　Translated into Japanese, 2001: Nankodo.

McCloskey, J.C., & Bulechek, G.M. (Eds.). (2000). *Nursing interventions classification (NIC)* (3rd ed). St. Louis: Mosby Year Book. (486 Interventions)
　　-Translated into Japanese, 2002: Nankodo.
　　-Translated into German, forthcoming: Hans Huber.
　　-Translated into Portugese, forthcoming: Artis Medicas.
　　-Translated into Dutch, 2002: Elsevier Gezondheidszorg.
　　-Translated into Spanish, 2001: Ediciones Harcourt, S. A.

B. The best introduction to NIC is to read the chapters in this current edition. In addition, we have included the following references for your interest.

Bibliography

1. Acello, B. (1997). Top Drawer: Nursing Interventions Classification (Book Review). *Computers in Nursing*, 15(5), 219, 230-231.
2. Alternative Link Systems, Inc. (2001). *The CAM and nursing coding manual*. Albany, NY: Delmar.
3. Arnold, J.M. (1999). Comparison of use of nursing language in documentation of rehabilitation nursing. In Rantz, M. J. & LeMone, P. (Eds.), *Classification of nursing diagnoses: Proceedings of the thirteenth conference* (pp. 285-290) Glendale, CA: CINAHL Information Systems.
4. Aquilino, M.L., & Keenan, G. (2000). Having our say: Nursing's standardized nomenclatures. *American Journal of Nursing*, 100(7), 33-38.
5. Barry-Walker, J., Bulechek, G.M., & McCloskey, J.C. (1994). A description of medical-surgical nursing. *Med-Surg Nursing*, 3(4), 261-268.
6. Beecroft, P. C. (1995). Differentiating advanced practice interventions and outcomes. *The Journal for Advanced Nursing Practice*, 9(5), 237.
7. Blegen, M.A., & Tripp-Reimer, T. (1997). Implications of nursing taxonomies for middle range theory development. *Advances in Nursing Science*, 19(3), 37-49.
8. Blegen, M.A., & Tripp-Reimer, T. (1997). Nursing theory, nursing research and nursing practice: Connected or separate? In J.C. McCloskey & H.K. Grace (Eds.), *Current issues in nursing* (5th ed.) (pp. 68-74). St. Louis: Mosby.

9. Bowker, G.C., Star, S.L., & Spasser, M.A. (2001). Classifying nursing work. *Online Journal of Issues in Nursing*, http://www.nursingworld.org/ojin/tpc7/tpc7_6.htm

10. Bowker, G.C., & Starr, S.L. (1999). *Sorting things out: Classification and practice.* Boston: MIT Press (2 chapters devoted to NIC).

11. Bowles, K.H., & Naylor, M.D. (1996). Nursing intervention classification systems. *Image: Journal of Nursing Scholarship, 28*(4), 303-308.

12. Bradley, V. (1995). NIC: What is it? *Journal of Emergency Nursing, 21*(4), 338-340.

13. Buckwalter, K.C. (1998). Interventions for specialty practice, *Journal of Gerontological Nursing, 24*(7), 5.

14. Bulechek, G.M., & McCloskey, J.C. (1990). Nursing intervention taxonomy development. In J.C. McCloskey & H.K. Grace (Eds.), *Current issues in nursing* (3rd ed.) (pp. 23-28). St. Louis: Mosby.

15. Bulechek, G.M., & McCloskey, J.C. (Eds.) (1992). The nursing clinics of North America: *Nursing interventions, 27*(2). Philadelphia: W.B. Saunders.

16. Bulechek, G.M. & McCloskey, J.C. (1993). Additional dialogue between Bulechek, McCloskey, and Grobe. In Canadian Nurses Association. *Papers from the Nursing Minimum Data Set Conference* (pp. 158-160). Ottawa, Ontario, Canada: Canadian Nurses Association.

17. Bulechek, G.M., & McCloskey, J.C. (1994). Nursing Interventions Classification (NIC): Defining nursing care. In J.C. McCloskey & H.K. Grace (Eds.), *Current issues in nursing* (4th ed.) (pp. 129-135). St. Louis: Mosby.

18. Bulechek, G.M., & McCloskey, J.C. (1999). Nursing diagnoses, interventions, and outcomes in effectiveness research, In G.M. Bulechek & J.C. McCloskey, (Eds.), *Nursing interventions: Effective nursing treatments* (3rd ed.) (pp. 1-26). Philadelphia: W.B. Saunders.

19. Bulechek, G.M., McCloskey, J.C., Denehy, J.A., & Titler, M. (1994). Report on the NIC project, Nursing interventions used in practice. *American Journal of Nursing, 94*(10), 59-66.

20. Bulechek, G.M., McCloskey, J.C., & Donahue, W. (1995). Nursing Interventions Classification (NIC): A language to describe nursing treatments. In N.M. Lang (Ed.), *Nursing data systems: The emerging framework* (pp. 115-131). Washington, DC: American Nurses Association. Reprinted as: Bulechek, G.M., McCloskey, J.C., & Donahue, W. Nursing Interventions Classification (NIC): A language to describe nursing treatments. In R.A. Mortensen (Ed.), *Proceedings of the First European Conference on Nursing Diagnoses: Creating a European Platform* (pp. 309-319). Copenhagen: Danish Institute for Health and Nursing Research.

21. Bulechek, G.M., McCloskey, J.C., & The Iowa Intervention Project Research Team (1997). Letter to the editor: All users of NIC encouraged to submit new interventions, suggest revisions. *Image: Journal of Nursing Scholarship, 29*(1), 10.

22. Bulechek, G.M. & McCloskey, J.C. (1999). *Nursing interventions: Effective nursing treatments* (3rd ed). Philadelphia: Saunders.

23. Burkhart, L. (2002). *An instance of knowledge representation: Measuring the domain completeness of the Nursing Interventions Classification system in parish nurse documentation.* Unpublished doctoral dissertation, Virginia Commonwealth University–Medical College of Virginia.

24. Carlson-Catalano, J. (1998). Nursing diagnoses and interventions for post-acute-phase battered women, *Nursing Diagnosis, 9*(3), 101-109.

25. Carter, J.K. (1995). *Implementation of the Nursing Interventions Classification in five clinical sites.* Unpublished doctoral dissertation, University of Iowa, Iowa City, Iowa.

26. Carter, J., Moorhead, S.A., McCloskey, J.C., & Bulechek, G.M. (1995). Using the Nursing Interventions Classification (NIC) to implement AHCPR Guidelines. *Journal of Nursing Care Quality, 9*(2), 76-86.

27. Cavendish, R., Lunney, M., Kraynyak-Luise, B., & Richardson, K. (1999). Nursing interventions in school settings. In M. J. Rantz & P. LeMone (Eds.), *Classification of nursing diagnoses: Proceedings of the thirteenth conference.* (pp 296-298) Glendale, CA: CINAHL Information Systems.

28. Center for Nursing Classification. (1996). *Nursing Interventions Classification (NIC) Publications: An Anthology.* Iowa City, IA: Center for Nursing Classification.

29. Center for Nursing Classification. (2000). Cox, R. Preparer. *Standardized nursing language in long term care.* Iowa City, IA: Center for Nursing Classification.

30. Center for Nursing Classification. (2000). *NIC interventions and NOC outcomes linked to the OASIS Information Set.* Iowa City, IA: Center for Nursing Classification.

31. Center for Nursing Classification. (2001). *Estimated time and educational requirements to perform 486 nursing interventions.* Iowa City, IA: Center for Nursing Classification.

32. Clarke, M. (1998). Implementation of Nursing Standardized Languages: NANDA, NIC & NOC [on-line] *On-line Journal of Nursing Informatics* (http://cac.psu.edu/~dxm12/OJNI.html) Vol.2, No.2.

33. Coenen, A., Ryan, P., & Sutton, J. (1997). Mapping nursing interventions from a hospital information system to the Nursing Interventions Classification (NIC). *Nursing Diagnosis, 8*(4), 145-151.

34. Cohen, M.Z., Kruckeberg, T., McCloskey, J.C., Bulechek, G.M., Craft, M.J., Crossley, J.D., Denehy, J.A., Glick, O.J., Maas, M.L., Prophet, C.M., Tripp-Reimer, T., Nelson, D.C., Wyman, M., & Titler, M. (1992). Inductive methodology and a research team. *Nursing Outlook, 39*(4), 162-165.

35. Contino, D.S. (2000) The ABCs of APCs. *Nursing Management*, 31(10), 12, 14-16.
36. Corbett, C.F., & Androwich, I.M. (1994). Critical paths: Implications for improving practice. *Home Healthcare Nurse*, 12(6), 27-34.
37. Craft-Rosenberg, M., & Denehy, J. (Eds.) (2001). *Nursing interventions for infants, children, and families.* Thousand Oaks, CA: Sage Publications, Inc.
38. Cullen, L.M., McCloskey, J.C., & Bulechek, G.M. (1994). Development and validation of circulatory nursing interventions. In R.M. Carroll-Johnson & M. Paquette (Eds.), *Classification of nursing diagnoses: Proceedings of the tenth conference* (pp. 307-310). Philadelphia: J.B. Lippincott.
39. Daly, J.M. (1997). How Nursing Interventions Classification fits in the patient information system patient core data set. *Computers in Nursing*, 15(Suppl. 2), S577-S581.
40. Daly, J.M., Button, P., Prophet, C.M., Clarke, M., & Androwich, I. (1997). Nursing Interventions Classification implementation issues in five test sites. *Computers in Nursing*, 15(1), 23-29.
41. Daly, J.M., Maas, M.L., & Buckwalter, K.C. (1995). Use of standardized nursing diagnoses and interventions in long-term care. *Journal of Gerontological Nursing*, 21(8), 29-36.
42. Daly, J.M., Maas, M.L., & Buckwalter, K.C. (1997). What interventions do nurses use in long term care? *The Director*, 5(3), 108-111.
43. Daly, J.M., McCloskey, J.C., & Bulechek, G.M.. (1994). Nursing Interventions Classification use in long term care. *Geriatric Nursing*, 15(1), 41-46
44. Daly, J.M., Maas, M.L., McCloskey, J.C., & Bulechek, G.M. (1996). A care planning tool that proves what we do. *RN*, June, 26-29.
45. Davis, K. A. (1995). AIDS nursing care and standardized nursing language: An application of the Nursing Intervention Classification. *Journal of the Association of Nurses in AIDS Care*, 6(6), 37-44.
46. Delaney, C., Mehmert, P.A., Prophet, C.M., Bellinger, S.L.R., Huber, D.G., & Ellerbe, S. (1992). Standardized nursing language for healthcare information systems. *Journal of Medical Systems*, 16(4), 145-159.
47. Delaney, C., & Moorhead, S. (1997). Synthesis of methods, rules, and issues of standardizing nursing intervention language mapping. *Nursing Diagnosis*, 8(4), 152-156.
48. Denehy, J. (2000). Measuring the outcomes of school nursing practice: Showing that school nurses do make a difference. *Journal of School Nursing*, 16(1), 2-4.
49. Denehy, J., & Poulton, S. (1999). The use of standardized language individualized healthcare plans. *Journal of School Nursing*, 15(1), 38-45.
50. Dougherty, C. M. (1999). Nursing interventions and outcomes for the nursing diagnosis decreased cardiac output. In M. J. Rantz & P. LeMone (Eds.), *Classification of nursing diagnoses: Proceedings of the thirteenth conference* (pp. 441-452). Glendale, CA: CINAHL Information Systems.
51. Eganhouse, D.J., McCloskey, J.C., & Bulechek, G.M. (1996). How NIC describes MCH nursing. *MCN, The American Journal of Maternal/Child Nursing*, 21, September/October, 247-252.
52. Engebretson, J. (1997). A multiparadigm approach to nursing. *Advances in Nursing Science*, 20(1), 21-33.
53. England, M. (1993). Classification of nursing interventions (Book Review). *Nursing Diagnosis*, 4(2), 79-80.
54. Finesilver, C., & Metzler, D. (Eds.), (2002). *Curriculum guide for implementation of NANDA, NIC, and NOC into an undergraduate nursing curriculum.* Iowa City: Center for Nursing Classification, the University of Iowa College of Nursing.
55. Fitzpatrick, M.J., McElroy, M.J., & DeWoody, S. (2001). Building a strong nursing organization in a merged service line structure. *JONA*, 31(1), 24-32.
56. Frederick, J., Scherb, C.A., Smith-Foremen, K., Witt, S., Quiram, J., Wagennar, J., Slama, C., Botemmak. K., Muilenburg, J., & Evans, K. (2001) Speaking a common language. *American Journal of Nursing*, 101(3), 2400.
57. Haddon, R. (1993). Bookshelf: Reviewed this month–Nursing Interventions Classification (Book Review). *RN* (May).
58. Hajewski, C., Maupin, J.M., Rapp, D. A., Sitterding, M., & Pappas, J. (1998). Implementation and evaluation of Nursing Interventions Classification and Nursing Outcomes Classification in a patient education plan. *Journal of Nursing Care Quality*, 12(5), 30-40.
59. Henry, S.B., Holzemer, W.L., Randell, C., Hsich, S., & Miller, T. J. (1997). Comparison of Nursing Interventions Classification with Current Procedural Terminology codes for categorizing nursing activities. *Image: Journal of Nursing Scholarship*, 29(2), 133-138.
60. Hoyt, K.S. (1997). President's message: Validating nursing with NANDA, NIC, and NOC. *Emergency Nurses Association*, 23, 507-509.
61. Hur, H.K., Kim, S., & Storey, M. (2000). Nursing diagnoses and interventions used in home care in Korea. *Nursing Diagnosis*, 11(3), 97-108.
62. Iowa Intervention Project—Daly, J.M. (Ed.). (1992). *NIC interventions linked to NANDA diagnoses.* Iowa City, IA: Iowa Intervention Project. (Out of Print.)
63. Iowa Intervention Project. (1992). *Taxonomy of nursing interventions.* Iowa City, IA: Iowa Intervention Project. (Out of Print.)

64. Iowa Intervention Project. (1993). The NIC taxonomy structure. *Image: Journal of Nursing Scholarship, 25*(3), 187-192. Reprinted as Iowa Intervention Project. (1995). NIC-domeinen en-klassen. Handboek Verpleegkundige Diagnostiek, interventies en resultaten (pp. A1550-1-A1550-3). Houten, The Netherlands: Bohn Stafleu Van Loghum; Iowa Intervention Project. (1995). De structuur van de NIC-taxonomie. Handboek Verpleegkundige dianostiek, interventies en resultaten (pp. A1500-1-A1500-12). Houten, The Netherlands: Bohn Stafleu Van Loghum.

65. Iowa Intervention Project (1995). Validation and coding of the NIC Taxonomy structure. *Image: Journal of Nursing Scholarship, 27*(1), 43-49.

66. Iowa Intervention Project—Bulechek, G.M., & McCloskey, J.C. (Eds.). (1996). *NIC implementation manual.* Iowa City, IA: Iowa Intervention Project. (Out of Print).

67. Iowa Intervention Project. (1996). *Core interventions by specialty.* Iowa City, IA: Iowa Intervention Project. (Out of Print).

68. Iowa Intervention Project. (1996). *NIC interventions linked to Omaha System problems.* Iowa City, IA: Iowa Intervention Project.

69. Iowa Intervention Project. (1996). *Nursing Interventions Classification (NIC) publications: An anthology.* Iowa City, IA: Iowa Intervention Project.

70. Iowa Intervention Project. (1997). Defining nursing's effectiveness: Diagnoses, interventions, and outcomes. In M. Rantz & P. LeMone (Eds.), *Classification of nursing diagnoses: Proceedings of the twelfth conference* (pp. 293-303). Glendale, CA: CINAHL Information Systems.

71. Iowa Intervention Project. (1997). Nursing interventions classification (NIC): An overview. In M.J. Rantz & L.P. LeMone (Eds.), *Classification of nursing diagnoses: Proceedings of the twelfth conference (NANDA)* (pp. 32-39). Glendale, CA: CINAHL Information Systems.

72. Iowa Intervention Project. (1997). Proposal to bring nursing into the information age. *Image: Journal of Nursing Scholarship, 29*(3), 275-281.

73. Iowa Intervention Project. (1998). *NIC interventions linked to NOC outcomes.* Iowa City, IA: Iowa Intervention Project. (Out of Print).

74. Iowa Intervention Project. (2001). Determining cost of nursing interventions: A beginning. *Nursing Economics, 19*(4), 146-160.

75. Jensen, B.A. (1999). You make the diagnosis: Case study: Family stress and Alzheimer's disease. *Nursing Diagnosis, 10*(4), 134, 148, 169-72.

76. Johnson, M., Bulechek, G., Dochterman, J. Maas, M., & Moorhead, S. (2001). *Nursing diagnoses, outcomes, interventions: NANDA, NOC, and NIC linkages.* St. Louis: Mosby.

77. Karolys, A. (1999). You make the diagnosis: Case study: The role of nurses in the protection of children and the importance of naming the phenomena of nursing concern. *Nursing Diagnosis, 10*(3), 92, 121-124.

78. Keenan, G.M., Stocker, J.R., Geo-Thomas, An. T., Soparkar, N.R., Barkauskas, V.H., & Lee, J.L. (2002). The HANDS project: Studying and refining the automated collection of a cross-setting clinical data set. *Computers in Nursing, 20*(3), 89-100.

79. Kirby, A. (1996). *Classification of advanced nursing functions using the Nursing Interventions Classification taxonomy.* Unpublished doctoral dissertation, University of Pennsylvania, Philadelphia, Pennsylvania.

80. LaDuke, S. (2002). Beyond the psychomotor realm. *Nursing Management,* March, 41-42.

81. LaDuke, S. (2000). Consider this...Competency assessments: A case for the Nursing Interventions Classification and the observation of daily work. *Journal of Nursing Administration, 30*(7/8), 339-340.

82. LaDuke, S. (2000). NIC puts nursing into words. *Nursing Management, 31*(2), 43-44.

83. LaDuke, S. (2001). Online nursing documentation: Finding a middle ground. *JONA, 31*(6), 283-286.

84. LaDuke, S. (2001). The role of staff development in assuring competence. *Journal for Nurses in Staff Development, 17*(5), 221-225.

85. Maas, M.L., Buckwalter, K.C., Hardy, M.D., Tripp-Reimer, T., Titler, M.G., & Specht, J.P. (2001). *Nursing care of older adults: Diagnoses, outcomes and interventions.* St. Louis: Mosby.

86. McCaskey, R. (1993). Nursing Interventions Classification (NIC): Iowa Interventions Project (Book Review). *Journal of Nursing Staff Development, 9*(3), 163.

87. McCloskey, J.C. (1994). Nurse executive: The NMDS is a trend, not a fad [Column]. *Journal of Professional Nursing, 10*(6), 332.

88. McCloskey, J.C. (1995). Help to make nursing visible. Guest editorial: *Image: Journal of Nursing Scholarship, 27*(3), 170, 175.

89. McCloskey, J.C. (1995). Nurse executive: The discipline hearts of a multidisciplinary team [Column]. *The Journal of Professional Nursing, 11*(4), 202.

90. McCloskey, J.C. (1995). Nursing interventions classification (NIC): Development and use (pp. 79-98). In Schwartz, R.P. (Ed.). *Advances in classification research.* Vol. 6. Medford, N.J. Information Today, Inc.

91. McCloskey, J.C. (1996). Standardizing nursing language for computerization (pp. 16-27). In M. Mills, C. Romano, & B. Heller (Eds.), *Information management in nursing and health care.* Springhouse, PA: Springhouse.

92. McCloskey, J.C. (1997). Nursing Interventions Classification program facilitates data gathering, study of nursing. *Clinical Data Management, 3*(12), 1,4-5.

93. McCloskey, J.C. (1998). Nursing Interventions Classification (NIC) (pp. 371-374). In J. Fitzpatrick (Ed.), *Encyclopedia of nursing research.* New York: Springer Pub.

94. McCloskey, J.C., & Bulechek, G.M. (1993). Defining and classifying nursing interventions. In P. Moritz (Ed.), *Patient outcomes research: Examining the effectiveness of nursing practice—Proceedings of the state of the science conference* (NIH Pub. No 93-3411) (pp. 63-69). Washington DC: National Institute of Nursing Research.

95. McCloskey, J.C., & Bulechek, G.M. (1993). Nursing intervention schemes (pp. 77-91). In Canadian Nurses Association. *Papers from the Nursing Minimum Data Set Conference.* Ottawa, Ontario, Canada: Canadian Nurses Association.

96. McCloskey, J.C., & Bulechek, G.M. (1994). Reply to Edward Halloran's letter to the editor. *Image: Journal of Nursing Scholarship, 26*(2), 93.

97. McCloskey, J.C., & Bulechek, G.M. (1994). Classification of nursing interventions: Implications for nursing diagnoses (pp. 113-125). In R.M. Carroll-Johnson & M. Paquette (Eds.), *Classification of nursing diagnoses: Proceedings of the tenth conference.* Philadelphia: J. B. Lippincott. Reprinted as: McCloskey, J.C., & Bulechek, G.M. (1993). Classification van verpleegkundige interventies: Implicaties voor de verpleegkundige diagnose. In G. Bruggink & L. Regeer (Eds.), *Verpleegkundige diagnostiek in Nederland* (pp. 49-61). Amsterdam: LEO Verpleegkundig Management.

98. McCloskey, J.C., & Bulechek, G.M. (1994). Classification of nursing interventions: Implications for nursing research (pp. 65-81). In J. Fitzpatrick, J. Stevenson, & N. Polis (Eds.), *Nursing research and its utilization.* New York: Springer Publishing.

99. McCloskey, J.C., Bulechek, G.M., & Members of the Iowa Intervention Project Group. (1994). Letter to the editor: Toward data standards for clinical nursing information: Reply to Ozbolt, Fruchtnicht, & Hayden. *Journal of the American Medical Informatics Association, 1*(6), 469-471.

100. McCloskey, J.C., & Bulechek, G.M. (1994). Standardizing the language for nursing treatments: An overview of the issues. *Nursing Outlook, 42*(2), 56-63.

101. McCloskey, J.C., & Bulechek, G.M. (1995). Nursing Interventions Classification (NIC): Development and use (pp. 79-98). In R. Schwartz (Ed.). *Advances in classification research.* Vol. 6. Medford, NJ: Information Today, Inc.

102. McCloskey, J.C., & Bulechek, G.M. (1995). Nursing Interventions Classification (NIC): Development and use (pp. 111-132). In R.P. Schwartz, C. Beghtol, E.K. Jacob, B.H. Kwasnik, & P.J. Smith (Eds.), *Proceedings of the Sixth ASIS SIG/CR (American Society for Information Science, Special Interest Group/Classification Research) Workshop.* Chicago: ASIS SIG/CR.

103. McCloskey, J.C., & Bulechek, G.M. (1998). Nursing Interventions Classification—Current status and new directions [on-line] *On-line Journal of Nursing Informatics, 2*(2) (http://cac.psu.edu/~dxm12/OJNI.html).

104. McCloskey, J.C., & Bulechek, G.M. (1998). Nursing Interventions Classification (NIC): Development and use. In R. Schwartz, C. Beghtol, B.H. Kwasnik, & P.J. Smith (Eds.), *Advances in Classification Research* (Vol. 6, pp. 79-98). Medford, NJ: Information Today.

105. McCloskey, J. & Bulechek, G. (1999). Nursing Interventions Classification (NIC): Current status and new directions. In M. Rantz & P. Lemone (Ed.), *Classification of nursing diagnosis: Proceedings of the thirteenth conference.* Glendale, CA: CINAHL Information Systems. (Same paper as in the 1998 *On line Journal of Nursing Informatics.*)

106. McCloskey, J.C., Bulechek, G.M., Cohen, M.Z., Craft, M.J., Crossley, D., Denehy, J.A., Glick, O.J., Kruckeberg, T., Maas, M.L., Prophet, C.M., & Tripp-Reimer, T. (1990). Classification of nursing interventions. *Journal of Professional Nursing, 6*(3), 151-157.

107. McCloskey, J.C., Bulechek, G.M., & Donahue, W. (1998). Nursing interventions core to specialty practice. *Nursing Outlook, 46*(2): 67-76.

108. McCloskey, J.C., Bulechek, G.M., & Eganhouse, D.J. (1997). Letter to the editor: Toward enhancing collaboration: Addressing the assumptions made by Toni Vezeau, MCN. *The American Journal of Maternal/Child Nursing, 22,* March/April, 1997, 104.

109. McCloskey, J.C., Bulechek, G.M., Moorhead, S., & Daly, J. (1996). Nurses' use and delegation of indirect care interventions. *Nursing Economics, 14*(1), 22-33.

110. McCloskey, J.C., Bulechek, G.M., & Tripp-Reimer, T. (1995). Reply to William K. Cody's letter to the editor. *Nursing Outlook, 43*(2), 93-94.

111. McCloskey, J.C., & Maas, M. (1998). Interdisciplinary team: The nursing perspective is essential. *Nursing Outlook, 46*(4):157-163.

112. Mitchell, E.R., & Lunney, M. (2000). You make the diagnosis. Case study: A case management plan for a chemically dependent homeless man. *Nursing Diagnosis, 11*(2), 46,80-3.

113. Mobily, P.C., Herr, K.A., & Kelley, L.S. (1993). Cognitive-behavioral techniques to reduce pain: A validation study. *International Journal of Nursing Studies, 30*(6), 537-548.

114. Moorhead, S., & Delaney, C. (1997). Mapping nursing intervention data into the Nursing Interventions Classification (NIC): Process and rules. *Nursing Diagnosis, 8*(4), 137-144.

115. Moorhead, S.A., McCloskey, J.C., & Bulechek, G.M. (1993). Nursing Interventions Classification (NIC): A comparison with the Omaha System and the Home Health Care Classification. *Journal of Nursing Administration, 23*(10), 23-29.

116. Moss, L. (Producer), & Donahue, W. (Associate Producer). (1994). *Meet NIC: The Nursing Interventions Classification (NIC)* [Video, 40 min.]. New York: National League for Nursing.

117. Nolan, P. (1998). Competencies drive decision-making. *Nursing Management, 29*(3), 27-29.

118. O'Connor, N.A. (2000). Application of standardized nursing language to describe adult nurse practitioner practice. *Nursing Diagnosis, 11*(3), 109-120.

119. O'Connor, N.A., Hameister, A.D., & Kershaw, T. (2000). Developing a database to describe the practice patterns of adult nurse practitioner students. *Journal of Nursing Scholarship, 32*(1), 57-63.

120. O'Connor, N.A., Kershaw, T., Hameister, A.D. (2001). Documenting patterns of nursing interventions using cluster analysis. *Journal of Nursing Measurement, 9*(1), 73-90.

121. Park, S., Park, J., Jung, M., & Yom, Y. (2001). Nursing Interventions Classification in Korea. In *ACENDIO Proceedings of the Third European Conference of the Association for Common European Nursing Diagnoses, Interventions and Outcomes in Berlin* (pp. 124-134) Bern, Germany: Verlag Hans Huber.

122. Parris, K.M., Place, P.J., Orellana, E., Calder, J., Jackson, K., Karolys, A., Meza, M., Middough, C., Nguyen, V., Shim, N.W., & Smith, D. (1999). Integrating nursing diagnoses, interventions, and outcomes in public health nursing practice. *Nursing Diagnosis, 10*(2), 49-56.

123. Pavelka, L., McCarthy, A., & Denehy, J. (1999). Nursing interventions used in school nursing practice. *Journal of School Nursing, 51*(1), 29-37.

124. Payne, J. (2000). The Nursing Interventions Classification: A language to define nursing. *Oncology Nursing Forum, 27*(1), 99-103.

125. Petterson, M. (2000). Competence assessment approach broadens view of nursing skills. *Critical Care Nursing, 20*(3), 112, 105-107.

126. Poulton, S. (1996). Use of NIC in individualized nursing care plans. *NIC Letter, 4*(2), 3.

127. Prophet, C. (1994). Nursing Interventions Classification (NIC). In S.J. Grobe & E.S.P. Pluyter-Wenting (Eds.), *Nursing informatics: An international overview for nursing in a technological era: Proceedings of the Fifth International Symposium on Nursing Informatics* (NI-94) (pp. 692-696). New York: Elsevier.

128. Prophet, C.M., Dorr, G.G., Gibbs, T.D., & Porcella, A.A. (1997). *Implementation of standardized nursing languages (NIC, NOC) in on-line care planning and documentation. Informatics: The impact of nursing knowledge on health care informatics* (pp. 395-400). Washington, DC: IOS Press.

129. Redes, S., & Lunney, M. (1997). Validation by school nurses of the Nursing Intervention Classification for computer software, *Computers in Nursing, 15*(6), 333-338.

130. Robbins, B.T. (1997). Application of Nursing Interventions Classification (NIC) in a cardiovascular critical care unit. *Journal of Continuing Education in Nursing, 28*(2), 78-82.

131. Scherb, C.A. (2001). *Describing nursing effectiveness through standardized nursing languages and computerized clinical data.* Unpublished doctoral dissertation, University of Iowa, Iowa City, Iowa.

132. Scherb, C.A. (2000). Standardized nursing language: A necessity for computer information systems. *Clinical Data Management, 7*(1), 4-7,12.

133. Shelton, J.M. (1996). *Professional nurse case manager interventions in patient care.* Unpublished master's thesis, The University of Arizona, Tucson, Arizona.

134. Sigsby, L.M., & Campbell, D.W. (1995). Nursing Interventions Classification: A content analysis of nursing activities in public schools. *Journal of Community Health Nursing, 12*(4), 229-237.

135. Steelman, V.M., Bulechek, G.M., & McCloskey, J.C. (1994). Toward a standardized language to describe perioperative nursing. *AORN Journal, 60*(5), 786-795.

136. Thoroddsen, A. (2001). Applicability of the Nursing Intervention Classsification (NIC) after translation to another culture and language. In *ACENDIO Proceedings of the Third European Conference of the Assoication for Common European Nursing Diagnoses, Interventions and Outcomes in Berlin* (pp. 139-140). Bern, Germany: Verlag Hans Huber.

137. Tillman, H. (1997). *Classification schemes for nursing language.* Unpublished doctoral dissertation, Virginia Commonwealth University–Medical College of Virginia.

138. Titler, M.G. (1994). Research for practice: Using NIC in nursing practice [Column] *Med-Surg Nursing, 3*(4), 300-302.

139. Titler, M.G., Bulechek, G.M., & McCloskey, J.C. (1996). Use of the Nursing Interventions Classification by critical care nurses. *Critical Care Nurse, 16*(4), 38-54.

140. Titler, M., & McCloskey, J.C. (Eds.). (1988). On the scene: University of Iowa Hospital and Clinics: Outcomes Management, *Nursing Administration Quarterly, 24*, 31-65.

141. Titler, M., Pettit, D., Bulechek, G.M., McCloskey, J.C., Craft, M.J., Cohen, M.Z., Crossley, J.D., Denehy, J.A., Glick, O.J., Kruckeberg, T.W., Maas, M.L., Prophet, C.M., & Tripp-Reimer, T. (1991). Classification of nursing interventions for care of the integument. *Nursing Diagnosis, 2*(2), 45-56.

142. Tripp-Reimer, T., Woodworth, G., McCloskey, J.C., & Bulechek, G.M. (1996). The dimensional structure of nursing interventions. *Nursing Research, 45*(1), 10-17.

143. Twohy, K.M., & Reif, L. (1997). What do public health nurses really do during prenatal home appointments? *Public Health Nursing, 14*(6), 324-331.
144. University of Michigan. (2000). *Standardized nursing language: A visible difference* (Video). Ann Arbor, MI: Medical Center Information Technology, University of Michigan.
145. Wakefield, B., McCloskey, J.C., & Bulechek, G.M. (1995). Nursing Interventions Classification: A standardized language for nursing care. *Journal for Healthcare Quality, 17*(4), 26-33.
146. Walker, K.P., & Prophet, C.M. (1997). *Nursing documentation in the computer-based patient record: Proceedings of Nursing Informatics 1997*. New York: Elsevier.
147. Welton, R. (1996). University of Maryland identifies nurse core competencies using NIC. *NIC/NOC Letter, 4*(3), 4.
148. Wu, S.H., & Thompson, C.B. (2001). Evaluation of the Nursing Intervention Classification for use by flight nurses. *Air Medical Journal, 20*(1), 33-37.
149. Yom, Y. (1995). *Identification of nursing interventions in Korea*. Unpublished doctoral dissertation, University of Iowa, Iowa City, Iowa.
150. Yom, Y. (1998). Translation and validation of Nursing Interventions Classification (NIC) in English and Korean. *Image: Journal of Nursing Scholarship, 30*(3): 261-264.
151. Yom, Y., Chi, S.A., & Yoo, H.S. (2002). Application of nursing diagnoses, interventions, and outcomes to patients undergoing abdominal surgery in Korea. *International Journal of Nursing Terminologies and Classifications, 13*(3), 77-87.

Abbreviations

A-aDO$_2$	Alveolar arterial Oxygen Pressure Difference
ABC	Airway, Breathing, Circulation
ABG	Arterial Blood Gas
ABO	Blood types A, B, O
ADH	AntiDiuretic Hormone
ADL	Activity of Daily Living
AICD	Automatic Implantable Cardioverter Defibrillator
AIDS	Acquired Immune Deficiency Syndrome
ARDS	Adult Respiratory Distress Syndrome
AST	ASpartate aminoTransferase
AV	AtrioVentricular
avDO$_2$	arteriovenous Oxygen Difference
BE	Base Excess
Bicarb	Bicarbonate
BP	Blood Pressure
BUN	Blood Urea Nitrogen
C	Centigrade
Ca	Calcium
CBC	Complete Blood Count
CC	Cubic Centimeter
CDC	Centers for Disease Control
CK	Creatinine Kinase
cm	centimeter
CNS	Central Nervous System
CO	Cardiac Output
CO$_2$	Carbon dioxide
CPAP	Continuous Positive Airway Pressure
CPP	Cerebral Perfusion Pressure
CPR	CardioPulmonary Resuscitation
Cr	Creatinine
CSF	CerebroSpinal Fluid
CVA	Cerbral Vascular Accident
CVP	Central Venous Pressure
C-Section	Cesarean Section
D$_5$W	Dextrose 5% in Water
DDVAP	Desmopressin Acetate
DNA	DeoxyriboNucleic Acid
ECG	ElectroCardioGram
ECT	ElectroConvulsive Therapy
EDC	Expected Date of Confinement
EEG	ElectroEncephaloGram
EKG	ElectroKardioGram

EMG	ElectroMyoGram
EOA	Esophageal Obturator Airway
EOM	ExtraOcular Movement
EPA	Environmental Protection Agency
ET	Endotracheal Tube
FEV_1	Forced Expiratory Volume in one second
FVC	Forced Vital Capacity
GI	GastroIntestinal
GIFT	Gamete IntraFallopian Transfer
gm	gram
H_2	Hydrogen
HCl	HydroChloric Acid
HCO_3	Bicarbonate
Hct	Hematocrit
Hg	Mercury
Hgb	Hemoglobin
HIV	Human Immunodeficiency Virus
HOB	Head Of Bed
HRT	Hormone Replacement Therapy
ICP	IntraCranial Pressure
ICU	Intensive Care Unit
IRB	Institutional Review Board
IM	IntraMuscular
I&O	Intake and Output
IV	IntraVenous
IVF	In Vitro Fertilization
IVF-ET	In Vitro Fertilization–Embryo Transfer
JVD	Jugular Venous Distention
K	Potassium
LDH	Lactate DeHydrogenase
LMDS	Low-Molecular-Weight Dextrans
mA	milliAmpere
MADD	Mothers Against Drunk Driving
MAP	Mean Arterial Pressure
MAST	Military AntiShock Trousers
mEq/hr	milliEquivalant per hour
mEq/l	milliEquivalant per liter
Mg	Magnesium
mg	milligram
mg/dl	milligram per deciliter
min	minute
ml	milliliter
ml/kg/hr	milliliter per kilogram per hour
mm^3	cubic millimeter
mm Hg	millimeters of mercury
MVV	Maximal Voluntary Volume
Na	Sodium
$NaHCO_3$	Sodium Bicarbonate
NG	NasoGastric
NPO	Non Per Os (Nothing by mouth)
NSAID	NonSteroidal AntiInflammatory Drug

OB/Gyn	Obstetrics/Gynecology
OR	Operating Room
OSHA	Occupational Safety and Health Administration
OT	Occupational Therapy
oz	ounce
P	Pulse
PAP	Pulmonary Artery Pressure
PAWP	Pulmonary Artery Wedge Pressure
PaCO$_2$	Partial arterial Carbon dioxide pressure
PaO$_2$	Partial arterial Oxygen pressure
PCA	Patient-Controlled Analgesia
PCO$_2$	Partial Carbon dioxide pressure
PCWP	Pulmonary Capillary Wedge Pressure
PEEP	Positive End Expiratory Pressure
PERF	Peak Expiratory Flow Rate
PFT	Pulmonary Function Tests
pH	Hydrogen ion concentration
PIC	Peripherally Inserted Central Catheter
PO	Per Os (orally)
PO$_4$	Phosphate
PRN	Pro Re Nata (as often as necessary)
PT	Physical Therapist
PT	Prothrombin Time
PTT	Partial Thromboplastin Time
PVC	Premature Ventricular Contraction
qid	four times a day
Q$_{sp}$/Q$_t$	physiologic blood flow per minute/cardiac output per minute
RAP	Right Atrial Pressure
REM	Rapid Eye Movement
Rh	Rhesus antigen
RH$_0$(D)	Rhesus antigen
ROM	Range Of Motion
RN	Registered Nurse
RT	Respiratory Therapist
SADD	Students Against Drunk Drivers
SaO$_2$	Saturation (arterial) Oxygen
SIADH	Syndrome of Inappropriate AntiDiuretic Hormone
SQ	Subcutaneous
SvO$_2$	Saturation (venous) Oxygen
SVR	Systemic Vascular Resistance
S$_3$	3rd heart sound
S$_4$	4th heart sound
TENS	Transcutaneous Electrical Nerve Stimulation
TPN	Total Parenteral Nutrition
UO	Urine Output
U/S	Ultrasound
VAD	Venous Access Devices
V$_d$/V$_t$	Physiological dead space/Tidal volume
V/Q scan	Ventilation-Perfusion scan
WBC	White Blood Cell/White Blood Count
WIC	Women, Infants, and Children
ZIFT	Zygote IntraFallopian Transfer

Index

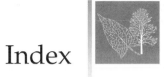

Figures denoted by *f*; tables denoted by *t*; boxes denoted by *b*.